AO Publishing

AO Principles of
Fracture Management

AO Publishing

Thomas P. Rüedi
William M. Murphy

AO Principles of
Fracture Management

with illustrations by Michael Renner and Kaspar Hiltbrand

Section Editors
Chris L. Colton
Alberto Fernandez Dell'Oca
Ulrich Holz
James F. Kellam
Peter E. Ochsner

Coordinating Editor
Gustave E. Fackelman

Illustration Editor
Yves Harder

Thieme
Stuttgart · New York

Design & typesetting: DynaPub, CH-8645 Jona
Concept: Egle Consulting, CH-8332 Russikon
Illustrations: Büro für Gestaltung, Michael Renner,
CH-4123 Allschwil, and
K. Hiltbrand, CH-4058 Basel
Illustration editing: Dr. med. Yves Harder,
Inselspital, CH-3010 Bern
Scans: ComArt, CH-6330 Cham, and
AO Media Services, CH-7270 Davos Platz
Video digitizing: AO Media Services, CH-7270 Davos Platz
Video editing: PD Dr. med. Dr. h.c. U. F. A. Heim,
CH-3073 Gümligen
Coordinating editor: Prof. Dr. med. vet G. E. Fackelman,
USA-Rockwood, ME 04478
Indexing: Jill Halliday, GB-Diss, Norfolk IP21 4QT

Library of Congress Cataloging-in-Publication Data

Rüedi, Thomas P., 1935-
AO Principles of Fracture Management/T.P. Rüedi, W.M. Murphy;
with illustrations by M. Renner and K. Hiltbrand.
p.; cm.
Includes bibliographical references and index.
ISBN 3131174412 — ISBN 0-86577-886-8
1. Fractures—Treatment. I. Title Principles of Fracture Management.
II. Title: Fracture management. III. Murphy, W.M. (William M.) IV.
Title.
[DNLM: 1. Fractures—therapy. WE 175 R918a 2000]
RD101, R84 2000
617.1'5—dc21   00-032598

Copyright © 2000, by AO Publishing
Clavadelerstrasse, CH-7270 Davos Platz
Exclusive distribution right by Georg Thieme Verlag,
Rüdigerstrasse 14, DE-70469 Stuttgart, Germany, and
Thieme New York, 333 Seventh Avenue, New York,
NY 10001, USA
Printed by G. Canale & C. S.p.A.,
IT-10071 Borgaro T.se Torino

ISBN 3-13-117441-2 (GTV)
ISBN 0-86577-886-8 (TNY)

Acknowledgement:
Photos in chapters 3.2.2 and 3.3.3 are reproduced by permission of Mathys Medical Ltd. and Stratec Medical.
Figure 3.2.3-1 is reprinted from Pauwels F, Biomechanics of the Locomotor Apparatus, (1980, Fig. 11a-f, page 157) with permission from Springer-Verlag Berlin Heidelberg.
Sequences of non-AO videos are reproduced by permission of the authors (see video index).

Contributors

Authors

Jorge E. Alonso, MD
University of Alabama
at Birmingham
1813 6th Avenue South MEB 509
US-Birmingham, AL 35233

George M. Babikian, MD
Orthopaedic Association of
Portland Maine Medical Center
University of Vermont
33 Sewall Street, PO Box 1260
US-Portland, ME 04104

Craig S. Bartlett, III, MD
Department of Orthopaedics and
Rehabilitation, University of
Vermont McClure Musculoskeletal
Research Center
R.T. Stafford Hall, Room 426
US-Burlington, VT 05405

Fred Baumgaertel, PD Dr. med.
Gesundheitszentrum Evang. Stift
Sankt Martin GmbH
Johannes Müller Str. 7
DE-56068 Koblenz

Flip P. Besselaar, MD
Academisch Medisch Centrum
Universiteit van Amsterdam
Meibergdreef 9
NL-1105 Amsterdam AZ

Editors/Authors

Thomas P. Rüedi
Prof. Dr. med., FACS
Kantonsspital
Chirurgisches Departement
CH-7000 Chur

William M. Murphy, FRCSI
Corbie Wood, 52 Copsem Lane
Oxshott, Leatherhead
GB-Surrey KT22 ONT

Chris L. Colton, FRCS, FRCSEd
The Maltings, Tofts Farm
GB-Bradmore NG11 6PE

Alberto Fernandez Dell'Oca, MD
British Hospital, Orthopaedic
Dept., Av. Italia 2420
UY-11600 Montevideo

Ulrich Holz, Prof. Dr. med.
Katharinenhospital
Klinik für Unfall- und
Wiederherstellungschirurgie
Kriegsbergstrasse 60
DE-70174 Stuttgart

James F. Kellam, MD, FRCS, FACS
Carolinas Medical Center
Dept. of Orthopaedic Surgery
PO Box 32861
US-Charlotte, NC 28232

Peter E. Ochsner, Prof. Dr. med.
Orthopädische Klinik
Kantonsspital Liestal
CH-4410 Liestal

Jochen Blum, PD Dr. med.
Johannes Gutenberg Universität
Klinik und Poliklinik für
Unfallchirurgie
Langenbeckstrasse 1
DE-55131 Mainz

Lutz Claes, Prof. Dr. rer. biol. hum
Institut für Unfallchirurgische
Forschung und Biomechanik
Universität Ulm
Helmholtzstr. 14
DE-89081 Ulm

R. Paul Clifford, FRCS
Jersey General Hospital
Gloucester Street
GB-St Helier, Jersey, JE2 3QS

Peter de Boer, FRCS
York District Hospital
Wigginton Road
GB-York YO3 7HE

Deborah M. Eastwood, FRCS
Royal Free Hospital
Pond Street
GB-London NW3 2QG

Donald P. Endrizzi, MD
Orthopaedic Association of Portland
Maine Medical Center University
of Vermont
33 Sewall Street, PO Box 1260
US-Portland, ME 04104

Diego L. Fernandez, PD Dr. med.
Lindenhofspital Bern
Bremgartenstrasse 119
CH-3012 Bern

Robert Frigg
Mathys Medical Ltd.
Güterstrasse 5, Postfach
CH-2544 Bettlach

Emanuel Gautier, Dr. med.
Department of Orthopaedic Surgery
Kantonsspital
CH-1708 Fribourg

Christoph W. Geel, MD, FACS
Orthopedic Trauma Service
Upstate Medical University
550 Harrison Center, Suite 100
US-Syracuse, NY 13202

Rene J. A. Goris, Prof. Dr. med.
University Hospital Nijmegen
PO Box 98101
NL-6500 Nijmegen HB

Norbert P. Haas, Prof. Dr. med.
Unfall- und Wiederherstellungs-
chirurgie, Universitätsklinikum
Charité, Humboldt Universität
Campus Virchow-Klinikum
Augustenburger Platz 1
DE-13353 Berlin

David M. Hahn, FRCS
University Hospital
The Queens Medical Centre
GB-Nottingham MG7 2UH

Markus Hehli, Dipl. Ing.
Spital Davos
Promenade 4
CH-7270 Davos Platz

Dominik Heim, PD Dr. med.
Spital Frutigen, Chirurgische Abt.
CH-3714 Frutigen

David L. Helfet, MD
Orthopaedic Trauma Service
Hospital for Special Surgery
535 East 70th Street
US-New York, NY 10021

Reinhard Hoffmann, PD Dr. med.
Städtische Kliniken Offenbach/Main
Klinik für Unfall- und Wiederher-
stellungschirurgie
Starkenburgring 66
DE-63069 Offenbach

Brian J. Holdsworth
BSc, MB, LRCP, FRCS
Nottingham University Hospital
Orthopaedic Department
The Queens Medical Centre
GB-Nottingham NG7 2UH

Dankward Höntzsch, Prof. Dr. med.
BG-Unfallklinik Tübingen
Schnarrenbergstr. 95
DE-72076 Tübingen

James B. Hunter, BA, FRCSEd Orth
Queen's Medical Centre
GB-Nottingham NG7 2UH

Ann E. Hunter, FRCP, MRCPath
Department of Haematology
Leicestershire Royal Infirmary
GB-Leicester LE1 5WW

Roland P. Jakob, Prof. Dr. med.
Hôpital Cantonal Fribourg
CH-1708 Fribourg

Eric E. Johnson, MD
University of California—Los Angeles,
UCLA School of Medicine
Depart. of Orthopaedic Surgery
10833 Le Conte Ave, 76-134 CHS
US-Los Angeles, CA 90095

Christoph Josten, Prof. Dr. med.
Zentrum für Chirurgie, Unfall-
und Wiederherstellungschirurgie
Liebigstrasse 20a
DE-04103 Leipzig

Jesse B. Jupiter, MD
Harvard Medical School
Massachusetts General Hospital
WAC 527, 15 Parkman Street
US-Boston, MA 02114

Lothar Kinzl, Prof. Dr. med.
Abt. für Unfall-, Hand- und
Wiederherstellungschirurgie
Universitätsklinikum Ulm
Steinhövelstrasse 9
DE-89075 Ulm

Christian Krettek, Prof. Dr. med.
Unfallchirurgische Klinik der
Medizinischen Hochschule Hannover
Carl-Neubergstrasse 1
DE-30625 Hannover

Dieter Leu, Dr. med.
Im Wiesengrund 3
CH-4613 Rickenbach

René K. Marti, Prof. Dr. med.
Academisch Medisch Centrum
Universiteit van Amsterdam
Meibergdreef 9
NL-1105 Amsterdam AZ

Alain C. Masquelet, MD
Service de Chirurgie Orthopédique
Hôpital Avicenne, Université Paris XIII
125, route de Stalingrad
FR-93009 Bobigny Cedex

Robert Mathys, jr., Dipl. Ing. ETH
Dr. h.c. Robert Mathys Stiftung
Bischmattstrasse 12, Postfach
CH-2544 Bettlach

Peter Matter, Prof. Dr. med.
AO Foundation
Clavadelerstrasse
CH-7270 Davos Platz

Michael D. McKee, MD
St. Michael's Hospital
55 Queen Street East, Suite 800
CA-Toronto, Ont. M5C 1R6

Gert Muhr, Prof. Dr. med.
Berufsgen. Krankenanstalt
"Bergmannsheil Bochum"
Gilsingstr. 14
DE-44789 Bochum

Urs Müller, Dr. med.
Orthopädische Klinik
Kantonsspital Liestal
CH-4410 Liestal

Michael Nerlich, Prof. Dr. med.
Klinikum der Universität
Abtl. Unfallchirurgie
Franz-Josef-Strauss-Allee 11
DE-93042 Regensburg

John O'Dowd, FRCS Orth
Orthopaedic Department
Guy's and St Thomas's Hospitals
St Thomas Street
GB-London SE1 9RT

Stephan M. Perren, Prof. Dr. med.
AO Zentrum
Clavadelerstrasse
CH-7270 Davos Platz

Tim Pohlemann, Prof. Dr. med.
Unfallchirurgische Klinik der
Medizinischen Hochschule
Hannover
Carl-Neubergstrasse 1
DE-30625 Hannover

Ortrun Pohler, Prof., PhD
STRATEC Medical
Eimattstrasse 3
CH-4436 Oberdorf

Jaime Quintero, MD
Depto. de Ortopedia y
Traumatologia
Hospital Clinica San Rafael
Carrera 8a. No. 17-45 Sur
CO-Santafe de Bogota

Ernst L.F.B. Raaymakers, MD
Academisch Medisch Centrum
Universiteit van Amsterdam
Meibergdreef 9
NL-1105 Amsterdam AZ

Pietro Regazzoni, Prof. Dr. med.
Kantonsspital
Chirurgische Abteilung
Spitalstrasse 21
CH-4031 Basel

Pol M. Rommens, Prof. Dr. med.
Johannes Gutenberg Universität
Klinik und Poliklinik für
Unfallchirurgie
Langenbeckstrasse 1
DE-55131 Mainz

Christian Ryf, Dr. med.
Spital Davos
Promenade 4
CH-7270 Davos Platz

Joseph Schatzker, MD, B.Sc., FRCSC
Sunnybrook Health
Science Centre
2075 Bayview Avenue, Suite A315
CA-Toronto, Ont. M4N 3M5

Michael Schütz, Dr. med.
Unfall- und
Wiederherstellungschirurgie
Universitätsklinikum Charité der
Humboldt Universität
Campus Virchow-Klinikum
Augustenburger Platz 1
DE-13353 Berlin

Christoph Sommer, Dr. med.
Kantonsspital
Chirurgisches Departement
CH-7000 Chur

Michael D. Stover, MD
Loyola University Medical Center
Department of Orthopaedic Surgery
2160 South 1st Avenue
US-Maywood, IL 60153

Norbert P. Südkamp, Prof. Dr. med.
Unfall- und
Wiederherstellungschirurgie
Klinikum Albert-Ludwig
Universität Freiburg
Hugstetterstrasse 55
DE-79106 Freiburg

Rudolf Szyszkowitz, Prof. Dr. med.
Landeskrankenhaus—
Universitätsklinikum Graz,
Klinik für Unfallchirurgie
Auenbruggerplatz 7a
AT-8036 Graz

Slobodan Tepic, Dr. sci.
Rigistrasse 27b
CH-8006 Zürich

Otmar L. Trentz, Prof. Dr. med.
Universitätsspital
Departement Chirurgie
CH-8091 Zürich

Lijckle van der Laan, MD, PhD
Department of Surgery
Saint Elisabeth Hospital
PO Box 90151
NL-5000 LC Tilburg

J. Tracy Watson, MD
Division of Orthopaedic
Traumatology, Wayne State
University School of Medicine
4201 St. Antoine Street
University Health Center 7-C
Detroit Medical Center
US-Detroit, MI 48201

Bernhard Weigel, Dr. med.
Klinikum der Universität
Abtl. Unfallchirurgie
Franz-Josef-Strauss-Allee 11
DE-93042 Regensburg

Andy Weymann, Dr. med.
AO International
Clavadelerstrasse
CH-7270 Davos Platz

Raymond R. White, MD
Orthopaedic Association of Portland
Maine Medical Center University
of Vermont
33 Sewall Street, PO Box 1260
US-Portland, ME 04104

Bernd Wittner, Dr. med.
Katharinenhospital
Klinik für Unfall- und
Wiederherstellungschirurgie
Kriegsbergstrasse 60
DE-70174 Stuttgart

Peter Worlock, DM FRCS
Oxford Radcliffe Hospital
Trauma Unit, Critical Care Centre
Headley Way
GB-Oxford OX3 9DU

Werner Zimmerli, Prof. Dr. med.
Medizinische Universitätsklinik
Kantonsspital
Rheinstrasse 26
CH-4410 Liestal

Foreword

Revolutions, and their leaders, that are successful and survive are rare—especially in medicine. The five founders of the AO were such, and like true revolutionaries they had to convince the proletariat that this revolution, though appealing to surgeons, was also based on scientific principles. To do this required careful documentation of all cases, from which evaluation and learning allowed them the full development of a method which culminated in the original AO Manual, the working treatise of this remarkable AO revolution.

Fortunately, the revolution continues even today—the principles remain the same, but the methods have evolved, as clearly they should. This, the fifth major publication, is no longer a manual, as its predecessors, but an interpretation of the AO philosophy and principles as they apply to the management of fractures for the new millennium. In addition, the baton has been passed and the message herein has been written by the many disciples of the founders—all of whom have benefited, as have their many patients worldwide, by their association with the AO revolution.

As befits the AO at the turn of the new century, the format is also revolutionary and high tech, including a written tome and a CD-ROM version with surgical techniques, videos and annotated references—a first for such a text, to my knowledge, in surgery, let alone for fractures. This yeoman task has been spearheaded by Thomas P. Rüedi and William M. Murphy, who with their associate editors and AO "in-house" Publication Department, under the direction of Rainer Egle, in collaboration with Thieme International, have produced this, the AO "Bible" for the new millennium—a truly remarkable achievement.

On behalf of all fracture surgeons, but especially those of the AO family, our thanks and congratulations to all those involved and may the revolution, started 40 years ago, continue to flourish and evolve.

David L. Helfet, MD
New York, March 2000

Source books

The editors have relied heavily on these texts throughout this book.

- **Müller ME, Allgöwer M, Schneider R, et al.** (1991) *Manual of Internal Fixation.* 3rd ed. Berlin Heidelberg New York: Springer-Verlag.

- **Müller ME, Nazarian S, Koch P** (1987) *Classification AO des fractures: les os longs.* Berlin Heidelberg New York: Springer-Verlag.

- **Müller ME, Nazarian S, Koch P, et al.** (1990) *The Comprehensive Classification of Fractures of Long Bones.* Berlin Heidelberg New York: Springer-Verlag.

- **Rüedi T, von Hochstetter AHC, Schlumpf R** (1984) *Surgical Approaches for Internal Fixation.* Berlin: Springer-Verlag.

- **Heim U, Pfeiffer KM** (1988) *Internal Fixation of Small Fractures.* 3rd ed. Berlin Heidelberg New York: Springer-Verlag.

- **Tile M** (1995) *Fractures of the Pelvis and Acetabulum.* Baltimore: Williams & Wilkins.

- **Schatzker J, Tile M** (1996) *The Rationale of Operative Fracture Care.* 2nd ed. Berlin Heidelberg New York: Springer-Verlag.

- **Texhammer R, Colton C** (1994) *AO/ASIF Instruments and Implants.* 2nd ed. Berlin Heidelberg New York: Springer-Verlag.

- **Mast J, Jakob R, Ganz R** (1989) *Planning and Reduction Technique in Fracture Surgery.* Berlin Heidelberg: Springer-Verlag.

- **Letournel E, Judet R** (1993) *Fractures of the Acetabulum.* 2nd ed. Berlin Heidelberg New York: Springer-Verlag.

- **Weber BG, Brunner C, Frueler F** (1980) *Treatment of Fractures in Children and Adolescents.* Berlin Heidelberg New York: Springer-Verlag.

Introduction to the AO Principles of Fracture Management

The first AO book appeared in 1963, four years after the founding of the Swiss AO group. The editors were the group's founders, Maurice E. Müller, Martin Allgöwer, and Hans Willenegger and what they were introducing was a new set of principles—at that time quite revolutionary—of fracture treatment by absolute stability obtained through interfragmentary compression which produced rigid fixation. The feature of the book was a consecutive, fully documented and illustrated series of 188 lower leg fractures that had been internally fixed during a four-month period (winter 1961/62) at the department of surgery in Chur under the chairmanship of Martin Allgöwer.

Their thesis was backed up by this unique series, which demonstrated the effectiveness of fracture treatment when rationally conceived and properly performed.

In 1969, the first edition of the "AO Manual of Internal Fixation" was published by the same authors, offering step-by-step guidance on how to perform operative fracture treatment when it was indicated. Due to the high demand, that book, originally in German, was immediately translated into English, French, Italian, and Spanish. Revised editions followed in 1977 and 1992, again translated into many languages, including Chinese, Japanese, and Russian. All in all, close to 110,000 AO books have been distributed in the past 35 years.

Today, 40 years after the founding of the Swiss AO group, with worldwide acceptance of operative fracture management and with a considerable evolution in the concepts of fracture healing, it seemed appropriate to perpetuate the tradition in a somewhat different format.

The new publication on "AO Principles of Fracture Management" is designed not to be a handbook of osteosynthesis, but rather to offer comprehensive recommendations, supported by clinical guidance, on the principles of how to treat fractures in the new millennium. This content is based on the current concepts of AO teaching, with more emphasis on the pathophysiology and biology of fracture healing and somewhat less on the mechanical aspects, important though these still remain. To assist the reader, the layout is based on the modular structures of the latest AO courses.

Completely new and most attractive is the fact that besides the printed version, the entire book will be also provided on CD-ROM and eventually DVD-ROM. The somewhat unconventional format of the book is designed to reflect the shape of a computer screen. The CD-ROM version allows the addition of video-clips, for example, the dynamics of reduction maneuvers and technical tricks and also the opportunity to access much of the bibliography for easier cross-referencing and personal study.

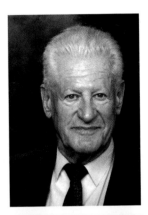

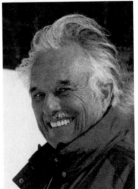

We offer our grateful thanks for their work, their tolerance and their patience, to more than 50 outstanding surgeons and scientists from across the world who have made contributions to this venture. It has been produced "in house" by the AO Publishing group under Rainer Egle and represents the efforts of a large and diverse team, as a glance at the acknowledgements section will confirm. Initiated two and a half years ago, the preparation of the manuscripts and illustrations, and the integration of the various innovations, took considerably longer than we had planned or anticipated, but hopefully the reader will find the end result worth the wait.

However, it is inevitable that not every statement will be agreed by all readers and that there will be some errors, the responsibility for which must lie with us, the editors, rather than the contributors. We do, however, invite constructive criticism, hoping to improve not only in a later edition, which we hope will be required, but before it. This invitation to make comments is something more than a standard editorial platitude.

We will be able to respond appropriately, because it is our intention regularly to reissue our CD-ROM in revised and improved form— first update in December 2001. This will allow us to correct any major errors and to enjoy the opportunity for regular up-dating with new references, techniques, implants, and instruments, while sparing our readers (and ourselves and successor editors) the burden and expense of over-frequent new editions.

All of the surgeons involved in producing this book have, to varying degrees, been able to rely on successive editions of the AO Manual of Internal Fixation during our training and in our day-to-day working lives. With respect and gratitude we offer the dedication of this new style book to all those pioneers, some now no longer with us, who began this series of AO books, and in particular to the two peerless masters, Martin Allgöwer and Maurice E. Müller, whose lively presence in AO circles we hope will long continue.

Thomas P. Rüedi, MD, FACS, and
William M. Murphy, FRCSI
Editors-in-Chief

Acknowledgements

William M. Murphy & Thomas P. Rüedi

We have already expressed our sincere thanks and appreciation to the many authors and co-authors who combined to write this book and we are grateful to our colleagues on the editorial board who put in many long hours of preparing texts and illustrations for publishing and who gave much support in a variety of other ways.

Apart from the writers and editors, a number of people have contributed to the production of this publication, and to mention them by name is only a very small token of thanks for much hard work.

First in this context is the small staff of AO Publishing under the guidance of Rainer Egle. Doris Straub Piccirillo, together with her assistant Martina Späti, have accomplished the enormous and almost impossible task to manage over 50 authors (to say nothing of the editors). They had to prepare and finalize the manuscripts to the very last details, and the layout work was then carried out with great expertise by Dr. Daniel Erni.

The illustrators Michael Renner and his team, as well as Kaspar Hiltbrand, have produced high quality work to meet our demands and deadlines.

AO Media Services under Dr. Andreas Affentranger were responsible for the preparation and scanning of the x-rays as well as for the video clips, which were selected with great care and discrimination by PD Dr. Urs Heim. Valuable editorial support was given by Prof. Peter Matter and Dr. Andy Weymann.

The AO TK and members of the Expert Groups have reviewed the manuscripts of sections 3 and 4 to check for any technical inaccuracies.

Finally, we would like to extend our thanks to the Board of Directors of the AO Foundation and Dr. Wolfram Einars who supported us in this ambitious project, originally initiated by Prof. Peter Matter and Rainer Egle and then entrusted to us.

As the finished manuscripts are delivered to Thieme Verlag for printing, marketing, and distribution, we can only hope that the readers' judgement will be favorable, thereby justifying the efforts of all involved.

1.1 AO philosophy and principles

Joseph Schatzker

1 AO philosophy

The philosophy of the AO group has remained consistent and clear, from its inception by a small group of friends and colleagues in 1958 to its current status as a worldwide surgical and scientific foundation. Seeing as its central concern all patients with skeletal injuries and related problems, the philosophy has been directed to providing for them a pattern of care designed to bring an early return to mobility and function. This philosophy has driven everything that has grown from the original aspirations and plans of the founding group, and remains the central inspiration of today's AO Foundation.

The key to its implementation has been effective and rational management of injured bones and soft tissues so as to foster rapid restoration of the patient's function. Management protocols have constantly been adapted to take account of the fresh understanding of the healing process gained from growing clinical expertise and expanding research.

2 Background

In the first half of the 20th century, fracture management was concentrated on the restoration of bony union, to the exclusion, largely, of other considerations seen today not only as relevant but essential.

The methods employed to manage fractures, mostly by immobilization in plaster or by traction, had the effect, too often, of inhibiting rather than promoting function throughout the healing period, which was itself frequently prolonged. The key concept of the AO was to give expression to its philosophy by safe and effective open reduction and internal fixation of fractures, intimately combined with early functional rehabilitation.

Long before the establishment of the AO, there had, of course, been keen championship and authoritative recognition of the value of open reduction and fixation of fractures. The innovative approaches and technical vision of early advocates of surgical fracture care are well documented. That their ideas were either not heard or failed to penetrate shows how arid was the ground on which these pioneering seeds first fell and, equally, what great technical and biological obstacles remainded to be overcome.

The list is formidable: infection, dubious metallurgy, poor biological awareness, ill-conceived implants, and an underdeveloped understanding of the role of fixation were all added to peer group scepticism often amounting to real hostility.

Thus, such highlights as the visionary innovations of the Lambottes, the technical achievements of Küntscher with the intramedullary nail, and the conceptual advances of Lucas-Championnière and his protagonist Perkins in introducing early motion (albeit on traction), were dimmed by an apparent inability to reconcile within one pattern of care the two concepts of effective splintage of the fracture and controlled mobility of the joints.

3 The role of the AO

What was needed—and what the AO provided—was a coordinated approach to identify these obstacles, to study the difficulties they caused, and to set about overcoming them. The chosen path was to investigate and understand the relevant biology, to develop appropriate technology and techniques, to document the outcomes and react to the findings, and, through teaching and writing, to share whatever was discovered.

This enormous challenge had an apparently small beginning. In the 1940's and 1950's, questions were being asked, not least by the Swiss state and commercial insurance companies, as to why, if it took some fractures 6–12 weeks to heal, it often took 6–12 months for the patients to return to work.

The story of how an encounter with Robert Danis, first through his writings and later by a personal visit, provided the inspiration for Maurice Müller and the group he subsequently gathered about him to begin developing answers to questions, has been well documented.

The essence of Danis' observation was that if he used a compression device to impart absolute stability to a diaphyseal fracture, healing without callus would take place and, while it was happening, the adjacent joints and muscles could safely and painlessly be exercised.

Inspired by this concept and driven by a determination not only to apply it but to establish how and why it worked, Müller and the AO group set in train a process of surgical innovation, technical development, basic research, and clinical documentation. This progressed as an integrated campaign to improve the results and minimize the problems of fracture care. They then set about propagating their message by writing and teaching. That work continues to this day, with involvement of many specialist groups working mostly, it should be said, in harmony to the common end of improving patient care world-wide, in greatly differing environments.

4 AO principles

Today, any statement of the key concepts—conventionally referred to as the AO "principles"—through which the AO philosophy was given expression, can be remarkably similar in wording to what appeared in the early AO publications from 1962 onwards. The essential feature, now as then, is the proper management of the fracture within the environment of the patient. The need was for a proper understanding of the "personalities" of the fracture and of the injury; from this all else would follow.

The original management objectives were restoration of anatomy, establishment of stability, while preserving blood supply, with early mobilization of limb and patient. These were at first presented as the fundamentals of good internal fixation. However, with increased understanding of how fractures heal, with acceptance of the supreme role of the soft tissues and with ever-expanding understanding of how implants and bones interact, they have undergone certain conceptual and technological changes while gaining their present status as the principles not just of internal fixation but of fracture management overall.

Central to the effective application of the AO's concepts was the understanding that articular fractures and diaphyseal fractures have very different biological requirements. Allied to this was the increasingly clear recognition that the type and timing of surgical intervention must be guided by the degree of injury to the soft-tissue envelope and the physiological demands of the patient.

5 Progress and development

The AO principles relating to anatomy, stability, biology, and mobilization still stand as fundamentals. How they have been expressed, interpreted, and applied over the past 40 years has gradually changed in response to the knowledge and understanding emerging from scientific studies and clinical observation.

It is now accepted that the pursuit of absolute stability, originally proposed for almost all fractures, is mandatory only for joint and certain related fractures (**chapter 2.3**), and then only when it can be obtained without damage to blood supply and soft tissues (**chapters 1.5** and **5.2**). Within the diaphysis, there must always be respect for length, alignment, and rotation.

When fixation is required, splintage by a nail is usually selected and this leads to union by callus. Even when the clinical situation favors the use of a plate, proper planning and the current techniques for minimal access and fixation have been designed to minimize any insult to the blood supply of the bony fragments and soft tissues.

It must be appreciated that simple diaphyseal fractures react differently to plating and to nailing, and if plating is employed, absolute stability must be achieved. In contrast, multifragmentary fractures can all be treated by splintage. Fractures of the forearm diaphyses, where long bone morphology is combined with quasi-articular functions, need special consideration (**chapter 4.3.1**). Articular fractures demand anatomical reduction and absolute stability to enhance the healing of articular cartilage and make early motion possible, which is necessary for good ultimate function.

The imperatives of soft-tissue care, originally expressed in the principle of preserving blood supply to bone, must be addressed in every phase of fracture management, from initial planning to how, if at all, the bone is to be handled. A clear understanding of the roles of direct and indirect reduction (**chapter 3.1**), together with informed assessment of how the fracture pattern and soft-tissue injuries relate to each other, will lead to correct decisions on strategy and tactics being made and incorporated into the preoperative plan. From this will follow the choice of implant compatible with the biological and functional demands of the fracture.

6 Philosophy and principles today

In earlier days, the AO principles appeared in a succinct, even dogmatic format. Thus expressed, they transformed not just internal fixation, but fracture management overall. Fracture care became a structured process, rooted in good science and technology and nourished by research and documented studies.

The importance of and the need for fracture fixation in such difficult situations as infection, joint injuries, and polytrauma has been validated and applied to patient care.

These same AO principles are here set out in a form believed to be valid today.

AO principles

1. Fracture reduction and fixation to restore anatomical relationships.
2. Stability by fixation or splintage, as the personality of the fracture and the injury requires.
3. Preservation of the blood supply to soft tissues and bone by careful handling and gentle reduction techniques.
4. Early and safe mobilization of the part and the patient.

These still embody the AO philosophy of patient care and they can still be quite briefly stated. However, it takes a book the size of this one to give full expression to all that they imply for dealing with the consequences of trauma.

Indeed, the continuing study of how the trauma patient's tissues and psyche respond to injury and its management brings the encouraging conviction that when the next formal restatement of the principles comes to be made, the knowledge and understanding on which they are based will once again have been expanded for the benefit of those to whom they are applied and those who apply them alike.

7 Suggestions for further reading

1. **Lucas-Championnère J** (1907) Les dangers de l'immobilisation des membres—fragilité des os—altérnation de la nutrition de la membre—conclusions pratiques. *Rev Med Chur Pratique;* 78:81–87.
2. **Müller ME, Allgöwer M, Willenegger H** (1965) *Technique of Internal Fixation of Fractures.* Berlin Heidelberg New York: Springer-Verlag.
3. **Schatzker J** (1998) M. E. Müller—on his 80th Birthday. *AO Dialogue;* 11 (1):7–12.

8 Updates

Updates and additional references for this chapter are available online at:
http://www.aopublishing.org/PFxM/11.htm

1.2 Biology and biomechanics in fracture management

Stephan M. Perren & Lutz Claes

1 Introduction—*Stephan M. Perren*

This chapter addresses anyone who is eager to appreciate the biological and biomechanical basis of fracture management—the why and how of the way bone reacts to intervention—thus facilitating the choice of the appropriate procedure for any fracture problem. It offers a review of the basic rationale for the interested clinical user, rather than precise data for scientists. The literature quoted contains data concerning the special features discussed. For more extensive references the scientific literature should be consulted. In spite of worldwide research, much remains unknown or controversial. We will, therefore, consider the facts and abstain from far-reaching interpretations.

The main goal of internal fixation is to achieve prompt and, where possible, full function of the injured limb with rapid rehabilitation of the patient. Although reliable fracture healing is only one element in functional recovery, its mechanics, biomechanics, and biology should be understood. For biological or bio-mechanical reasons it is often necessary to sacrifice some strength and stiffness. **For internal fixation, neither the strongest nor the stiffest implant is necessarily optimal.** Internal fixation cannot permanently replace a broken bone but provides temporary support.

Under critical conditions, the mechanical requirements may be more demanding than the biological advantages. Every surgeon must determine which combination of technology and procedure best fits his experience, environment, and in particular the demands of the patient.

Before choosing an implant material, several aspects have to be considered. Depending on the requirements, the stronger and more forgiving stainless steel may be preferable to the electrochemically inert and biologically superior and more deformable but less strong titanium. In other situations it may be more favorable to use titanium, especially in its pure c.p. titanium form.

For internal fixation, neither the strongest nor the stiffest implant is necessarily optimal.

2 Bone as a tissue

The intact bone serves as a scaffold that supports and protects the soft parts and enables locomotion and mechanical functioning of the limbs. The important mechanical characteristics of bone are its stiffness (bone deforms only a little under load) and strength (bone tolerates high load without failure). In considering a fracture and its healing, the brittleness of bone is of special interest: **bone is strong but it breaks under very small deformation [1].** This means that bone behaves more like glass than like rubber. Therefore, at the onset of fracture healing, bone cannot bridge a fracture gap which is continually subject to displacement. For an unstable or flexibly fixed (see **section 4.2**) fracture, a sequence of biological events, mainly the formation of soft and hard callus, helps to reduce the mobility and deformation of the repair tissues. Resorption of the fragment-ends further reduces tissue deformation. These reactions ultimately promote biological stabilization of the fracture. Finally, internal remodeling restores the original bone structure.

Bone is strong but it breaks under very small deformation.

The role of surgery should be to guide and support this healing process.

3 Fracture of bone

A fracture is the result of single or multiple overload. The fracture occurs within a fraction of a millisecond. It results in appreciable damage to soft tissue due to rupture and an implosion-like process. Rapid separation of fracture surfaces creates a void resulting in severe soft-tissue damage (**Video AO51013**).

3.1 The mechanical and chemical effects of the fracture

The mechanical effect of a fracture consists primarily in a loss of bony continuity, resulting in pathological mobility and loss of the support function of bone, and leading ultimately to pain. Surgical stabilization may restore the function immediately. Thus, the patient regains pain-free mobility and avoids such sequelae of disturbed or abolished function as algodystrophy (see **chapter 6.5**).

Traumatic discontinuity of bone ruptures blood vessels within and without the bone. Spontaneously released chemical agents help to induce bone healing. In fresh fractures these agents are very effective and scarcely need any boost. **The role of surgery should be to guide and support this healing process.**

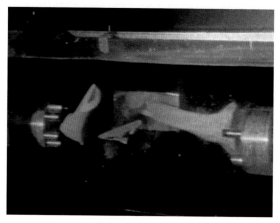

 Video AO51013

3.2   Fracture and blood supply

Although a fracture is a purely mechanical process, it triggers important biological reactions such as bone resorption and bone (callus) formation. These two processes depend on the blood supply. The following factors may almost always damage the blood supply and have an immediate bearing on the surgical procedures:

- The accident: As a result of the displacement of the fragments, periosteal and endosteal blood vessels are ruptured and periosteum is stripped. Furthermore, the implosion damages the soft tissues which are essential for the repair process as well.
- The transportation: If rescue and transportation take place without prior fracture stabilization, motion at the fracture site will add to the initial damage.
- The surgical approach: All surgical exposures of the fracture will invariably result in additional damage, as shown by recent work on ligation of the perforating arteries in the femoral diaphysis [2].
- The implant: Considerable damage to bone circulation may result not only from the retraction and periosteal stripping required to apply an implant, but also from the interface between that implant and the bone (**Fig. 1.2-1**) [3].
- Elevated intra-articular pressure reduces the epiphyseal bone circulation, especially in young patients.

Dead bone can only be revitalized by removal and replacement (creeping substitution), a process which takes a long time to be completed. It is generally accepted that necrotic tissue (especially bone) disposes to and sustains infection (see **chapter 6.1**). Another effect of necrosis also studied is the induction of internal (Haversian) remodeling. This allows replacement of dead osteocytes but results in temporary weakening of the bone due to the temporary porosis which is part of the remodeling process. Under certain combinations of damage and loading, sequestration of a dead bone fragment may ultimately occur with long-lasting consequences.

A fracture is a purely mechanical process, but triggers important biological reactions.

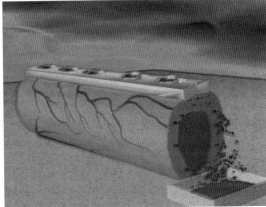

Fig. 1.2-1: The effect of implant contact upon bone blood supply. The blood supply within the area immediately deep to the plate is damaged. This area will undergo remodeling that removes the dead bone. During the second and third month after onset of necrosis, the induced remodeling results in temporary porosis. Such porosis corresponds to the tunneling activity of the Haversian osteons. It will subsequently be filled up. Occasionally, in the presence of an infection the temporary porosis may lead to sequestration.

4 Biomechanics and bone healing in different situations

4.1 Fractures without surgical stabilization

4.1.1 Mechanics

Fracture of a bone in most cases produces a completely unstable situation.

Fracture of a bone in most cases produces a completely unstable situation. Obvious exceptions to this statement are impaction fractures of the metaphyses. Non-displaced fractures with intact periosteum, as well as abduction fractures of the proximal end of the femoral neck and green-stick "fractures", are relatively stable.

Fractures without treatment

Nature tries to stabilize mobile fragments by muscle contraction.

Without treatment, **nature tries to stabilize the mobile fragments by pain-induced contraction of the surrounding muscles**, which may lead to shortening. At the same time, hematoma and swelling increase the hydraulic-pressure effect, although only temporarily, and may also have a transient stabilizing effect.

Observations made of bone healing without treatment are a help in understanding the positive and negative effects of medical intervention. It is surprising to observe how well initial mobility is compatible with solid bone healing (**Fig. 1.2-2**). In such cases the residual problem is lack of alignment and, consequently, impairment of function.

Fractures with conservative treatment

As in any fracture treatment, conservative management consists first in closed reduction to restore gross alignment. Subsequent stabilization maintains reduction and reduces mobility of the fragments which enable them to "unite" readily. In conservative treatment stabilization is achieved by the following means.

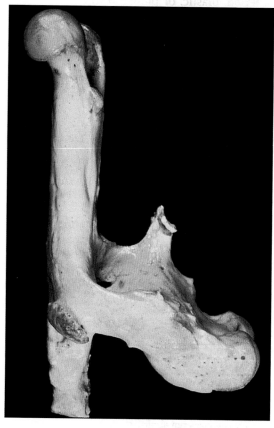

Fig. 1.2-2: Spontaneous healing of a fracture without treatment. Solid healing has been achieved but there is a severe degree of malalignment.

Traction (Fig. 1.2-3)

Application of traction along the long axis of the bone not only aligns the bone fragments, by, for example, "ligamentotaxis", but provides some stabilization as well.

External splinting

Application of externally applied splints made of wood, plastic, or plaster results in a certain

a)

b)

c)

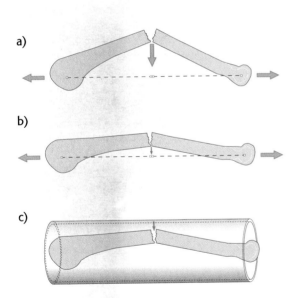

Fig. 1.2-3: Fracture reduction and stabilization by means of traction. a/b) Figures illutrate that the force reducing the fracture perpendicularly to the long axis decreases with alignment. Thus gross mobility is reduced while micro-motion persists. c) Stabilization of a fracture using a plaster cast. The plaster cast acts like a splint, it reduces mobility but does not abolish it. The cast represents a very stiff splint. The mobility stems from the fact, that the plaster cast is only loosely coupled to the bone through soft tissues.

amount of fracture stabilization. **The splint dimensions are the most important mechanical element.** Therefore, circular external splints are very stiff and strong, based on their large diameter. The strength of an external splint is mainly a function of its dimensions. A circular splint with its large outer diameter is very stiff, but its poor coupling to bone, because of interposed soft tissue, reduces its efficiency. Externally applied splints (plastic cast) result in restoration of gross anatomy and maintenance of reduction under conditions of relative mobility. In diaphyseal fractures, correct fragment alignment is all that is needed for proper function of the limb or for prompt healing of the fracture. In articular fractures, however, precise anatomical reduction is important to avoid incongruency which would give rise to excessive local strain (see also **chapter 3.1**).

4.2 Fractures with flexible surgical fixation—*Lutz Claes*

With flexible fixation, the fracture fragments displace in relation to each other when load is applied across the fracture site. A typical example is "splinting" by nail or bridging plate, in contrast to compression plating which is non-flexible. Displacement increases with the applied load and decreases with the rigidity of the splint. The two types of behavior under flexible fixation are:

- Elastic: The load results in reversible deformation of the splint. After unloading, the fragments of the fracture spring back into their former relative position.

The splint dimensions are the most important mechanical element.

With flexible fixation, the fracture fragments displace in relation to each other when load is applied across the fracture site.

- Plastic: The load results in an irreversible deformation of the splint, and the fracture fragments maintain permanent displacement. Plastic deformation occurs immediately following a variable amount of elastic deformation.

4.2.1 Mechanics

Mechanics of flexible fixation

There is no exact definition of required or tolerated flexibility or relative stability. In general, a fixation method is labeled as flexible if it allows an appreciable interfragmentary movement under functional weight bearing. **Therefore, all fixation methods with the exception of compression techniques may be seen as flexible fixations.** Devices for fracture fixation such as external fixators, internal fixators, or intramedullary nails possess various degrees of stiffness and lead to fixations of gradually differing flexibility depending on how they are applied and loaded. However, all of them allow interfragmentary movement, which can stimulate callus formation or inhibit bony union.

Intramedullary nail

The classical Küntscher nail, implanted after reaming, achieves good stability against bending moments and shear forces perpendicular to its long axis, but it is rather inefficient against torque and is unable to prevent axial shortening (telescoping). The torsional stiffness of slotted nails is low and the torsional and axial coupling between the nail and bone is loose. Therefore, the effective application of this nail was mainly limited to simple transverse or short oblique fractures (i.e., fractures that provide buttress and spontaneously lock against torsion). Additionally, the Küntscher nail is flexible in bending, which promotes callus formation.

Progress in nail design, notably the introduction of locking, which, in turn, made possible the development of the solid nail, overcame the limitations of the Küntscher nail. Due to interlocking, such nails are better able to withstand torsional moments and axial loading [4]. The stability under these loads is dependent on the diameter of the nail and the geometry and number of the locking bolts and of their spatial arrangement. The bending flexibility depends on the fit of the nail within the medullary canal and the extent of the fracture area, and can be as small as the bending flexibility of the nail itself. Intramedullary nails are located within the mechanical center of the bone and, therefore, have similar mechanical behavior in the frontal and lateral plane. This differs from what occurs with plate fixation (for more information see **chapter 3.3.1**).

External fixators

External fixators provide fixation based on the principle of splinting. Today's external fixators are commonly used as unilateral (or monolateral) devices. These are splints which are eccentrically located, in contrast to the nails, and exhibit an asymmetric mechanical behavior. They are stiffer when loaded in the plane of the Schanz screws than when perpendicular to them. An exception to this statement concerns ring fixators which display almost uniform behavior in all planes, so that displacement of the bone fragments in relation to one another is mainly axial.

All fixation methods with the exception of compression techniques may be seen as flexible fixations.

External fixators provide fixation based on the principle of splinting.

The stiffness of fracture stabilization by external fixation depends on a number of factors, such as:

- The type of implants used, for example, screws and bars.
- The geometrical arrangements of these elements in relation to the bone.
- The characteristics of the coupling of the device to the bone [5] (see **chapter 3.3.3**).

The most important factors with respect to the stability of the fixation are:

- Stiffness of the connecting rods.
- Distance between the rod (or rods) and the bone axis. The stiffer the rod (or tube) and the nearer it is to the bone axis, the more rigid is the fixation.
- Number, spacing, and diameter of the Schanz screws or of the wires, and their tension.

Usually, two Schanz screws of proper diameter in each main fragment are sufficient for a flexible fixation of a long bone fracture. The interfragmentary movement of a fracture fixation by a unilateral fixator under loading is a combination of axial, bending, and shearing displacement. A conventional application such as AO-double-tube arrangements results, under partial loading of 200–400 N, in interfragmentary movements of several millimeters and stimulates callus formation. **The external fixator is the only system which allows the surgeon to control flexibility of the fixation.**

This technique can also be used to modify the loading of the fracture area as healing progresses. This can be done by extending the distance between the bar (fixator body) and the bone, or by reducing the number of bars (or tubes in case of a double-tube fixator). In ad-dition, some types of external fixators allow axial telescoping, to stimulate the healing process (see **chapter 3.3.3**).

Internal fixators, bridging plates

Plates which span a comminuted fracture in the manner of the external fixator, provide elastic splinting. The stiffness of such an osteosynthesis depends on the dimensions of the fixator or the plate and the quality of coupling to the main fragments (see **chapter 3.3.2**).

4.2.2   Bone healing in unstable conditions

General remarks concerning bone healing under unstable conditions

Fracture healing under unstable or flexible fixation typically occurs by callus formation that mechanically unites the bony fragments. The sequence of callus healing can be divided into four stages: inflammation, soft callus, hard callus, and remodeling. The stages overlap and are determined arbitrarily. Although different investigators have described various graduations, the cascade of the healing processes is basically the same [6].

Inflammation

After the fracture, inflammation soon starts, and lasts until cartilage or bone formation begins to occur (1–7 days post-fracture). Initially there is hematoma formation and inflammatory exudate from ruptured blood vessels. Bone necrosis is seen near the ends of the fracture fragments. Vasodilatation of vessels and hyperemia in the soft tissues surrounding the

Fracture healing under flexible fixation typically occurs by callus formation.

Only the external fixator allows the surgeon to control flexibility.

fracture take place. Ingrowth of vasoformative elements and capillaries into the hematoma then occurs and cellular proliferation is enormously enhanced. Cells involved during this inflammatory period are polymorphonuclear neutrophils, macrophages, and, later on, fibroblasts. Within the hematoma there is a network of fibrin and reticulin fibrils; collagen fibrils are also present. The fracture hematoma is gradually replaced by granulation tissue. Osteoclasts in this environment remove necrotic bone at the fragment ends [6].

Soft callus

Eventually, pain and swelling decrease and soft callus is formed. This corresponds roughly to the time when the fragments are no longer freely moving, approximately 3 weeks postfracture. By the end of this stage, the stability present is adequate to prevent shortening, although angulation at the fracture site can still occur. The soft-callus stage is characterized by an increase in vascularity and ingrowth of capillaries into the fracture callus and by a further increase in cellularity. Fibrous tissue replaces the hematoma. New bone formation starts subperiosteally, and chondroblasts appear in the callus between the bone fragments [6, 7].

Hard callus

When the fracture ends are linked together by soft callus, the stage of hard callus starts and it lasts until the fragments are firmly united by new bone (3–4 months). The soft callus is converted by enchondral ossification and intramembranous bone formation into a rigid calcified tissue.

Chronological analysis shows that bony callus proliferation begins in areas remote from the fracture which are mechanically idle, and slowly progresses towards the fracture (**Fig. 1.2-4**). Two

a)
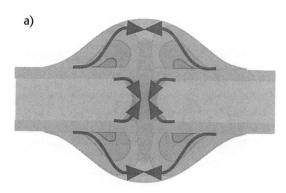

b)
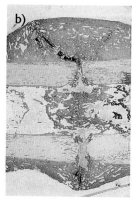
c)
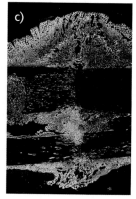

Fig. 1.2-4: a) New bone formation starts periosteally far from the fracture line and progresses towards the fracture level. Callus wedges unite most frequently peripherically and endosteally, whereas cortical healing occurs after bridging by callus.

b) Histological section of a callus healing in sheep tibia after osteotomy and external fixation (9 weeks postoperatively). c) Fluorescent labeling of the progress of new bone formation in sheep tibia 9 weeks postoperatively (green 4 weeks, yellow 8 weeks staining).

different types of bone formation occur at the same time:

- Enchondral ossification, mainly in the late phase of periosteal callus formation,
- Intramembranous bone formation periosteally and endosteally.

Bony bridging of the callus normally occurs at the periphery of the periosteal callus and endosteal bone and precedes the remodeling phase.

Remodeling

The stage of remodeling begins once the fracture has solidly united. The process may take from a few months to several years. It lasts until the bone has completely returned to its original morphology, including restoration of the medullary canal. The woven bone is slowly replaced by lamellar bone.

Biomechanics of callus healing

When bone fractures are splinted, movement of the fragments in relation to one another depends on the amount of external loading, stiffness of the splints, and the stiffness of the tissues bridging the fracture.

Initial postoperative interfragmentary movement decreases [8–10] healing time in relation to the increasing size and rigidity of the callus. When the interfragmentary movement is sufficiently reduced, "hard" bony callus bridging can occur (**Fig. 1.2-5**). For cell and tissue differentiation within the healing zone, the local tissue strain and hydrostatic pressure are more important than the interfragmentary movement. In an early stage of healing, when mainly fibrous tissue is present, the fracture tolerates a

deformation or tissue strain greater than in a later stage when the callus contains mainly calcified tissue. **Strain conditions will have to be taken into account when judging under which clinical conditions bony bridging will occur or a non-union develop.** Bony bridging between the distal and proximal callus formations can only occur when the local strain, i.e., relative deformation, is below that of the newly formed bone [11]. Even for the most simple fracture pattern and interfragmentary movement, the tissue strain shows an inhomogeneous distribution in the callus and in the cortical fracture gap [12]. Furthermore, the structure of the bridging element (direct connection or "woven" bone) is an essential factor. However, as long as the local mechanical conditions allow the cells to produce bone by enchondral ossification and/or intramembranous bone formation, the stiffness of the callus can be increased and the local tissue strain reduced to values which then allow for bony bridging.

Strain conditions will have to be taken into account when judging whether bony bridging or non-union will occur.

After union the stage of remodeling may take from a few months to several years.

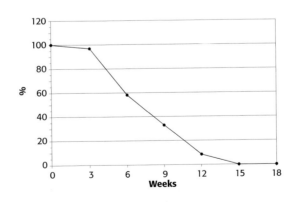

Fig. 1.2-5: Typical course of interfragmentary movement monitored for human tibial shaft fractures. The postoperative initial interfragmentary movements under 300 N axial load (normalized to 100% at the outset) decrease with the passage of time. After about 13 weeks, the callus healing has stabilized the fracture.

Bone forming cells such as osteoclasts and chondrocytes are located at the surface of the cortex or the existing callus. They experience the local surface strain and hydrostatic pressure which may be different from the strain between the bony surfaces [12, 13].

Multifragmentary fractures seem to tolerate more motion between the two main fragments because the overall movement is shared by several serial fracture planes, which reduces the tissue strain or deformation locally.

Today there is clinical experience and experimental proof that flexible fixation can stimulate callus formation, thereby accelerating fracture healing [10, 14]. This can be observed in diaphyseal fractures splinted by intramedullary nails, external fixators, or bridge plating. However, if the interfragmentary strain is excessive (instability), or the fracture gap is too wide, bony bridging by callus is not obtained in spite of good potential callus formation (hypertrophic non-union) [15].

The capacity to stimulate callus formation seems to be limited and may be insufficient when large fracture gaps are to be bridged [16]. In such cases "dynamization" by allowing axial shortening of the fixation device (nail or external fixator) can reduce the fracture gap and permit bony bridging. On the other hand, interfragmentary movement (loading) may also be too small to stimulate the necessary callus formation if the fixation device is too stiff, or if the fracture gap is too wide (low strain) [11].

Again dynamization may be the solution to the problem. If a patient is too immobile to load the operated leg, an externally applied load might be the way to stimulate callus formation [17].

Callus healing and blood supply

An immediate reduction of total bone blood flow has been observed following a fracture or osteotomy, the cortical circulation being reduced by nearly 50% [18]. This reduction has been attributed to a physiological vasoconstriction in both the periosteal and the medullary vessels as a response to trauma [19]. During the repair of a fracture, however, the adjacent intraosseus and extraosseus arterial circulation proliferates. After 2 weeks, a peak of blood supply can be observed. Thereafter, during healing, blood flow in the callus area gradually decreases again. There is also a temporary inversion of the normally centripetal blood flow after disruption of the medullary system. Microangiographic [20, 21] studies have demonstrated that **much of the vascular supply to the callus area derives from the surrounding soft tissue (Fig. 1.2-6) [20, 21], a reason not to strip any soft tissues!**

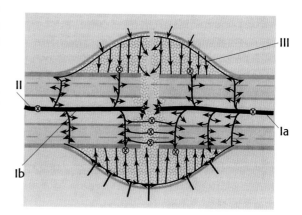

Fig. 1.2-6: Blood supply of callus formation. Top: before bony bridging. Bottom: after bony bridging. Ia) Nutrient artery ascending, Ib) nutrient artery descending, II) metaphyseal arteries, III) periosteal arteries (adapted from Rhinelander).

Complex multifragmentary fractures tolerate more motion between the main fragments than simple ones.

Much of the vascular supply to the callus area derives from the surrounding soft tissue.

Stimulation of callus formation seems limited and may be insufficient if too large a fracture gap persists.

The early vascular response seems to be extremely sensitive to the prevailing mechanical conditions. The vascular response in the cortex and in the bone marrow appears to be greater after more flexible fracture fixation than when rigid fixation is employed. However, large tissue strains, caused by instability, reduce the blood supply, especially to the fracture gap [22].

Internal fixation of fractures alters the biology of fracture healing because the fracture hematoma and soft-tissue blood supply are affected by the operative procedure. Following considerable intramedullary reaming, endosteal blood flow is reduced, but if reaming has been moderate, is rapidly restored.

Reaming does result in a delayed return of blood flow in cortical bone, which depends on the extent of reaming and the size of nail [23, 24]. Overall, endosteal blood perfusion is less affected by nailing without reaming than by "reamed nailing". Histological investigations showed that bone healing was faster after nailing without reaming and that the area of avascularity was reduced. However, the presence or absence of reaming did not affect the blood flow within the fracture callus, because the callus was mainly vascularized from the surrounding soft tissues [25].

The least damage to the blood supply, however, is done by the use of external or internal fixators with minimal fragment manipulation and little contact between implant and bone [26, 27].

4.3 Fractures with absolute stability of surgical fixation—*Stephan M. Perren*

4.3.1 General comments concerning absolute stability

If a fracture is bridged by a stiff splint, its mobility is reduced and little displacement occurs under functional load. This is often called rigid fixation. Although rigidity of the implants contributes to reducing fracture mobility, the only technique which will effectively abolish motion at the fracture site is interfragmentary compression (i.e., compression acting between the fragments).

Absolute stability diminishes the strain at the fracture site to such an extent that allows for direct healing without visible callus. Direct healing of this kind is rather a consequence of the existing biomechanical conditions than a goal in itself. When cortical bone is avascular due to trauma, long-lasting stability is required and this is where absolute stability offers the best conditions and chances for healing. In case of complications, disturbance of bone biology or vascularity is by far more serious than a mechanical condition arising from too flexible a fixation–high strain–possibly resulting in delayed union or nonunion. It takes much more experience and greater skill to treat a complication due to disturbed vitality than to fix a simple reactive (hypertrophic) non-union which just needs added mechanical stability (see chapter 6.3).

Early vascular response is influenced by local mechanical conditions.

Internal fixation of fractures alters the biology of fracture healing.

Reaming does result in a delayed return of blood flow in cortical bone.

Absolute stability reduces strain at the fracture site that allows direct bone healing.

Blood supply is least damaged by using external or internal fixators.

Treating complications due to disturbed vitality–vascularity–requires great skill.

4.3.2 Basic aspects of mechanics

The tools to achieve absolute stability are:

- **Compressive preload**
  Compression maintains close contact between two fragments, as long as compression at the fracture site exceeds the traction forces acting at the fragment ends. Studies using the sheep as an experimental animal showed that compressive pre-load does not produce pressure necrosis, neither in plate screws nor in axially compressing plates [6, 28]. Rahn [29] could show that even overloaded bone does not undergo pressure necrosis provided overall stability is maintained (**Fig. 1.2-7**).

- **Production of friction**
  When fracture surfaces are compressed against each other, friction is installed. Friction counteracts shear forces that act tangentially so sliding displacement is avoided (**Fig. 1.2-8**). Shearing stems, in most cases, from torque applied to the limb and is more important than forces acting perpendicular to the long axis of the bone. The amount of friction depends on the compression between the surfaces. For smooth bony surfaces the normal forces produce somewhat less than 40% of friction [30–32]. Rough surfaces allow a form fit and interdigitation of the fragments, which additionally counteract displacement due to shear.

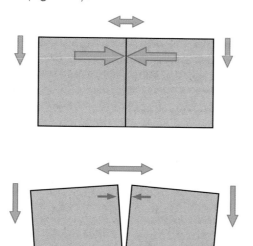

Fig. 1.2-7: Stabilization through application of compression. The compressive preload abolishes displacement of the fracture fragments and results in absolute stability as long as the compression produced is larger than the traction produced by function.

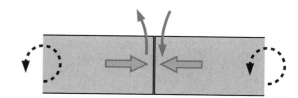

Fig. 1.2-8: Stabilization through application of compression producing friction. As long as the amount of friction is larger than the force that tends to displace the fracture along the fracture plane, absolute stability is maintained. Screw fixation of a plate relies on the same mechanism.

4.3.3   Implants providing absolute stability of fixation

Lag screws and interfragmental compression (see chapter 3.2.1)

The lag screw is a good example of an implant which relies heavily upon compression. The lag screw is applied to have purchase only in the remote cortex, and approximation between the thread and the head of the screw results in interfragmentary compression between the cortices. The fracture located between the remote and near cortices is thereby compressed and absolute stability by pre-load and friction is obtained.

In vivo experiments have shown that with lag screws not only can high amounts of forces (> 2,500 N) be produced [6, 33] (Fig. 1.2-9), but moreover, that such forces are maintained over a period which exceeds the time required for fracture healing. Compression produced by a lag screw is not only large, but it acts optimally from within the fracture in contrast to the compression produced by plates (see chapter 3.2.2).

Special biomechanical aspects and limitations

There are two relative disadvantages of compression fixation by lag screw alone. Lag screws provide a high amount of compression, but the lever arm of such compression is, in most instances, too limited to resist functional loading. This applies similarly for bending and torque, because the range of action of the compression is limited to a small diameter viewed from the center of the screw. This explains why long oblique fractures may be fixed by two to three lag screws only, while short oblique or transverse fracture cannot.

When a screw thread strips under a single overload, it loses its compressive action and is unable to recover its function. Therefore, **lag screws and plate screws should not be tightened to a level where they start to give way. Under such application the bone threads are partially damaged and/or the screws are plastically deformed. The more the screw is tightened, the greater the risk that it will lose resistance, i.e., its holding power.**

Do not over-tighten a screw, it may become loose.

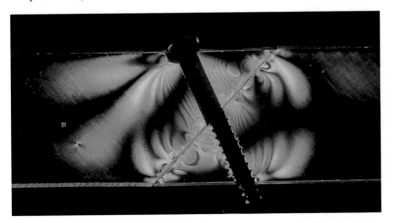

Fig. 1.2-9: Photoelastic model showing the compression exerted upon an oblique osteotomy. The lag screw produces forces of around 2,500 to 3,000 N.

Plates and their different functions

A fracture fixed with one or more lag screws provides rigid fixation without motion (absolute stability), but in general such fixation resists only minimal loading. A splint bridging the fracture site can reduce the load placed on a fracture site. Therefore, lag screws are usually combined with plates acting as splints to protect against or neutralize additional forces (**Fig. 1.2-10** and **Fig. 1.2-11**). When the fracture is closely adapted and compressed, the splint does not reduce motion but it reduces loading across the fracture.

Different plate functions

Compression is but one of many functions of a plate which can be achieved singly or in combination with other implants. The plate applied on the tension side of a bone acts optimally as a tension band. A plate may also be applied under tension so that it compresses the bone along its long axis (**Fig 1.2-12**). When used alone, this application is effective in certain transverse or short oblique fractures.

When a plate bridges a bone defect, it supports the bone fragments and keeps them in proper alignment. The plate then has a buttress function (see **chapter 3.2.2**). Under such conditions the plate initially carries full functional load (**Fig 1.2-13**).

Fig. 1.2-10: Compression by a plate. This classical picture shows that by applying tension to the plate, compression of the plated bone segment can be produced. Thus, compression acts within the bone along its long axis. Such compression is effective only in transverse fractures and, as shown using photoelasticity, is effective only in the near cortex underlaying the plate.

Fig. 1.2-11: Compression by a prebent plate. Symmetrical compression may be achieved by prebending the plate. The slightly curved plate is applied to the bone surface with the middle part elevated. When the screws are tightened, the far cortex opposite to the plate is compressed as well.

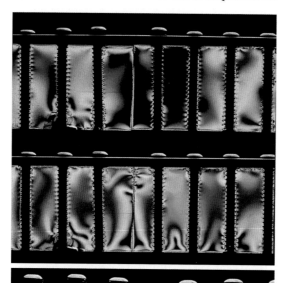
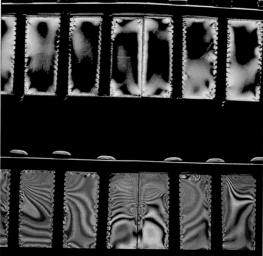

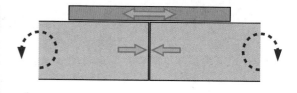

Fig. 1.2-12: Tension band plate. The plate is applied to the convex surface of the long bone, preferably on the opposite side to the muscle mass. Thus, the plate is loaded in tension and the bone in compression.

Compression using other implants

Nails are not suited to provide compression, because their spring constant, i.e., the deformation to force ratio, is very small. Thus, minute amounts of adjustment of the fracture result in shortening or creeping of the locking bolts within metaphyseal bone. This would abolish long-term stability. Still, there is a place, in the early stages, for short-term compression to reduce fracture mobility, and consequent pain, in locked nailing. **Fixators are very well suited for compression fixation in metaphyseal bone,** for example, in osteotomies. This does not necessarily apply for the diaphysis where asymmetry and flexibility must be considered together with compression. Cerclage wires lose their compression after application when the wires are released (elastic recoil) or bent over to the bone surface.

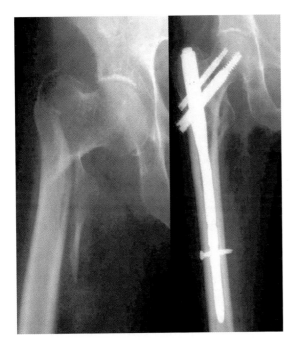

Fig. 1.2-13: Implant functioning as a buttress. The buttress function of the PFN (proximal femoral nail) provides support to the bone mainly by maintaining the original shape of the bone where the latter is not able to provide resistance to axial load. Such load would result in shortening of the bone. Buttressing is an important technique around the metaphyseal ends of the long bones.

4.3.4 Bone healing under absolute stability

Bone healing is different for cortical and cancellous bone. The basic elements correspond qualitatively, but the volume to surface ratio being very different, the speed and reliability of healing are generally better in cancellous bone.

Diaphyseal fractures

In the diaphysis, stable or rigid fixation is achieved by means of interfragmentary compression to maintain the fracture fragments in close apposition (see **chapter 3.2.2**). Pain due to motion will subside and allow for early functional after-treatment within a few days (**Fig.1.2-14**).

Radiologically, only minor changes can be observed: Under absolutely stable fixation, there is minimally visible callus formation or none at all. The fact that the fragment ends are closely apposed means that there is no actual fracture gap to be seen on the x-ray (**Fig. 1.2-15**). This renders the judgement of fracture healing difficult. **A gradual disappearance of the fracture gap, with trabeculae growing across it, is a good sign, while a widening of the gap may be an indirect sign of instability.** The surgeon judges the progress of healing based on

External fixators are very suited for compression fixation in metaphyseal bone.

In stable fixation disappearance of the fracture gap is a good sign, while widening of the gap may be an indirect sign of instability.

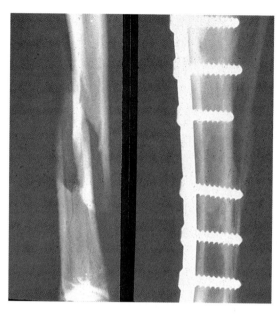

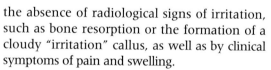

Fig. 1.2-14: Direct healing of a plated diaphysis in a German shepherd dog with unrestricted weight bearing. When the fracture fragments are held together, for instance by interfragmentary compression, no displacement between the fragment surfaces occurs. Under these conditions direct bone healing is achieved by internal remodeling of the lamellar bone.

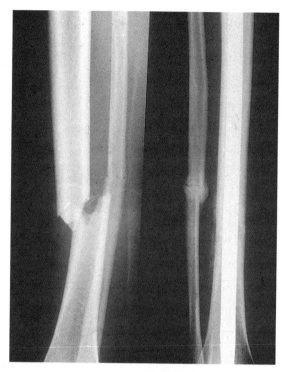

Fig. 1.2-15: Direct bone healing is not the rule after medullary nailing, but can occasionally be observed under conditions of stability. Transverse tibial fracture in a human 7 weeks postoperatively.

the absence of radiological signs of irritation, such as bone resorption or the formation of a cloudy "irritation" callus, as well as by clinical symptoms of pain and swelling.

The histological sequence of healing under conditions of absolute stability:

- In the first few days after surgery there is minimal activity within bone near the fracture. The hematoma is then resorbed and/or transformed into repair tissue. The swelling subsides while the surgical wound heals.
- After a few weeks the Haversian system starts to remodel the bone internally as

shown by Schenk and Willenegger [34] (**Fig. 1.2-16** and **Fig. 1.2-17**). At the same time "stable" gaps between imperfectly fitting fragments start to fill with lamellar bone whose orientation is transverse to the long axis of the bone.

- In the subsequent weeks, the cutter heads of the osteons reach the fracture and cross it wherever there is contact or only a minute gap [35], thus producing an interdigitation of newly formed osteons bridging the gap.

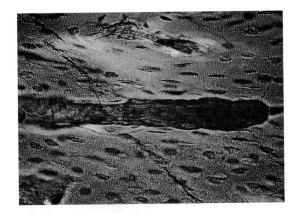

Fig. 1.2-16: Histological appearance of direct cortical bone healing. The areas of dead and damaged bone are replaced internally by Haversian remodeling. The fracture line has been graphically enhanced.

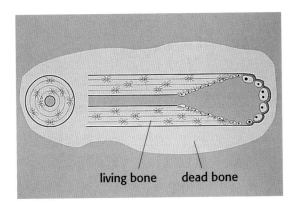

living bone   dead bone

Fig. 1.2-17: Schematic diagram of Haversian remodeling. The osteon carries at its tip a group of osteoclasts that drill a tunnel into the dead bone. Behind the tip, osteoblasts form new bone with living cells and connection to the capillaries within the canal.

Fractures in cancellous bone

Mechanically, fractures about the metaphysis are characterized by a comparatively large fracture surface. This offers good fixation in terms of bending and torque, and thus these fractures tend to be more stable, while healing occurs more rapidly. Radiological evaluation is somewhat impeded by more complex 3-D structure of the cancellous bone. The main histological activity seen in fracture healing of cancellous bone occurs at the level of the trabeculae. Healing is—due to the larger surface per volume—more likely to occur faster than in cortical bone. **Because vascularization of the cancellous bone is better, necrosis is less likely to occur.**

Necrosis in cancellous bone is less likely because of its better vascularization.

4.3.5   Biomechanics and biology of stable fracture fixation

Induction of fracture healing

Stable fixation reduces and holds the fracture so that it behaves like intact bone. It appears likely that fracture instability is the most important mechanism triggering or inducing callus in the non-stable situation. It is, therefore, difficult to understand why a stably fixed fracture would heal at all. It could be assumed that under absolute stability the effect of necrosis of the fragment ends induces internal remodeling of the bone which eventually crosses the fracture line and thus repairs the fracture. If this mechanism is to be accepted as being of importance, the treatment of choice for a fracture with extended damage to the blood supply consists in absolute stability produced by interfragmentary compression.

Precision of reduction

Today, in diaphyseal fractures, we refrain from exact reduction of a complex fracture pattern to avoid surgical damage to the blood supply. However, in articular fractures, "precise" reduction is still considered essential.

Recovery of blood supply

Absolute stability also has positive effects on blood supply, in that under stable conditions the blood vessels may more easily cross a fracture site. Despite the deleterious effects of some surgical procedures used to achieve absolute stability, once obtained, it supports the repair of blood vessels (**Fig. 1.2-18**).

In plate fixation, the comparably large contact area (footprint) of conventional plates is considered as a disadvantage. Bone tolerates mechanical loading quite well and protects the blood vessels within its structures from being affected by it. The blood vessels entering the

bone from the periosteal and endosteal sides are, however, very sensitive to any external contact. When plates are placed onto the bone surface, they are likely to disturb this periosteal blood supply. In conventional plating, part of the stability is obtained by friction between the plate and bone, which requires a minimum area of contact. Extended and continuous contact between any implant and bone results in

Absolute stability has positive effects on vascular ingrowth.

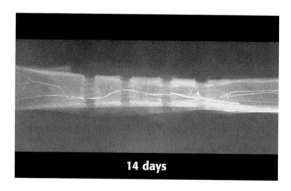

14 days

Fig. 1.2-18: The effect of stability on revascularization. The osteotomy of a rabbit tibia has been reduced and stably fixed. As early as 2 weeks after the complete transection of the bone and medullary cavity the blood vessels appear reconstructed and are functioning, as this angiography at 14 days shows.

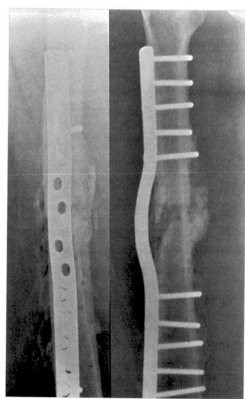

Fig. 1.2-19: Bridging plate: the plate spans a critical fracture area and is fixed only near its two ends. Thus, contact at the fracture site that could impede circulation is avoided and there is a possibility for including a bone graft under the "bridge".

areas of bone necrosis in the cortex directly underneath, for instance, a plate. This may lead to temporary porosis of the bone and, exceptionally, to sequestration. Recent studies have shown that reduction of the interface between implant and bone may improve resistance to local infection and enhance fracture healing [36] (**Fig. 1.2-19**).

4.4   Special implants

These observations have led to the development of the new LC-DCP (limited contact dynamic compression plate), but also to different concepts like the internal fixator, where the plate barely touches the cortex, while the screws lock in the plate holes (see **chapters 3.2.1** and **3.4**).

LC-DCP and internal fixators

For a reduced contact between the "plate body" and the bone and in order to reduce vascular damage, the plates were first undercut as far as safe application of screw compression would allow [37]. The next step consisted in minimizing the plate-bone contact to isolated points only [27, 38–44]. With the PC-Fix (point contact fixator) the splinting body is not pressed towards the bone due to a specially designed conical interlocking screw hole. While the LC-DCP still acts like a plate, the PC-Fix resembles a plate but acts, completely differently, as an internal fixator, i.e., a splint.

Locked screws

When the plate is used like a splint, it may take advantage of screws which are locked within the plate (**Fig. 1.2-20** and **Fig. 1.2-21**). An early example of such a device is the so-called

Schuhli, i.e., a washer-nut between the plate undersurface and the bone surface. When the nut is tightened against the plate, the screw is positioned perpendicularly to the plate body and firmly held in place [45]. A modification of this technique allows the screw to be stabilized in a selected inclination [46].

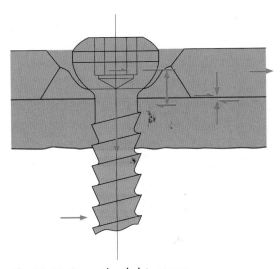

Fig. 1.2-20: Conventional plate screws

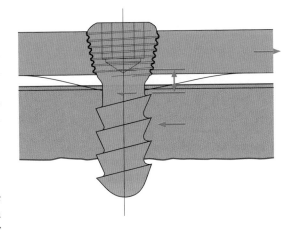

Fig. 1.2-21: Locked plate screws.

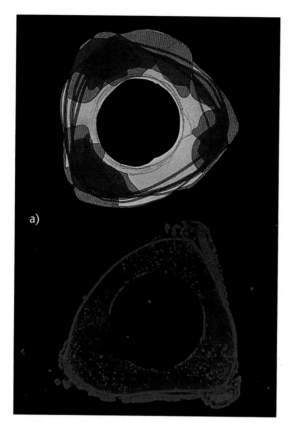

a)

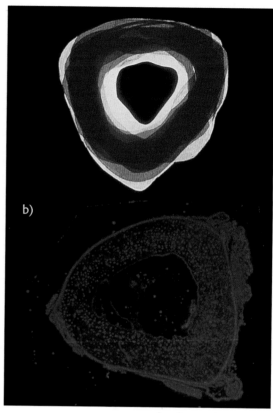

b)

4.5 Recent developments in internal fixation technology

The most important recent advance in internal fixation of fractures consists mainly in the realization of minimally invasive techniques [47] (see **chapters 3.3.2** and **3.4**). In the area of medullary nailing research has shown that the damage to endosteal blood supply can be reduced by avoiding reaming [48] (**Fig. 1.2-22**).

A further advance in nailing is the development of nails of variable flexibility. The nails are flexible at insertion and then are stiffened

Fig. 1.2-22: Effect of reamed (a) and unreamed (b) nails on the blood supply of the tibia in a group of dogs. The blood supply after the unreamed procedure is markedly better.

The lower part of each picture is a sample cross-section of the dog tibia 7 hours after surgery and preterminal application of procion red. Active blood vessels are shown as small red dots. The upper part of each picture is a composite with all cross-sections of the relevant group superimposed. The inner white area of the superimposed picture is an artifact.

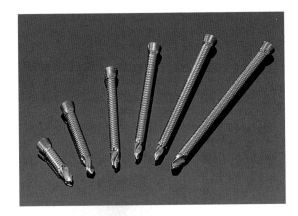

Fig. 1.2-23: Tip of a self-drilling and self-tapping screw. Such screws can be used especially with unicortical fixation. In bicortical fixation the sharp tip of the screw will likely cause irritation of the periosteal soft tissues. Self-drilling unicortical screws do not produce this problem. Furthermore, with self-drilling screws the required length cannot be measured. This is, however, not a problem for unicortical screws of predetermined length.

by a special mechanism. These nails are presently undergoing clinical testing. In external fixation, the development of the "seldrill" screw, as a radially preloading Schanz screw, has contributed to solving the problem of micro-motion-induced loosening (**Fig. 1.2-23**).

Conventional plating is being increasingly replaced by using internal fixators (**Fig. 1.2-24**). These devices, like the PC-Fix, are splints which do not require being pressed "plate-like" to bone. Thus, the area of contact can be reduced to small points isolated from each other. When developing these implants it was realized, at the same time, that by fixing the screw heads within the plate of the PC-Fix, the length of the screws could be reduced to unicortical dimensions only. This allows safe use of self-drilling self-tapping screws because the sharp drill bit tip of the screw no longer protrudes from the remote

cortex. The same principle of bolting rather than compressing implants to bone has shown its advantages in hand and maxillofacial surgery.

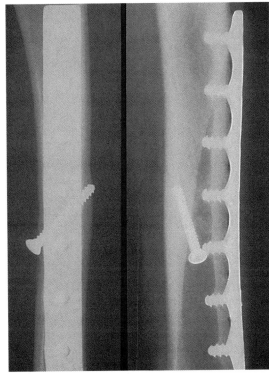

Fig. 1.2-24: Internal fixators consist of a "plate-like" body and screws but they function in a different way than the conventional plates: The conventional plate is pressed to the bone surface with high forces producing friction that prevents shear between the plate undersurface and the bone. Internal fixators forego the need for interface compression. The screws are locked within the fixator body and they act more like bolts than screws. The screw thread serves only to prevent stripping but does not produce interface compression. Thus, the contact surface between fixator and bone can be abolished or consist of small points only (point contact).

5 Outlook

Today's state-of-the-art technology of surgical fracture treatment offers interesting possibilities but it is wide open to improvement both in terms of surgical technique and of instruments and implants. The goal is well defined as being simple and cost-effective technology to achieve reliable healing and early return to full function of the limb and the patient. The technology must be of appropriate quality and its application must be safe and simple, as well as easy to learn and understand for surgeons of all levels of skills. Basic research and basic development need to cooperate with practically-oriented research and development. Once again, we face the need for intense communication and collaboration.

6 Bibliography

1. **Yamada H** (1970) *Strength of biological materials.* Baltimore: Williams & Wilkins.
2. **Farouk O, Krettek C, Miclau T, et al.** (1999) The topography of the perforating vessels of the deep femoral artery. *Clin Orthop;* (368):255–259.
3. **Gautier E, Cordey J, Mathys R, et al.** (1984) *Porosity and remodeling of plated bone after internal fixation: Result of stress shielding or vascular damage?* Amsterdam: Elsevier Science Publishers: 195–200.
4. **Schandelmaier P, Krettek C, Tscherne H** (1996) Biomechanical study of nine different tibia locking nails. *J Orthop Trauma;* 10 (1):37–44.
5. **Claes L, Burri C, Gerngross H** (1982) Biomechanische Untersuchungen zur Stabilität verschiedener Fixateur externe Osteosynthesen. *Unfallheilkunde;* 32–36.
6. **Bluemlein H, Cordey J, Schneider U, et al.** (1977) Langzeitmessung der Axialkraft von Knochenschrauben in vivo. *Med Orthop Tech;* 97 (1):17–19.
7. **Sarmento A, Latta LL** (1995) *Functional Fracture Bracing.* Berlin Heidelberg New York: Springer-Verlag.
8. **Claes L, Augat P, Suger G, et al.** (1997) Influence of size and stability of the osteotomy gap on the success of fracture healing. *J Orthop Res;* 15 (4):577–584.
9. **Claes L, Schmickal T, Kisse B, et al.** (1998) Monitoring and Analyses of Bone Healing of 100 Tibia Fractures. 72 (Abstract). *6th Meeting of the International Society for Fracture Repair.*
10. **Claes L, Wilke HJ, Augat P, et al.** (1995) Effect of dynamization on gap healing of diaphyseal fractures under external fixation. *Clin Biomech;* 10:227–234.
11. **Perren SM, Cordey J** (1980) *The concept of interfragmentary strain.* Berlin Heidelberg New York: Springer-Verlag.
12. **Claes LE, Heigele CA** (1999) Magnitudes of local stress and strain along bony surfaces predict the course and type of fracture healing. *J Biomech;* 32 (3):255–266.
13. **Claes LE, Heigele CA, Neidlinger-Wilke C, et al.** (1998) Effects of mechanical factors on the fracture healing process. *Clin Orthop;* (355 (Suppl)):132–147.
14. **Goodship AE, Kenwright J** (1985) The influence of induced micromovement upon the healing of experimental tibial fractures. *J Bone Joint Surg [Br];* 67 (4):650–655.

15. **Schenk R, Müller J, Willenegger H** (1968) [Experimental histological contribution to the development and treatment of pseudarthrosis]. *Hefte Unfallheilk;* 94:15–24.

16. **Brighton CT** (1984) The biology of fracture repair. *Instr Course Lect;* 33:60–82.

17. **Kenwright J, Goodship AE** (1989) Controlled mechanical stimulation in the treatment of tibial fractures. *Clin Orthop;* (241):36–47.

18. **Grundnes O, Reikeras O** (1992) Blood flow and mechanical properties of healing bone. Femoral osteotomies studied in rats. *Acta Orthop Scand;* 63 (5):487–491.

19. **Kelly PJ, Montgomery RJ, Bronk JT** (1990) Reaction of the circulatory system to injury and regeneration. *Clin Orthop;* (254):275–288.

20. **Brookes M, Revell WJ** (1998). *Blood Supply of Bone. Scientific aspects.* London: Springer-Verlag.

21. **Rhinelander FW** (1974) Tibial blood supply in relation to fracture healing. *Clin Orthop;* 105 (0):34–81.

22. **Eckert-Hübner K, Claes L** (1998) Callus Tissue Differentiation and Vascularization under Different Conditions. 11 (Abstract). *6th Meeting of the International Society for Fracture Repair.*

23. **Danckwardt Lilliestroem G, Lorenzi G, Olerud S** (1970) Intramedullary nailing after reaming. An investigation on the healing process in osteotomized rabbit tibias. *Acta Orthop Scand;* 134 (Suppl):1–78.

24. **Smith SR, Bronk JT, Kelly PJ** (1990) Effect of fracture fixation on cortical bone blood flow. *J Orthop Res;* 8 (4):471–478.

25. **Pfister U** (1983) [Biomechanical and histological studies following intramedullary nailing of the tibia]. *Fortschr Med;* 101 (37):1652–1659.

26. **Claes L, Heitemeyer U, Krischak G, et al.** (1999) Fixation technique influences osteogenesis of comminuted fractures. *Clin Orthop;* (365):221–229.

27. **Perren SM, Buchanan JS** (1995) Basic concepts relevant to the design and development of the Point Contact Fixator (PC-Fix). *Injury;* 26 (Suppl):1–4.

28. **Perren SM, Huggler A, Russenberger M, et al.** (1969) Cortical bone healing. *Acta Orthop Scand;* 125 (Suppl):3–63.

29. **Rahn BA, Gallinaro P, Schenk R, et al.** (1971) Compression interfragmentaire et surcharge locale de l'os. In: Boitzy A, editor. *Ostéogenèse et compression.* Bern: Huber.

30. **Enzler M** (1977) *Die Reibung zwischen Metallimplantat und Knochen.* (Thesis).

31. **Mikuschka Galgoczy E** (1977) *Die Kraftübertragung zwischen Osteosyntheseplatte und Knochen: Anteil der Reibung in vivo.* (Thesis).

32. **von Arx C** (1975) *Schubübertragung durch Reibung bei Plattenosteosynthesen.* 1–34 (Thesis).

33. **Cordey J, Widmer W, Rohner A, et al.** (1977) Dosierung des Drehmoments beim Einsetzen von Knochenschrauben. (Experimentelle Studie an Kortikalisschrauben mit Hilfe elektronischer Drehmomentschraubenzieher). *Z Orthop;* 115:601–602.

34. **Schenk R, Willenegger H** (1963) Zum histologischen Bild der sogenannten Primärheilung der Knochenkompakta nach experimentellen Osteotomien am Hund. *Experientia;* 19:593–595.

35. **Rahn BA, Gallinaro P, Baltensperger A, et al.** (1971) Primary bone healing. An experimental study in the rabbit. *J Bone Joint Surg [Am];* 53 (4):783–786.

36. **Eijer H** (1997) *Einfluss des Implantat-designs auf die lokale Infektentstehung – Experimentelle Untersuchung von DCP und PC-Fix Osteosyntheseplatten an Kaninchen.* Med. Fakultät der Rheinischen Friedrich-Wilhelms-Universität. Bonn: 1–70.

37. **Perren SM** (1991) The concept of biological plating using the limited contact-dynamic compression plate (LC-DCP). Scientific background, design and application. *Injury;* 22 (Suppl 1):1–41.

38. **Auer JA, Lischer C, Kaegi B, et al.** (1995) Application of the Point Contact Fixator in large animals. *Injury;* 26 (Suppl 2):37–46.

39. **Bishop N, Tepic S, Bresina SJ** (1995) A distractor for fracture reduction with minimal subsidiary handling forces. *Injury;* 26 (Suppl 2):24–27.

40. **Bresina SJ, Tepic S** (1995) Finite Element Analysis (FEA) for the PC-Fix screw drive, plate design, overcuts. *Injury;* 26 (Suppl 2):20–23.

41. **Savoldelli D, Montavon PM** (1995) Clinical handling: small animals. *Injury;* 26 (Suppl):47–50.

42. **Schatzker J** (1995) Changes in the AO/ASIF principles and methods. *Injury;* 26 (Suppl):51–56.

43. **Tepic S, Perren SM** (1995) The biomechanics of the PC-Fix internal fixator. *Injury;* 26 (Suppl):5–10.

44. **van Frank Haasnoot E, Münch T, Matter P, et al.** (1995) Radiological sequences of healing in internal plates and splints of different contact surface to bone. (DCP, LC-DCP and PC-Fix). *Injury;* 26 (Suppl):28–36.

45. **Kolodziej P, Lee FS, Patel A, et al.** (1998) Biomechanical evaluation of the schuhli nut. *Clin Orthop;* (347):79–85.

46. **Klaue K, Knothe U, Perren SM, et al.** (1998) The interlocking plate screw. Further development for increasing versatility in osteosynthesis by plates. *10th Conference of the ESB;* Leuven.

47. **Farouk O, Krettek C, Miclau T, et al.** (1999) Minimally invasive plate osteosynthesis: does percutaneous plating disrupt femoral blood supply less than the traditional technique? *J Orthop Trauma;* 13 (6):401–406.

48. **Klein MP, Rahn BA, Frigg R, et al.** (1990) Reaming versus non-reaming in medullary nailing: interference with cortical circulation of the canine tibia. *Arch Orthop Trauma Surg;* 109 (6):314–316.

7 Updates

Updates and additional references for this chapter are available online at:
http://www.aopublishing.org/PFxM/12.htm

1.3 Implants and materials in fracture fixation

Stephan M. Perren, Robert Mathys, Ortrun Pohler

1 General requirements

In internal fixation, the implant material of choice is still metal, which offers high stiffness and strength, good ductility and is biologically well tolerated. Today's metal implants are made either of stainless steel or titanium. Apart from metals, ceramics, polymers, and carbon composites, degradable materials are also used, although mainly for special applications as is the case for biologically derived materials [1].

Implant materials used for internal fixation must conform to certain basic requirements, amongst which reliable function and minimal side effects are obviously and equally important. Less evident is the need for appropriate handling qualities. The selection of material properties and implant design must respond to several often conflicting requirements, which will be used as guidelines as the different implants are discussed. Our discussion is intended to offer a logical basis for proper selection of materials rather than to provide detailed technical and biological knowledge.

2 Special requirements

2.1 Stiffness

Stiffness characterizes the relation between load applied and resulting elastic deformation. Fracture of a bone can be understood as discontinuity of bone stiffness. **Osteosynthesis restores bone stiffness temporarily, while fracture healing restores it permanently.**

When we consider an implant (nail, plate, or external fixator) spanning a fracture, for example in the lower limb, the stiffness of the implant must prevent buckling at the fracture site. To allow proper healing the device must, furthermore, reduce fracture mobility to below the critical level at which repair tissue will form.

The stiffness of the implant results from the stiffness of the material (modulus of elasticity), but even more importantly from the stiffness that is determined by the shape and dimensions of the implant itself. As an example, we may consider the modulus of elasticity of titanium which is about half that of stainless steel (**Fig. 1.3-1**). Yet an increase of the thickness of a standard titanium plate by a few of tenths of a millimeter will restore its

Only metal offers high stiffness and strength, good ductility, and biocompatibility at the same time.

Today's metal implants are made either of stainless steel or titanium.

Osteosynthesis restores bone stiffness temporarily, while fracture healing restores it permanently.

Stiffness of an implant depends not only on the material, but even more on the design and the dimensions of the device.

bending stiffness. In the past, several propositions have been made to use implants with more "bone-like" material stiffness than metals such as plastic or carbon reinforced composites [2, 3]. Still, implants with very low material stiffness do not as a rule offer an acceptable balance between biological and mechanical advantages. Such **less stiff implants reduce but do not abolish stress shielding**. Research has shown that early temporary porosis of bone in contact with implants does not depend upon the degree of unloading (or so-called stress shielding) but rather on the amount of direct vascular damage caused by the implant [4].

> Less stiff implants reduce but do not abolish stress shielding.

2.2 Strength

The term strength defines the limit of stress that a material or structure can withstand without deformation or rupture. Thus, strength determines the level of load up to which the implant remains intact.

Before a metal ruptures, it may irreversibly deform. Here again, the dimensions of the implant are often more important than strength of the material. The strength of c.p. (commercially pure) titanium is about 10% less than that of steel (**Table 1.3-1**), but an increase of implant cross-section will compensate for the difference in material strength. Strength may characterize the limit of stress (force per unit area) which results in an immediate rupture. **In internal fixation the resistance to repeated load,**

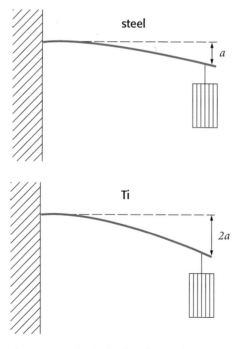

Fig. 1.3-1: Under similar bending condition and cross-sections, the titanium plate deforms nearly twice as much as the steel plate. This is due to the lower modulus of elasticity of titanium (Ti ~110 GPa, steel ~200 GPa).

Table 1.3-1: Typical mechanical properties of implant materials as used for bone screws.

	International Standards	Ultimate Tensile Strength (UTS) MPa	Elongation %
Unalloyed (c.p.) titanium grade 4B (cold-worked)	ISO 5832-2	860	18
Ti-6Al-7Nb	ISO 5832-11	1060	15
Implant quality stainless steel (cold-worked)	ISO 5832-1	960	15

which may result in failure by fatigue, is more important than strength. Compared to steel, c.p. titanium is somewhat less resistant to single loads but superior when high cycle repeated loads are acting (**Fig. 1.3-2**) [5].

2.3 Ductility

The ductility of an implant material characterizes the degree of plastic deformation it tolerates before rupture. **The ductility of a material determines the degree to which a plate, for instance, can be contoured.** As a general rule, materials of high strength such as titanium alloys and highly cold-worked pure titanium offer less ductility than steel.

Ductility provides some forewarning of impending failure, for instance during insertion of a screw. According to international standards, a 4.5 mm cortex screw (ISO 6475) must tolerate more than 180° of elastic and plastic angular deformation before breakage (**Fig. 1.3-3**). Titanium, having a lower ductility, therefore provides less of a prewarning, which means that the surgeon should first acquire some bench experience leading to a different handling technique (**Fig. 1.3-4**). The possible problems due to lower ductility of titanium may be overcome by the design of the implant: In an ongoing clinical test series with more than 2,000 locked PC-Fix screws, failure was observed neither at insertion nor thereafter [6].

Resistance to repeated loading is more important in internal fixation than ultimate strength.

Ductility of a material determines the degree to which a plate can be contoured.

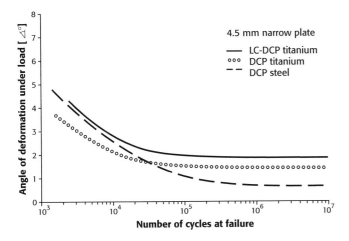

Fig. 1.3-2: Fatigue resistance—the influence of material and design. Fatigue tests of DC-plates comparing AO stainless steel and AO c.p. titanium under conditions of controlled angular deformation. Under low cycle conditions steel is better. In internal fixation where high cycle fatigue conditions are more relevant c.p. titanium is superior. The influence of the design was demonstrated, whereby the LC-DCP with its continuous stiffness along the plate proved to be superior to the DCP.

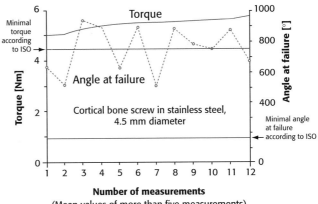

Fig. 1.3-3: Torque testing of 4.5 mm bone screws made of stainless steel. The maximum torque at failure ranges from 5–6 Nm. The angle at failure ranges from 500° to nearly 1,000°.

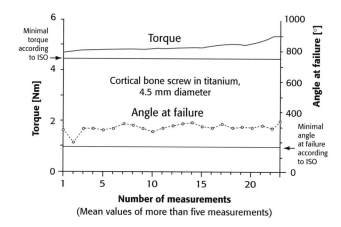

Fig. 1.3-4: Torque testing of 4.5 mm bone screws made of pure titanium. The maximum torque at failure is above 4.6 Nm. The angle at failure ranges from 200° to nearly 350°. The variance of the angle at failure is smaller than with stainless steel.

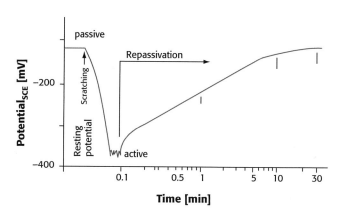

Fig. 1.3-5: Repassivation behavior of titanium in 0.9 % NaCl solution after scratching the surface with a needle.

2.4   Corrosion resistance

Corrosion determines how much "metal" is released into the surrounding tissue.

Corrosion determines how much "metal" is released into the surrounding tissue. Corrosion is different in implants made of one single component and in implant systems with several components. Stainless steel (ISO 5832-1), if tested as a single element (i.e., only as plate or as screw and not in combination of the two) is highly corrosion resistant even in the aggressive environment of the body fluids. This is due to a protecting passive layer which forms on the surface. However, when a screw head is moving in relation to the plate hole, or in relation to a nail, the passive layer is repeatedly destroyed and there is "fretting" and local corrosion in the area of contact. In contrast to stainless steel, c.p. titanium does not show such behavior [7]. Its passive layer is formed very quickly, is electrically isolating, and the implant shows literally no corrosion (**Fig. 1.3-5**). Nevertheless, when two implants made of titanium are moved against each other under load, metal debris from abrasion may be observed, and it may, though rarely, lead to harmless discoloration of the tissues. Therefore, for biological internal flexible fixation, titanium is the material of choice.

2.5   Surface structure

The surface of an implant comes into close contact with the surrounding tissues. As has been shown for titanium, the structure of metal surfaces may be made differently. The surface structure of an implant in contact with bone is of interest in respect to interface force transmission. In conventional applications, the force transmission of a plate or nail relies on friction between the implant and the bone. Strong adhesion between the screw thread and bone may be a disadvantage when considering removal of screws.

The implant surface in contact with the soft tissues has received basic consideration lately [8]. A stable interface to the soft tissues is of importance in respect to tissue adherence which may prevent formation of fluid-filled dead spaces surrounding the implant. Such dead spaces promote the growth of bacteria, while the fibrous capsule around the fluid-filled space prevents access of any of the body's cellular defense mechanisms. It is therefore of interest to promote or support the adherence of the soft tissues to the implant surface by selecting an appropriate material and surface structure. On the other hand there are situations, for example, in hand surgery, where adherence of implant surfaces to tendons and capsules is undesirable.

3 Biocompatibility

An implant material which corresponds to international standards generally manifests an adequate level of biocompatibility. There are, however, differences as shown in studies of metal applications in humans [9]. **Better behavior of an implant in respect to resisting infection may be achieved by appropriate selection of the implant material [10, 11].**

3.1 Local toxic reactions

Tissue cultures and organ cultures with bone specimens have been used to assess the toxicity of soluble corrosion products [12]. Such tests are used for screening prior to implantation in the animal. *In vivo* studies on animals [13] and from retrieved tissue samples in humans [9] indicate biological reasons for favoring c.p. titanium over stainless steel (**Fig. 1.3-6**).

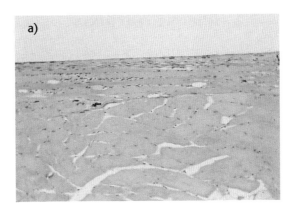

Fig. 1.3-6:
a) Histological appearance of the contacting tissue in the vicinity of a cylinder of AO pure titanium. The micrograph corresponds to 3 weeks of implantation. After an initial, non-specific reaction, little inflammation and minimal encapsulation were seen.

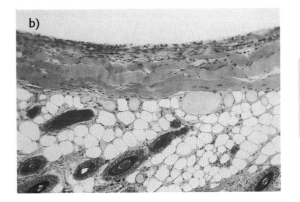

Appropriate selection of the implant material may help to improve resistance to infection of a specific implant.

b) Histological appearance of the contacting tissue in the vicinity of a cylinder of AO stainless steel. The reaction of the tissue to a single implant of steel was comparably good. If different components of implants (plate and screws) are fretting against each other, the reaction is more pronounced for steel because of "fretting" corrosion.

3.2 Allergic reactions

Some studies report that up to 20% of healthy young females are sensitive to nickel. Similar allergic reactions to skin contact are known for cobalt and chromium. **Relevant allergic reactions to nickel-containing stainless steel implants after internal fixation are estimated to be around 1 to 2%. Exact data is, however, not available. On the other hand, we do not know of any allergic reactions to c.p. titanium.** So-called "nickel-free steel" is under development and seems promising, but is not yet ready for clinical use.

Allergic reactions to stainless steel implants are rare and completely unknown for c.p. titanium devices.

3.3 Induction of tumors?

Continuous irritation of tissues may, exceptionally, lead to a neoplastic reaction. This is known from scar tissue as well as from heavily corroding metal, such as particles of ammunition. The incidence of carcinogenesis from internal fixation material, i.e., primary tumors induced by an implant, seems to be extremely low in humans, given the millions of such implants that are not removed after fracture healing. Dogs have been reported to produce sarcomas near stainless steel implants, although infection and physical irritation were contributing factors [14].

4 "New" metallic implant materials

4.1 High strength alloys

We have seen many materials being proposed to solve special problems, such as avoiding implant failure under extreme mechanical load. Improved strength may be achieved by using alloy components for titanium (e.g., vanadium) which are less biocompatible than nickel. The good overall corrosion resistance of titanium alloys neutralizes part of this potential disadvantage. The choice of an implant material depends on the priority given to mechanical advantages over biological tolerance.

4.2 Shape memory alloys

An attractive proposition seems to be to use metal alloys with a so-called shape memory effect [15]. Today's material with "shape memory" has not seen general use because of the following problems:

- The memory effect must be reliably inducible.
- The amount of force developed must be controllable.
- The material must be properly machineable.
- The cost must be appropriate in view of the advantages offered.
- The biocompatibility must be good.
- Where implant removal is considered the shape memory effect should be reversible.

Today's shape memory implant materials are very hard and thus difficult to machine. Their effect is more or less an "all or nothing" mechanism, while costs are above average. Furthermore, the presently available memory alloy contains about 50% nickel.

5 Biodegradable implants

Many implants are recommended for removal after fracture healing especially in the weight-bearing bones of the lower limb. Biodegradable materials are after a certain period of implantation resorbed or dissolve to form harmless by-products, such as H_2O and CO_2-like polylactides, which offer fair tissue tolerance. **Due to limited mechanical properties they are of interest for implants which must resist only minor loading and where surgical removal is a major undertaking.** Examples of such implants are pins for the fixation of chondral or osteochondral small defects of articular surfaces, or thin plates and screws used for fracture treatment in the maxillofacial area, including the orbit [16, 17] and skull defects, especially in children [18].

Presently, resorbable membranes are being tested for the treatment of bone defects with or without the potential for "drug" release.

An ideal sterilization process is not yet available [19]. Some caution is advised in situations susceptible to infection, as degradable material seems to exhibit a reduced resistance to infection if compared to the best metal implants [20].

6 Methods and materials for filling bone defects

The surgeon is frequently confronted with the need to treat a bone defect which may stem from the initial trauma or is the result of infection and/or avascularity. Bone may be replaced immediately or after an interval during which the host site is prepared. Common methods and materials are:

- Autogenous cancellous, corticocancellous or cortical bone, either as free or vascularized bone grafts. Though autogenous bone is superior to any other substitute, the supply for grafting is limited and the donor site is often painful. To take optimal advantage of autogenous cancellous bone, the graft may be protected using different types of bioresorbable membranes [21, 22]. As studied by Klaue et al. [23], the formation of a biological envelope may be induced by the membranes and thereafter the autogenous bone graft is inserted.
- The ingenious and successful technique of distraction osteogenesis as presented by Ilizarov [24] can be understood as being an optimally vascularized autogenous bone graft of ideal shape and dimension. The technique is quite reliable but demanding for the patient in respect of limitation of mobility, patience, and the risk of pin track infections. To cope with some of these problems other techniques have been proposed (see **chapters 6.2** and **6.3**).

Due to their mechanical properties biodegradable implants have only limited indications.

- The use of allograft bank bone requires great caution in respect to infection resistance and immunological behavior.
- Deproteinized bone (Kiel bone) behaves rather like an inert filler conducting only limited bone formation [25].

6.1 Replacement of bone by synthetic fillers

These substitutes appear attractive; they must, however, provide an appropriate combination of reliable mechanical strength, minimal impedance to bone healing, bone conductivity and/or induction. Bioresorption must occur without compromising the healing process including local resistance to infection.

The synthetic materials most commonly used for filling bone defects are hydroxyapatite (HA), β-tricalcium phosphate (β-TCP), and HA/β-TCP composites (biphasic calcium phosphate = BCP). These materials have an excellent osteoconductivity. However, they are also brittle, which reduces their field of application to low or non-load-bearing applications.

The bioresorption rate of HA is counted in decades, so HA has to be considered as non-resorbable. The solubility of β-TCP is very close to that of the mineral part of bone. Therefore, β-TCP granules or blocks are generally resorbed within 1 or 2 years *in vivo*. The biological properties of BCP are intermediate between those of β-TCP and HA.

Calcium phosphate materials are normally made porous during manufacture. Two types of pores have to be distinguished: micropores and macropres. Micropores have a size smaller than 10–30 micrometers, typically close to 1 micrometer. Micropores are too small to enable bone ingrowth. Macropores have a size larger than 30–50 micrometers. Bone can penetrate macropores and hence provide a good mechanical anchoring. Porous materials have much lower mechanical properties in terms of compression strength than dense materials. However, their resorption rate is much faster, particularly for interconnected macroporous materials.

Injectable bone substitutes, such as so-called calcium phosphate cements, have good handling properties, are mechanically stable (up to about 50 MPa in compressive strength), and are very porous (close to 50% volume). However, the small average pore size (typically 1 micrometer) prevents cell migration within the material. Additionally, these calcium phosphate cements are resorbed layer by layer rather than uniformly.

A combination of fillers with bone-inducing substances such as BMPs, and slow drug release, seems to offer an attractive potential for the future. The choice of the proper filler material depends largely upon the surgical priority to reach a proper individual balance of biological and mechanical advantages.

7 Glues

In many situations, especially in intra-articular fractures, the surgeon is confronted with the need to add and fix fragments. The use of even very small implants for this is not only difficult but also questionable. A degradable glue would solve the problem provided

- it offered proper strength under difficult conditions (saline environment),
- it were reliably and easily applicable,
- it did not impede healing i.e., were biodegradable,
- it were biocompatible (among others did not reduce local resistance to infection).

8 Bibliography

1. **Perren SM, Gasser B** (2000) Materials in Bone Surgery. *Injury;* 31 (Suppl 4).

2. **Tonino AJ, Davidson CL, Klopper PJ, et al.** (1976) Protection from stress in bone and its effects. Experiments with stainless steel and plastic plates in dogs. *J Bone Joint Surg [Br];* 58 (1):107–113.

3. **McKibbin B** (1980) Carbon Plates. In: Uhthoff HK, editor. *Current Concepts of Internal Fixation of Fractures.* Berlin: Springer-Verlag. 146–148.

4. **Gautier E, Cordey J, Mathys R, et al.** (1984) Porosity and Remodelling of Plated Bone after Internal Fixation: Result of Stress Shielding or Vascular Damage. In: Ducheyne P, Van der Perre G, Aubert AE, editors. *Biomaterials and Biomechanics:* Elsevier Science Publisher. 195–200.

5. **Perren SM, Pohler O, Schneider E** (2001) Titanium as Implant Material for Osteosynthesis Applications. *Titanium in Medicine.* Berlin: Springer-Verlag.

6. **Haas NP, Hauke C, Schütz M, et al.** (In prep.) The principles of the internal fixator applied to diaphyseal fractures of the forearm using the Point Contact Fixator (PC-Fix): Results of 387 fractures of a prospective multicentric study. *J Orthopaedic Trauma.*

7. **Steinemann SG** (1985) Corrosion of titanium and titanium alloys for surgical implants. In: Luejering G, Zwicker V, Bunk W, editors. *Titanium, Science and Technology,* 1373–1379.

8. **Richards RG, Owen GR, Rhan BA, et al.** (1997) A quantitative method of measuring cell-substrate adhesion areas. *Cells and Materials;* 7 (1):15–30.

9. **Ungersboeck A, Geret V, Pohler O** (1995) Tissue reaction to bone plates made of pure titanium: a prospective, quantitative clinical study. *Journal of Materials Science;* Materials in Medicine 6:223–229.

10. **Hauke C, Schlegel U, Melcher GA, et al.** (1996) Einfluss des Implantatmaterials auf die lokale Infektionsresistenz bei der Tibiamarknagelung. Eine experimentelle Vergleichsstudie am Kaninchen mit Marknägeln aus rostfreiem Stahl und Reintitanium. *Swiss Surgery;* 1 (Suppl 2):45.

11. **Arens S, Schlegel U, Printzen G, et al.** (1996) Influence of materials for fixation implants on local infection. An experimental study of steel versus titanium DCP in rabbits. *J Bone Joint Surg [Br];* 78 (4):647–651.

12. **Gerber H, Burge M, Cordey J, et al.** (1975) [Quantitative determination of tissue tolerance to corrosion products in organ culture]. *Langenbecks Arch Chir;* 389–394.

13. **Geret V, Rahn BA, Mathys R, et al.** (1980) A Method for Testing Tissue Tolerance for improved Quantitative Evaluation through Reduction of relative Motion at the Implant–Tissue Interface. In: Winter GD, Leray JL, de Groot K, editors. *Evaluation of Biomaterials:* John Wiley & Sons Ltd.

14. **Stevenson S, Hohn RB, Pohler OE, et al.** (1982) Fracture-associated sarcoma in the dog. *J Am Vet Med Assoc;* 180 (10):1189–1196.

15. **Baumgart F, Bensmann G, Haasters J** (1980) *Memory Alloys – New Material for Implantation in Orthopaedic Surgery.* Berlin Heidelberg New York: Springer-Verlag: Part 1, 122.

16. **Claes L, Burri C, Kiefer H, et al.** (1986) [Resorbable implants for refixation of osteochondral fragments in joint surfaces]. *Aktuelle Traumatol*; 16 (2):74–77.

17. **de Roche VR, Kuhn A, de Roche-Weber P, et al.** (1996) [Development of a resorbable implant: experimental reconstruction of the orbits with polylactate membranes. Animal model and preliminary results]. *Handchir Mikrochir Plast Chir*; 28 (1):28–33.

18. **Illi OE, Stauffer UG, Sailer HF, et al.** (1991) [Resorbable implants in craniofacial surgery in childhood. A contribution to the development of poly(lactide) implants]. *Helv Chir Acta*; 58 (1–2):123–127.

19. **Gogolewski S, Mainil-Varlet P** (1996) The effect of thermal treatment on sterility, molecular and mechanical properties of various polylactides. I. Poly(L-lactide). *Biomaterials*; 17 (5):523–528.

20. **Hauke C, Mainil-Varlet P, Printzen G, et al.** (1997) Lokale Infektresistenz bei experimenteller Kontamination resorbierbarer Osteosyntheseimplantate aus Poly(L-Lactid) und Poly(L/DL-Lactid). In: Oestern HJ, Rehm KE, editors. *Hefte zu Der Unfallchirurg. 61. Jahrestagung der Deutschen Gesellschaft für Unfallchirurgie e.V., Kongressbericht.* Springer Verlag: 852.

21. **Gerber AS, Gogolewski S** (1996) The treatment of large diaphyseal bone defect using polylactide membranes in combination with autogenenic cancellous bone. *5th World Biomaterials Congress*; Toronto. Transactions; 19, 32.

22. **Gugala Z, Gogolewski S** (1999) Regeneration of segmental diaphyseal defects in sheep tibiae using resorbable polymeric membranes: a preliminary study. *J Orthop Trauma*; 13 (3):187–195.

23. **Klaue K, Knothe U, Anton C, et al.** (1996) Biological implementation of autologous foreign body membranes in consolidation of massive cancellous bone graft. *OTA Orthopedic Trauma Association*; Boston; 71.

24. **Ilizarov GA** (1988) The principles of the Ilizarov method. *Bull Hosp Jt Dis Orthop Inst*; 48 (1):1–11.

25. **Hutzschenreuter P** (1972) [Accelerated healing of alloplastic bone grafts through presensitization of the recipient and stable osteosynthesis]. *Langenbecks Arch Chir*; 331 (4):321–343.

9 Updates

Updates and additional references for this chapter are available online at:
http://www.aopublishing.org/PFxM/13.htm

1.4 Fracture classification: biological significance

William M. Murphy & Dieter Leu

1 Introduction

The **basis of all clinical activity, be it assessment and treatment, investigation and evaluation, or learning and teaching, must be sound data, properly assembled, clearly expressed, and readily accessible.** Recognizing this, the AO group in its early days sought to document all the fracture cases treated by its members. Obviously, quality control, by whatever name it was then known, was a principal reason for this major effort at the outset of the AO's work. There was a need, during this pioneering phase, to assess the efficacy and the risks of what were, at that time, often viewed as very aggressive methods of fracture management. However, it became clear, as the volume of information built up, that some means must be found of codifying it, so that data could readily be added and extracted. This meant the development of a workable system of fracture classification [1].

Of course, the concept of classifying fractures was not new. On the contrary, almost every fracture had attracted at least one classification of its own, which was often of considerable value in actual management. However, these groupings were usually free-standing and uncoordinated and proved quite unhelpful for comparisons between the outcomes of different treatment regimes [2, 3]. What was needed was a classification protocol which would be not only universally applicable but also universally acceptable. Maurice E. Müller and his associates set about this monumental task and it is a measure of its complexity that it was not until 1990 that the third edition of the AO Manual [4] carried an extended account of the AO Classification of Long Bones, based on the achievements of Müller's group as published in 1987 and 1990 [5, 6]. Work on classification of fractures of the axial skeleton as well as of the foot and hand followed and still continues.[1]

---

[1] Notes from the editors-in-chief T.P. Rüedi and W.M. Murphy:
The AO Classification has been variously published and titled. Elements of it appeared in the first and second AO Manuals. The first complete version of the Long Bone Classification appeared in French as the AO Classification (1987) and shortly afterwards in English (1990) as the Comprehensive Classification, both by Müller et al. This modification, deriving from a SICOT Commission chaired by Professor Müller, was subsequently expanded by the addition of Pelvic and Spinal Classification, with work on the latter, as well as on foot and hand fractures, still developing. Various helpful leaflets presenting the classification in summary form and in CD format have also appeared and some have been or are now being updated. The latest "comprehensive" publication in print came in 1996 in the form of a supplement to Volume 10 of the Journal of the Orthopaedic Trauma Association. The numbering of the smaller bones is more complete in this than in the Comprehensive version and so we have adhered to it in this Volume. The AO Foundation has established a Committee to cooperate with Professor Müller in maintaining the quality and consistency of the Classification, which is henceforth named the Müller AO Classification.

"A classification is useful only if it considers the severity of the bone lesion and serves as a basis for treatment and for evaluation of the results."
Maurice E. Müller

The basis for all clinical activity must be sound data.

A fracture classification must be adaptable.

Within the AO, a decentralized documentation process has been developed, with the additional option of pooling the locally collected data from different centers. The AO clinical investigation and documentation department now provides guidelines and assistance in co-ordinating such multi-center clinical investigations from the planning phase to the final evaluation and publication. Underpinning this activity is the system on which Müller based his comprehensive fracture classification of the long bones, and on which other groups related to the AO Foundation have built or are building classifications of other skeletal areas. **The system presents a way not just to document fractures but to understand them in biomechanical and biological terms.** Needless to say, the state of the relevant soft tissues must also be diligently observed for incorporation into the decision-making process and recorded following the systems set out in **chapter 1.5.**

The system presents a way not just to document fractures but to understand them in biomechanical and biological terms.

Any classification system should offer competence in the acquisition, storage, and retrieval of data; what distinguishes Müller's system is that it provides a framework within which a surgeon can recognize, identify, and describe the injury to the bone. Thereafter, the other attributes of classification as defined by Müller at the head of this chapter can follow. **The discipline of the alpha-numeric notation serves to guide the surgeon's assessment of the fracture** to whatever depth the situation requires and afterwards to record and store his observations. However, it is the surgeon's description of the fracture which is central to the exercise. It is needed to permit good decision making in the light of the structured observations required by the classification protocol, and also to generate the code.

The discipline of the alpha-numeric notation serves to guide the surgeon's assessment of the fracture.

The key which unlocks this fracture classification is accurate description.

It follows, given the evolving and progressive nature of our understanding of fractures, and the consequent development of new treatment techniques which may influence outcomes, that **a fracture classification, while remaining consistent, must be adaptable.** This is of importance in the face of dynamic developments in treatment which, in particular, may influence the prediction and evaluation of outcomes [7]. The founding generation of AO surgeons has bequeathed, in the AO Comprehensive Classification, a very potent means to maintain the quality of our fracture management [8]. The present generation must rise to the challenge of maintaining its unique value while keeping it sufficiently flexible to accommodate new techniques and instruments and widening perceptions.

2 The principles of the fracture classification

If the surgeon is to make full use of this system, the first aim must be to identify what Müller has called as the "essence" of the fracture. This is the attribute which gives the fracture its particular identity and enables it to be assigned to one particular type rather than another. After this comes the process of putting into words what the surgeon understands as prime characteristics of the fracture, the challenges it brings, how it is to be managed, and what outcome may be anticipated with proper treatment.

The key which unlocks this fracture classification, therefore, is accurate description. Each bone or bone region is numbered and the long bones are each divided into three segments (**Fig. 1.4-1** and **Fig. 1.4-2**).

2.1 The plan of the classification

The fractures of each bone segment are then divided into three types and with further subdivision into three groups and their subgroups (**Fig. 1.4-2**) generating a hierarchical organization in triads.

The definitive subdivision of each group into subgroups may often be possible only after surgery, when the finer fracture details have been established.

These groups and subgroups are then arranged in an ascending order of severity according to the morphological complexities of the fractures, the difficulties inherent in their treatment, and their prognosis.

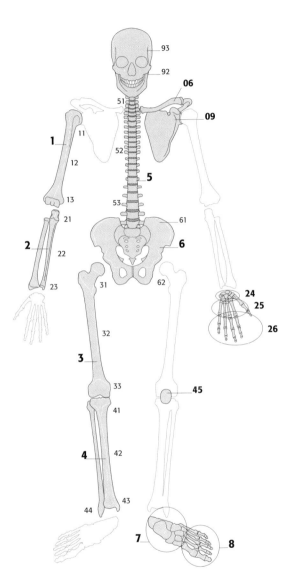

Fig. 1.4-1: Numbering, according to the OTA system for the anatomical location of a fracture, in three bone segments (proximal 1, diaphyseal 2, distal 3).

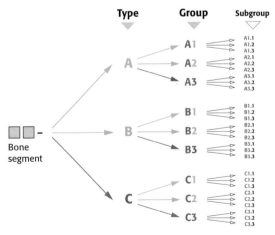

Fig. 1.4-2: To express the morphological characteristics of the fracture three types are labeled A, B, and C. Each type is then divided into three groups A1, A2, A3, B1, B2, B3, C1, C2, C3.

Within this classification, the identity of any fracture emerges from the answers to the following questions:

- Which bone?
- Which bone segment?
- Which fracture type?
- Which group?
- Which subgroup?

2.2 Bones, segments, types, and groups

The subgroups represent three characteristic variations within one group. As each group can itself be further subdivided into three subgroups, denoted by number .1, .2, .3, the result is 27 subgroups for each bone segment and 81 subgroups for each bone.

Müller and his co-workers have recently [9] refined the process by which, once the bone and the segment have been identified, the surgeon "interrogates" (for want of a better word) the fracture to establish not just its identity, but its essence.

Within this "binary" concept, the triad-based arrangement remains, but at each hierarchical level the surgeon asks a question to which the reply must be one of only two possible answers.

Thus, in a fracture identified as diaphyseal in a long bone, the first "binary" question relates to severity "Is it simple or multifragmentary?" (**Fig. 1.4-3**).

If the fracture is identified as simple, type A, the next question relates to mechanism "Was it spiral or bending?" (**Fig. 1.4-4**).

If the fracture is identified as spiral, it is then classified as A1.

Within the "binary" concept, the surgeon asks a question to which the reply must be one of only two possible answers.

Fig. 1.4-3:

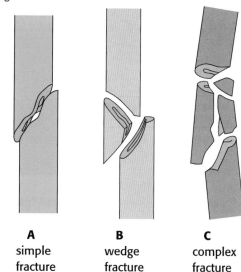

A	B	C
simple fracture	wedge fracture	complex fracture

Fig. 1.4-4:
Type A: simple fractures

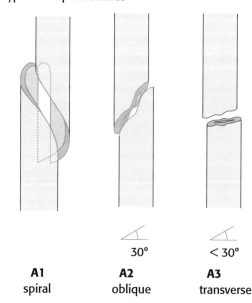

A1	A2	A3
spiral	oblique 30°	transverse < 30°

Binary questioning has the additional benefit that **if a choice from two answers cannot be identified, the imaging is probably inadequate and more information is needed.** The process may be continued to whatever depth is appropriate for the particular occasion. Obviously, in certain situations additional refinements, known as "modifiers" and "qualifications", are required to give complete expression to the complexities of the fractures encountered.

However, the goal of this chapter is to explain the rationale and process of the classification system, not to provide a detailed guide to implementing it. Therefore, discussion of the classification is confined largely to bones, segments, types, and groups as this is what is normally needed for everyday clinical application and communication. Further division into subgroups is explained and discussed as appropriate elsewhere in the book and in the Müller AO Electronic Long Bone Fracture Classification [10].

In illustrating the classification, the colors green, orange, and red denote progressive severity. Therefore, A1 indicates the fracture with the best prognosis and C3 the fracture with the worst prognosis. Thus, in identifying the information necessary to classify a fracture, one has already gone some way to establishing its mechanism, severity, and prognosis.

3 The coding of the fracture diagnosis

The diagnosis of a fracture is obtained by combining its anatomical location with its morphological characteristics. The answers to the questions described above will produce a five-element alpha-numeric code for the fracture:

□□–□□.□ . This is made up of the two "location" numbers (bone and segment) followed by the letter, indicating the fracture type, and two numbers that express the morphological characteristics of the fracture. To use the system one needs to be clear about what these abbreviations mean.

The numbering of the bones has been decided simply by convention and is self-evident from **Fig. 1.4-1**.[2] It should again be noted that the pairings of radius and ulna, and tibia and fibula are each regarded as one long bone. The identification of the segments needs a little more consideration [11].

3.1 Bone segments

Fig. 1.4-5

Each long bone has three segments:
  1 = the proximal segment
  2 = the middle (diaphyseal) segment
  3 = the distal segment
and for the distal tibia/fibula
  4 = malleolar segment

The malleolar segment is an exception, related to the complexity of its fractures and is classified as the fourth segment of the tibia/fibula.

A long bone is usually divided into one diaphyseal, two epiphyseal, and two metaphyseal segments. To determine the limits between the middle (diaphyseal) segment and the end segments, the segments are defined by a square whose sides are the same length as the

If a choice from two answers cannot be identified, the imaging is probably inadequate and more information is needed.

---

[2] Regrettably, there are differences in the numbering of some of the smaller bones between the Comprehensive and OTA versions of the Müller AO Classification. These will need to be resolved.

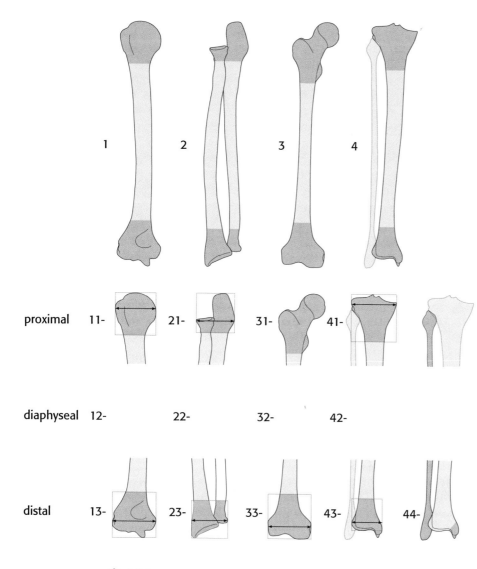

1	2	3	4	
proximal	11-	21-	31-	41-
diaphyseal	12-	22-	32-	42-
distal	13-	23-	33-	43-	44-

Fig. 1.4-5:
Anatomical location is designated by two numbers: one for the bone and one for its segment (ulna and radius, tibia and fibula are considered as one bone). The malleolar segment (44-) is an exception. The proximal and the distal segments of long bones are defined by a square whose sides are the same length as the widest part of the epiphysis (exceptions 31- and 44-).

widest part of the epiphysis (exceptions: 31- and 44-, see caption of **Fig. 1.4-5**).

In this classification no distinction is made between the epiphysis and the metaphysis. They are considered as one segment because the morphology of the fracture in the metaphysis influences the treatment and the prognosis of the articular fracture.

At this point, the important concept of the "center" of the fracture needs to be addressed. This is relevant because if a fracture is associated with a non-displaced fissure which reaches the joint, it could still be classified as a middle segment fracture (diaphyseal) depending on its center, which must be established before a fracture can definitively attached to any given segment.

4   Center of the fracture

In the context of fracture description, the term center means what it says. However, while the center of a simple fracture is apparent, and in a wedge fracture it lies where the wedge is broadest, the center of a complex fracture is usually identifiable only after reduction.

When all the features are listed, the fracture can be coded, but while the type and group may be readily identified, clarifying the final details of subgroups and qualifications may, again, only be possible after reduction.

5   The long bones

Two numbers designate the anatomical location, one for the bone and one for the bone segment.

Fig. 1.4-6:

a) Example of the coding of a fracture without subgroup: **32-B2**

b) Example of the coding of a fracture with subgroup: **33-C3.3**

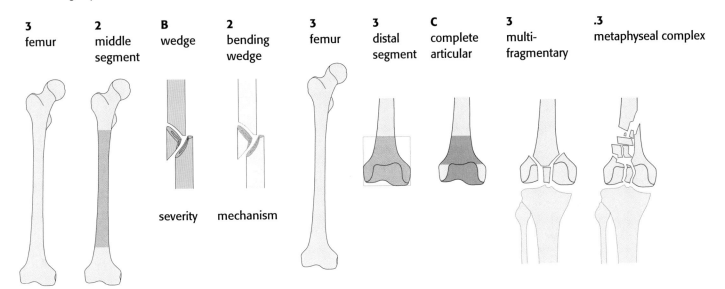

| **3** femur | **2** middle segment | **B** wedge | **2** bending wedge | **3** femur | **3** distal segment | **C** complete articular | **3** multi-fragmentary | **.3** metaphyseal complex |

severity   mechanism

5.1 Bones

As has been noted, ulna and radius, as well as tibia and fibula are each considered as one bone, making four long bones in all.

    1 = humerus
    2 = radius/ulna
    3 = femur
    4 = tibia/fibula

5.2 Types

In the proximal (-1) or distal (-3) segments all fractures are either type A, type B, or type C.

Fig. 1.4-7:

Type A   extra-articular fractures, or
Type B   partial articular fractures, or
Type C   complete articular

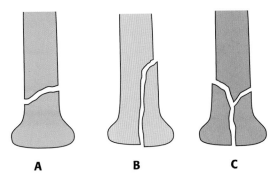

    A   **B**   **C**

Exceptions:

Fig. 1.4-8a:
proximal humerus (11-):

Type A	extra-articular unifocal
Type B	extra-articular bifocal
Type C	articular

Fig. 1.4-8b:
proximal femur (31-):

Type A	trochanteric area
Type B	neck
Type C	head

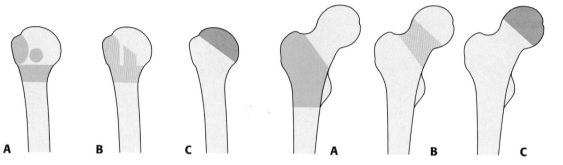

A   B   C   A   B   C

Fig. 1.4-8c:
malleolar segment (44-):

Type A	infrasyndesmotic level
Type B	transsyndesmotic level
Type C	suprasyndesmotic level

A fracture at transsyndesmotic level will destabilize the syndesmosis.

Fig. 1.4-9:
All fractures of the middle (2) segment are either "simple" fractures (type A) or multifragmentary fractures. Thus, multifragmentary fractures are split into "wedge" (type B) fractures and "complex" fractures (type C).

Type A	simple fractures
Type B	wedge fractures
Type C	complex fractures

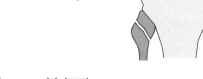
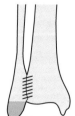
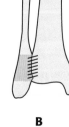
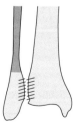
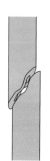
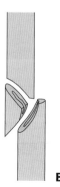
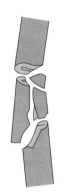

A   B   C   A   B   C

Fig. 1.4-10: Example of classification of distal femur (33-) fractures into groups (1–3)

33-A extra-articular fracture

33-B partial articular fracture

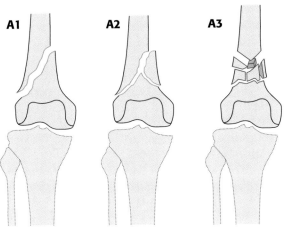
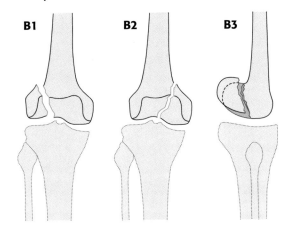

33-A1 simple
33-A2 metaphyseal wedge
33-A3 metaphyseal complex

33-B1 lateral condyle, sagittal
33-B2 medial condyle
33-B3 frontal

33-C complete articular fracture

5.3 Groups, subgroups, and qualifiers or modifiers

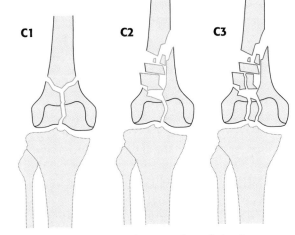

Once a fracture, whatever its bone segment, has been recognized as one of three fracture types (A, B, C), then each type may be further divided in three fracture groups (1, 2, 3), a process facilitated by binary questioning. For more specialized requirements, these groups are further divisible into three subgroups (.1, .2, .3), and in areas of particular complexity the further sub-categories known as qualifiers may be applied. These must also be known when the fracture has to be fixed and, where relevant, they are discussed in the appropriate sections of the text (**Fig. 1.4-10**).

33-C1 articular simple, metaphyseal simple
33-C2 articular simple, metaphyseal multifragmentary
33-C3 articular multifragmentary

6 Classification of soft-tissue injuries

Many different variables must be included when grading an open or closed fracture including the skin injury (IC, IO), the underlying muscle and tendon injury (MT), and the neurovascular injury (NV).

This soft-tissue classification is fully discussed in **chapter 1.5**.

7 Classification of spinal injuries

(see **chapter 4.11**)

Within this classification the spine injuries are hierarchically ranked according to severity and anatomical location corresponding to the Müller AO Classification of long bones (**Fig. 4.11-11**).

Severity progresses from type A to type C and similarly within each type, group, and further subdivision. Ranking of the spine injuries was primarily determined by the degree of instability. Prognostic aspects were taken into consideration as far as possible.

This classification needs to cater for the varying anatomical characteristics prevailing at different levels of the spine. There are four main segments of the spine (to which the number 5 had been assigned) with each vertebra having its own identity as a subsegment, except in the sacrum which is regarded as a single entity. Within this arrangement, the three main categories, the types, have their typical fundamental injury pattern, which is defined by (usually) recognizable radiological criteria. Three different mechanisms can be identified as common dominators of the types:

- Compressive force, which causes compression and burst injuries, type A;
- Tensile force, which causes injuries with transverse disruption, type B;
- Axial torque, which causes rotational injuries, type C.

The exception to this is the lower cervical spine 51.03 to 51.05, where injury caused by distraction is more severe than that from rotation and is, therefore, assigned to type C, with rotation injuries falling into type B.

The application of the AO Classification to the principles of managing spinal fractures is discussed in **chapter 4.11**.

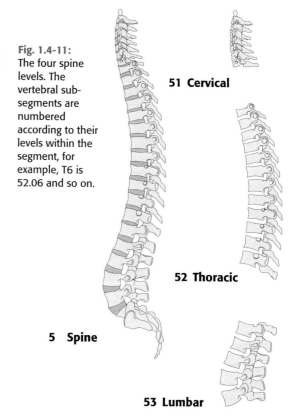

Fig. 1.4-11: The four spine levels. The vertebral sub-segments are numbered according to their levels within the segment, for example, T6 is 52.06 and so on.

51 Cervical

52 Thoracic

5 Spine

53 Lumbar

8 Classification of pelvic ring and acetabular injuries

8.1 Pelvic ring

(see **chapter 4.4**)

This classification of pelvis injuries is based on and is adapted to the universal AO Classification nomenclature suggested by M. E. Müller et al. and the classification nomenclature suggested by M. Tile et al. This classification is also divided into **bone** (6), **segments** (1,2), **types** (A, B, C), and **groups** (1, 2, 3). For a scientific classification for specialized surgeons or clinical investigators each of the three groups can be further subdivided into three **subgroups** (.1, .2, .3) and qualifications.

Anatomically, pelvic ring injuries can be described as anterior lesions or posterior lesions and as a combination of both types [12].

Anterior lesions or lesions of the anterior arch may be
- a disruption of the symphysis pubis, or
- a fracture of one or both pubic rami, possibly in combination with a disruption of the symphysis, or
- avulsion of the insertion of the rectus abdominis muscle, or
- combined lesions.

Posterior lesions or lesions of the posterior arch may be unilateral or bilateral injuries and may involve the
- Ilium: An iliac fracture usually extends from the greater sciatic notch to the iliac crest, but it can also extend into the posterior column of the acetabulum.

- Sacroiliac joint: A sacroiliac lesion may be a pure dislocation, but more commonly it includes a portion of the ilium or the sacrum.
- Sacrum: Fractures of the sacrum may be vertical or transverse below the sacrogluteal line. Vertical fractures are common in pelvic ring injuries. Transverse fractures are really spinal injuries.

Displacement of the posterior complex is most important in estimating the stability of the pelvic ring injuries. All the pelvic ring injuries, depending on the degree of posterior bony or ligamentous damage, can be classified as stable, rotationally unstable but vertically stable, or unstable both rotationally and vertically. Any break in the continuity of the sacrogluteal line represents displacement of the posterior complex.

The following terms are particularly relevant to pelvic injuries:

bilateral: both sides are involved.
contralateral: the other side, secondary lesion.
high variety: upper end of the fracture reaches the iliac crest.
ipsilateral: injury of the same side as the more severe lesion.
low variety: upper end of the fracture reaches the anterior border of the iliac crest.
partial unstable: (pelvic fractures) rotationally unstable but vertically and posteriorly stable. Posterior displacement less than 1 cm.
stable: able to withstand normal physiological stresses without displacement.
unilateral: only one side is involved.
unstable: (pelvic fractures) complete disruption of the posterior complex with a three-dimensional translational and rotational instability.

8.2 Acetabulum

(see **chapter 4.5**)

Our understanding of acetabular fractures and their classification derives mainly from the pioneering work of Judet and Letournel [13]. The particular scheme of classification employed by Letournel [14] is extensively used in the day-to-day management of these complex injuries.

Anatomically, acetabular injuries may be divided, on the one hand, into partial articular and complete articular fractures and, on the other hand, into fractures of one column or both columns (the anterior and posterior), and into transversely oriented fractures.

9 Classification of foot fractures

The AO Foot & Ankle Expert Group is close to completing its work on establishing a classification for fractures of the foot.

10 Classification terminology

The main glossary is to be found in the last section of the book. The following list of terms used in classification may be helpful in understanding this chapter.

articular: fractures which involve the articular surface. They are subdivided into partial articular and complete articular fractures.

articular-partial: these fractures involve only part of the articular surface, while the rest of that surface remains attached to the diaphysis.

articular-complete: fractures in which the articular surface is disrupted and completely separated from the diaphysis. The severity of these fractures depends on whether their articular and metaphyseal components are simple or multifragmentary.

complex: a fracture with one or more intermediate fragment(s) in which, after reduction, there is no contact between the main proximal and the distal fragments. The complex fractures are spiral, segmental, or irregular.

extra-articular: these fractures do not involve the articular surface, also they may be intracapsular. They include apophyseal and metaphyseal fractures.

impacted: a stable and usually simple fracture of the metaphysis or epiphysis in which the fragments are driven one into the other.

multifragmentary: a term used to characterize any fracture with one or more completely separated intermediate fragment(s) in the diaphyseal segment and the metaphysis. It includes the wedge and the complex fractures.

multifragmentary depression: a fracture in which part of the joint is depressed and the fragments are completely separated.

pure depression: an articular fracture in which there is pure depression of the articular surface without a split. The depression may be central or peripheral.

pure split: a fracture, resulting from a shearing force, in which the direction of the spilt is usually longitudinal.

simple: a term used to characterize a single circumferential fracture of a diaphysis or metaphysis, or a single disruption of an articular surface. Simple fractures of the diaphysis or metaphysis are spiral, oblique, or transverse and have only two fragments.

wedge: a fracture with one or more intermediate fragment(s) in which, after reduction, there is some contact between the main fragments. The spiral or bending wedge may be intact or fragmented.

11 Bibliography

1. **Colton CL** (1991) Telling the bones [editorial]. *J Bone Joint Surg [Br]*; 73(3):362–364.

2. **Bernstein J, Monaghan BA, Silber JS, et al.** (1997) Taxonomy and treatment— a classification of fracture classifications. *J Bone Joint Surg [Br]*; 79(5):706–707; discussion 708–709.

3. **Colton CL** (1997) Fracture classification. *J Bone Joint Surg [Br]*; 79(5):706–707; discussion 708–709.

4. **Müller ME, Allgöwer M, Schneider R, et al.** (1991) *Manual of Internal Fixation.* 3rd ed. Berlin Heidelberg New York: Springer-Verlag.

5. **Müller ME, Nazarian S, Koch P** (1987) *Classification AO des fractures: les os longs.* Berlin Heidelberg New York: Springer-Verlag.

6. **Müller ME, Nazarian S, Koch P, et al.** (1990) *The Comprehensive Classification of Fractures of Long Bones.* Berlin Heidelberg New York: Springer-Verlag.

7. **Burstein AH** (1993) Fracture classification systems: do they work and are they useful? [editorial]. *J Bone Joint Surg [Am]*; 75(12):1743–1744.

8. **Orozco R, Sales JM, Videla M** (2000) *Atlas of Internal Fixation. Fractures of Long Bones.* Berlin Heidelberg New York: Springer-Verlag.

9. **Müller ME** (1994) *CCF Comprehensive Classification of Fractures. Pamphlet I and II.* Bern: M. E. Müller Foundation.

10. *Müller AO Electronic Long Bone Fracture Classification.* (2002) AO Publishing/ Thieme. (in preparation).

11. **Spiegel PG, et al.** (1996) *Fracture and Dislocation Compendium. Journal of Orthopaedic Trauma. Official Journal of the Orthopaedic Trauma Association and the International Society for Fracture Repair;* 10 (Suppl 1). Philadelphia: Lippincott–Raven.

12. **Tile M** (1995) *Fractures of the Pelvis and Acetabulum.* Baltimore: Williams & Wilkins.

13. **Judet R, Judet J, Letournel E** (1964) Fractures of the acetabulum: classification and surgical approaches for open reduction. *J Bone Joint Surg*; 46:1615–1646.

14. **Letournel E, Judet R** (1993) *Fractures of the Acetabulum.* 2nd ed. Berlin Heidelberg New York: Springer-Verlag.

12 Updates

Updates and additional references for this chapter are available online at:
http://www.aopublishing.org/PFxM/14.htm

1.5 Soft-tissue injury: pathophysiology and its influence on fracture management
Evaluation/classification of closed and open injuries

Norbert P. Südkamp

Introduction

Fractures with a soft-tissue injury must be considered as surgical emergencies. They need a sophisticated management protocol as well as an excellent grading system in order to achieve the goal of uncomplicated healing with complete restitution of function.

Open fractures and fractures with concomitant closed soft-tissue damage are very often associated with additional injuries, where the primary care and priorities of multiply injured patients must be considered. As far as the fracture itself is concerned, the difficulty is to make a correct analysis of the extent of the soft-tissue injury, as well as to determine what steps and procedures should be instituted, and in which sequence. The surgeon needs not only to be familiar with the pathophysiology of a soft-tissue injury, but also with the timing, risks, and benefits of the different treatment options, and must consider both the local injury and the whole patient.

Immediately after resuscitation, and as soon as the vital parameters appear stable, assessment of the musculoskeletal system is undertaken. This must include the history of the injury and a complete diagnostic work-up of the bony and the soft-tissue lesions. These provide the surgeon with the data required to classify the limb injury, a prerequisite for the subsequent decision-making process.

1 Pathophysiology and biomechanics

1.1 Open soft-tissue injury

The condition of the wound after injury is determined by the following factors:
- Type of insult and area of contact (blunt, penetrating, pointed, sharp, crush, etc.).
- Force applied.
- Direction of force (vertical or tangential).
- Area of body affected.
- Contamination of the wound (sterile surgical wound, degree of dirt, foreign bodies, etc.).
- General physical condition of the patient (age, associated illness, immune response, etc.).

Fractures with soft-tissue injuries are surgical emergencies.

Table 1.5-1: Types of wounds.

Type of force	Type of injury
Sharp, pointed	Dash, stab wound
Blunt	Contusion injury, cut
Extension, twist	Laceration
Shear	Degloving, wound defect, avulsions, abrasion
Combination of forces	Wounds from blows, impaling, bites, and gunshot
Crushing	Traumatic amputation, rupture, crush injury
Thermal	Burns

A combination of these factors will produce different types of wounds, as shown in **Table 1.5-1**. The wounds differ not only in their shape, but also in the type of treatment required and the prognosis for healing [1].

Any injury causes bleeding and tissue destruction. This activates humoral and cellular mechanisms to stop bleeding and to resist infection. **The sequential healing processes starting immediately after trauma can be divided into three phases: the exudative or inflammatory phase, the proliferative phase, and the reparative phase.**

The healing process has three phases: exudative, proliferative, and reparative.

2 Pathophysiological responses in healing

2.1 Inflammatory phase

In the initial inflammatory phase, there is a massively increased interaction between the leukocytes and the injured microvascular endothelium. The traumatically induced exposure of the subendothelial collagen structures leads to the aggregation of thrombocytes. These, in addition to vasoconstriction (serotonin), secrete adrenaline and thromboxane-A and, above all, cytokines such as PDGF and TGF-β, which have a strong chemotactic and mitogenic effect on macrophages, neutrophilic granulocytes, lymphocytes, and fibroblasts. Vasoconstriction, thrombocyte aggregation, and the cascade-like activation of the clotting and complement systems act together with fibrin to stop the bleeding. As a side effect, the damaged tissue is under-perfused, leading to subsequent hypoxia and acidosis. The first cells to move from the small vessels into the damaged tissue are neutrophilic granulocytes and macrophages. While the leukocytes are responsible for non-specific resistance to infection, the main function of the macrophages lies in the removal of necrotic tissue and microorganisms (phagocytois and secretion of proteases) and in the production and secretion of cytokines (PDGF: mitogenic and chemotactic; TNF-α: pro-inflammatory and angiogenic; (β-FGF, EGF, PDGF, and TGF-β: mitogenic [2, 3]).

Besides the cytokine-induced early activation of immunocompetent cells, the macrophages are responsible for the inhibition and destruction of contaminating bacteria and the removal of cell debris from the damaged tissue. However, the capacity of the macrophages for phagocytosis is limited. If their capacity is overloaded by an excessive amount of necrotic tissue, this will decrease the antimicrobial activities of the mononuclear phagocytes. Since these phagocytic activities are associated with high oxygen consumption, areas of hypoxia and avascular areas are especially at risk of infection. **The pathophysiological rationale for performing radical surgical débridement in areas of dead tissue [4] lies, therefore, in helping or supporting the phagocytic process of the macrophages.**

Individual chemotactic substances, such as kallikrein, improve vascular permeability and exudation by releasing the nonapeptide bradykinin from α_2-globulin fraction. Prostaglandin originating from tissue debris stimulates the release of histamine from the mast cells and causes local hyperemia, which is necessary for the metabolic processes of wound healing. In addition, highly reactive oxygen and hydroxyl radicals are also released during the peroxidation of membrane lipids [5], which cause a further destabilization of the cell membranes. These mechanisms result in an impairment of endothelial permeability in the capillary system, which again promotes hypoxia and acidosis in the damaged areas.

The infiltrating granulocytes and macrophages, with their capacity to resist infection and to engulf cell debris and bacteria (physiological wound débridement), play a key role in the inflammatory response of traumatized tissue and therefore have a decisive effect on the subsequent reparative processes [6].

2.2 Proliferative and reparative phases

After successful occlusion of the vessels, the proliferative phase begins, followed by a smooth transition to the reparative phase. Stimulated by the mitogenic growth factors, fibroblasts, followed by endothelial cells, migrate into the area of the wound and proliferate there. These cells have a series of growth factor receptors on their surfaces and, by paracrine and autocrine processes, release several cytokines and synthesize the structural proteins of the extracellular matrix (collagen). Fibronectin—proteins cleft from the surface of the fibroblasts by hydrolases—facilitate the bonding of type I collagen to α_1-chains, an important prerequisite for progressive reparative cell proliferation. Parallel to this activity, the proliferating endothelial cells are forming into in-growing capillaries, the typical characteristic of granulation tissue. At the end of the reparative phase, water content is reduced and the collagen initially formed is replaced by cross-linked collagen type III [7]. Fibrosis and scarring follow. The role of the growth factors in scar formation is as yet unclear, but it seems that TGF-β plays a decisive role [8–10].

The pathophysiological rationale for radical débridement is to support phagocytosis.

3 Diagnosis and treatment in closed soft-tissue injuries

3.1 Problems of diagnosis and assessment

In open soft-tissue injuries, contamination and infection of the wound have a negative effect on pathophysiological processes, whereas **in closed injuries the principal diagnostic and therapeutic difficulties lie in the inaccessibility of the subcutaneous soft tissues.** This particular situation, in which the problem of assessment is combined with progressive secondary loss of tissue, is a central issue in the clinical management of closed soft-tissue injuries [11]. Although almost all modern imaging procedures permit qualitative assessment of posttraumatic closed soft-tissue injuries, clinically useful test procedures for the quantitative assessment of damage are not yet available. There are, as yet, no clear diagnostic criteria, which would allow definitive preoperative differentiation between reversibly (living) and irreversibly (dead) damaged tissue, as a guide to selecting options for treatment and prognosis.

3.2 Damage mechanisms

The pathomorphological correlate for progressive myonecrosis of initially vital, marginal areas, (i.e., those not directly affected by the trauma) of skeletal muscle (secondary tissue loss) is prolonged breakdown of the microvascular blood supply. Concurrently with the damage arising from ischemia itself, resulting from damage to vessels, there occurs a massive, trauma-induced, inflammatory reaction in both the damaged areas and those immediately adjacent. This is characterized by a drastic increase in leukocyte-endothelial interaction and subsequent loss of endothelial integrity (increased microvascular permeability). This situation leads to massive transendothelial leakage of plasma and consequently to interstitial edema [12].

3.3 Compartment syndrome

A compartment syndrome is defined as an increase within a fascial or osteofascial space of interstitial fluid pressure sufficient to compromise microcirculation and neuromuscular function [14, 20].

3.3.1 Mechanism and local pathology

In closed fractures with soft-tissue injury, the threat posed by compartment syndrome is not to be underestimated. It is triggered by an increase in intramuscular pressure, either exogenous (restrictive plaster casts) or endogenous (ischemia, hematoma), within a closed osteofascial space at a level above a critical microvascular perfusion pressure [13, 14]. If impairment of microcirculation resulting from increased tissue pressure persists, severe and irreversible neuromuscular dysfunction due to hypoxia will occur, with muscle necrosis and axonotmesis. In contrast to previous opinions, it has been shown that for compartment syndrome to become manifest, it is the relationship (ΔP, muscular perfusion pressure) of the mean systemic blood pressure to the intramuscular compartment pressure which is critical rather than the constant threshold value of 30 mmHg. Thus, it has become apparent that for a ΔP of less than 40 mmHg, obvious dysregulation in nutritive perfusion, in tissue oxygenation, and in the aerobic cell metabolism are already occurring [13]. The aim of any therapeutic procedure must, therefore, be the immediate decompression of the soft tissue by dermatofasciotomy to achieve revascularization of the capillary bed.

3.3.2 Compartment syndrome— clinical manifestations and management

A compartment may be defined as an anatomical space, bounded on all sides either by bone or deep fascial envelope, which contains one or more muscle bellies. In addition, the surrounding epimysium, the skin, or a constricting dressing can create such an envelope with limiting boundaries. The relative inelasticitiy of the envelope's wall means that if the muscle tissue swells, the pressure in the osseofascial envelope can increase.

The diagnosis of a compartment syndrome is usually made by the clinical manifestations of unrelenting and bursting ischemic muscle type pain that is unrelieved by the expected amounts of analgesia. There is usually some numbness and tingling in the involved nerve distribution, assuming that one has an alert, conscious patient whose perceptions or response have not been changed by distracting injury or environmental circumstance, such as alcohol.

Clinical signs show a tense swollen compartment where palpation will reproduce the pain and passive stretch of the digits of the muscle of the involved compartment will also increase the pain. This sign may be helpful, although not very specific. A sensory deficit in the nerve traversing the compartment may or may not be present. Motor weakness is a late change. Pulses are always palpable in a compartment syndrome, because in a normotensive patient, the muscle pressures rarely exceed the systolic level.

If the magnitude and duration of this interstitial pressure increase are great enough, irreversible tissue necrosis will occur. Patients who suffer from an untreated or overlooked compartment syndrome may suffer ischemic contracture, as described by Volkmann, which clinically corresponds to a contracted non-functional limb. In order to preserve function in severe extremity trauma, the surgeon must have thorough knowledge of the symptoms and causes of a potential or impending compartment syndrome.

The rise of pressure may also result from an increase in volume within a given compartment by hemorrhage, perivascular infusions, and edema due to abnormal capillary permeability in prolonged ischemia.

There is agreement that the blood flow to the muscles is determined by the relationship of the intracompartmental to the intravascular blood pressure and not by the absolute pressure within a fascial compartment. Hypotension can equally result in a compartment syndrome, as different authors [13, 21] have shown. **Multiply injured patients with hypovolemia and hypoxia are therefore predisposed to develop compartment syndromes.** Other injuries carrying a high risk of developing compartment syndrome include: vascular injuries with peripheral ischemia, high-energy trauma, severe soft-tissue crush, and comminuted fractures of the tibia [22].

3.3.3 Diagnosis

The differential diagnosis is between arterial injury and peripheral nerve injury. This can be determined by the fact that absent pulses point to arterial injury, while peripheral nerve injury is the diagnosis of exclusion.

Compartment syndromes can also be diagnosed by tissue-pressure measurements. The

Severe pain—especially on passive motion—is often the first sign for a compartment syndrome.

Multiply injured patients with hypovolemia and hypoxia are predisposed to compartment syndrome.

tissue pressure is usually elevated before signs and symptoms develop, and this attribute can be used to diagnose an impending compartment syndrome, or to clarify in situations where clinical examination may be unreliable, such as the head injury or the drug patient. Tissue measurements can be done by a variety of techniques. The infusion technique is simple and continuous, but may worsen the syndrome, and usually has a higher pressure threshold than other methods. The wick technique uses some fine material inside the catheter to maintain the opening to allow continuous monitoring. Finally, the stick technique is usually a reliable, simple system to use but requires one to buy the appropriate equipment.

3.3.4 Management

The treatment of choice is the dermatofasciotomy, since the skin, as long as it remains intact, acts as a limiting membrane, sustaining the compartment syndrome. There are several techniques, and those most commonly used are the double-incision technique of Mubarak [23] and the parafibular dermatofasciotomy described by Matsen [20]. Both techniques provide a release of all four compartments in the lower leg. Even if the pressure is increased in only one or two compartments, it is mandatory to release all. This is true for every possible location of compartment syndrome in the upper or lower extremity. The fibulectomy fasciotomy as popularized in the vascular surgical literature is contraindicated for trauma patients.

3.4 Systemic response to soft-tissue injury

Apart from the local microvascular and cellular damage associated with traumatic soft-tissue injury, severe damage can also lead to a marked systemic inflammatory response (MOD, multiorgan dysfunction syndrome) with the release of proinflammatory cytokines (TNF-α, IL-1, IL-6, IL-10) and damage to central organs away from the injury site (remote organ injury) [15–17].

Thus, the pathophysiological changes in damaged tissue after soft-tissue trauma are the product of a vicious circle (**Fig. 1.5-1**) made up of:

1. Impairment of microvascularity with hypoxia.
2. Acidosis.
3. Permeability damage.
4. Edema.
5. Increase in interstitial pressure due to edema in the presence of constriction of the swelling tissue by fasciae or skin with secondary disturbance to perfusion.
6. Metabolic dysfunction of the tissue and necrosis.
7. Greater vulnerability to infection of the damaged tissue. Acidosis of the polytraumatized patient.
8. Protraction of all mechanisms in the presence of generalized hypoxia and acidosis of the polytraumatized patient.

3.5 Emergency evaluation of soft-tissue injury

3.5.1 History

Tscherne [18] and Yaremchuk et al. [19] have emphasized the importance of a complete patient history. To determine the appropriate choice and

Fig. 1.5-1: Pathophysiology of the soft-tissue injury.

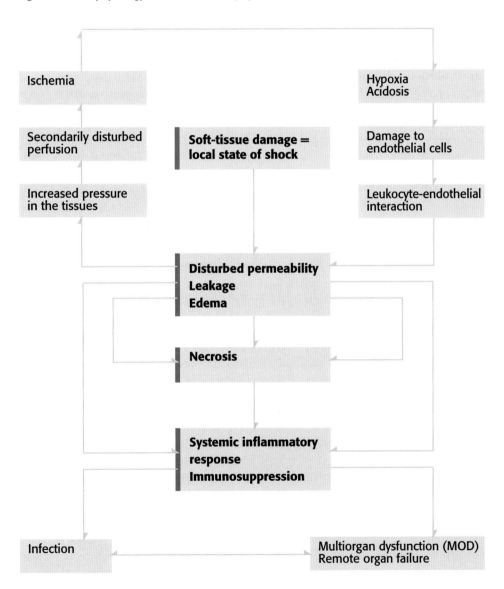

timing of treatment the surgeon needs to know when, where, and how the injury occurred. For instance, prolonged entrapment in a car suggests the possibility of a compartment syndrome, and barnyard accidents have a high risk of infection. **Most important of all is the knowledge of the amount and direction of force or energy causing the injury.** This determines both the extent of the injury and the necessary steps in treatment. The greater the force, the more serious will be the damage and sequelae.

Knowledge of the direction and the amount of force or energy causing the injury is essential.

Concomitant soft-tissue injuries are most important not only in open but also in closed fractures.

3.5.2 Vascular status

For the assessment of an injured limb it is mandatory to determine its vascular status. The peripheral pulses as well as the temperature and the capillary refill must be checked and compared with the uninjured side. Although the absence of a palpable pulse is an important pointer to potential vascular damage, the presence of a pulse or a good capillary refill does not necessarily guarantee an intact vascular supply. We advocate Doppler examination of the injured and unharmed extremity for screening. In all cases of doubt or where the history of trauma, the physical examination, or the radiographic fracture patterns are suggestive of vascular damage, angiography should be performed.

3.5.3 Neurological status

Neurological assessment can be difficult in the multiply injured patient because of unconsciousness, with lack of response to tests for motor function and sensation. However, examination of the reflexes and the response to strong, painful stimuli give some indications of major deficits. These examinations have to be performed repeatedly, because the confirma-

tion of a major nerve deficit can be decisive in the choice between salvage versus amputation in severely injured extremities.

3.5.4 Soft-tissue conditions

Although less evident than in open fractures, concomitant soft-tissue injuries have an enormous importance also in closed fractures. Their exact evaluation and determination can be much more difficult than in open fractures and their severity is easily underestimated. Simple abrasions represent an injury of the physiological barrier of the skin and can allow the development of deep infection. If this occurs, it is usually therapeutically much more challenging and difficult compared to a simple perforation of the skin.

In open fractures, the wound is covered by sterile dressing at the site of the accident and this should not be removed before the patient is brought to the operating theater. Only there and under sterile conditions is the full extent of the soft-tissue damage assessed. (Some authors allow one removal for a Polaroid photograph to facilitate planning.)

The degree of wound contamination is important in that it influences the course and outcome of the injury. Foreign bodies and dirt particles give useful information about the level of contamination and allow this to be correctly graded. High-velocity shotgun wounds and farming accidents have to be considered as severely contaminated.

After formal surgical skin preparation, with washout of dirt and debris, the traumatic wound is excised and, if necessary, extended. Gentle manipulation and inspection give best information about the condition of the bone and the extent of soft-tissue damage. The surgical débridement becomes a diagnostic exercise as skin edges, subcutaneous fat, muscles, and fascial elements are checked for viability and bleeding. **The definitive assessment of a soft-tissue injury requires an experienced surgeon as it determines the treatment protocol as well as the choice of the implant for fracture fixation.**

A compartment syndrome is seen mostly in the lower leg but can also occur in the thigh, forearm, buttock, and foot. Compartment syndromes may occur at any time during the first few days after trauma.

3.5.5 Assessment of the fracture

At the time of débridement careful inspection of bony fragments, their relationship to the soft-tissue envelope and blood supply, as well as the information obtained from the x-rays, combine to optimize the assessment of the damage. **The radiographic fracture pattern provides indirect information about the soft-tissue injury**, and shows foreign bodies, dirt, soft-tissue density, or entrapped air around and/or distal to the fracture site.

3.5.6 Management algorithm

Fig. 1.5-2 shows a flow chart of considerations and actions required in the management of fractures with concomitant soft-tissue damage.

3.6 Classification of fractures with soft-tissue injury

A classification of the concomitant soft-tissue injury, considering all essential factors, offers the best support in choosing the appropriate management of fracture treatment and guides the surgeon's attention to the necessary issues and measures (for an alternative view on classification systems, see **chapter 5.2**). It also **effectively decreases complications by preventing avoidable treatment errors and it may even be of some prognostic value.** There is also the possibility to monitor and compare standardized treatment protocols with classification systems, reminding the surgeon to consider the value of additional measures.

The most commonly used classifications of open fractures are the one by Gustilo and Anderson [24, 25] and by Tscherne [26].

3.6.1 Gustilo and Anderson classification

On the basis of a retrospective and prospective analysis of 1,025 open fractures Gustilo and Anderson [24] developed their classification, initially describing three types (I–III). Clinical practice led Gustilo to extend and subdivide his classification of the type III injury into subgroups A, B, and C [25].

Gustilo type I: Fractures of this type have a clean wound of less than 1 cm in size with little or no contamination. The wound results from a perforation from the inside out by one of the fracture ends. Type I fractures are simple fractures, like spiral or short oblique fractures.

Gustilo type II injuries have a skin laceration larger than 1 cm, but the surrounding tissues have minor or no signs of contusion. There is no dead musculature present and the fracture instability is moderate to severe.

Gustilo type III open fractures have extensive soft-tissue damage, frequently with compromised vascularity with or without severe wound contamination, and marked fracture instability due to comminution or segmental

The assessment of soft-tissue injuries requires a lot of experience.

The fracture pattern provides indirect information about potential soft-tissue injuries.

Soft-tissue classification decreases complications by preventing therapeutic errors and can have prognostic value.

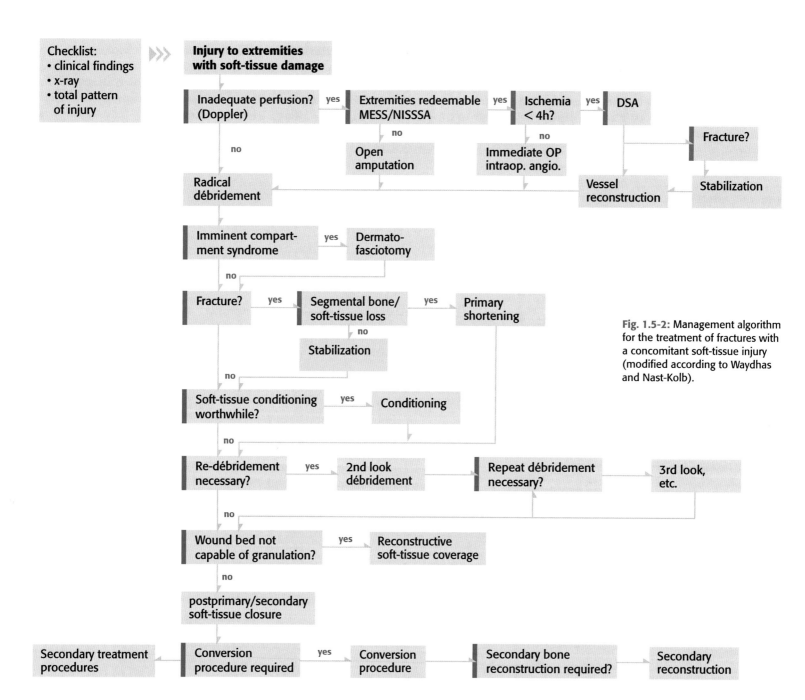

Checklist:
• clinical findings
• x-ray
• total pattern of injury

Injury to extremities with soft-tissue damage

Inadequate perfusion? (Doppler) — yes → Extremities redeemable MESS/NISSSA — yes → Ischemia < 4h? — yes → DSA

no (Extremities redeemable) → Open amputation

no (Ischemia) → Immediate OP intraop. angio.

DSA → Fracture?

no (Inadequate perfusion) → Radical débridement

Vessel reconstruction

Stabilization

Radical débridement → Imminent compartment syndrome — yes → Dermato-fasciotomy

no → Fracture? — yes → Segmental bone/soft-tissue loss — yes → Primary shortening

no (Segmental) → Stabilization

no (Fracture) → Soft-tissue conditioning worthwhile? — yes → Conditioning

no → Re-débridement necessary? — yes → 2nd look débridement → Repeat débridement necessary? → 3rd look, etc.

no → Wound bed not capable of granulation? — yes → Reconstructive soft-tissue coverage

no → postprimary/secondary soft-tissue closure

Secondary treatment procedures ← Conversion procedure required — yes → Conversion procedure → Secondary bone reconstruction required? → Secondary reconstruction

Fig. 1.5-2: Management algorithm for the treatment of fractures with a concomitant soft-tissue injury (modified according to Waydhas and Nast-Kolb).

defects. Because of the many different factors occurring in this group, Gustilo decided to form the subtypes III A, III B, and III C.

Gustilo type III A usually results from high-energy trauma, but there is still adequate soft-tissue coverage of the fractured bone, despite extensive soft-tissue laceration or flaps.

Gustilo type III B in contrast to the type III A has an extensive soft-tissue loss with periosteal stripping and bone exposure. These injuries are usually associated with massive contamination.

Gustilo type III C includes any open fracture associated with arterial injury requiring repair, independent of the fracture type.

3.6.2 Tscherne classification of soft-tissue injuries

In Tscherne's classification, soft-tissue injuries are grouped according to severity into four different categories. Along with this the fracture is labeled as open or closed by an "O" or a "C".

Open fracture grade I (Fr. O I): Fractures of this group are represented by skin lacerated by a bone fragment from the inside. There is no or only little contusion of the skin, and thus fractures are the result of indirect trauma (type A fractures according to the AO classification). However, cases with a minor skin wound, or even with no visible soft-tissue damage, but with a fracture resulting from direct trauma, as type B and type C fractures in the AO classification, must be classified as grade II open.

Open fracture grade II (Fr. O II): Grade II open fractures are characterized by any type of skin laceration with a circumferential skin or soft-tissue contusion and moderate contamination. This injury can be accompanied by any type of fracture. Any severe soft-tissue damage without injury to a major vessel or peripheral nerve is categorized in this group.

Open fracture grade III (Fr. O III): To classify a fracture as grade III the fracture must have an extensive soft-tissue damage, often with an additional major vessel injury and/or nerve injury. Every open fracture that is accompanied by ischemia and severe bone comminution belongs in this group. Furthermore, farming accidents, high-velocity gunshot wounds, and manifest compartment syndromes are graded as third degree open because of their extremely high risk of infection.

Open fracture grade IV (Fr. O IV): Grade IV open fractures represent the subtotal and total amputations. Subtotal amputations are defined by the "Replantation Committee of the International Society for Reconstructive Surgery" as separation of all important anatomical structures, especially the major vessels with total ischemia. The remaining soft-tissue bridge may not exceed 1/4 of the circumference of the limb. Any case of revascularization can only be classified as grade three open.

3.6.3 Tscherne classification of closed fractures

Closed fracture grade 0 (Fr. C 0): No or minor soft-tissue injury. The fracture C 0 includes simple fracture types with an indirect fracture mechanism. A typical example is the spiral fracture of the tibia in a skiing injury.

Closed fracture grade I (Fr. C I): Superficial abrasion or contusion, the fragment pressure from within, simple or medium severe fracture types. A typical injury is the unreduced pronation–dislocation fracture of the ankle joint; the soft-tissue damage occurs through fragment pressure at the medial malleolus.

Closed fracture grade II (Fr. C II): Deep contaminated abrasions and localized skin or muscle contusions through an adequate direct trauma. The imminent compartment syndrome also belongs into this group. Usually the injury results from direct trauma with medium to severe fracture types. A typical example is the segmental fracture of the tibia from a direct blow by a car fender.

Closed fracture grade III (Fr. C III): Extensive skin contusions, destruction of musculature, subcutaneous tissue avulsion. Manifest compartment syndromes and vascular injuries are also graded Fr. C III. The fracture types are severe and mostly comminuted. The soft-tissue treatment of this fracture grade is usually much more difficult than a type III open fracture.

3.6.4 Hannover fracture scale

As long ago as 1980 Tscherne published for the first time a soft-tissue classification not only for open but for closed fractures, as he had realized that closed injuries to soft tissue were quite frequently underestimated. From this original classification [26] evolved the much more elaborate Hannover fracture scale.

More and more problems in the treatment of complex open fractures are due to high-velocity injury patterns. The above-mentioned and most frequently used classifications have shown limitations for these types of injuries. Horn [27] and Brumback [28] have furthermore shown in different studies that there is only a moderate interobserver reliability in classifying open fractures using the Gustilo and Anderson classification.

For these reasons, the Hannover group [29] developed the Fracture Scale (HFS) from an analysis of approximately 1,000 open fractures from 1980 to 1989 (**Table 1.5-2**).

This considers every detail of the injury to the involved extremity and is made up as a checklist. The fracture type according to the AO classification, the skin laceration, the underlying soft tissues, the vascularity, the neurological status, the level of contamination, a compartment syndrome, the time interval between injury and treatment, and the overall severity of the injury to the patient are added up to prove the total score.

"Bone loss" represents bone fragments that have been lost at the site of the accident. The longest axis of the missing piece of bone is measured and graded either as smaller or greater than 2 cm, for example, in a missing butterfly fragment the length on the outside and not the thickness would be the value considered.

For the evaluation of soft-tissues the score provides three different categories: the size of the skin wound, the area of skin loss, and the damage to deep soft tissues such as muscles and tendons. Due to different diameters and thickness of different levels in the involved extremities, the extent of soft-tissue damage is related to the circumference of the level of injury. This allows a comparison of injuries to the different levels of the upper and lower extremity. The three different categories of soft-tissue damage allow evaluation of both superficial and deep injury.

The category "amputation" serves as a primary judgement of the mechanism of the amputation in respect of a possible replantation.

An exact evaluation of the neurological status at the time of admission is often difficult, but monitoring of reflexes allows a gross estimation of possible neurological damage. This can be

A   Fracture type

Type A	1
Type B	2
Type C	4

Bone loss

< 2 cm	1
> 2 cm	2

B   Soft tissues

Skin (wound, contusion)

no	0
< 1/4 circumference	1
1/4–1/2	2
1/2–3/4	3
> 3/4	4

Skin defect

no	0
< 1/4 circumference	1
1/4–1/2	2
1/2–3/4	3
> 3/4	4

Deep soft tissues (muscle, tendon, ligaments, joint capsule)

no	0
< 1/4 circumference	1
1/4–1/2	2
1/2–3/4	3
> 3/4	6

Amputation

no	0
Subtotal/total guillotine	20
Subtotal/total crush	30

Fr. O 1:	2–3 points
Fr. O 2:	4–19 points
Fr. O 3:	20–69 points
Fr. O 4:	> 70 points

C   Ischemia/compartment syndrome

no	0
Incomplete	10
Complete	
< 4 hours	15
4–8 hours	20
> 8 hours	25

D   Nerves

Palmar-plantar sensations

yes	0
no	8

Finger-toe motion

yes	0
no	8

E   Contamination

Foreign bodies

none	0
single	1
multiple	2
massive	10

F   Bacteriologic smear

aerobe, 1 germ	2
aerobe, > 1 germ	3
anaerobe	2
aerobe-anaerobe	4

G   Onset of treatment

(only if soft-tissue score > 2)

6–12 hours	1
> 12 hours	3

Fr. C 0:	1–3 points
Fr. C 1:	4–6 points
Fr. C 2:	7–12 points
Fr. C 3:	> 12 points

Table 1.5-2: Hannover fracture scale with correlation of the fracture scale score to Tscherne's classification of open and closed fractures.

important in the process of making a decision between salvage and amputation.

At the time of admission a bacteriologic evaluation of smears may not yet be available, but the bacterial contamination is still a part of the score to remind the treating surgeons to take it into account.

The score supports injury management and therapy control. Partial scores, particularly "bone score" or the "soft-tissue score", are valuable for treatment decisions and estimation of possible complications.

Table 1.5-2 also shows the relationship of the fracture scale scores to Tscherne's classification of closed and open fractures.

3.6.5 The soft-tissue grading system of the AO

The AO also, because of the limitations of the existing classifications systems including moderate interobserver reliability and the grading of many different injuries into the same subgroup, was moved to develop a more detailed and precise grading system for fractures with concomitant soft-tissue damage.

This grading system identifies injuries to the different anatomical structures and assigns them to different severity groups. The skin (integument), the muscles and tendons, and the neurovascular system are the targeted anatomical structures; the fracture is classified according to the AO classification of fractures.

The grading of the skin lesion is done separately for open or closed fractures, the letters "O" and "C" designate these two categories. In closed fractures there are five different severity groups. IC1 represents the injury of the integument in a closed fracture, the digit "1" indicates the least and the digit "5" the highest soft-tissue damage.

Fig. 1.5-3 shows and **Table 1.5-3** describes the different severity grades of closed soft-tissue injuries while **Fig. 1.5-4** and **Table 1.5-4** explain and illustrate those of open soft-tissue injuries.

Although there may be considerable damage to the muscle envelope, there is rarely an injury to tendons except in severe injuries. The involvement of the neurovascular system always

AO soft-tissue classification

Skin lesions IC (closed fractures)

IC 1	No skin lesion
IC 2	No skin laceration, but contusion
IC 3	Circumscribed degloving
IC 4	Extensive, closed degloving
IC 5	Necrosis from contusion

Table 1.5-3:
Description of skin lesions (IC) in closed fractures.

Skin lesions IO (open fractures)

IO 1	Skin breakage from inside out
IO 2	Skin breakage from outside in < 5 cm, contused edges
IO 3	Skin breakage from outside in > 5 cm, increased contusion, devitalized edges
IO 4	Considerable, full-thickness contusion, abrasion, extensive open degloving, skin loss

Table 1.5-4:
Description of skin lesions (IO) in open fractures.

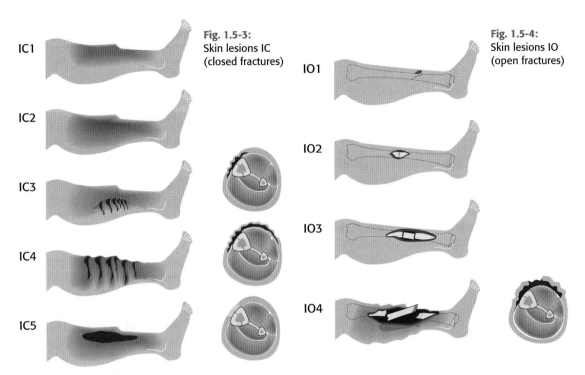

IC1

IC2

IC3

IC4

IC5

Fig. 1.5-3:
Skin lesions IC
(closed fractures)

IO1

IO2

IO3

IO4

Fig. 1.5-4:
Skin lesions IO
(open fractures)

indicates most severe injuries of the kind represented by the Gustilo types IIIB and IIIC and they also usually indicate a high complication rate. Both muscle and tendon injuries as well as neurovascular injuries and their respective extents are—if they occur—highly prognostic for the fate of the extremity. Therefore, a grading of the extent of the injury of these structures is essential. **Fig. 1.5-5** illustrates and **Tables 1.5-5** and **1.5-6** explain the involvement of the different severity groups of muscle/tendon injury and neurovascular structures.

Examples

A simple, closed spiral midshaft tibial shaft fracture with no relevant lesions of skin, muscle/tendons, nerves, and vessels is graded: 42-A1.2/IC1-MT1-NV1.

Muscle/tendon injury (MT)

MT 1	No muscle injury
MT 2	Circumscribed muscle injury, one compartment only
MT 3	Considerable muscle injury, two compartments
MT 4	Muscle defect, tendon laceration, extensive muscle contusion
MT 5	Compartment syndrome/crush syndrome with wide injury zone

Table 1.5-5: Description of muscle and tendon injuries.

Neurovascular injury (NV)

NV 1	No neurovascular injury
NV 2	Isolated nerve injury
NV 3	Localized vascular injury
NV 4	Extensive segmental vascular injury
NV 5	Combined neurovascular injury, including subtotal or even total amputation

Table 1.5-6: Description of neurovascular injuries.

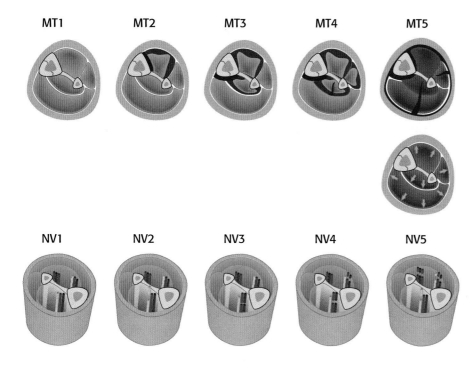

MT1   MT2   MT3   MT4   MT5

NV1   NV2   NV3   NV4   NV5

Fig. 1.5-5: Muscle/tendon injury (MT) and neurovascular injury (NV).

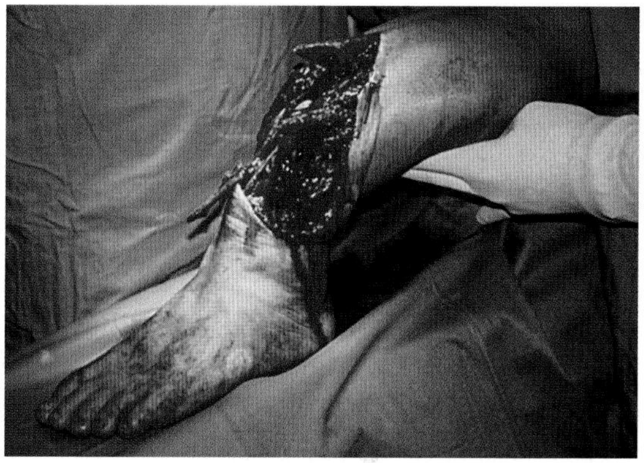

Fig. 1.5-6: Example of a 42-C3.3/IO4-MT5-NV1

In contrast, **Fig. 1.5-6** shows a severe open complex irregular distal tibial shaft fracture with extensive skin and bone loss, muscle and tendon damage, but no neurovascular injury. This injury will be graded as 42-C3.3/IO4-MT5-NV1.

3.6.6   Usage of classification systems[1]

Fractures with a concomitant soft-tissue injury have become more frequent. In particular, the higher grades in the Gustilo and Anderson classification of open fractures and in the Tscherne classification of closed fractures are most challenging from the therapeutic standpoint. These injuries have the highest complication rates and can cause severe disability to the patient.

We should keep in mind that classification systems have several objectives, namely to:
- assist the surgeon with decision making,
- identify treatment options,
- anticipate problems,
- suggest the course of treatment,
- predict the outcome,
- enable an analysis and a comparison of similar cases,
- assist documentation,
- facilitate communication.

3.6.7   Conclusion

Against this background, the Gustilo and Anderson classification of open fractures and the original Tscherne classification of closed

[1] For another viewpoint on soft-tissue classification see chapter 5.2.

fractures which were published in 1984 and 1982 respectively are no longer sufficient and will not be able to meet the required objectives of today. For **adequate treatment of a fracture with a concomitant soft-tissue injury it is mandatory to use a more sophisticated and detailed grading system,** currently available in the Hannover fracture scale or the AO soft-tissue grading system.

For adequate treatment of a fracture with a concomitant soft-tissue injury it is mandatory to use a sophisticated and detailed grading system.

4 Bibliography

1. **Levin SL** (1995) Personality of soft-tissue injury. *Tech Orthop;* 10:65–73.

2. **Leibovich SJ, Polverini PJ, Shepard HM, et al.** (1987) Macrophage-induced angiogenesis is mediated by tumor necrosis factor-alpha. *Nature;* 329 (6140):630–632.

3. **Steenfos HH** (1994) Growth factors and wound healing. *Scand J Plast Reconstr Surg Hand Surg;* 28 (2):95–105.

4. **Dorow C, Markgraf E** (1997) [Therapy of soft tissue injuries—biological strategies]. *Zentralbl Chir;* 122 (11):962–969.

5. **van der Vusse GJ, van Bilsen M, Reneman RS** (1994) Ischemia and reperfusion induced alterations in membrane phospholipids: an overview. *Ann NY Acad Sci;* 723:1–14.

6. **Cromack DT, Porras-Reyes N, Mustoe TA** (1990) Current concepts in wound healing: growth factor and macrophage interaction. *J Trauma;* 30 (Suppl 12):129–133.

7. **Lynch SE** (1991) Interactions of growth factors in tissue repair. Clinical and experimental approaches to dermal and epidermal repair in normal and chronic wounds. *Prog Clin Biol Res;* 365:341–357.

8. **Schmid P, Itin P, Cherry G, et al.** (1998) Enhanced expression of transforming growth factor-beta type I and II receptors in wound granulation tissue and hypertrophic scar. *Am J Pathol;* 152 (2):485–493.

9. **Servold SA** (1991) Growth factor impact on wound healing. *Clin Podiatr Med Surg;* 8 (4):937–953.

10. **Wu L, Siddiqui A, Morris DE, et al.** (1997) Transforming growth factor beta 3 (TGF beta 3) accelerates wound healing without alteration of scar prominence. Histologic and competitive reverse-transcription-polymerase chain reaction studies. *Arch Surg;* 132 (7):753–760.

11. **Levin SL, Condit DP** (1996) Combined injuries—soft tissue management. *Clin Orthop;* (327):172–181.

12. **Mittlmeier T, Schaser K, Kroppenstedt S, et al.** (1997) Microvascular response to closed soft-tissue injury. *Trans Orthop Res Soc;* 44:317–318.

13. **Heppenstall RB** (1997) Compartment syndrome: pathophysiology, diagnosis and treatment. *Techniques Orthop;* 12:92–108.

14. **Shrier I, Magder S** (1995) Pressure-flow relationships in in vitro model of compartment syndrome. *J Appl Physiol;* 79 (1):214–221.

15. **Gullo A, Berlot G** (1997) Ingredients of organ dysfunction failure. *World J Surg;* 20 (4):430–436.

16. **Kirkpatrick CJ, Bittinger F, Klein CL, et al.** (1996) The role of the microcirculation in multiple organ dysfunction syndrome (MODS): a review and perspective. *Virchows Arch;* 427 (5):461–476.

17. **Smail N, Messiah A, Edouard A, et al.** (1995) Role of systemic inflammatory response syndrome and infection in the occurrence of early multiple organ dysfunction syndrome following severe trauma. *Intensive Care Med;* 21 (10):813–816.

18. **Tscherne H, Gotzen L** (1984) *Fractures With Soft Tissue Injuries.* Berlin Heidelberg New York: Springer-Verlag.

19. **Yaremchuk MJ, Gotzen L** (1984) Acute management of severe soft-tissue damage accompanying open fractures of the lower extremity. *Clin Plast Surg;* 13 (4):621–624.

20. **Matsen FA,III, Winquist RA, Krugmire RB, Jr.** (1980) Diagnosis and management of compartmental syndromes. *J Bone Joint Surg [Am];* 62 (2):286–291.

21. **Zweifach SS, Hargens AR, Evans KL, et al.** (1980) Skeletal muscle necrosis in pressurized compartments associated with haemorrhagic hypertension. *J Trauma;* 20 (11):941–947.

22. **Blick SS, Brumback RJ, Poka A, et al.** (1986) Compartment syndrome in open tibial fractures. *J Bone Joint Surg [Am];* 68 (9):1348–1353.

23. **Mubarak SJ, Owen CA** (1977) Double incision fasciotomy of the leg for decompression in compartment syndromes. *J Bone Joint Surg [Am];* 59:184–187.

24. **Gustilo RB, Anderson JT** (1976) Prevention of infection in the treatment of one thousand and twenty-five open fractures of long bones: retrospective and prospective analyses. *J Bone Joint Surg [Am];* 58 (4):453–458.

25. **Gustilo RN, Mendoza RM, Williams DN** (1984) Problems in the management of type III (severe) open fractures: a new classification of type III open fractures. *J Trauma;* 24 (8):742–746.

26. **Tscherne H, Ouster HJ** (1982) [A new classification of soft-tissue damage in open and closed fractures (author's transl)]. *Unfallheilkunde;* 85 (3):111–115.

27. **Horn BD, Rettig ME** (1993) Interobserver reliability in the Gustilo and Anderson classification of open fractures. *J Orthop Trauma;* 7 (4):357–360.

28. **Brumback RJ, Jones AL** (1994) Interobserver agreement in the classification of open fractures of the tibia. The results of a survey of two hundred and forty-five orthopedic surgeons. *J Bone Joint Surg [Am];* 76 (8):1162–1166.

29. **Südkamp N, Haas NP, Flory PJ, et al.** (1989) [Criteria for amputation, reconstruction and replantation of extremities in multiple trauma patients]. *Chirurg;* 60 (11):774–781.

5 Updates

Updates and additional references for this chapter are available online at:
http://www.aopublishing.org/PFxM/15.htm

2.1 The patient and the injury
Decision making in severe soft-tissue trauma

Peter Worlock

1 Introduction

In fracture management **assessment and decision making must focus on the patient as a whole**.

It is tempting to use the fracture in isolation as the basis for making decisions about the method and timing of treatment. After all, a fracture is easily identified on an x-ray and it can then be described and classified (see **chapter 1.4**). However, it must be remembered that the fracture occurs in the limb of a patient, so there is a need for an overall philosophy of assessment, expressed through a relatively standardized and accessible system which enables appropriate decisions to be taken and which can be modified for the individual patient and the individual injury or combination of injuries.

Musculoskeletal injuries frequently occur in association with injuries to other parts of the body and, therefore, **must be considered in the context of polytrauma**, treating the patient as a whole (see **chapter 5.3**).

There are a number of systems of initial assessment and management of the polytrauma patient. One in widespread use is the Advanced Trauma Life Support system, developed by the American College of Surgeons.

In musculoskeletal trauma surgery, as in any branch of acute medicine, there is a hierarchy which determines the priority of surgical procedures (**Table 2.1-1**).

Table 2.1-1:

Priorities in surgical management of musculoskeletal injury

1) Save life
2) Save limb
3) Save joints
4) Restore function

First in priority are those procedures necessary to save life, such as packing the retroperitoneal space or applying an external fixator to an unstable pelvic fracture to stop (or at least to control) bleeding and the early stabilization of femoral shaft fractures to help prevent adult respiratory distress syndrome (ARDS) (see **chapter 5.3**). Next in priority are procedures needed to save a limb. Into this category fall restoration of the vascular supply, surgical management of open fractures, and reconstruction of the soft-tissue envelope. Third in line are procedures necessary to save a joint, which

Assessment and decision making must focus on the patient as a whole.

First in priority are those procedures necessary to save life.

Musculoskeletal injuries frequently occur in association with injuries to other parts of the body and must be considered in the context of polytrauma.

The treating hospital must be looked at and the facilities available weighed against the care and skills required to carry out optimum treatment. By bringing these factors together, the treating surgeon is able to define the "personality of the injury".

It is not only necessary to assess the fracture itself, but also to define the degree of soft-tissue injury.

include surgical exploration and débridement of open joint injuries, together with the reduction and stabilization of intra-articular fractures, allied to tendon and ligament reconstruction, to allow early movement.

Finally, in order of priority, come procedures designed to restore optimal limb function. These include surgical techniques to limit deformity and to facilitate bone and soft-tissue healing.

In forming a management plan, **it is not only necessary to assess the fracture itself, but also** to carry out a careful clinical examination of the affected limb **to define the degree of soft-tissue injury**. A number of patient factors must be assessed and related to specific injury factors. Then, the "environmental factors" of **the treating hospital must be looked at**

and the facilities available weighed against the care and skills required to carry out optimum treatment. By bringing these factors together, the treating surgeon is able to define the "personality of the injury" (**Fig. 2.1-1**)[1].

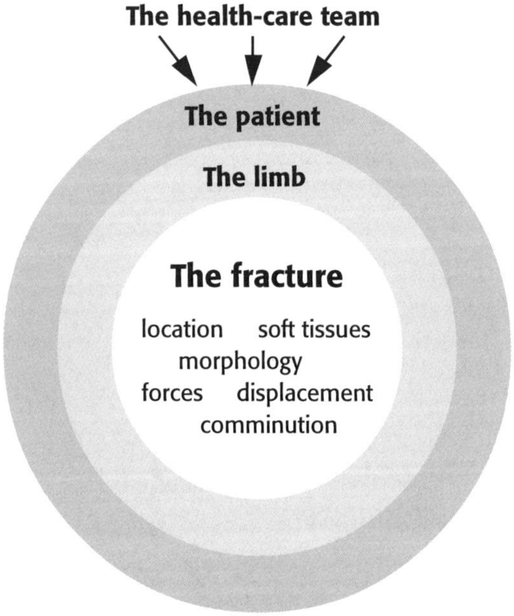

2 Injury factors

At the time of injury, external forces make contact with the body, and energy is transferred from the external object to living tissue. The damage inflicted is directly proportional to kinetic energy and this in turn is proportional to its velocity and mass ($K_\varepsilon = {}^1/_2\, mv^2$). Because kinetic energy increases with the square of the velocity, high-speed impacts produce significantly greater damage in living tissue than due low velocity impacts (**Table 2.1-2**).

Fig. 2.1-1: The personality of the injury is determined by careful assessment of the patient, the injury, and the environment (the expertise of the health-care team).

Table 2.1-2: Energy dissipated in injuries

Injury	Energy dissipated [ft-lbs]
Fall from kerb	100
Skiing injury	300–500
High-velocity gunshot wound	2,000
Car bumper collision	100,000

2.1   Injury patterns

Important information can be gleaned from the pattern of injuries—for instance, the patient with blunt chest injury and bilateral femoral shaft fractures has clearly been the recipient of significant energy transfer and in this situation it is unlikely that the abdomen/pelvis have escaped injury. **The magnitude of the injury** also **depends on the type of tissue and the site of force application**.

An external force applied to the anterior shin would be dissipated through thin skin and then through the tibia, creating an open tibial fracture (a significant problem with considerable morbidity). The same magnitude of force applied to the posterior calf would be dissipated through the local musculature and perhaps not cause a fracture at all. The application of a direct force perpendicular to the axis of the limb causes greater localized injury than an axial force applied remotely.

It is important to recognize that **there is a zone of soft-tissue injury which is larger than the area of the fracture site** (**Fig. 2.1-2**). The situation is similar to that seen in a burn; there is a central zone of necrosis surrounded by a zone of stasis (**Fig. 2.1-3**). Within the zone of stasis, tissue that is marginally viable at the time of initial injury is likely to die in the hours/days following the insult. Even the healthy

The magnitude of the injury also depends on the type of tissue and the site of force application.

There is a zone of soft-tissue injury, which is larger than the area of the fracture site.

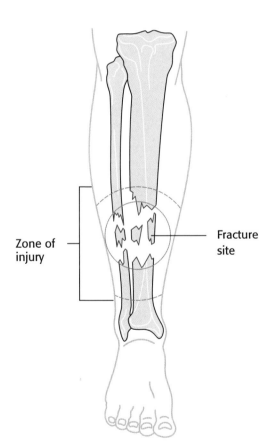

Fig. 2.1-2: Diagram representing zone of injury—an area greater than the fracture site.

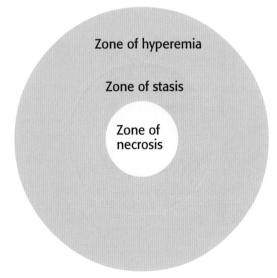

Fig. 2.1-3: The zones of injury in a burn are analogous to the concept of a soft-tissue zone of injury.

living tissue surrounding the zone of necrosis and the zone of stasis will not remain unaffected, as it is here that blood flow will initially increase, producing the so-called zone of hyperemia.

Defining the extent of the zone of injury remains a difficult but critical task in both open and closed fractures and the evaluation and classification of both closed and open injuries (see **chapter 1.4** and **chapter 1.5**) are essentially concerned with defining the extent of the zone of injury.

The assessment and management of polytrauma patients has been said to comprise the "three Rs" of Resuscitation, Reconstruction and Rehabilitation. Rather than breaking these phases down into distinct and separate groups, modern care focuses on producing a treatment plan to deal with the patient as a whole, aiming for optimum recovery. These phases will therefore overlap.

2.2 Resuscitation

Based on the ATLS protocol, initial assessment and management of the polytrauma patient is divided into four phases:
- primary survey,
- resuscitation phase,
- secondary survey,
- definitive care.

In practice, the primary survey and resuscitation phase take place simultaneously. As life-threatening injuries are identified, they are managed. The primary survey consists of "ABCDE" (Airway, Breathing, Circulation, Disability, and Exposure). **The first objective in the primary survey is to obtain and maintain a secure airway.** This may require simple or complex airway management techniques, but the cer-

vical spine must be immobilized during these maneuvers, to prevent possible further damage.

After establishment of an airway, maintenance of adequate ventilation of the lungs with oxygen is the next priority. It may be necessary to deal with conditions such as tension pneumothorax and massive open pneumothorax at this stage. The key objective in management of the polytrauma patient is ensuring perfusion of the living tissues with adequately oxygenated blood. Therefore, the prevention or treatment of shock takes place as the "circulation" phase. Two large-bore intravenous lines should be established and fluid resuscitation commenced with Hartmann's solution (Ringer's lactate). The patient should receive an infusion of two liters as rapidly as possible. If hemodynamic instability persists after infusion of two liters of crystalloid, then blood transfusion should be commenced. Patients with persistent hemodynamic instability will require surgical intervention to control hemorrhage. An ultrasound eximination of the abdomen in the emergency room may be helpful at this time. In cases of unstable pelvic fracture, the orthopedic surgeon must be prepared to play his part in saving life by decreasing pelvic volume and producing some pelvic stability.

After the "ABCs" have been performed, with life-threatening conditions identified and managed, a simple neurological assessment is performed in the "disability" (D) phase. At this stage, an attempt is made to try and define the level of consciousness and whether there is any major neurological deficit in any of the four limbs. The patient is then exposed (E) so that a full examination is performed. When not being examined, the patient should be covered with a warm blanket to prevent hypothermia.

The secondary survey takes place after the "ABCs" have been completed. It involves a

The first objective in the primary survey is to obtain and maintain a secure airway.

head-to-toe and back-to-front clinical evaluation of the patient, followed by appropriate radiological assessment, to define the full and complete pattern of injuries. Any individual limb injuries will need more detailed assessment, to define the precise pattern of each. The limbs should be carefully inspected externally for wounds, bruising, and swelling. Any deformity should be gently corrected. Dislocated joints should be reduced as rapidly as possible; they may be hampering the circulation and venous return or producing pressure on nerves and skin. **As a general rule, no harm will come in re-aligning the limbs into the normal anatomical position.** Continuing damage occurs when dislocated joints and widely displaced fractures are not corrected.

2.3   **Fracture management**

In respect of musculoskeletal injury, the following three questions need to be asked on each occasion:
1. What needs to be done?
2. When does surgery need to be performed?
3. How much can be safely performed?

Using the hierarchy already described (see **section 1**), the first priority will be to carry out any procedures that are necessary to save life. The most common reason for involvement of the orthopedic surgeon at this stage is in the management of a major pelvic fracture. An assessment must be made of both mechanical and hemodynamic instability during the primary and secondary survey. The pelvis is examined to see if there is any obvious movement suggesting instability. If a major pelvic fracture is seen on the AP x-ray, then inlet and outlet views should be taken in the resuscitation room

(see **chapter 4.4, Fig. 4.4-1**). These will allow prompt and rapid clarification of the injury and show whether there is any significant posterior or vertical shift.

The patient will then fall into one of five categories and appropriate decisions about emergency management can be made (see **chapter 4.4, Fig. 4.4-4**).

Other life-saving orthopedic interventions may include early stabilization of long bone fractures. In the 1980's, a number of retrospective studies suggested improved outcome after early femoral fracture stabilization in multiple trauma (with a reduced incidence of ARDS). Prospective studies in this field [2, 3] produced contradictory results. Pulmonary complications were found to parallel the frequency of chest injury.

During this resuscitative phase of life-saving surgery, the primary principle must be to "do no further harm". If the patient is hemodynamically stable, normothermic, has normal clotting and no ventilatory problems, then definitive stabilization of long bone fractures can be undertaken. However, in patients with persisting problems of this nature, surgical procedures on the limbs should be limited to exploration/excision of major wounds and simple stabilization of lower limb diaphyseal fractures. Half-pin external fixators with two pins above and two pins below the fracture can provide good provisional stability for shaft fractures. Using such minimal techniques, it is often possible to carry out surgery for the lower limbs while thoracic, maxillofacial, or neurosurgical procedures are simultaneously performed.

Complex intra-articular and periarticular fractures can be managed at this stage with bridging external fixators to restore length and alignment. If the patient's condition permits,

As a general rule, no harm will come in re-aligning the limbs into the normal anatomical position.

percutaneous screw fixation can be performed to maintain reduction of articular surfaces.

Continual monitoring is required during this resuscitative surgery phase. If the patient's condition deteriorates (coagulopathy, hypoxia, hypothermia, raised intracranial pressure), then major surgery should be halted. **Unless surgery is life saving, the patient is better off on the intensive care unit than in the operating room**.

High-energy open fractures, particularly of the lower limb, are common in polytrauma patients. The decision between salvage and amputation becomes especially important in the critically ill polytrauma patient. The impact of limb salvage procedures (in terms of both continuing metabolic load and the possible effect of multiple, long surgical procedures) must be considered. In order to save life, it may be necessary to amputate a mangled extremity [4] (see **chapter 1.5**).

2.4　Reconstruction

With time, and as the patient's condition stabilizes on the intensive care unit, windows of opportunity will arise for further reconstructive procedures. It is at this secondary stage (from day five to day ten—"window of opportunity" as outlined in **chapter 5.3**) that consideration is given to reconstruction of intra-articular/periarticular fractures and of upper limb injuries—part of the "reconstruction" phase of treatment.

Whatever the patient's status, each area of injury requires careful clinical and radiological assessment as part of the decision-making process. **Continuing to view the patient as a whole is essential**.

Assessment of the extent of swelling/bruising can help to determine the zone of injury. How-

ever, if assessment takes place soon after injury, then the extent of soft-tissue damage may not be apparent or appreciated. Assessment must be made of the neurovascular status, distal to the injury. Skin perfusion and the status of peripheral pulses can be assessed in all patients (using the Doppler probe if necessary). However, it should be remembered that the **presence of peripheral pulses and adequate skin circulation distally will not exclude a more proximal compartment syndrome.** In the conscious patient, it is usually possible to perform a relatively thorough assessment of motor and sensory function in the limb, once analgesia has been administered. All such details must be recorded.

The possibility of compartment syndrome must always be considered. This is most common in the forearm and lower leg, but can occur at other sites. This is discussed in detail in **chapter 1.5**.

In circumstances where there is any clinical suspicion of compartment syndrome, it is best to carry out formal and wide fasciotomy to decompress the suspected compartments. If fasciotomy is undertaken, some form of surgical stabilization of the fracture will become necessary, as **the very act of fasciotomy reduces stability and the operation will convert a fracture from closed to open**.

2.5　Classification issues

There are classification systems described for soft-tissue injuries—both open and closed (see **chapter 1.5**). With open fractures, where surgical exploration is undertaken, it is relatively easy to define the precise and complete extent of the soft-tissue injury by exploring the wound thoroughly. Accurately grading the severity of the soft-tissue injury in closed fractures is diffi-

Unless surgery is life saving, the patient is better off on the intensive care unit than in the operating room.

Presence of peripheral pulses and adequate skin circulation does not exclude a compartment syndrome.

Fasciotomy reduces stability and will convert a fracture from closed to open.

Continuing to view the patient as a whole is essential.

cult. **The value of a classification system [5] is to alert the surgeon to** the complexity and magnitude of **possible soft-tissue problems.**

Considerable information can be gained from radiological assessment. Plain x-rays should be obtained, with a minimum of two films taken at 90° to each other. These will allow an initial attempt to classify the fracture (see **chapter 1.4**). However, x-rays taken acutely after injury are frequently of poor quality because of difficulty in positioning the limb correctly for standard views. The use of **traction films taken in the operating theatre under general anesthetic** is **invaluable for more exact delineation of the fracture pattern**. Although taking such x-rays may seem to add to the operation time, the information gained is frequently so valuable that the procedure overall is shortened.

The x-rays must also be scrutinized for clues about soft-tissue injury, as well as for what they tell about bony injury. Obviously, a multifragmentary fracture implies that significant energy has been dissipated through the limb and is a pointer to significant soft-tissue damage. It is frequently possible to see the degree of swelling of the soft tissue on the plain x-rays. After open injury, foreign bodies and air may be seen in tissues, while their presence at some distance away from the fracture site will give a further clue as to the overall extent of the soft-tissue damage.

Accurate classification of the fracture itself will allow the surgeon to identify potential hazards in its management and to develop strategies both to avoid problems and to prevent complications. Of particular importance is analysis of the fracture pattern to assess the inherent stability. The **final stability after operative intervention is a mixture of the inherent stability of the fracture and the stability imparted by surgery. Particular attention must be paid to fracture lines that extend**

into the metaphysis or joint. These may be small and not show up clearly on plain x-rays taken at right angles to each other. They could readily be disturbed by use of an inappropriate technique (such as an intramedullary nail). **Time invested in obtaining good-quality x-rays is seldom wasted**, especially as accident and emergency-unit x-rays are of poor quality. They can often be bettered when repeated in the operating room, with the patient anesthetized and traction applied to the limb.

Consideration should also be given to the use of CT scanning in metaphyseal and intra-articular fractures. This will allow detailed planning of the definitive fixation technique and frequently allows use of a more limited exposure.

2.6 Amputation

The key issue in management of severe open fracture of the limbs (particular the tibia) is whether or not salvage is possible. Modern techniques of surgical reconstruction (bone, vessel, nerve, tendon) make it attractive to try and salvage every limb. However, **the patient may be better served by an early amputation as definitive treatment,** allowing rapid functional rehabilitation to commence. Millstein et al. [6] reviewed 72 patients with lower limb fractures, with associated vascular injury. Revascularization was performed in 28 patients and primary amputation in 44 patients. Overall, good function was achieved in only 32% of the revascularizations; the rate for primary amputees was 70%.

In the last 10 years, a number of scoring systems have been proposed to try and ease decision making in this area. One of the most widely used is the Mangled Extremity Severity Score (MESS), reported by Helfet et al. [7]. The

The value of classification is to alert the surgeon to possible soft-tissue problems.

Time invested in obtaining good quality x-rays is seldom wasted.

Traction films under general anesthetic are invaluable for a more exact diagnosis.

The patient may be better served by an early amputation as definitive treatment.

Stability after operative fixation is a mixture of inherent fracture stability and surgical stability. Pay attention to fracture lines that extend into the metaphysis or joint.

system assigns scores to the severity of the skeletal and soft-tissue injury, the degree of limb ischemia, the presence or absence of systemic hypotension, and the age of the patient. A score of seven or more was initially reported to be predictive of non-viability, and amputation was advised. However, Robertson [8] reviewed 152 patients with severely injured limbs and carried out retrospective scoring by MESS. He found that all patients with a score of seven or more on admission required amputation. However, in 49 patients with a MESS of less than seven, delayed amputation was required. He concluded that the MESS lacked sensitivity, but could be used as a guide (see **chapter 1.5**).

Inevitably, it is necessary to fall back on clinical judgment and assessment of the "personality of the injury". Patient factors (see **section 3**) to be considered include age, presence or absence of pre-existing disease, other injuries, the patient's work and hobbies, desires of the patient and family, and consideration of pre-existing psychological problems.

The limb factors to be considered include the mechanism of injury, the degree of damage to the bone and soft tissues, the presence or absence of any injury to the ipsilateral foot, the quality of distal sensation, and the ischemic time before successful revascularization.

Environmental factors (see **section 4**) include whether or not there are facilities available for optimum reconstruction/rehabilitation, what is going to be the socio-economic cost to the patient and his family, and what is the cost to society and the healthcare system.

The key decision—whether to reconstruct or amputate—does not have to be made on day one. A "primary" amputation in this situation is one performed within the first 5–7 days. Initial exploration and débridement performed as an emergency will allow precise definition of the injury and a preliminary reconstruction (vascular, bone, and joint) can be performed. Then, if the outlook is felt to be poor and amputation required, this can be discussed with the patient and family over the next 24–48 hours. During this time, the artificial limb and appliance center can be involved. This can be very helpful in planning a definitive amputation. It is also possible to allow patient and family to meet others who have undergone successful amputation in the past.

There will always be debate on the absolute and relative indications for amputation in severe lower limb trauma. However, by way of example, the current indications as used in the Oxford Trauma Unit are shown in **Table 2.1-3** and **Table 2.1-4**.

3 Patient factors

As well as assessing the injury in some detail, it is also necessary to look at the patient as a whole in order to build up the "personality" of the injury. Clearly, there will be differences in emphasis between those patients with polytrauma and those patient with isolated injuries. The objective in polytrauma management is to save life, then to save the limb, then to try to save joints in order to restore limb function.

In contrast, the patient with an isolated limb injury or even multiple limb injuries, needs to be seen as a surgical emergency only if the fracture is open, or if there is an associated vascular injury. In such circumstances, management must proceed as rapidly as possible. The objective with open fractures is to deal with these within 6 hours of injury, as surgical management within this time window has been shown, both clinically and experimentally, to reduce complication rates.

There will always be debate on the absolute and relative indications for amputation in severe lower limb trauma.

Table 2.1-3:

Suggested indications for amputation in the lower limb: absolute

1) Complete amputation at time of accident.

2) Irreparable sciatic or posterior tibial nerve injury in association with a type IIIc open fracture.

3) Ischemic time > 6–8 hours in a type IIIc open fracture.

4) Associated life-threatening injuries with prolonged shock, DIC, or ARDS.

5) Cadaveric foot at initial examination.

Table 2.1-4:

Suggested indications for amputation in the lower limb: relative

1) Type IIIc open fracture.

2) Crush injury to lower limb and ipsilateral foot.

3) Significant tibial bone loss or associated severe damage to knee/ankle joints.

4) Type IIIc open fracture in patient > 50 years.

5) Isolation/complete major nerve injury.

6) Inadequate facilities.

3.1   Vascular injuries

After vascular injuries, the earlier the revascularization, the better the outcome. It is usually not wise to delay surgical intervention by attempting conventional arteriography in the radiology department. If there is a fracture at single level with an absent pulse distally, then it can be assumed that arterial injury will be at the site of the fracture, although **the effect of a joint dislocation at another level, which has reduced spontaneously, must be excluded.** If there is doubt, on-table arteriography can be performed rapidly to identify the site of problem, while screening by Doppler may be even more rapid and convenient, but not as reliable.

Conventional arteriography in the radiology department may be of some use where there are multiple level injuries within a limb, since arterial damage can occur at more than one site. It is in such circumstances that formal arteriography may be of value. However, if the patient is to have arteriography in a radiology depart-ment, every effort must be made to carry out the examination as quickly as possible, so as to reduce the ischemic time.

Apart from fractures with an open wound or a vascular injury, the other type of injury requiring emergency orthopedic surgical management is a dislocation or fracture/dislocation of a joint. The vast majority of closed limb injuries can be treated initially by splintage and elevation, while the fracture pattern is defined and the patient's background investigated.

Exclude a spontaneously reduced joint dislocation at another level.

3.2   Concurrent problems

It is essential to know of any pre-existing medical problems, especially those requiring long-term medication. Patients with ischemic heart disease and chronic lung disease represent a significant anesthetic challenge. Conditions such as insulin-dependent diabetes pose problems both from a local point of view,

Any pre-existing medical problems, especially those requiring long-term medication, must be known.

in terms of potential infection, and from a systemic point of view in terms of controlling the patient's metabolic environment. Potential complications from other medication, classically exemplified by corticosteroid use, may, after fracture surgery, include poor healing, an increased risk of infection, and delayed union. Clearly, previous vascular bypass surgery in an injured limb greatly enhances the hazards of the situation. Systemically, the patient may not cope well with major surgery and will require increased steroid cover.

The patient's own lifestyle is also a major factor. Quite apart from the respiratory and cardiovascular effects of tobacco smoking, there is known to be a specific association between cigarette smoking and delayed or non-union of fractures. Patients who consume large quantities of alcohol may have abnormal liver function, with consequent coagulation problems, and alcohol abusers are frequently non-compliant and intolerant of the specific rehabilitation regimes that may be required. It could prove pointless to involve such a patient in a technique where compliance is essential.

Intravenous drug abuse is an increasing problem carrying an increased risk of HIV, hepatitis B, and hepatitis C infections. In an acute situation, universal precautions should be applied to reduce the risk for operating room personnel. It is also important, with planned reconstructive surgery, to be able to advise affected patients how they can appropriately weigh the risks against the benefits of what may be proposed.

It is important that the patient's pre-injury level of function is clearly known. It is clearly pointless to aim at high-quality limb function in an already disabled patient who cannot make use of it. **Treatment should be tailored to the patient's functional needs**.

Conversely, in the professional athlete or sportsman, a high level of limb function may be required rapidly and this may influence the choice of method.

3.3 Psychological factors

The psychological aspect of injury must not be neglected, with consideration for both the patient's preinjury psychological/psychiatric status and the possible reactions to the current injury. Complex injuries may require demanding and staged reconstructive procedures. It is important to consider the pre-injury psychological status and to respect it in producing a management plan. Some patients with established psychiatric conditions may have difficulty complying with weight-bearing instructions and may tolerate external fixators poorly.

In addition, it must be remembered that every patient will have some sort of psychological reaction to the physical injury sustained. This can be very marked in previously normal individuals who, literally within a moment, find themselves severely disabled. Time spent in explaining the nature of the injury and the available options for treatment will inevitably be repaid in the long run if it builds confidence in the surgeon and the treatment program. It **is important to try to promote positive involvement by members of the patient's family** at this stage (see below).

When the patient cannot give a detailed account of his occupation, hobbies, and of his functional requirements, consultation and discussion with the family is essential to establish the patient's pre-injury status. A management plan for an unconscious patient will have to be formed, at least at the outset, with close relatives.

Promote involvement of members of the patient's family.

It is important that the patient's pre-injury level of function is clearly known.

Treatment should be tailored to the patient's functional needs.

It is essential that the patient and, where appropriate, the patient's family should have a clear understanding of the nature of the injury and realistic expectations of what can be achieved by surgical reconstruction/rehabilitation, so that what the patient expects of the outcome matches what the surgeon knows he can deliver (barring unforeseen complications). This is approached by a "contract" between the patient and the surgeon. **One of the main reasons for litigation is a breakdown in communication and understanding between the patient and the surgeon**.

4 Environmental factors

Firstly, there is the issue of physical facilities. Access to both adult and pediatric intensive care will be required for those with serious injuries or major concurrent medical problems, given that trauma can strike anyone from the very young to the very old. Complex injuries often require complex assessment and lack of such facilities as MRI and CT may make it impossible to reach an accurate diagnosis in some cases.

4.1 Facilities

Modern fracture surgery should be performed in a modern operating theatre. The use, for surgical fixation of fractures, of the ultra clean-air and laminar flow facilities which have become routine for joint replacement surgery, has been questioned in some quarters. However, biologically, there is no real difference between implanting a metal total joint replacement or a metal plate through a surgical wound. The consequences of infection are disastrous in either case. Additionally, **a full range of im-plants and instruments to carry out appropriate surgery in all areas of the body must be available**.

High-quality image intensification is essential and the lack of it in the operating theatre will make it impossible to perform some types of surgery, for instance, intramedullary nailing.

The skills and training of the personnel involved in the surgery are also important. Trauma very often happens at unsociable hours. Senior and experienced staff (both surgical and anesthetic) must be available round the clock to provide experienced input into its management.

From the point of view of operative fracture surgery, the operating room personnel are clearly critical. **It is the responsibility of the surgeon**, by producing a proper preoperative plan/surgical tactic, **to ensure that his/her team knows what is going to happen** and what will be needed.

Achieving such skills—both for surgeons and operating-room personnel—is not easy. Ideally, **all those involved in the provision of surgical care for trauma patients**, (surgeons, anesthetists, and operating-room personnel) should spend the greater part of their time working in this field and **have regular exposure to structured training**. Those who are called upon to work only occasionally in trauma care can find it a stressful and demoralizing experience, and it is certainly not ideal for the patient.

4.2 Rehabilitation

Finally, with regard to environmental factors, it must be remembered that the **care of the patient does not stop once the surgery is completed.** In musculoskeletal trauma, per-

A full range of implants and instruments must be available.

Reasons for litigation include breakdown in communication and understanding between the patient and the surgeon.

It is the responsibility of the surgeon to ensure that his/her team knows what is going to happen.

All those involved in the provision of surgical care for trauma patients must have regular training.

Care of the patient does not stop once the surgery is completed.

haps more than any other surgical specialty, rehabilitation is of critical importance. The best osteosynthesis can be rendered useless without appropriate postoperative care and rehabilitation. It remains a matter of concern that in many parts of the world such skilled rehabilitation teams are not available and to establish them must be a major priority in the years to come.

Successful rehabilitation not only includes the traditional physical therapy but also will involve the input of occupational therapists, speech therapists, dietitians, social workers, psychologists, and (sometimes) psychiatrists. In addition, there must be close and meaningful liaison between the hospital-based rehabilitation team and those who carry on once the patient returns home. Regrettably, the provision of appropriately skilled rehabilitation personnel within primary care facilities is frequently worse even than in hospitals.

It is absolutely essential that those responsible for provision of musculoskeletal injury care take a long, critical and honest look at their own working environment. Without sophisticated facilities and highly trained personnel, it may not be safe to carry out complex reconstruction surgery and patients should be transferred (as rapidly and safely as possible) to an institution where these are available. **When the patient's needs exceed the resources available in the treating institution, such a transfer is mandatory**.

When the patient's needs exceed the available resources a transfer is mandatory.

5 Summary

Table 2.1-5:

Summary of system of assessment/decision making in fracture surgery

1) History: Initially to define direction/magnitude of force.

2) Examination: Estimate extent of zone of injury by assessment of bruising/abrasions/degloving/wounds. Assess (if possible) neurovascular status and muscle/tendon function.

3) Radiology: Define site/type of fracture (Comprehensive Classification of Fractures). Will give additional information on energy dissipation (zone of injury).

4) Patient: Further history to define pre-existing conditions, occupation/hobbies/psychological status and expectations.

5) Needs: Define optimum treatment for individual patient (i.e., what resources are required?).

6) Environment: Are all necessary resources available for providing optimum treatment? If not, transfer patient to where resources are available.

7) Contract: What the patient expects and what the surgeon can achieve must be the same. This may require negotiation.

The objective of management of musculo-skeletal injury is to achieve a full return of patient and limb function. Within such management the first priority is to save life. Initial assessment and resuscitation of the patient with life threatening injuries proceed simultaneously, without attempting full and formal assessment of all the factors outlined above.

When the polytrauma patient has been physiologically stabilized or if there are isolated/multiple fractures (when life is not at risk), then a more comprehensive and formal assessment is made in an attempt to define personality of the injury. This will allow logical decision making using the principles outlined in **section 2.2** and **section 2.3**. An outline of the system of assessment/decision making used in fracture surgery is given in **Table 2.1-5.**

6   Bibliography

1. **Tile M** (1984) Fractures of the pelvis and acetabulum. In: Tile M, editor. *Pelvic Fractures.* Baltimore: Williams & Wilkins.
2. **Bone LB, Johnson KD, Weigelt J, et al.** (1989) Early versus delayed stabilization of femoral fractures. A prospective randomized study. *J Bone Joint Surg [Am];* 71 (3):336–340.
3. **Reynolds MA, Richardson JD, Spain DA, et al.** (1995) Is the timing of fracture fixation important for the patient with multiple trauma? *Ann Surg;* 222 (4):470–478; discussion 478–481.
4. **Herve C, Gaillard M, Andrivet P, et al.** (1987) Treatment in serious lower limb injuries: amputation versus preservation. *Injury;* 18 (1):21–23.
5. **Oestern HJ, Tscherne H** (1984) Pathophysiology and classification of soft tissue injuries associated with fractures. In: Tscherne H, Gotzen L, editors. *Fractures with Soft Tissue Injuries.* Berlin Heidelberg New York: Springer-Verlag.
6. **Millstein SG, Hunter GA, Kellam JF** (1990) Injuries of the lower limb leading to revascularisation and/or amputation in polytrauma. *Orthopaedic Trauma Association, Annual Meeting.* Lippincott-Raven, Philadelphia.
7. **Helfet DL, Howey T, Sanders R, et al.** (1990) Limb salvage versus amputation. Preliminary results of the Mangled Extremity Severity Score. *Clin Orthop;* (256):80–86.
8. **Robertson PA** (1991) Prediction of amputation after severe lower limb trauma. *J Bone Joint Surg [Br];* 73 (5):816–818.

7   Updates

Updates and additional references for this chapter are available online at:
http://www.aopublishing.org/PFxM/21.htm

2.2 Diaphyseal fractures: principles

Peter de Boer

1 Introduction

The management of diaphyseal fractures is evolving and progressing. New reduction and fixation concepts are emerging, based on better understanding of the biology of fracture repair and of the role of the soft tissues in the healing process [1]. It is appreciated that **anatomical reduction of every fracture fragment is not necessary for normal limb function.** With more treatment options available, decision making has become more complex. The factors relevant to the correct management of an individual diaphyseal fracture must constantly be kept up to date.

2 Functional considerations

The diaphysis of a long bone has many functions. The two most important are to maintain its proximal and distal joints in their correct spatial relationship and to provide attachment for muscles which move them. **In the leg the normal mechanical axis of the limb should be restored** [2]. This requires union without

shortening, angulation, or rotational deformity. Good function can then be expected even if the individual fracture fragments are not anatomically reduced (**Fig. 2.2-1**).

Some residual deformity can be tolerated in the lower limb without causing functional problems, e.g., shortening of up to 1 cm or minimal angular deformities in the plane of adjacent joints. Up to 10° of anterior or posterior bowing of a healed tibial fracture is compatible with good ankle function, despite severe cosmetic deformity. However, valgus or varus deformity of even 5° may subject the joint to abnormal forces and lead to posttraumatic osteoarthritis [3].

Shortening of the humeral shaft produces little functional disability and because the shoulder has the largest range of joint movement in the body, some malrotation or angular deformity is tolerated as well. **Conversely, the diaphyses of the radius and ulna, being part of a complex articulation that includes the proximal and distal radioulnar joints, require anatomical reduction for normal limb function.**

Exact anatomical reconstruction of the diaphysis is not necessary for normal limb function.

Radius and ulna demand anatomical reduction similar to a joint.

Joints must be in their original axial relationship.

3 Incidence

While in most parts of the world improved car design and the use of seat belts have reduced the incidence of diaphyseal fractures [4], in the developing countries the sharp increase of mechanized transport, particularly motorcycles, is producing more diaphyseal injuries. Many of these injuries are open and present late because of delay in transporting victims to hospital.

Pedestrian trauma figures are, however, static and the incidence of open fractures, as a percentage of injuries, is rising. An increasingly aging population [5] has raised the incidence of osteoporotic diaphyseal injuries.

4 Mechanism

Patterns of injury

Fractures can be caused by direct or indirect forces. Indirect trauma usually dissipates less energy than a direct blow and causes proportionately less fragment displacement and soft-tissue damage or open fractures [6]. The differing injury patterns are recognized in the various AO classifications [7] (**chapters 1.4, 1.5, 5.1**).

Spiral (type A1) and butterfly (type B1) fractures result from indirect rotational forces. They have large areas of bone surfaces in contact, and minimal soft-tissue damage. Fracture healing is therefore usually swift and uneventful, although holding the reduction without fixation may be difficult.

Wedge fractures (type B2) are produced by bending forces. The force applied to the limb is considerable and the resulting damage to soft tissue and periosteum is significant. Union may

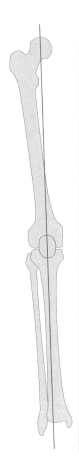

Fig. 2.2-1:
Diagram of the mechanical axis of the lower limb showing correct alignment of femur and tibia (according to Pauwels [3]).

take a long time and direct surgical approaches to the fracture site will further devitalize the bone.

Transverse fractures (type A3) or shattered bone (type C) are usually also caused by direct forces which are often enormous, especially in the femur. If the bone is of normal quality and the fracture is widely displaced, the degree of soft-tissue damage will be extensive. Even with intact skin, direct exposure of the fractures results in further insult to the soft tissues already compromised by injury.

It follows that fracture type and displacement are good predictors of soft-tissue damage. This insight should guide the surgeon towards suitable methods of reduction and fixation. The greater the anticipated soft-tissue damage, the more important the choice of implant, reduction technique, and gentle overall management (chapter 3.3.2).

5   Initial evaluation

5.1   Patient status

The protocol for assessing a patient on first contact is described in chapter 2.1. Problems relating to children's fractures are to be found in chapter 5.4.

A well-taken **history is of foremost importance in assessing a diaphyseal fracture, particularly to discover the mechanism and forces which caused the fracture.** The force generated in motor vehicle injury is approximately one hundred times that generated by a simple fall. Although the x-rays may look similar, the consequent soft-tissue injury will be very different.

Most displaced fractures are identified by observation only. Palpation is also useful to elicit tenderness. The most important elements of the physical examination concentrate on any arterial or neurological damage. Certain fractures, including displaced fractures of the distal femur or proximal tibia, should attract a high level of suspicion of arterial injuries. **An arterial injury will dominate the decision-making process because of the immediate need for reconstruction with appropriate stabilization of the fracture.**

Another most urgent condition concerns the development of a compartment syndrome, which is seen mostly in the lower leg, but can also occur in the thigh, forearm, buttock, and foot [8]. The clinical picture and the management are fully described in chapter 1.5. Compartment syndromes may occur at any time during the first few days after trauma. They are commonest in widely displaced fractures, but can occur in open fractures and also following closed intramedullary nailing.

5.2   Radiographic evaluation

X-rays are the mainstay of diagnosis. **AP and lateral views that must include the adjacent joints** will serve in most cases, while oblique projections may be helpful in the metaphysis. Standard views of the opposite side are very useful for preoperative planning, especially for nailing (chapter 2.4). CT and MRI scanning have no role in the assessment of acute diaphyseal injuries, although they may be useful in planning reconstructive surgery in cases of complex malunions.

C fracture pattern

Radiography allows accurate classification of diaphyseal fractures. Fractures which are widely displaced, multifragmentary, or transverse have usually been caused by higher energy than those that are minimally displaced, simple, or spiral.

In the lower extremity, load-sharing implants (intramedullary nails) which splint the bone and allow early weight bearing are therefore preferable to implants such as plates and screws, which are more prone to fatigue failure if healing is prolonged [6].

Fracture type and displacement are good predictors of soft-tissue damage.

A compartment syndrome is as serious as arterial disruption.

AP and lateral views must include adjacent joints.

History of accident indicates the amount of energy involved.

Arterial injury dominates decision making.

Bone quality influences the choice of fixation technique.

Shaft fractures in the same limb all need fixation.

Soft-tissue conditions dictate fracture management.

Absolute indications:
• saving life
• saving limb

However, shaft fractures with metaphyseal or intra-articular extensions may not be suitable for nailing and require direct reduction and rigid internal fixation to maintain the anatomical relationships of articular fracture components.

Bone quality is also highly relevant. Severe osteoporosis diminishes the holding power of screws or pins. External fixation [9] and plating of fractures in osteoporotic bone may fail. The treatment of pathological fractures may also demand special considerations. In a patient with a limited life expectancy it may be more sensible to aim for mobility and pain relief, rather than perfect reduction or the use of an adjuvant technique which may retard bone healing, i.e., the use of bone cement [9].

5.3 Associated injuries

Soft-tissue injuries always influence and may frequently dictate the management options of a diaphyseal fracture. A closed, simple, displaced transverse fracture of the shaft of the tibia can be managed by intramedullary nailing, plating, or external fixation. Severe skin contusion excludes the standard plating option because the surgical approach might further compromise the soft tissues. A badly contaminated wound might be a deterrent to primary nailing because of the risk of sepsis. In this situation preliminary treatment with an external fixator would be the treatment of choice.

Similarly, both the acute arterial disruption and the compartment syndromes need emergency management. In cases requiring vascular repairs or extensive release of the muscle compartments, the associated fracture must be stabilized at the same time. Thus the associated injury not only dictates the need for stabilization, but also determines its timing and the approach. Plating of the fracture through the exposure used for the vascular repair may be the treatment of choice, as there may not be time for anything else.

Management of life-threatening injuries always takes precedence over that of a diaphyseal injury. The overall approach described in **chapter 2.1** should be followed.

The presence of more than one fracture in the same limb may make it desirable to fix all of them, particularly if the combination has produced a "floating" joint. Additional fractures in other limbs, e.g., bilateral humeral shaft fractures, can render a patient almost helpless. This situation may dictate operative stabilization of a fracture that might well be treated non-operatively, if isolated.

6 Indications for operative fracture fixation

The indications for internal or external fixation of diaphyseal fractures vary throughout the world depending on the available facilities. **There are several absolute indications which can be grouped around two headings— saving life and saving limb.**

6.1 Absolute indications

Saving life

Immediate stabilization of femoral shaft fractures in polytraumatized patients has been shown to decrease morbidity and mortality considerably (**chapter 5.3**) [10]. However, there are conflicting reports as to the use of intramedullary nails or plates, while external fixation may always be applied as a temporary expedient [11, 12].

Saving limb

Stabilization of diaphyseal fractures is part of an emergency operation to save a limb in the case of an acute vascular injury, compartment syndrome, as well as in open fractures (**chapters 1.5 and 5.1**). Moving fracture ends compromise not only the vascular repair but also the healing of any severe soft-tissue injury.

6.2 Relative indications

Inability to reduce or hold a fracture by conservative means:

Fractures of the shaft of the femur are very difficult to reduce and hold in traction. Non-operative treatment is indicated only exceptionally, usually if proper operating facilities do not exist.

Fractures of the shaft of the tibia are often easy to reduce by manipulation, but the stability of the reduction depends on the fracture pattern. Well reduced transverse fractures may be stable to axial loading, but union is often slow. Non-operative treatment of unstable multifragmented fractures carries a high risk of shortening and malalignement, although fracture healing may be relatively fast.

Humeral shaft fractures are often difficult to reduce and hold by non-operative means, but since significant degrees of malunion are compatible with good limb function, surgical fixation is indicated only in special cases.

Fractures of the forearm bones are difficult to reduce and hold anatomically by non-operative means. As even minimal malalignment impedes normal limb function, surgery is usually indicated.

6.3 Early mobilization of patients

Early mobilization carries enormous benefits for patients, especially the aged. Stabilization of shaft fractures allows early movement of adjacent joints and avoids the "fracture disease" or algodystrophy seen with prolonged immobilization (**chapter 6.5**). Successful fracture fixation is also associated with earlier return to work, shorter hospital stays, and possibly reduced costs for compensation/invalidity.

There are also economic aspects; for example a femoral shaft fracture treated non-operatively usually needs many weeks in hospital, compared to a few days after intramedullary nailing. This makes the cost of non-operative treatment of femoral shaft fractures prohibitive in many developed countries. In case of a severe complication this may, however, change drastically [13].

Relative indications:
Inability to reduce or hold a fracture by non-operative means.

7 Non-operative treatment

Non-operative treatment, usually by traction and/or cast, may be used for temporary or definitive management. This usually avoids the risk of infection and the equipment needed is minimal. Time to union is, however, longer and there are higher risks of malunion, malalignment, and stiffness of the adjacent joints.

In adults, some fractures are best managed non-operatively. Undisplaced or minimally displaced fractures of the tibia and humerus can very well be treated non-operatively in a cast. This requires regular follow-up, since secondary displacements before bony union are quite frequent.

Femoral shaft fractures should not be managed non-operatively if adequate facilities and know-how exist for safe surgical care. Non-operative management is very time consuming and the incidence of shortening and angular deformity is high.

Operative management of displaced diaphyseal fractures usually produces better functional results than conservative treatment in all bones apart from the humerus [14]. If appropriate operating facilities and instrumentations do not exist locally, conservative treatment is still indicated even for femoral shaft fractures. It is probably better to end up with a malunion than with chronic osteomyelitis.

The two main non-operative methods available are traction and plaster casting. Both require skill, experience, and supervision. Traction is time consuming and may cause delayed union in the tibia. However, it is an excellent form of provisional fixation while waiting for definitive surgery.

Casting, if properly applied, is very safe, although the frequent need to include adjacent joints may cause stiffness. This can be minimized by the use of hinged braces [15]. Angulation may be controlled by a well applied cast; it may, however, be difficult to control rotation and shortening. Casts in adults are therefore largely confined to those diaphyseal fractures which are initially hardly displaced and therefore quite stable.

8 General principles of operative treatment

For specific and more detailed information see **chapter 4**.

8.1 Timing

The timing of operative treatment of diaphyseal injuries can be complex. No operative treatment should be contemplated until the patient's general condition has been assessed. Vascular injuries and open fractures are special cases requiring emergency management.

In general terms, if direct open reduction and internal fixation are indicated, the sooner it happens the better. Swelling will develop, and operating through swollen tissues leads to difficulty in wound closure and the risk of subsequent breakdown. For direct open reduction, surgical intervention within 6 hours is recommended [16]. If, as sometimes happens, significant swelling occurs sooner than this, it is usually safer to establish provisional stabilization and wait 7–10 days for the swelling to subside.

Shaft fractures of the tibia and the femur are mostly treated by indirect reduction and intramedullary nailing. In this situation, swelling around the fracture site is less of a problem because the soft tissues are not invaded. Timing is therefore less critical. Every procedure demands a complex surgical set-up and may need to await an experienced surgical team and backup. If, for any reason, it is not carried out in the first 48 hours, it is probably best delayed for 7–10 days, because of the increased incidence of adult respiratory distress syndrome (ARDS) occurring in patients operated on between 3 and 7 days from the accident.

8.2   Preoperative planning and approaches

All operative fixations of diaphyseal fractures should be planned carefully. The details of available techniques are covered in **chapter 2.4**. **Effective planning should ensure that the surgeon does not embark on a surgical procedure unless the required personnel and equipment are available.**

In open fractures it is vital to look beyond the first operation to plan how definitive soft-tissue cover will ultimately be obtained. Otherwise an external fixator, used for provisional stabilization, may obstruct the placement of a soft-tissue flap.

The surgical approach to a fracture clearly depends on the site, soft-tissue conditions, and choice of fixation device. Knowledge of the anatomy is essential, while dissection must be gentle. When the planned approach is unfamiliar, reference to a standard work on surgical approaches is mandatory [17, 18] and dissection of cadaveric material is desirable.

Adoption of minimally invasive techniques calls for percutaneous access, usually carried out with x-ray control. These techniques may possibly minimize soft-tissue trauma, but are technically quite demanding. The need to master the relevant anatomy is even greater, as the surgeon cannot see the tissues and structures beneath which the operation is being carried out.

8.3   Reduction and fixation techniques

Diaphyseal fractures can be reduced directly or indirectly; the principles are described in **chapter 3.1**. Independent of the technique, any reduction maneuver should be as gentle as possible to the soft parts and periosteum surrounding the fracture, the aim being to preserve all existing blood supply.

In the treatment of diaphyseal fractures the fixation techniques used most commonly are intramedullary nailing, plating, and external fixation.

Intramedullary nails are internal splints which are load sharing and allow early weight bearing. Because they permit a degree of movement at the fracture site, their use is associated with callus formation and early bone union [7]. Locked intramedullary nails allow multifragmentary fractures to be held out to length.

Plates and screws may be a good option for shaft fractures extending to the metaphyseal area or into a joint. They can be inserted either with direct or indirect reduction techniques. In simple fractures that can easily be reduced anatomically, the classical interfragmentary lag screw, combined with a neutralization plate, is still an excellent way of fixation. Plating of complex, multifragmentary diaphyseal fractures should be done by minimally invasive techniques, with indirect reduction and the plate acting as bridge, leaving the fracture focus untouched (**chapters 3.2.2, 3.3.1, 3.3.2,** and **3.4**).

External fixators are still the gold standard in case of severe soft-tissue problems and in those parts of the world where nails and plates are more difficult and risky to use for logistical and technical reasons, e.g., image intensi-

Preoperative planning must include thinking ahead.

Timing of surgery depends on the patient, soft-tissue conditions, logistics, and facilities.

fication. However, fracture healing may be delayed and pin track problems (infection, loosening) are common. External fixators are therefore not a popular choice for definitive fixation and a change of method is often considered once the early problems have been mastered (**chapter 3.3.3**).

9 Postoperative care

Immediate postoperative management

Good preoperative planning is the key.

General principles relating to observations, drains, dressings, etc. are addressed in **chapter 5.7**, but the following points, specific to diaphyseal fractures, should be noted.

The mobilization of a given patient is often influenced by the presence of other injuries and how patients are mobilized depends not only on their fractures but their overall state.

Mobilization depends on the surgeon's assessment of the stability.

The most important single factor in deciding about mobilization and functional loading is the surgeon's assessment of the stability of the fixation. The fracture anatomy and the fixation technique must be considered together. When there is doubt, activity may need to be delayed and carefully monitored.

Physiotherapy aimed at muscle rehabilitation should commence as soon as possible after surgery and continue until normal function of the limb is obtained. Early active movements of the muscles and joints are best, but can be painful. Continuous passive motion [19], if used, should always be combined with active muscle exercises.

The most stable combination for weight bearing is a perfectly reduced transverse fracture of the middle of a lower limb bone fixed anatomically with a tight-fitting dynamically locked intramedullary nail.

The most unstable combination would be a multifragmented fracture, extending almost from metaphysis to metaphysis, treated by an external fixator.

Whenever possible, a fracture/implant combination should allow some load transmission through the fracture site on mobilization. Load transmission is a good stimulus for bone growth, and prolonged non-weight bearing is associated with profound disuse osteopenia, atrophy of articular cartilage, and muscle wasting. **Good preoperative planning is the key to avoiding fixations that are not strong enough to allow partial weight bearing.**

10 Outcome

Patient outcomes vary with the severity of the injury; so do the complications, which are covered in **part 6** of the book. Low-velocity injuries without associated soft-tissue damage should regain full function as a matter of course with appropriate treatment. High-velocity injuries with soft-tissue loss will not regain normal function, but careful assessment, preoperative planning, meticulous operative technique, stressing preservation of soft tissues, combined with diligent postoperative rehabilitation will ensure the optimum result for any patient.

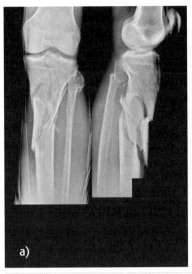

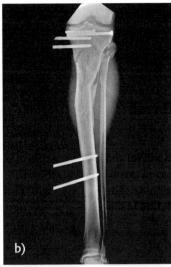

Fig. 2.2-2: High-velocity injury (MVA) to the proximal tibia in a 30-year-old man.
a) The closed injury is a multifragmentary fracture of the shaft of the tibia with proximal metaphyseal and intra-articular extension. The complex fracture pattern suggests extensive soft-tissue damage despite the fact that the fracture is closed.
b) The intra-articular fracture component was treated by closed reduction and percutaneous cannulated screws, while the shaft fragments were bridged with a unilateral external fixator. Both procedures avoided any further soft-tissue damage to the zone of injury. The knee was then mobilized on a continuous passive motion (CPM) machine.

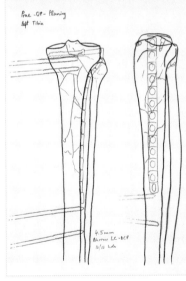

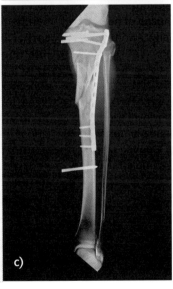

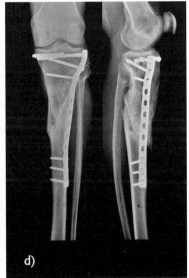

c) Ten days after the accident, when the soft tissues had recovered, a bridge plate was planned and applied to the lateral side of the tibia through stab incisions planned at the upper and lower ends of the chosen plate. Because the plate alone would not have provided enough stability to prevent varus deformation, the bridging external fixator was kept *in situ* to allow mobilization of the patient. The external fixator was removed at 8 weeks when callus formation was seen at the fracture site.

d) The fracture went on to uneventful union at 16 weeks. Note: the correct axis, length, and rotation have been preserved.

11 Bibliography

1. **McKibbin B** (1978) The biology of fracture healing in long bones. *J Bone Joint Surg [Br];* 60-B (2):150–162.
2. **Kenwright J, Richardson K, Spriggins AJ** (1986) Mechanical healing patterns of tibial fractures treated using different mechanical environments. *EUR SOC Biomech;* 5:173.
3. **Pauwels F** (1980) *Biomechanics of the locomotor apparatus. Contributions of the functional anatomy of the locomotor apparatus.* Berlin: Springer-Verlag.
4. **Wallace WA** (1983) The increasing incidence of fractures of the proximal femur: an orthopaedic epidemic. *Lancet;* 1 (8339):1413–1414.
5. **Melton LJI, Riggs BL** (1983) Epidemiology of Age Related Fractures. In: Alveoli LV, editor. *The Osteoporotic Syndrome: Detection, Prevention and Treatment.* New York: Grene and Straton: 45-721.
6. **Perren SM** (1989) The biomechanics and biology of internal fixation using plates and nails. *Orthopedics;* 12 (1):21–34.
7. **Müller ME, Nazarian S, Koch P, et al.** (1990) *The Comprehensive Classification of Long Bone Fractures.* Berlin Heidelberg New York: Springer-Verlag.
8. **McBroom RJ, Cheal EJ, Hayes WC** (1988) Strength reductions from metastatic cortical defects in long bones. *J Orthop Res;* 6 (3):369–378.
9. **Bone LB** (1992) Emergency Treatment of the Injured Patients. In: Browner B, Jupiter JB, Levine AM, editors. *Skeletal Trauma.* Philadelphia: WB Saunders Co: 127-1451.
10. **Bone LB, Johnson KD, Weigelt J, et al.** (1989) Early versus delayed stabilization of femoral fractures. A prospective randomized study. *J Bone Joint Surg [Am];* 71 (3):336–340.
11. **Pape HC, Remmers D, Regel G, et al.** (1995) [Pulmonary complications following intramedullary stabilization of long bones. Effect of surgical procedure, time and injury pattern]. *Orthopade;* 24 (2):164–172.
12. **Boulanger BR, Stephen D, Brenneman FD** (1997) Thoracic trauma and early intramedullary nailing of femur fractures: are we doing harm? *J Trauma;* 43 (1):24–28.
13. **Bonatus T, Olson SA, Lee S, et al.** (1997) Nonreamed locking intramedullary nailing for open fractures of the tibia. *Clin Orthop;* (339):58–64.
14. **Wallny T, Sagebiel C, Westerman K, et al.** (1997) Comparative results of bracing and interlocking nailing in the treatment of humeral shaft fractures. *Int Orthop;* 21 (6):374–379.
15. **Sarmiento A, Latta LL** (1995) *Closed Functional Tretment of Fracture Bracing.* Berlin Heidelberg New York: Springer-Verlag.
16. **Rogers FB, Shackford SR, Vane DW, et al.** (1994) Prompt fixation of isolated femur fractures in a rural trauma center: a study examining the timing of fixation and resource allocation. *J Trauma;* 36 (6):774–777.
17. **Hoppenfeld S, de Boer P** (1994) *Surgical approaches in Orthopaedics. The Anatomy Method. Ed. 2.* Philadelphia: Lippincott.

18. **Rüedi T, von Hochstetter AHC, Schlumpf R** (1984) *Surgical Approaches for Internal Fixation.* Berlin: Springer-Verlag.

19. **Salter RB** (1994) The physiologic basis of continuous passive motion for articular cartilage healing and regeneration. *Hand Clin;* 10 (2):211–219.

12   Updates

Updates and additional references for this chapter are available online at:
http://www.aopublishing.org/PFxM/22.htm

2.3 Articular fractures: principles

Michael D. Stover & James F. Kellam

1 Introduction

Diarthrodial joints provide a smooth, stable capacity for motion of the appendicular skeleton to perform specialized tasks. Joints vary widely in their structure, but share common features essential to their function. A synovial joint consists of two end segments of bone bound together by a fibrous capsule. In certain areas, this capsule is specialized into discrete ligaments. The articulating end segment of bone is covered with resilient, elastic, and avascular hyaline cartilage, which helps to distribute force to the underlying subchondral bone [1].While the articulating surface of each bone is smooth, opposing joint surfaces may be incongruous, thus limiting contact between them to a small area for much of the range of joint motion. Joint stability relies upon the passive stabilizers, namely bone and joint morphology, and the surrounding ligaments. Active stabilization is provided by the muscles which cross the joint. The capsule is lined with a membrane that produces a dialysate of blood, rich in hyaluronic acid, which provides lubrication and nutrition for the articular cartilage surfaces. Maintenance of a healthy articular segment is dependent on joint motion and repetitive loading. Disruption of any component of the joint can result in

altered joint function through the pathological processes of arthrofibrosis or osteoarthrosis. For example, displaced intra-articular fractures are associated with gaps or steps at the joint surface. This alteration in joint morphology can immediately affect stability, cause pain, and disrupt effective motion of the joint. The inflammatory response associated with such an injury can lead to extensive fibrosis within an injured joint, exacerbated by unskilled immobilization or inappropriate surgical procedures. For these reasons, closed reduction and external immobilization failed in the early treatment of intra-articular fractures. The early result following fracture consolidation was commonly a bony deformity with associated stiffness, pain, and functional disability. Overall motion was later improved using traction and joint mobilization, but instability and incongruity of the joint persisted. In order to avoid the complications of closed treatment, **Charnley [2] proposed that perfect anatomical restoration and freedom of joint movement could be obtained simultaneously only by internal fixation.** However, he and others were dissatisfied with the outcome of early attempts at open reduction and internal fixation of intra-articular

Perfect anatomical restoration and freedom of joint motion can only be obtained by internal fixation (Sir John Charnley).

fractures. Available implants were unable to achieve fixation sufficiently rigid to allow early motion and prevent displacement. Therefore, patients received the worst possible combination of the risks of open reduction together with the complications of long-term external immobilization. With the advent of antibiotics, improved soft-tissue handling, new implant designs, and a better understanding of the injuries by surgeons experienced in fracture care, open reduction and internal fixation of intra-articular fractures became reliably safe and more widely accepted. The initial results, following protocols for treatment set forth by the AO group, confirmed that rigid internal fixation and early joint motion improved x-ray and clinical results [3]. This has set the precedent for the current philosophy of operative treatment of these injuries.

Review of the experimental and clinical studies led Schatzker in 1987 to enunciate the principles of intra-articular fracture treatment as follows:

- Immobilization of intra-articular fractures results in joint stiffness.
- Immobilization of articular fractures treated by open reduction and internal fixation results in much greater stiffness.
- Depressed articular fragments, which do not reduce as a result of closed manipulation and traction, are impacted and will not reduce by closed means.
- Major articular depressions do not fill with fibrocartilage, and instability, which results from their displacement, is permanent.
- Anatomical reduction and stable fixation of articular fragments is necessary to restore joint congruity.

- Metaphyseal defects must be bone grafted to prevent articular fragment redisplacement.
- Metaphyseal and diaphyseal displacement must be reduced to prevent joint overload.
- Immediate motion is necessary to prevent joint stiffness and to ensure articular healing and recovery. This requires stable internal fixation.

2 Mechanism of injury

There are two common mechanisms of injury for articular fractures. The most common is the **indirect application of force, producing a bending moment through the joint, which drives a part of the joint into its opposing articular surface. Usually the ligaments are strong enough to resist this eccentric load, converting the bending moment to direct axial overload, fracturing the joint surface. Typically, this results in a partial articular fracture** (**Fig. 2.3-1a**). The second mechanism is the direct application of force, either directly to the metaphyseal-diaphyseal component of the joint, or through axial transmission of force from one end segment of bone to the opposing surface. **This direct crushing or axial application of force commonly causes an explosion of the bone and a dissipation of force into the soft tissues. Complete multifragmentary articular fractures, with associated severe soft-tissue injuries, are the result.** The bone quality, the position of the limb, and the exact vector of the force applied will determine the fracture pattern (**Fig. 2.3-1b**).

Indirect bending forces to a joint typically result in a partial articular fracture.

Direct axial forces produce crushing or explosions of the joint components, so-called complete articular fractures.

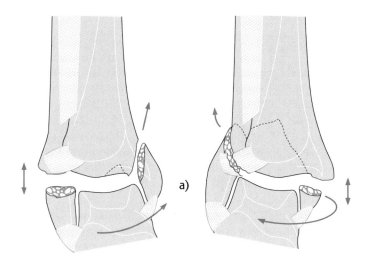

Fig. 2.3-1: There are two mechanisms that commonly cause an articular fracture: a) An eccentric load or indirect force which causes a pronation or supination, varus or valgus mechanism to any joint. Loading one side of the joint usually produces a split or shearing fracture, while a pull on the ligamentous insertion on the opposite side results in an avulsion fracture or torn ligament.

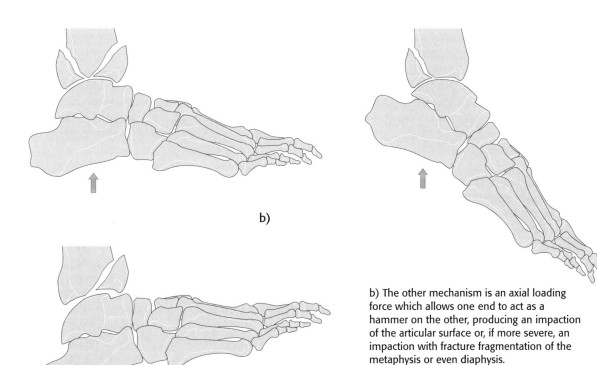

b) The other mechanism is an axial loading force which allows one end to act as a hammer on the other, producing an impaction of the articular surface or, if more severe, an impaction with fracture fragmentation of the metaphysis or even diaphysis.

Knowing the mechanism of injury helps in predicting the amount of soft-tissue damage.

Articular fracture dislocations have associated neurovascular injuries.

3 Evaluation of patient and injury

Because the etiology of many of these injuries is a high-energy mechanism, it is important to evaluate the patient fully for associated musculo-skeletal and nonorthopedic injuries. It is not uncommon for patients to have concomitant fractures of the calcaneus, tibial plateau, acetabulum, spine, or long bones, due to the shared mechanism of injury.

In assessing a specific joint injury, close attention should be paid to the soft tissues. Intra-articular fractures may cause gross mal-alignment of the limb, articular surface incongruity, or an associated joint subluxation or dislocation. **All have the potential to compromise the circulation to the surrounding skin, or even the limb itself, and so the vascular status distal to injury should be checked. This is best done by palpation of the pulses distal to the injury.** If there are no palpable pulses or a discrepancy exists from the contralateral side, the use of a Doppler monitor and assessment of capillary refill, color, and skin temperature are necessary. A careful neurological examination of the limb should also be completed and documented. Prompt realignment of the limb should be followed by a repeat neurological and vascular examination. Extensive open wounds, lacerations, or de-gloving are easily identified in the zone of injury, but a small disruption of the integument near a fracture must be considered an open fracture, or joint injury, until proven otherwise. Inspection for leakage of bloodstained synovial fluid, fat globules in blood, or a leakage of intra-articular injected fluid indicate whether a fracture or joint injury communicates with the wound.

In the absence of open wounds extensive injury to the surrounding tissues can still occur. **Determining the exact mechanism that caused the injury can help to predict the extent to which the soft tissues may be damaged.** The presence and location of any abrasions, joint effusion, skin blistering, and soft-tissue swelling should be noted. Point tenderness at ligamentous insertions may be the only clue to ligamentous disruption. Muscular compartments should be evaluated for any evidence of compartment syndrome. Both the AO and the Tscherne classification systems for closed injuries quantify the extent of soft-tissue damage (**chapter 1.5**). This is helpful in the development of a treatment plan. Following full evaluation, the limb can be immobilized temporarily in a well-padded splint, or by traction, to reduce further swelling and potential additional soft-tissue compromise.

4 Evaluation of the bone injury

Plain x-rays can provide a wealth of information regarding the injury to bone and offer clues to associated soft-tissue injury. They have traditionally been the most important tool available to the fracture surgeon for the assessment and treatment of fractures. Initial x-ray analysis includes two views obtained in planes 90° to each other and centered over the injury zone (**Fig. 2.3-2a**). The remainder of the limb will be examined by x-rays if clinically indicated. To ensure adequate detail, the area of interest should not be covered by dense bandaging or

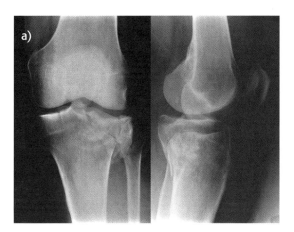

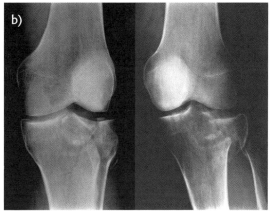

Fig. 2.3-2: X-ray evaluation of the bony injury:
a) Standard AP and lateral x-rays usually demonstrate the major fracture pattern but show no details. Impaction of the joint surface can be assumed when looking at the subchondral lines and double densities in the metaphysis.

b) Oblique views in two planes may give even better evidence of the articular involvement and help to determine more precisely the extent and location of the lesion.

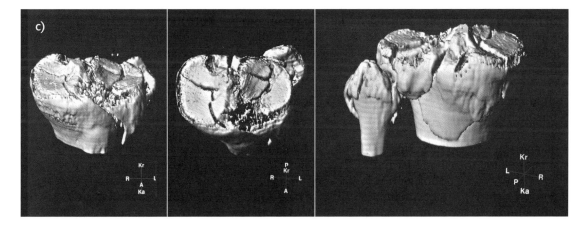

c) Axial CT-scans and (even more so) 3-D reconstruction give the complete picture of a damaged joint and thereby facilitate preoperative planning. If these are not available, the "old" technique of tomography certainly provides sufficiently adequate information.

In displaced articular fractures "traction views" help planning.

Impacted articular fragments require operative reduction.

Axial malalignment accelerates joint degeneration.

splintage. **If extensive fragmentation and deformity are present, traction applied to the extremity during the x-ray examination may improve understanding of the injury. Therefore, initial x-rays may require a physician in attendance to stabilize the limb in order to ensure that adequate images are obtained. For simple fractures, AP and lateral x-rays will suffice.**

For more complex fractures, oblique x-rays taken at 45° to the coronal plane will help to identify fracture fragments (**Fig. 2.3-2b**). Displacement and fragmentation of the articular and metaphyseal bone, identified by the plain films, can provide information about the amount of energy absorbed by the limb. Free articular fragments impacted into the supporting cancellous bone of the metaphysis can be identified by the density of their subchondral cortical bone (**Fig. 2.3-2a/b**). As mentioned, these depressed fragments, without soft-tissue attachments, cannot be reduced by closed manipulation to their original position. **The identification of such impacted fragments can have implications for the subsequent treatment of the fracture, since they require operative reduction.**

The Müller AO Classification of fractures (**chapter 1.4**) categorizes fractures of the end segment of bone using a standard glossary of terms to improve communication, to develop treatment protocols, and to determine the outcome for specific injuries. The addition of computed tomography along with 2-D and 3-D reconstruction provide additional information about the number and position of the articular fragments, the presence of impacted articular segments, the location of metaphyseal fracture lines, and the overall morphology of the injury. This can be helpful in planning screw placement and implant position prior to surgery (**Fig. 2.3-2c**).

5 Scientific basis of treatment of articular fractures

Although the amount of energy absorbed by the bone can be evaluated with x-rays, the degree and extent of injury to the overlying hyaline cartilage cannot be so judged. Studies on the effects of impact load reveal that hyaline cartilage may fracture prior to bone, and a single impact can alter the biochemical composition of the cartilage matrix [4, 5]. Nevertheless, ample evidence suggests that articular cartilage can remain viable after blunt trauma [6, 7] and that reconstruction of the articular surface and restoration of the axial alignment of the limb offer the joint the best possible chance of recovery. Pauwels [8] proposed that there exists an equilibrium between articular cartilage regeneration and degeneration, depending on the biomechanical environment of the joint. Articular cartilage is able to withstand a specific amount of force (F) per unit area (A), better defined as stress (S), where $S = F/A$. If this stress exceeds a certain level for a period of time, articular cartilage may not be able to adapt and degeneration will follow. Increases in stress at the articular cartilage can be secondary to axial malalignment of the bone or unreduced articular surfaces following injury [9]. **Axial malalignment alters load transmission across a joint and has been associated with accelerated joint degeneration** (**Fig. 2.3-4**). Instability, caused by fracture or internal derangement, can also lead to cartilage degeneration and may be important too in determining outcome [10, 11]. Pauwels [8] proposed that anatomical restoration of the joint surfaces and mechanical axes are necessary for a successful outcome following a displaced articular fracture.

Repair of adult articular cartilage injury following fracture depends on early anatomical reduction, rigid fixation, and early motion. Cartilaginous defects associated with fracture of the subchondral bone receive repair messages and undifferentiated mesenchymal cells from the underlying bone. Small gaps, or steps, in the articular surface can repair, but with a higher percentage of fibrocartilage, which has inferior mechanical properties and durability [12]. **Mitchell and Shepard [13] demonstrated experimentally that anatomical reduction and interfragmentary compression fixation of an intra-articular fracture, followed by continuous motion, can lead to true hyaline cartilage healing.** Llinas [14]

showed that articular cartilage and subchondral bone surfaces exhibit adaptive mechanisms that may partially restore congruity and load transmission to a joint with a step-off of less than 10% of the local articular cartilage thickness. This provides a guide to the minimal acceptable joint reduction. Salter et al. [12] demonstrated that immobilization of an injured joint leads to stiffness and articular cartilage degeneration, due to lack of nutrition and the formation of pannus. Further experiments revealed that the use of continuous passive motion (CPM) facilitated the repair of full-thickness articular cartilage defects in immature rabbits.

The longer surgical reduction and stabilization of an articular fracture are delayed, the

Repair of adult articular cartilage depends on exact reconstruction, rigid fixation, and early motion.

Continuous passive motion after anatomical reduction and rigid fixation of an articular fracture can lead to hyaline cartilage healing.

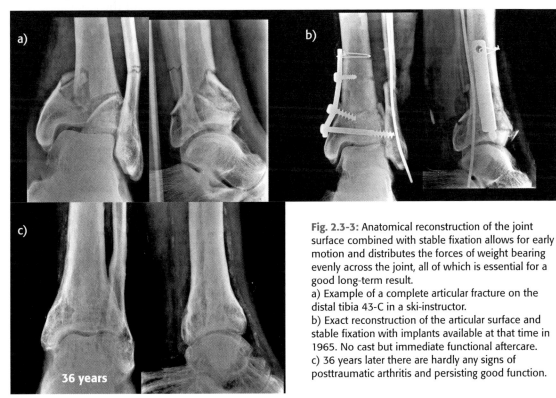

Fig. 2.3-3: Anatomical reconstruction of the joint surface combined with stable fixation allows for early motion and distributes the forces of weight bearing evenly across the joint, all of which is essential for a good long-term result.
a) Example of a complete articular fracture on the distal tibia 43-C in a ski-instructor.
b) Exact reconstruction of the articular surface and stable fixation with implants available at that time in 1965. No cast but immediate functional aftercare.
c) 36 years later there are hardly any signs of posttraumatic arthritis and persisting good function.

more hazardous and the worse the healing of the cartilage injury and the more likely that a later degeneration will result. Injury to hyaline cartilage without fracture of the underlying subchondral bone is not associated with an inflammatory response, due to its avascularity, and therefore does not repair spontaneously. The effect of isolated cartilage injury on long-term outcome of joint trauma is yet to be determined.

There seems to be little tolerance for alterations in joint morphology in experimental animal models. This has been confirmed in humans through clinical studies, which have demonstrated that final functional and x-ray results depend on anatomical reduction and early active joint motion [**3**, **15**, **16**]. On the other hand, exact reconstruction and stable fixation may give functionally excellent and long-lasting results (**Fig. 2.3-3**).

The preoperative plan prevents hazards, is educational, and helps quality control.

6 Principles of treatment

6.1 Understanding of the injury

A thorough history of the mechanism of injury, preinjury functional and work status, and patient expectations is required. Physical examination of the patient and limb is mandatory. Soft-tissue injury, especially swelling, blisters, abrasions, and/or lacerations must be assessed and documented. X-ray evaluation is performed so that the surgeon may understand the fracture pattern.

Exact history, clinical and x-ray assessment are mandatory for preoperative planning.

6.2 Preoperative planning

Preoperative planning is an important prerequisite for contemplating open reduction and internal fixation of intra-articular fractures. Adequate x-ray analysis (see **Fig. 2.3-2**) will allow the surgeon to understand both the totality of the injury (what Nicol called the "personality" of the fracture) and what will be needed during operation to accomplish the goal of anatomical restoration. Deciding the details of the procedure, the operating table, patient position, approach, specific instruments, the implants, and the need for intraoperative x-ray, prior to commencing, will likely allow the surgery to proceed more effectively and without the "ambush" of unforeseen problems. **A detailed plan and surgical tactics are mandatory prior to starting any osteosynthesis of an intra-articular fracture, as well as serving as an educational tool and a quality control exercise for the surgeon.**

6.3 Timing of operation

Following full evaluation of the patient and the specific injury, certain factors may influence a surgeon's ability to intervene at a given time. In a patient with an isolated injury to a joint, the rapid onset of excessive swelling after injury to a subcutaneous joint is usually the result of hemorrhage into the joint and surrounding tissues. Immediate surgery may allow evacuation of such a hematoma, while reduction and fixation will reduce further bleeding and allow resolution of the swelling. Therefore, a window of opportunity for early fracture fixation may be present immediately following the injury.

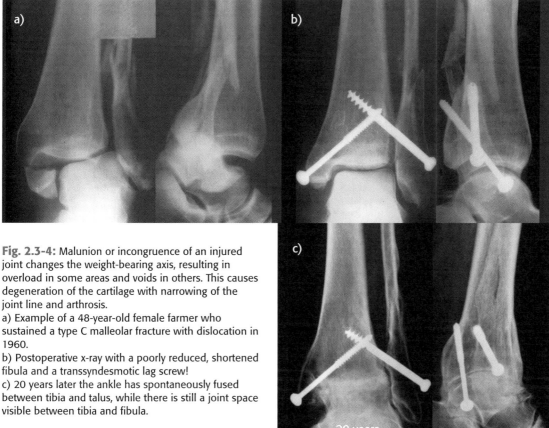

Fig. 2.3-4: Malunion or incongruence of an injured joint changes the weight-bearing axis, resulting in overload in some areas and voids in others. This causes degeneration of the cartilage with narrowing of the joint line and arthrosis.
a) Example of a 48-year-old female farmer who sustained a type C malleolar fracture with dislocation in 1960.
b) Postoperative x-ray with a poorly reduced, shortened fibula and a transsyndesmotic lag screw!
c) 20 years later the ankle has spontaneously fused between tibia and talus, while there is still a joint space visible between tibia and fibula.

If the soft-tissue envelope around the joint is swollen or traumatized with abrasions or degloving injuries on presentation, early surgery within the first few days may be contraindicated. It is known that fixation of long bones may decrease the morbidity and mortality associated with prolonged bed rest, but no such data exist on the early fixation of intra-articular injuries.

Complex intra-articular reconstruction may require prolonged operative time, and therefore the immediate treatment of these injuries may be contraindicated in the multiply injured patient. Exceptions to this would be open intra-articular fractures, which require at least a formal operative débridement, wound excision, and irrigation. During the procedure, all osteochondral fragments should be retained, unless severely contaminated (**chapter 5.1**).

Reduction and temporary or definitive stabilization of the joint surface should be accomplished during the same operation as the operative débridement, so that when formal reconstruction is undertaken all the articular

In articular fractures timing of surgery depends on soft-tissue condition.

Temporary joint bridging by external fixation helps to resolve swelling.

fracture fragments will be available to guide the final reduction. **Early temporary stabilization of the fracture by external fixation to span the joint, or traction, may be helpful in preventing further soft-tissue injury by controlling the fractured limb and by maintaining bone and soft-tissue alignment during resolution of the acute hemorrhage and inflammation. Any delay in definitive fixation will be determined by the condition of the patient and the soft-tissue envelope. It is safe to operate when the skin has regained its creases and wrinkles over the operative site with motion.**

Abrasions and blisters need to be epithelialized and dry. Where there is a closed subcutaneous degloving and crushing of the subcutaneous fat, early operative débridement and a possible delayed articular reconstruction are likely to be required. By assessing the inflammatory mediators, Trentz (**chapter 5.3**) has shown that the reduced endocrine response at 7–10 days after injury corresponds to the clinical resolution of the swelling and inflammation. Finally, if surgery is delayed for more than 2–3 weeks, reconstruction may be more difficult and complicated by reorganization of the injured tissues, limiting the ability to obtain anatomical restoration of the articular surface and axial alignment of the bone, thereby prejudicing the long-term results [**17**].

6.4 Surgical approach

For most appendicular skeletal injuries, skin incisions should be longitudinal, perpendicular to the axis of the joint, and not directly over any bony prominence. They should not be so liberal as to lead to desiccation of sensitive structures (e.g., nerves, tendons). The possibility of future procedures should be kept in mind while planning the approach, although this consideration should not limit the access necessary for reduction and fixation. Skin incisions should be extensile for further exposure, so as to limit tension on the skin during wound retraction. Although skin has a rich vascular supply derived from the underlying fascia, in areas of traumatized tissue large cutaneous flaps should be avoided. Full-thickness fasciocutaneous flaps can be raised to allow mobilization of the soft tissues for improved access to the bone. Once down to bone, care should be taken to avoid unnecessary stripping of any capsular or soft-tissue attachments of cortical fragments. Access to the joint can be accomplished either through fracture planes and associated rents in the articular capsule or through planned arthrotomies. Extensive stripping of capsule from articular bony fragments must be avoided in order to maintain their blood supply. Evacuation of hemarthrosis and any intra-articular debris is facilitated by copious irrigation of the joint. Manual or mechanical traction applied to the limb can improve the view of the joint surfaces.

6.5 Articular reduction

All fracture surfaces must be thoroughly cleared of hematoma and any early callus. At this stage, loose osteochondral fragments can be removed from the wound, but impacted fragments should not yet be elevated from their underlying cancellous beds. Regardless of their size, all articular fragments should initially be retained as keys to the final reduction. Once debris has been cleared, traction is removed from the limb to allow the intact portions of the joint to resume an anatomical position. If inadequate stability exists, the large distractor,

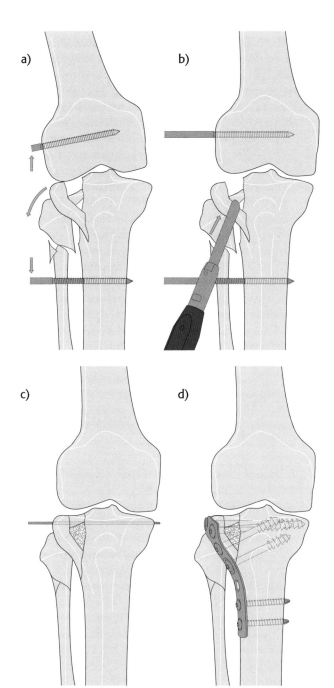

Fig. 2.3-5: Reconstruction of a tibial plateau 41-B3 fracture, through a straight lateral parapatellar approach:
a) Indirect reduction and axial alignment by ligamentotaxis with a joint bridging distractor.
b) The large, impacted articular fragment is elevated with a curved impactor, introduced through the fracture or through a cortical window in the metaphysis.
c) After temporary fixation of the reduced fragment with a K-wire, the meta-physeal/epiphyseal bone defect is filled with autogenous cancellous bone or a cortico cancellous block acting as a strut.
d) The reconstructed lateral plateau is finally buttressed by a L-plate or T-plate. The K-wire has been replaced by a (cannulated) 6.5 mm cancellous bone lag screw.

or an external fixator, may be used to maintain distraction and axial alignment and to allow a degree of indirect reduction of fracture fragments (**Fig. 2.3-5a**). The intact joint surfaces and the opposing articular surfaces are used to judge the reduction of displaced or impacted articular fragments. **Working through the fracture or through a window created in the metaphyseal cortex, central depressed fragments can be elevated and reduced. Impacted osteochondral fragments should be elevated from the underlying metaphyseal bone along with an adequate block of cancellous bone by an osteotome or elevator.** This technique maintains the impacted zone between the subchondral cortical bone and its underlying cancellous bone, facilitating possible future fixation (**Fig. 2.3-5b**).

Impacted fragments must be elevated and fixed in the reduced position.

Although free cartilage or osteochondral fragments without cancellous bone support, will be helpful in positioning major articular fragments, it would be difficult to fix and maintain their position later, while their long-term viability is questionable. They are therefore discarded after aiding in the reduction. **Bone defects left behind within the metaphysis are filled with an autogenous cancellous or corticocancellous graft for early support of the articular surface and to stimulate reconstitution of metaphyseal bone stock.** Cortical reduction and soft-tissue attachments will guide the repositioning of peripheral fracture fragments and their associated articular surfaces. Self-locking bone holding forceps or K-wires are used to hold the fracture in position provisionally while the reduction is confirmed (**Fig. 2.3-5c**).

Special circumstances exist which require deviation from the usual reconstructive protocol. In simple fractures, with a single large fragment split from the joint and causing instability, closed reduction can be performed in the operating suite. Using fluoroscopy, the reduction can be confirmed, followed by stabilization of the fracture using guide wires and cannulated screws [18]. In the presence of intra-articular and metaphyseal fragmentation (C3 injuries), no portion of the articular surface is in continuity with the metaphysis. If initial cortical reduction of the metaphysis will provide a stable framework upon which the articular reduction can be built, then the order of the procedure is reversed and the metaphysis is first reconstructed to the intact diaphysis.

Direct inspection of the joint surface, either through arthrotomies or arthroscopically, will evaluate the reduction of the cartilaginous surfaces [19, 20]. **Intra-operative fluoroscopy or x-rays will provide information on reduction of the bone. Once the reduction is satisfactory, fixation of the intra-articular portion can be completed.** Lag screw fixation causes compression between cancellous surfaces and results in stable fixation of the fragment. If multiple small fragments are present, reduction of the fracture and support of small fragments can be maintained with fully threaded position screws. In this instance, absolute stability may not be obtained due to the small areas of fragment contact. Care must be taken not to overcompress these fragments. Techniques have recently been described in which multiple screws are placed in the proximity of the subchondral surface to support fracture fragments (rafting technique), but the effect on the local biological and mechanical environment of the bone and cartilage is not yet clear.

6.6 Metaphyseal/ diaphyseal reduction and fixation

The primary goal for reduction and fixation of the extra-articular component is restoration of axial alignment with adequate stability to start early motion. In simple partial fractures extending into the metaphysis (B1), lag screw fixation may be sufficient [21]. With fragmentation of the metaphysis or joint surface, gaps and defects in cancellous or cortical bone can remain following reduction. The reduced area of contact decreases the amount of stability contributed to the construct by the bone itself, while only some of the force can be borne by a

Metaphyseal bone defects must be grafted with autogenous bone or a substitute.

Joint surface restoration must be checked intraoperatively.

buttress plate. **Comminution of the metaphysis or diaphysis may tempt a surgeon to precisely reduce and internally fix all of the non-articular cortical fragments. Such exact reductions may result in improved stability, however, at the cost of possible devascularization of fragments. Exact reduction of cortical fragments in the metaphysis is not necessary as long as axial alignment of the limb is maintained** (**Fig. 2.3-5d**). Large fragments can be positioned with clamps and held with screws. **A buttressing device, usually a plate, is then used to fix the articular block to the intact portion of the diaphysis. Currently, external fixators and hybrid ring fixators are becoming more popular, due to their ability to reduce indirectly and protect the fracture zone without surgical dissection [22–24].** However, absolute stability is not obtained. A significant part of the force is transmitted through the fixator and relative stability of the entire construct will be sufficient to allow controlled early motion (**chapters 4.8.1** and **4.8.3**).

6.7   Soft-tissue reconstruction

Ligament injury occurs in 20–30% of intra-articular fractures around the knee. Intra-substance tears of the cruciate ligaments are commonly left untouched due to the risk of knee stiffness following early reconstruction and poor results following primary repair. Medial collateral injuries are usually not repaired, but require bracing and early motion. Avulsion injuries of the collateral and cruciate ligaments can be dealt with during surgery of the intra-articular fracture. Regardless of the treatment, early motion should be started soon after repair. Unless it appears that ligament repair will improve stability to facilitate postoperative mobilization, it should be delayed [25, 26].

Following bony reconstruction, suction drains should be placed to prevent fluid collection and reduce postoperative swelling. Deep layers are loosely approximated and the skin closed with atraumatic technique (**chapter 1.5**). **To avoid complications of skin necrosis and wound dehiscence, it is vital to avoid tension on skin closure.** If this cannot be achieved, the wound should be left open beneath sterile, non-desiccating dressings and the patient scheduled for further surgical inspection and possible soft-tissue cover in 2–5 days. The timing of this "second look" will depend on the nature of the soft-tissue injury. Preoperative consultation with surgeons trained in soft-tissue transfers may be prudent, as local or distant soft-tissue transfers can reliably cover remaining defects (**chapter 5.2**).

6.8   Postoperative care

The joint should be placed in a soft bulky bandage postoperatively. If stable fixation has been achieved, early postoperative CPM or active assisted and active range of motion exercises can be started under the supervision of a therapist.

A short period of immobilization, to maintain optimal position of the extremity until muscle control of joint motion is regained, will help to prevent soft-tissue deformity. Although the importance of early motion on cartilage and ligament healing has been demonstrated, if the

In the metaphysis axial alingment is more important than anatomical reduction.

Skin closure without tension is vital for uneventful healing.

The metaphysis can be buttressed by plate or external fixators.

surgeon is unable to achieve adequate operative stability of the fracture, postoperative immobilization may need to be continued until early signs of consolidation are noted on x-rays, indicating that postoperative stiffness is likely. Frequent x-ray surveillance is important for fractures treated non-operatively or by internal fixation. Early detection of loss of reduction or fixation will allow timely corrective intervention. Limited weight bearing (10–15 kg) is tolerated. Isometric muscle exercises are started on day one following the operation. With the start of weight bearing, strengthening of the muscles crossing the joint can begin.

7 Summary

Because of the uniqueness of the articular end segment of a bone, the treatment is different from that of diaphyseal fractures. The principles of articular fracture management are designed to assure an anatomical reduction of the joint surface as the most crucial step. Axial realignment of the limb is imperative, to be achieved as permitted by the condition of the patient and of the soft tissues. The overall management of an articular fracture requires a well-designed preoperative plan and a skillfully executed surgical tactic, followed by appropriate aftercare, in order to guarantee the best possible outcome.

8 Bibliography

1. **Askew M, Mow VC** (1978) The biomechanical function of the collagen fibril ultrastructure of articular cartilage. *J Biomech Eng;* 100:105–115.
2. **Charnley J** (1961) *The Closed Treatment of Common Fractures.* Edinburgh: Livingstone.
3. **Schatzker J, Lambert DC** (1979) Supracondylar fractures of the femur. *Clin Orthop;* (138):77–83.
4. **Borrelli J Jr, Torzilli PA, Grigiene R, et al.** (1997) Effect of impact load on articular cartilage: development of an intra-articular fracture model. *J Orthop Trauma;* 11 (5):319–326.
5. **Mankin HJ** (1986) The response of articular cartilage in mechanical injury. *J Bone Joint Surg [Am];* 64 (3):460–466.
6. **Thompson RC, Oegema TR, Jr., Lewis JL, et al.** (1991) Osteoarthrotic changes after acute transarticular load. An animal model. *J Bone Joint Surg [Am];* 73 (7):990–1001.
7. **Milgram JW** (1986) Injury to articular cartilage joint surfaces: II. Displaced fractures of underlying bone. A histopathologic study of human tissue specimens. *Clin Orthop;* (206):236–247.
8. **Pauwels F** (1961) Neue Richtlinien für die operative Behandlung der Coxarthrose. *Verh Dtsch Orthop Ges;* 48:322–366.
9. **Brown TD, Anderson DD, Nepola JV, et al.** (1988) Contact stress aberrations following imprecise reduction of simple tibial plateau fractures. *J Orthop Res;* 6 (6):851–862.
10. **Davis W, Moskowitz RW** (1988) Degenerative joint changes following posterior cruciate section in a rabbit. *Clin Orthop;* 93:307–312.

11. **McDevitt C, Gilbertson E, Muir H** (1977) An experimental model of osteoarthritis; early morphological and biochemical changes. *J Bone Joint Surg [Br]*; 59 (1):24–35.

12. **Salter RB, Simmonds DF, Malcolm BW, et al.** (1980) The biological effect of continuous passive motion on the healing of full-thickness defects in articular cartilage. An experimental investigation in the rabbit. *J Bone Joint Surg [Am]*; 62 (8):1232–1251.

13. **Mitchell N, Shepard N** (1980) Healing of articular cartilage in intra-articular fractures in rabbits. *J Bone Joint Surg [Am]*; 62 (4):628–634.

14. **Llinas A, McKellop HA, Marshall GJ, et al.** (1993) Healing and remodeling of articular incongruities in a rabbit fracture model. *J Bone Joint Surg [Am]*; 75 (10):1508–1523.

15. **Matta JM** (1996) Fractures of the acetabulum: accuracy of reduction and clinical results in patients managed operatively within three weeks after the injury. *J Bone Joint Surg [Am]*; 78 (11):1632–1645.

16. **Knirk JL, Jupiter JB** (1986) Intra-articular fractures of the distal end of the radius in young adults. *J Bone Joint Surg [Am]*; 68 (5):647–659.

17. **Johnson EE, Matta JM, Mast JW, et al.** (1994) Delayed reconstruction of acetabular fractures 21–120 days following injury. *Clin Orthop*; (305):20–30.

18. **Koval KJ, Sanders R, Borrelli J, et al.** (1992) Indirect reduction and percutaneous screw fixation of displaced tibial plateau fractures. *J Orthop Trauma*; 6 (3):340–346.

19. **Cooney WP, Berger RA** (1993) Treatment of complex fractures of the distal radius. Combined use of internal and external fixation and arthroscopic reduction. *Hand Clin*; 9 (4):603–612.

20. **Fowble CD, Zimmer JW, Schepsis AA** (1993) The role of arthroscopy in the assessment and treatment of tibial plateau fractures. *Arthroscopy*; 9 (5):584–590.

21. **Koval KJ, Polatsch D, Kummer FJ, et al.** (1996) Split fractures of the lateral tibial plateau: evaluation of three fixation methods. *J Orthop Trauma*; 10 (5):304–308.

22. **Marsh JL, Smith ST, Do TT** (1995) External fixation and limited internal fixation for complex fractures of the tibial plateau. *J Bone Joint Surg [Am]*; 77 (5):661–673.

23. **Tornetta Pd, Weiner L, Bergman M, et al.** (1993) Pilon fractures: treatment with combined internal and external fixation. *J Orthop Trauma*; 7 (6):489–496.

24. **Stamer DT, Schenk R, Staggers B, et al.** (1994) Bicondylar tibial plateau fractures treated with a hybrid ring external fixator: a preliminary study. *J Orthop Trauma*; 8 (6):455–461.

25. **Bennett WF, Browner B** (1994) Tibial plateau fractures: a study of associated soft-tissue injuries. *J Orthop Trauma*; 8 (3):183–188.

26. **Delamarter RB, Hohl M, Hopp E,** (1990) Ligament injuries associated with tibial plateau fractures. *Clin Orthop*; (250):226–233.

9 Updates

Updates and additional references for this chapter are available online at:
http://www.aopublishing.org/PFxM/23.htm

2.4 Preoperative planning

Joseph Schatzker

1 Introduction

Prior to an operation, the time that a surgeon devotes to a careful preoperative plan is of critical importance and often determines the success or failure of the procedure. It is at this point that the surgeon can take all the time needed to define the surgical problem, to identify fully all the anatomical and technical aspects of the procedure, and then carefully plan the solution.

In order to define the surgical problem the surgeon must first establish the diagnosis. This requires a detailed history, a careful physical examination, all necessary laboratory tests, together with appropriate x-rays and whatever ancillary imaging studies, such as CT scans, 3-D reconstructions, or MRI, that the clinical situation dictates.

The diagnosis alone is not enough to guide the surgeon to the correct choice of a procedure. Proper decision making must also take into account the patient's physical state (see **chapter 2.1**), and the patient's expectations of the proposed treatment. In addition, the surgeon must have a thorough knowledge of the relevant operative procedures and the relative dangers and success rates of each. The decision to operate and the choice of the

procedure must be made, if at all possible, in consultation with the patient, once all the benefits and risks of the procedure have been carefully explained. Failure to communicate all these matters to the patient often stems from a failure to prepare a detailed preoperative plan.

The central feature of a careful preoperative plan of a procedure is first to identify the desired end result and then to add a detailed list of all the surgical steps involved in getting there.

The advantages of careful graphic preoperative planning are numerous and the requirements are simple. They are:
a) Good x-rays, including views of the normal side when appropriate and possible.
b) Transparencies or good tracing paper.
c) A full set of relevant implant templates of correct scale.
d) A goniometer.
e) Colored felt-tipped pens and a sharp pencil.

Using drawings, the surgeon can arrive at the best method or methods of solving a problem. The surgical process is worked out and performed on paper. It can be repeated as many times as necessary until the surgeon has grasped the full magnitude of the problem and has

The time that a surgeon devotes to a careful preoperative plan often determines the success or failure of the procedure.

The diagnosis alone is not enough to guide the surgeon to the correct choice of a procedure.

found the best solution. This process of trial and error allows the surgeon to get a feel for the dynamics and intricacies of the problem to be solved. The ability to shift the tracings around, to superimpose one on the other, to lengthen, to shorten, to angulate or displace, all aid in developing a 3-D image of the problem, of its associated soft-tissue implications, and of the ultimate solution.

The important landmarks for implant insertion are located, and distances, angles, and sizes of wedges can all be measured, leading to selection of the implant and its correct size. With a carefully executed plan the surgeon will never commence the operation lacking the necessary implants or instruments, and never attempt an inappropriate approach on an improperly positioned patient. The graphic plan forms a permanent record of the thought process and of the solution. If properly done it should eventually be seen to correspond to the post-operative x-ray, allowing an immediate quality control of the surgeon's efforts.

The plan should list also all the steps necessary for the procedure, numbered in the order in which they are to be carried out. This provides a step-by-step guide to the operation and allows the surgeon to concentrate on the procedure free from the distraction of having to improvise each stage as it arises. This results in surgery becoming not only faster but much safer. Unforeseen situations, however, can and do arise during the procedure, and the surgeon must always be prepared to adapt in response.

The plan should list also all the steps necessary for the procedure, numbered in order.

2 Planning in the acute situation

The tracing of the different fracture fragments from x-rays in different planes allows the surgeon to recognize details of previously unnoticed features of the fracture. In addition, considering the same fragment in different planes helps in forming a three dimensional concept of the fracture. Reduction of the fracture at the time of surgery results from manipulation of the fragments. Manipulating them on paper first often discloses not only latent angulation and shortening, but also rotational displacement. All of these need to be corrected.

In the early years of the AO method of operative fracture care, the same principles of reduction and stabilization applied to all fractures, diaphyseal as well as articular. Developments which have occurred over the years, in both the principles and the techniques used to treat fractures, are the result of biomechanical and biological research. Today's dictum is that in dealing with diaphyseal fractures the requirement is to restore length, rotation, and alignment, without seeking detailed anatomical reconstruction. In dealing with articular fractures, on the other hand, one must achieve anatomical reduction of the articular surface and reduction of the metaphyseal deformity in order to overcome axial malalignment and joint overload. The type of reduction and fixation of the metaphyseal deformity will be determined by the fracture morphology and the associated soft-tissue factors. Thus, the choice of a procedure, with all the associated details, is made on the basis of the patient factors and of fracture factors such as the status of the soft tissues, the bone, the segment, and the fracture morphology. Decisions made on the basis of these factors must always be tempered by the personal experience of the individual surgeon.

For diaphyseal fractures, which are to be stabilized with locked intramedullary nails, little detailed graphic preoperative planning is required. The issues which have to be decided are: which size and length of intramedullary nail—with or without reaming—and what type of interlocking, if choices are available. Plating, however, demands more detailed planning.

Simple fractures, if they are to be treated with screws and plates, require absolutely stable fixation. This can be achieved only with anatomical reduction and fixation by interfragmentary compression. Therefore, the issues to be addressed in planning are the type of fixation, lag screws alone or lag screws in combination with a plate, or compression applied with a plate alone as is often the case in transverse or very short oblique fractures. One must pay attention to the specifics of the fixation, and these include the type of reduction to be employed, direct or indirect, the order in which the devices are to be inserted, and, of course, the surgical approach.

In using plates to treat wedge and complex fractures, particularly the latter, the surgeon may strive for relatively stable fixation, which implies that the plate is applied as a bridging device or "bridge plate". The issues to preplan here are:

- The correct length, alignment, and rotation of the bone.
- The type and length of the plate.
- The number of screws.
- The function of the screws (as some may still be inserted as lag screws even in bridge plating).

Under these circumstances, indirect reduction is required in order to preserve the viability of all fragments. For this the surgeon must decide between using a distractor, or the plate and a distracting device. In addition, the surgical approach must be decided upon as well as the degree of invasiveness. Will the plate be slid under the muscle envelope with minimal exposure of the fracture, or to what degree will it be necessary to expose the fragments in order to apply and fix the plate?

Articular fractures present different challenges. The articular components require accurate anatomical reduction. The decision to be made is whether this will require direct exposure of the fragments or whether, as in tibial plateau fractures, reduction might be achieved with the aid of an arthroscope or an image intensifier. In dealing with articular fragments one has to aim for absolute stability to facilitate union and articular cartilage regeneration. Therefore, one has to rely on lag screws for fixation. These may be inserted under direct vision, or percutaneously as cannulated screws.

In complete articular fractures, for example, type C1 or C2 fractures of the distal femur, the articular reduction poses less of a challenge than does the re-establishment of axial alignment, which may be accomplished simply with the proper insertion of an angled blade plate or the compression screw of a DCS. The fixed angle of the device will automatically restore axial alignment. In type C3 fractures the task becomes much more difficult because a fixed angle device may not be appropriate. Here the surgeon may use a tracing of an x-ray of the normal side as a template of the desired end result, or else may use a template of the knee

Planning for plating needs to be more detailed than for nailing.

Articular fractures present different challenges than diaphyseal fractures.

joint axes as an aid in the plan for re-establishing normal axial alignment after reduction. The preoperative plan may first involve the cutting out of the outlined fragments, their numbering for identification, and their arrangement along the knee joint axis. Then come the specifics of fixing an appropriate plate to the reconstructed epiphyseal block, before undertaking an indirect reduction of the metaphyseal component of the fracture.

If there is a defect in the metaphysis because of compression of the cancellous bone, as is the case in axial impaction fractures, then one may plan for a bone graft and indicate this on the sketch. At times, the damage to the soft tissues will dictate bridging of the metaphysis with an external fixator as the first step, and a delayed final reconstruction would follow at 2–3 weeks, depending on the status of the soft tissues.

3 The surgical tactic

While the rehearsal of the operative procedure and its expression in the form of a drawing of the proposed final result are the central features of good preoperative planning, the surgical tactic by which the result is to be achieved must now be developed and recorded.

This might be considered under the following main headings.

The patient

- Type of anesthesia
- The need for a tourniquet
- Positioning
- Fracture table or radiolucent table

The procedure

- Approach
- Implants and instruments
- Special equipment for reduction
- Types of implants
- Need for bone graft or bone substitutes
- Cell saver or special blood substitutes

Support services

- X-rays or C-arm
- Other forms of aids to vision, for example, arthroscopic or computer-assisted guidance

Postoperative care

- CPM device
- Traction
- Splinting

Information on these matters will ensure that the OR staff have had time to prepare for their patient and to identify and remedy potential difficulties.

4 Planning techniques

4.1 Direct overlay

In a straight bone, each component may be traced onto a separate transparency and the bone is then rebuilt over its central axis, represented by a straight line (**Fig. 2.4-1**). An appropriate template is used for selection and placement of the implant(s).

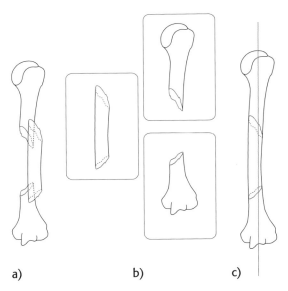

4.2 Overlay using the normal side

A tracing is made of the normal side. The fracture is drawn on another sheet and may be "exploded" for greater ease in identifying the fragments. The fragments may then be drawn into, or cut out and reassembled, on the normal drawing, which must be reversed to match the fractured side (**Fig. 2.4-2**).

4.3 Drawing a fracture adjacent to a joint using the physiological axes

Fig. 2.4-1: The direct overlay technique is a quick method for planning in a straight bone. The various components of the segmental fracture should be traced on individual pieces of paper. A straight line is drawn and the fragments are then assembled on this axis.

An outline of each physiological axis is made using a template or a drawing from the opposite side (**Fig. 2.4-3**). If the fracture involves the joint surface, this is first "re-assembled" using the

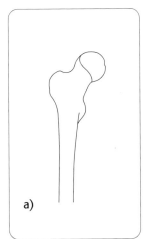 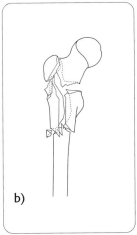 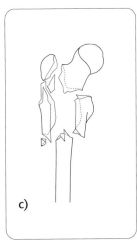 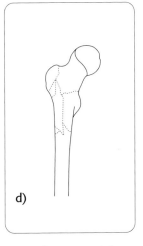

Fig. 2.4-2: Overlay using normal side.
a) Tracing of the normal side—rotated to serve as template. b) Tracing of the fracture.

c) The fracture fragments can be cut out or drawn separately.
d) These fragments are then re-assembled on the drawing of the intact side which has been reversed to match the fractured side.

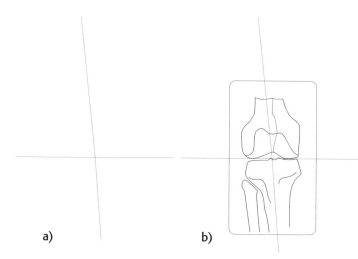

a)   b)

Fig. 2.4-3: b) An outline of each phyosiological axis is made using a template (a) or a drawing from the opposite side.

technique described in **section 4.2** (**Fig. 2.4-4a**). The assembled block is then drawn in, respecting the physiological axes and the mechanical axis of the joint. Any additional metaphyseal components are reassembled around the appropriate mechanical axis (**Fig. 2.4-4b/c**).

The principles of using the mechanical axis in the diaphysis are detailed in the osteotomy example (see **section 7**).

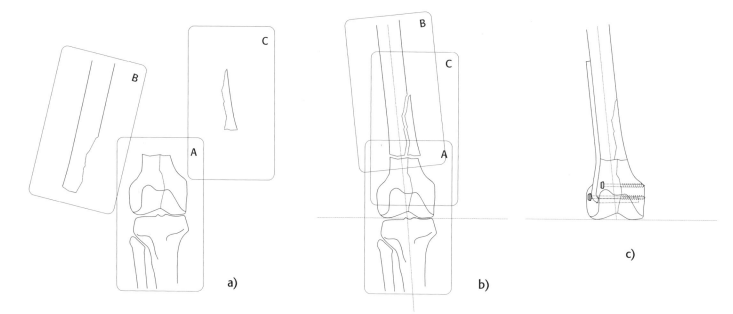

a)   b)   c)

Fig. 2.4-4: a) Each major fracture fragment is drawn on a separate sheet.
b) The bone is reassembled around the physiological axes.
c) By the use of templates the appropriate implants are drawn in.

5 Planning the correction of deformities

In order to define a deformity one requires an AP and a lateral x-ray of the bone. Frequently, x-rays of the normal side are also helpful as they help in establishing the normal anatomical axes which are an essential prerequisite in defining angular deformities. The x-rays of the normal side also provide a template of the desired end result of corrective surgery, which is usually the restoration of the normal relationships.

In dealing with deformities of the lower extremities, one should also obtain a three-foot standing film. This is important for two reasons. First it permits the establishment of the mechanical axis, which is an imaginary line drawn from the center of the hip to the center of the ankle joint (see **chapter 2.2**, **Fig. 2.2-1**). Under normal circumstances it passes through the center of the knee joint. Secondly, the **standing film allows one to see deformities under load. These may be present as a result of ligamentous laxity or loss of bony substance.** If one comes to suspect that a lax ligament is contributing to a deformity, a true stress x-ray should supplement the study. Similarly, if a ligamentous laxity exists on the concave side of a deformity, this must be determined by an appropriate stress film. To avoid overcorrection, the degree of correction obtained as a result of the laxity has to be accounted for and subtracted from the proposed amount of axial correction which was calculated on the basis of the anatomical axes.

When dealing with intra-articular deformities, in order to image their full complexity one must supplement the AP and lateral x-rays with special projections (e.g., Judet views of the acetabulum). There may be a need for CT scans with coronal and sagittal reconstructions, and frequently also for 3-D reconstruction and often for MRI. **The MRI will show fracture lines many months after the accident, when they are no longer easily discernible on a CT scan.**

Rotational deformities can often be determined, up to a point, by means of a careful physical examination. An accurate measurement, however, can be obtained only by comparing CTs of both the abnormal and normal extremity. To determine rotational deformities, one must order cuts through the joints proximal and distal to the bone so that one can select appropriate reference points to carry out the measurements.

Type of deformities

Deformities are either simple or complex. A simple deformity is a deformity in one plane only. A complex deformity occurs in at least two planes. Thus, a complex deformity may have angular deformities in two planes, a rotational deformity, and shortening.

Evolving the rationale of the procedure

Before one can correct a deformity one must go through a number of essential steps:
- Define the deformity.
- Define the procedure designed to correct the deformity.
- Decide whether the soft-tissue envelope will allow the procedure to be carried out without undue risks.
- Evaluate whether its risks and its potential benefits make the procedure justifiable.

The MRI will show fracture lines when they are no longer easily discernible on a CT scan.

CTs are needed for precise measurement of the rotational deformity.

Long standing films are important in dealing with lower limb deformity.

An angular deformity of a long bone is best corrected through the apex of the deformity.

6 The drawing of the preoperative plan

The drawing of the preoperative plan begins with a tracing of the outline of both the AP and lateral x-ray of the normal side. On these one marks in the anatomical axes, the joint axes where indicated, and in the lower extremity, the mechanical axis wherever possible.

Next one traces out the outlines of the AP and lateral x-ray of the deformed bone. One should then mark in the anatomical axes. The angles of correction are obtained by simply superimposing the tracing of the normal side over the tracing of the deformed side and by tracing in the normal anatomical axes on the deformed side. The intersection of the anatomical axes of the deformed side with the anatomical axes of the normal side gives one the angle of correction.

In a complex deformity it may be extremely difficult to draw in the anatomical axes because of the misshapen bone. In such a case it can be helpful to superimpose the tracing of the abnormal side over the tracing of the normal bone. One can begin with either the proximal or distal part of the bone. By superimposing the joint surfaces and as much of the metaphyses as possible, one can then draw in the anatomical axes of the normal side onto the deformed side and in this way establish the proximal and distal anatomical axes of the deformed bone. By extending the axes till they intersect one can obtain the angle of deformity and, thus, the angle of correction. The same steps are repeated for the lateral projections.

It is not possible to draw in the rotational deformity, but the degrees of malrotation should be marked in on the preoperative plan.

6.1 Where to do the correction?

An angular deformity of a long bone is best corrected through the apex of the deformity. In the past, surgeons attempted to correct diaphyseal angular deformities through the metaphysis, hoping for better healing from the cancellous bone. Such corrections, particularly if the corrective osteotomy was at a distance from the deformity, resulted in new complex deformities which rarely addressed the problem they were designed to correct. Usually the result was a further deformity which not only failed to correct the initial deformity, but resulted also in additional serious problems. These might include an undesirable angulation of a weight-bearing surface, which was now no longer at 90° to the weight-bearing axis, or in an undesirable translocation of the bone which led to abnormal loading of the articulations.

6.2 What type of osteotomy?

In planning a corrective osteotomy, the surgeon must realize the corrections which are possible.

One can carry out angular corrections in the coronal and sagittal planes, one can shorten or lengthen, rotate in or out, and lastly translocate medially, laterally, anteriorly, or posteriorly.

Osteotomy cuts can be transverse, oblique, or stepwise.

Whenever a rotational correction is necessary, it is best to begin with a transverse osteotomy at 90° to the long axis of the bone. This will allow for rotational corrections regardless of what wedges are cut from the other fragment. If the initial cut is oblique, and then one tries to correct a rotational deformity, one ends up with the very difficult task of having to cut a pyramidal wedge. Lastly, in correcting angular deformities the surgeon must remember that the wedges can be either open or closed, depending on whether one wishes to shorten or lengthen the bone. Closing wedges unite faster and rarely require bone grafting, but they sacrifice length. Opening wedges add length, but it is best to reserve them for children and younger teenagers, because in adults they heal very slowly or not at all. In adults, the defects can be grafted, if indicated, even if it means using allograft blocks.

Similar considerations apply to some degree to the mode of fixation. Opening wedges of diaphyses in the adult should not be attempted, if plate fixation is planned. If one uses an intramedullary nail for fixation, and if the osteotomy is done with an intramedullary saw leaving the soft-tissue envelope undisturbed, the usual result is good healing without any need for additional bone grafting. An exception would be an opening wedge where a plate might be used over a block allograft.

Progressive corrections of complex deformities are possible with the Ilizarov technique. The principles of such corrective procedures are different and the two techniques should not be confused.

Examples of osteotomies intended to correct deformities are to be found in **chapter 6.4** and what follows is a detailed description of the steps involved in planning such procedures.

7 Example of a preoperative plan

As an illustrative example of the preoperative plan of the correction of a simple deformity I have chosen a malunion of the proximal femur. It is the result of a fracture through the base of the neck which united with a 30° varus deformity.

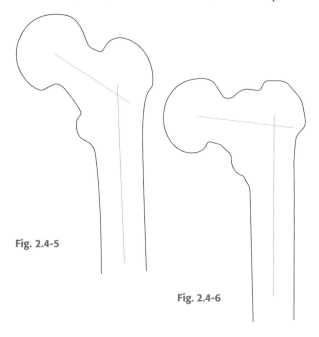

Fig. 2.4-5

Fig. 2.4-6

X-rays of the normal and the deformed sides should be at hand. The preoperative plan begins with the drawing of the outline of the normal bone (which is then reversed) (**Fig. 2.4-5**) and of the deformed bone (**Fig. 2.4-6**). Next the anatomical axes are marked in. The neck axis is found by joining the center of the head with the center of the neck. The shaft axis is found by joining the midpoint of the femur at two or three levels.

To find the difference between the neck shaft angles of the two bones we superimpose the two tracings. Because the deformity is

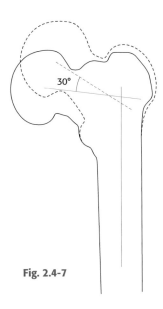

Fig. 2.4-7

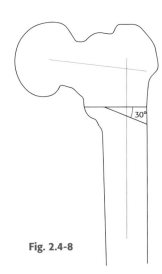

Fig. 2.4-8

An osteotomy at the level of the femoral neck is technically difficult and could result in an avascular necrosis of the head.

One must strive for a compromise between leg length and stability.

through the base of the neck, the outlines of the shafts and of the greater and lesser trochanters superimpose accurately. The angle formed between the axes of the necks is the angle of the deformity or the angle of correction (**Fig. 2.4-7**).

On the tracing of the deformed bone mark in the osteotomy. The corrective osteotomy would be best at the level of the apex of the deformity, which in this instance is the base of the neck. **An osteotomy at the level of the femoral neck is technically difficult and could result in an avascular necrosis of the head.** For this reason the correction will be done in the intertrochanteric area. As a general rule it is best to begin with an osteotomy at right angles (90°) to the long axis of the bone, since this facilitates any rotational correction, and makes the calculation of the angular corrections easier. Thus, at the level of the lesser trochanter draw a line at 90° to the anatomical axis of the femur (**Fig. 2.4-8**). We need to carry out a 30° valgus

osteotomy to correct the deformity. In the proximal femur a valgus correction requires the resection of a closing wedge with its base along the lateral cortex. Experience has shown that, up to 30°, the wedge can be cut from the distal fragment alone. If the desired correction exceeds 30°, the amount exceeding the 30° should be cut from the proximal fragment. Thus, if one were doing a 50° valgus osteotomy, 30° would be cut from the distal fragment and 20° from the proximal. The size of the wedge in width as compared to the diameter of the bone affects both the length of the leg and the stability of the reduction. Thus, the greater the wedge, the greater will be the loss of length and the greater will be the stability of the reduced fragments. **One must strive for a compromise between leg length and stability.** Thus, one should strive to cut a wedge which is just slightly greater than half of the diameter of the bone. This wedge is now marked in. Its base is

Make a tracing which shows the two fragments (**Fig. 2.4-11**) reduced. Take templates (**Fig. 2.4-12**) of the angled blade plates and see which angled blade plate fits best. We can readily see that the 120° angled blade plate, also referred to as the repositioning plate, fits best because its blade lines up along the anatomical axis of the neck and the plate lines up along the lateral cortex of the shaft. Many surgeons are tempted to use the DHS to carry out these corrections because of their familiarity with the implant. The 135° angle of the DHS, and more importantly its design, would lead to a medialization of the distal fragment with a resultant valgus load on the

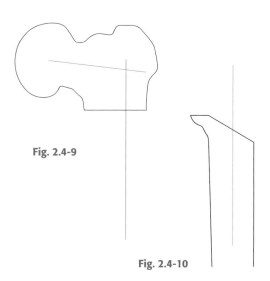

Fig. 2.4-9

Fig. 2.4-10

the lateral cortex and its apex subtends an angle of 30° with the line drawn at 90° to the long axis of the femur.

The next steps consist of tracing out the proximal and distal fragments. This will give us **Fig. 2.4-9** of the proximal fragment and **Fig. 2.4-10** of the distal fragment. Take these tracings and line them up on the tracing of the normal side. Make sure that the anatomical axes of the two distal fragments overlap. This will ensure that the anatomical axis of the distal fragment is restored to its normal distance from the weight-bearing axis, which is the imaginary line going through the center of the femoral head and the middle of the knee and ankle joints. This is important if one wishes to make certain that no abnormal varus or valgus loading of the knee takes place.

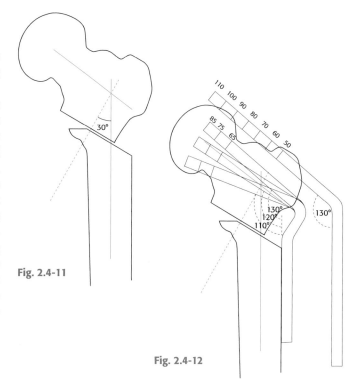

Fig. 2.4-11

Fig. 2.4-12

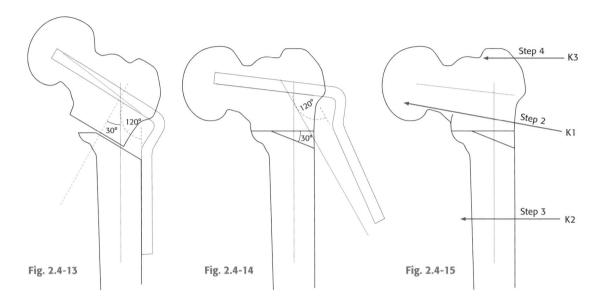

Fig. 2.4-13   Fig. 2.4-14   Fig. 2.4-15

knee. In a valgus osteotomy of the proximal femur, in order to restore the normal relationship of the distal fragments to the weight-bearing axis, it is generally necessary to lateralize the distal fragment which is impossible to achieve with the DHS. Mark in the 120° angled blade plate (**Fig. 2.4-13**).

Take the tracing with the outline of the malunion and overlap it with the tracing with the outline of the desired end result. Line up first the head and neck fragment and mark in the position of the angled blade plate in the neck and note carefully where it enters the greater trochanter in relationship to the rough line which marks the boundary between the tendons of the gluteus medius and vastus lateralis. This point of entry is called the window. Also note the distance between the window and the osteotomy (**Fig. 2.4-14**). The

distance must not be less than 1.5–2 cm or one runs the risk of fracture of the lateral cortex of the proximal fragment. This would be a very grave complication, since it would lead to loss of fixation and loosening of the blade in the proximal fragment. Mark in the osteotomy and the wedge to be resected. Measure the distance between the window and the rough line, the distance between the osteotomy and the rough line, the height of the wedge, and the distance where the wedge intersects the horizontal osteotomy line. These distances will serve for intraoperative references and guides.

One is now ready to mark in the guide wires and the operative steps (**Fig. 2.4-15**). Mark in guide wire K1. This is the guide wire which is positioned along the anterior inferior aspect of the femoral neck and serves to indicate the anteversion of the neck and the inclination of the neck axis.

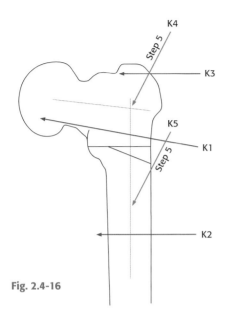

K4

Step 5

K3

K5

K1

Step 5

K2

Fig. 2.4-16

Next mark in K2. This guide wire is inserted at 90° to the anatomical axis of the distal fragment at a point sufficiently far removed from the osteotomy not to interfere with surgery. It serves as the reference K-wire for any angular corrections.

Next draw in K3. This will serve as the guide to the insertion of the seating chisel and subsequently the blade plate into the neck. The angle it subtends with its reference wire (K2) is determined by the implant one is going to use and the angular correction which is to be executed. If we were going to use a 90° angled blade plate to achieve a 30° valgus osteotomy, K3 would be inserted at 30° to K2. We are going to use, however, a 120° angled blade plate. Therefore, the angled blade plate must be inserted with its blade parallel to the reference guide wire K2 (120 – 90 = 30). This will ensure

that once the side plate is brought in line with the distal fragment, the proximal fragment will be rotated into valgus through an arc of 30°. K3 must also be inserted parallel to the axis of the femoral neck. Therefore, it must be inserted parallel to K1. Thus, K3 must be inserted in such a way that it is parallel to K2, when seen from the front and to K1 when seen from the side.

K4 and K5 are two guide wires which should be inserted parallel to one another, at 90° to the long axis of the bone in the sagittal plane, and one on each side of the osteotomy. They serve as rotational guides (**Fig. 2.4-16**). The practice of notching the cortex with an osteotome at the osteotomy or marking it with electro-cautery is a very imprecise guide to rotation because the marks are easily lost. K4 and K5 can also serve as guides to correction in the sagittal plane. This becomes important if one is going to do a flexion or an extension osteotomy. As we are going to do only a valgus osteotomy, K4 and K5 will serve only as guides to the correct rotational alignment of the fragments after the osteotomy is completed. Since they are inserted parallel to one another they must remain parallel. Any rotation about the anatomical axis would be reflected by an angle developing between these two guide wires. This fact can be used, of course, in doing a rotational correction. Under these circumstances K4 and K5 would serve as guides to the rotational correction. K6 is a K-wire inserted at an angle of 30° to K2 and distal to it.

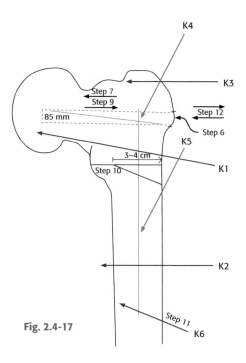

Fig. 2.4-17

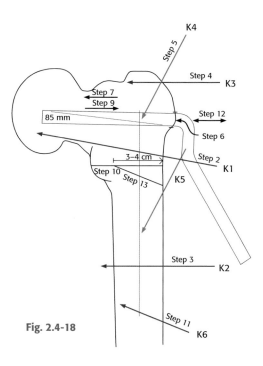

Fig. 2.4-18

Note the position of the window in the lateral cortex of the greater trochanter and the position of the seating chisel (**Fig. 2.4-17**), which assumes the same position in the neck as the blade of the angled blade plate.

One is now ready to mark in the operative steps on the plan in their sequential order (**Fig. 2.4-18**).

Step 1: Exposure

Standard anterolateral exposure. An anterior capsulotomy is done to expose the neck and to determine its axis. The vastus lateralis is reflected forwards together with the inferior capsule and the first perforating vessels are ligated and cut.

Step 2: K1

Insert this K-wire anteroinferiorly parallel to the neck axis in both planes.

Step 3: K2

Insert this K-wire at 90° to the anatomical axis of the shaft. It serves as the reference for angular corrections.

Step 4: K3

Insert this K-wire into the greater trochanter above the window and parallel to K1 and at such an inclination to K2 that the desired angular correction will be achieved when the angled blade plate is inserted and the osteotomy cut. In this case, the wires are parallel to K2 and in line with the axis of the neck.

Step 5: K4 and K5

Insert these two K-wires in the sagittal plane so that they come to lie parallel to one another, with one above and the other below the planned osteotomy. They will serve as the rotational control.

Step 6: Prepare the window

Drill three 4.5 mm holes parallel to K3 and to a depth of 3–4 cm in the area determined to be the window in the greater trochanter. Enlarge the holes with a router and join them with an osteotome. Bevel the caudal cortex to receive the shoulder of the angled blade plate.

Step 7: Insertion of seating chisel

Insert the seating chisel parallel to K3. Make sure that its guide is parallel to the long axis of the femur. Any angulation between the seating chisel guide and the long axis of the femur will result in either a flexion or an extension of the proximal fragment. One makes use of this fact if a flexion or an extension of the proximal fragment is desired.

Step 8: Intraoperative x-ray

Take an intraoperative x-ray or use an image intensifier to check the position of the seating chisel in the proximal fragment in both planes (AP and lateral). To get an intraoperative lateral view of the neck flex the hip to 90° and abduct the leg 20°. Take an AP x-ray. This will give you a perfect lateral projection of the femoral neck with the implant in situ.

Step 9: Back out the seating chisel about 1 cm

This loosens the seating chisel and makes its extraction much easier once the osteotomy is cut. If the seating chisel is not loosened before the osteotomy is cut, it becomes extremely difficicult to extract it.

Step 10: Cut osteotomy

Cut the transverse osteotomy parallel to K2 and at 90° to the long axis of the shaft.

Step 11: K6

This K-wire will serve as the guide for the cutting of the 30° wedge. It is inserted at 30° to K2 and distal to it so as not to interfere with the cutting of the wedge.

Step 12: Remove seating chisel

Remove the seating chisel and insert the 120° angled blade plate of predetermined length. It should be pushed in by hand with its handle parallel to K3. Do not hammer it in. If the seat has been properly cut with the seating chisel, the blade should slide in under pressure without the need to hammer it in. Hammering could easily change its course and result in a major malalignment.

Step 13: Cut wedge

Cut the 30° wedge. Make sure that before the wedge is cut the distal fragment is in proper rotational alignment with respect to the proximal fragment. Cut the wedge so that equal amounts are resected from the anterior and posterior portions of the lateral cortex. If the wedge is not properly centered, a rotational malalignment can result.

Step 14: Reduce osteotomy

Check the rotational alignment. Clamp the plate to the distal fragment with a Verbrügge clamp. Flex the hip to 90° and check the rotational alignment by noting the internal and external rotation of the hip.

Step 15: Compress the osteotomy

a)   This can be done with the help of a
tension device. The obliquity of the
osteotomy makes compression difficult
because the distal fragment has a
tendeny to displace medially and
proximally as compression is generated.

b)   An easy way to overcome this difficulty
is to allow the distal fragment to displace
slightly proximally and medially. One
then fixes the plate to the shaft with the
most distal screw. As the rest of the
screws are inserted, working in a distal
to proximal direction, the oblique
osteotomy is brought under compression.

Step 16: Bone graft

Cut the wedge into small pieces and bone
graft the osteotomy medially opposite the plate
(**Fig. 2.4-19**).

Step 17: Closure

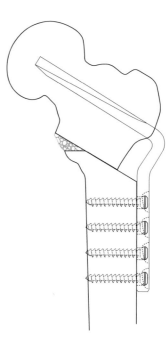

Fig. 2.4-19: Drawing of intended final result.

8   Suggestions for further reading

1. **Holdsworth BJ** (1989) Planning in fracture surgery. In: Bunker TD, editor. *Frontiers in Fracture Surgery.* London: Martin Dunitz.

2. **Mast J, Jakob R, Ganz R** (1989) *Planning and Reduction Technique in Fracture Surgery.* Berlin Heidelberg: Springer-Verlag.

3. **Müller ME, Allgöwer M, Schneider R, et al.** (1991) *Manual of Internal Fixation.* 3rd ed. Berlin Heidelberg New York: Springer-Verlag.

4. **Wade RH, Kevu J, Doyle J** (1998) Preoperative planning in orthopaedics: a study of surgeons' opinions. *Injury;* 29 (10):785–786.

9   Updates

Updates and additional references for this chapter are available online at:
http://www.aopublishing.org/PFxM/24.htm

3.1 Surgical reduction

Emanuel Gautier & Roland P. Jakob

1 Displacement of fragments, deformation (impaction) of bone

A diaphyseal fracture usually separates the bone into two main fragments—proximal and distal—with their adjacent joints. There are six ways in which these main fragments can displace in relation to each other: three pairs of displacements and three rotations along and around the x-, y-, and z-axes (**Fig. 3.1-1**).

Regardless of whether the fracture between these main fragments is simple, or multifragmentary, segmental, or showing even bone loss, **the aim of reduction in the diaphyseal bone is to reposition the epiphyses into correct relationship to each other**. This means restoring the bone length, the bone axis in both planes, and the rotation (**Fig. 3.1-2**).

The degree of fragmentation in any fracture depends exclusively upon the velocity of impact and the magnitude of forces and moments by which the bone was loaded. The degree and direction of displacement reflect the vectors of such external forces and moments, and the pull of the muscles that remained attached.

In young diaphyseal bone, plastic deformation can occur without complete discontinuity of the cortex. In the epiphyseal zones, deformation of the outer shape and inner structure can occur due to impaction of cancellous bone.

Displacement in diaphyseal and metaphyseal bone can readily be detected with conventional x-rays taken in at least two planes (anteroposterior and lateral). In the metaphysis and epiphysis, oblique views, often supplemented by conventional or computed tomography, may be needed to allow complete analysis of deformation, fragmentation, impaction, and fragment displacement.

Careful analysis of the site and extent of bone deformation as well as of the direction and degree of displacement is critical in the process of making the choice between the different treatment options. Furthermore, it is the basis for the selection of the best approach, reduction technique, and the most effective implant or fixation device.

The aim of reduction is correct alignment of adjacent joints.

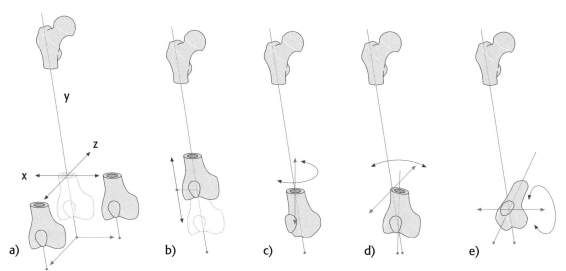

Fig. 3.1-1: Translational and rotational displacement. a/b) Displacement can occur along the three axes of the 3-D space, the x-, y-, and z-axis. Displacements along the z-axis are anterior or posterior (*dislocatio ad latus*), along the x-axis medial or lateral (*dislocatio ad latus*), and along the y-axis shortening or lengthening (*dislocatio ad longitudinem*).

c) Rotational displacement occurs around the y-axis. d/e) Angular displacement from the y-axis (in the transverse plane) is called internal or external angular malalignment (*dislocatio ad peripheriam*). From the y-axis or in the frontal plane it is called an axial malalignment in abduction or adduction (*dislocatio ad axim*) and around the x-axis or in the sagittal plane it is an axial malalignment in flexion or extension.

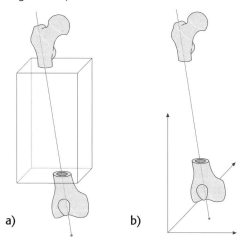

Fig. 3.1-2: Fracture zone and reduction. The fracture zone is like a box, whose content is of major importance with regard to the primary aim of reduction. After reduction, the proximal and the distal main fragments should be relocated into their correct former positions in the 3-D space.

2   Fracture reduction

Reduction is the act of restoring the correct position of the fragments, including the process of reconstruction of cancellous bone by disimpaction. Thus, it reverses the process which created the fracture displacement during the injury. Logically, it calls for forces and moments in directions opposite to those which produced the fracture. Preliminary analysis of the displacement and deformation helps to plan the tactical steps needed to achieve this goal [1]. This holds true for all methods, be they operative or non-operative, or closed or open (**Fig. 3.1-3**).

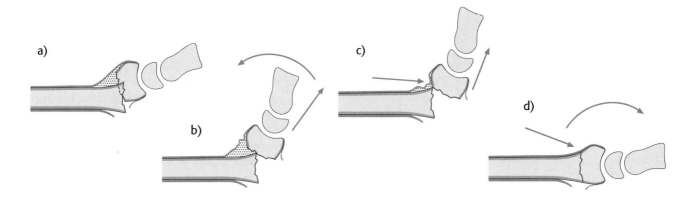

Fig.3.1-3: Closed reduction.
a) Distal radius fracture with shortening, posterior displacement and dorsal angulation. The intact periosteum on the dorsal side may act as an obstruction to reduction by traction, because the fragments are interlocked.
b) The first step to reduce this fracture consists in disengaging of the bone ends by extension of the wrist and dorsally angulated traction to relax the soft-tissue hinge.

c) Under dorsal traction the distal fragment is pushed (arrow) into its correct position, with the dorsal fragment ends reduced into contact.
d) With a flexion force and continuing push the distal fragment will realign.

2.1 Aim of reduction

In the diaphysis and metaphysis, the correct alignment of the two main fragments carrying the joint surfaces is important. The aim is to restore, as precisely as possible, the overall length of the bone, as well as the axial and rotational alignments.

In the articular segment, to avoid post-traumatic osteoarthrosis [1–3], anatomical reduction of the joint surface, with elevation of the impacted areas, is mandatory. Ideally no residual displacement should be tolerated. However, a widely accepted convention defines as acceptable any reduction in which residual displacement is less then half the thickness of the articular cartilage. Occasionally during surgery the problem may come up that a better reduction of a given joint cannot be achieved without additional risks like the need for a second surgical approach with prolongation of the operation ("le mieux est l'ennemi du bien"). Sometimes a less than perfect reduction has to be accepted for the sake of respecting biology. **Thus, there is a need for flexibility and for having a variety of surgical tactics and reduction and fixation techniques at hand.**

2.2 Reduction techniques

Reduction techniques must be gentle and atraumatic. They must preserve any remaining vascularity, since an adequate tissue response is a prerequisite for healing. Adequate blood supply to the repair tissues is crucial. Bone healing will be delayed or come to a stop if one or both of the following factors are impaired: the mechanical conditions at the fracture (strain) and the capacity for biological reaction [4–9].

Fracture reduction requires a variety of techniques and flexibility of approach.

In joints anatomical reduction is mandatory!

Reduction techniques must be gentle and atraumatic.

With indirect reduction the fracture is not exposed.

Indirect reduction is demanding and requires careful planning.

In simple shaft fractures direct reduction is acceptable.

Repeated use of reduction clamps endangers the vitality of bone fragments.

The accuracy of reduction at the joint level and the stability achieved by implants are the mechanical prerequisites for the biological response, i.e., type of healing. The healing process in turn is modulated by the additional surgical damage (exposure and implants) to the bone and surrounding soft-tissue envelope during the process of reduction and fixation.

There are two fundamentally different techniques for fracture reduction: direct or indirect.

The term direct reduction implies that the fracture area is exposed surgically or is already widely open. The fragments are grasped by surgical instruments and preferably not by hand. Reduction of the fracture fragments is achieved by applying forces and moments directed to the vicinity of the fracture zone.

In simple diaphyseal fracture patterns, direct reduction is technically straightforward and the result easy to control. With the exact local approximation of the two main fragments, length, axial, and rotational alignment of the bone itself are re-established. Biologically, in such easy fracture situations the surgical exposure should not add substantial vascular damage to the bone or soft tissues. However, this is only true if surgery is done carefully, with meticulous soft-tissue handling, and with limited, epiperiosteal exposure of the bone.

In more complex diaphyseal fractures the classical approach of direct reduction techniques may induce misguided attempts to expose and fix each individual fragment. In doing so the surgeon sequentially devascularizes every fragment. **The repeated use of bone clamps and other reduction tools or implants may completely devitalize the fragments in the comminuted area, which may have disastrous consequences for the healing process, including delayed union, non-union, infection, or implant failure.** Thus, only by understand-ing bone and soft-tissue biology and knowing the bad results after excessive devascularization, can the surgeon avoid failures after open reduction and internal fixation [10].

The term indirect reduction implies that the fracture lines are not directly exposed and seen, and that the fracture area remains covered by the surrounding soft tissues. Reduction is accomplished by using instruments or implants introduced away from the fracture zone, or through minimal incisions. Some specific implants, like the intramedullary nail, act simultaneously as a reduction tool and as a stabilization system.

In practice, correct reduction by indirect techniques is much more difficult to achieve. **It requires accurate assessment of the soft-tissue lesion, understanding of the fracture pattern, and meticulous preoperative planning.** Furthermore, the actual process of reduction is more demanding and necessitates the use of an image intensifier or intraoperative x-ray. Nevertheless, in biological terms, indirect reduction techniques offer enormous advantages because they add minimal surgical damage to tissues already traumatized by the fracture. All the instruments needed for reduction act away from the fracture zone, compromising the tissue perfusion only in an area where trauma has not already disturbed the blood supply.

Most of the available instruments or implants can be used in either technique of fracture reduction and the surgeon's success in preserving the biology of the tissues is not dependant on the specific instrument or implant used for the reduction. A presumably indirect technique which deviates into direct exposure of the fracture may not be detectable on the postoperative x-ray and may never be mentioned in the operation record; it may, however, end in disaster!

To achieve reduction, traction is normally applied in the long axis of the limb. This works only when the fragments are still connected to some soft tissues (**Video AO20163**). Traction may be applied manually, through a fracture table, or by the use of a distractor. The fracture table has the disadvantage that traction must be applied across at least one joint. The limb can not be moved by the surgeons and the surgical approach is frequently compromised. The distractor, applied directly to the main fragments, permits maneuvering of the limb during surgery. With the distractor under load, angular or rotational corrections are difficult and the construct may be cumbersome. As there is an inherent tendency for curved bone to straighten during the distraction procedure, the eccentric force produced by the unilaterally mounted distractor may produce additional deformity.

2.3 Instruments for reduction

2.3.1 Standard and pointed reduction forceps

The standard reduction forceps is typically an instrument used for direct fracture reduction. The fracture lines are exposed and the forceps are placed on each main fragment. In an oblique diaphyseal fracture, lengthening can be obtained with a rotational movement of the clamp while exerting some compression. The advantage of this technique is the ability to see that the desired reduction has been achieved. The disadvantage

Some form of traction is best for indirect reduction.

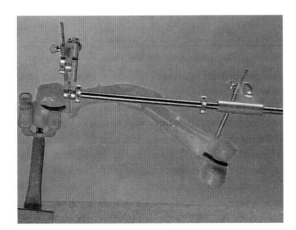

Video AO20163

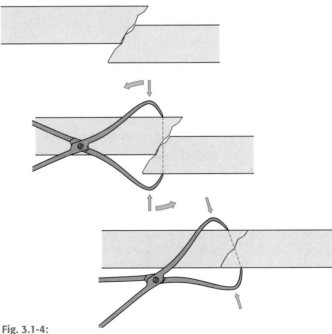

Fig. 3.1-4:
Direct reduction with standard reduction forceps. One branch of the clamp is positioned on each main fragment. With some pressure and simultaneous rotation of the handles the bone is lengthened and the fragments are reduced.

is the tendency of the forceps to slip on the bone surface, further damaging the periosteal envelope (**Fig. 3.1-4**).

The clamp is also useful when, for example, a femoral shaft fracture is plated and a residual

axial malalignment in the sagittal plane (flexion-extension) requires correction. With the plate applied and fixed to one fragment and with the fracture grossly aligned, one limb of the clamp grasps the bone (anterior or posterior) while the other limb engages on the border of the plate. By closing the clamp, such a flexion or extension malalignment is easily corrected (**Fig. 3.1-5**).

The pointed reduction forceps may be used for direct and indirect reduction as it is more gentle to the periosteal sleeve.

One application consists in grasping each of the two main fragments of a transverse fracture with reduction forceps (**Video AO20194a**). Reduction can be achieved by manual distraction, and in case of a simple fracture configuration, primary intrinsic stability ensues, allowing removal of the clamps without loss of reduction (**Fig. 3.1-6**).

> The pointed reduction forceps tends to be more gentle to the periosteum.

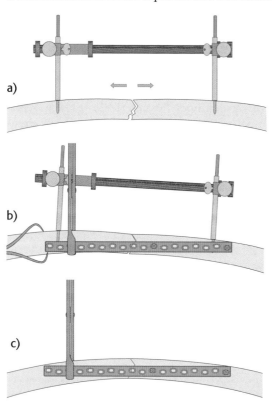

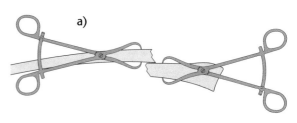

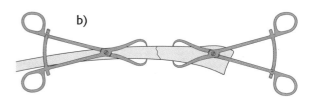

Fig. 3.1-5: Correction of axial malalignment.
a) Simple distraction of a femoral shaft fracture results in straightening of the femur, but with loss of its anterior bow.
b) To correct this deformity, the plate is first fixed to one main fragment with two screws, then a reduction forceps holds the plate in position on the other fragment. Axial alignment is achieved by means of compression with a standard reduction forceps holding the femoral shaft anteriorly and the plate posteriorly.
c) Reduction is provisionally secured by tightening the reduction forceps and correct rotational alignment is tested clinically.

Fig. 3.1-6: Direct manual reduction with the pointed reduction forceps.
a) Each main fragment is held with a pointed reduction forceps.
b) Lengthening is achieved by manual distraction while proper axial alignment can be controlled with the forceps.

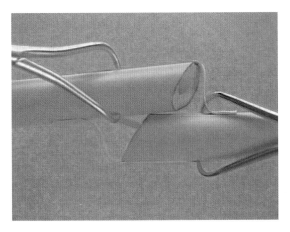

Video AO20194a

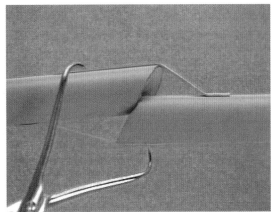

Video AO20194b

In case of an oblique fracture plane needing some lengthening, the pointed reduction forceps engages on the main fragments on each side, with a slight tilt of the forceps. By combining compression with a rotational movement of the clamp, correction of length can be obtained (**Video AO20194b**). To keep the fragments reduced, the first forceps has often to be replaced by a second one perpendicular to the fracture plane (**Fig. 3.1-7**).

For "closed" indirect reduction, for example, in the tibia, one or both points of this forceps can be inserted percutaneously through stab incisions. Depending on the size of the bone and the fragments to be reduced, a small or large pointed reduction forceps is utilized (**Fig. 3.1-8**).

In the tibia, the large pointed reduction forceps may be applied percutaneously.

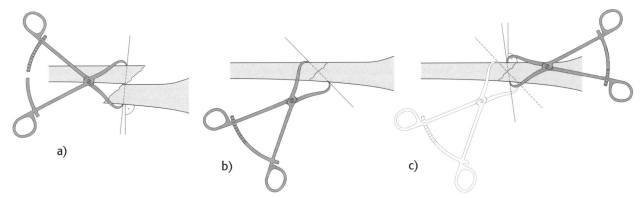

a)

b)

c)

Fig. 3.1-7: Direct reduction of an oblique diaphyseal fracture.
a) Both fragments are held with the slightly tilted pointed reduction forceps.
b) By gently rotating and compressing the forceps the bone is lengthened and the fracture reduced.
c) To secure the reduction, a second forceps in a position more or less perpendicular to the fracture plane is applied.

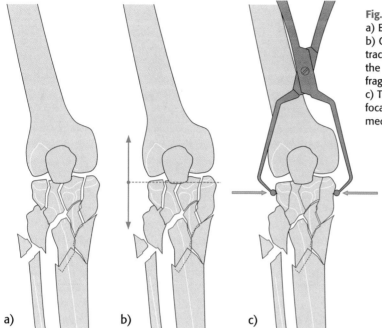

a)   b)   c)

Fig. 3.1-8: Indirect reduction with a pointed reduction forceps.
a) Example of a comminuted fracture of the tibial plateau.
b) Gross restoration of axial alignment and length can be achieved with traction by means of the femoral distractor or an external fixator across the knee joint. Ligamentotaxis leads to some reduction of the articular fragments.
c) The position of the articular fragments can be improved by a point-focal reduction with a large pointed reduction forceps grasping the medial and lateral fragments through small stab incision.

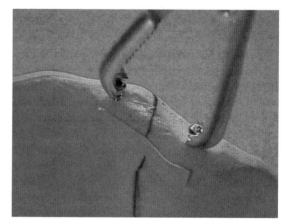

 Video AO20194c

2.3.2 Special reduction clamps

The Farabeuf clamp is designed to grasp screw heads introduced on either side of a fracture line (3.5 or 4.5 mm screws) (Fig. 3.1-9). Manipulation of the clamp allows one to apply compression and also permits limited lateral displacement in two different planes (Video AO20194c). However, distraction of the fracture gap is not possible. Nevertheless, this can be done with the pelvic reduction forceps (Jungbluth clamp), which is actually fixed on both fragments with a 4.5 mm cortex screw, allowing the fragments to be moved and reduced in three planes (distraction and compression, as well as lateral displacement in two planes) (Fig. 3.1-10) (Video AO20194d).

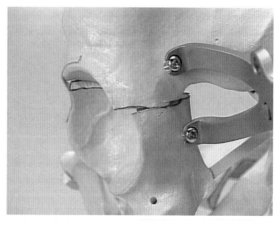

 Video AO20194d

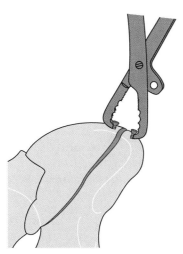

Fig. 3.1-9:
The Farabeuf clamp is mainly used for fracture reduction in the area of the iliac crest. It is anchored on both sides of the fracture with either 3.5 or 4.5 mm cortex screws. Distraction of the fracture is not possible using this technique. The clamp helps only to reduce side-to-side displacement and to close a fracture gap.

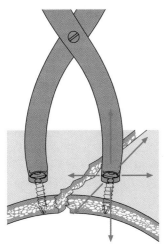

Fig. 3.1-10:
The pelvic reduction forceps (Jungbluth clamp) is fixed to the fragments with 4.5 mm cortex screws. This firm connection allows translational and reduction movements in all three planes.

2.3.3 Other instruments useful for reduction

In cortical bone, the small-tipped Hohmann retractor can be used as a lever or pusher to achieve reduction. The tip of the retractor is placed between the two cortices of a diaphyseal fracture. It is then turned through 180° to engage the cortex of the opposite fragment. With a bending force applied by the Hohmann retractor, the two cortices can be both opposed and realigned, allowing gentle reduction of the fracture. Another turn of the retractor is commonly needed to remove it [1] (**Fig. 3.1-11**) (**Video AO20194e**).

A further application of the Hohmann retractor is to reduce a translational displacement in the cancellous bone of an iliac wing fracture. First the tip of the Hohmann is lightly hammered into the bone. Then it is turned and, with some hammer blows, reduction can be achieved with

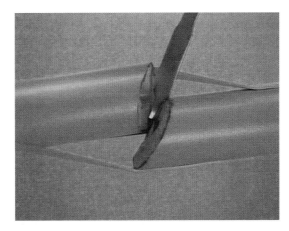

Video AO20194e

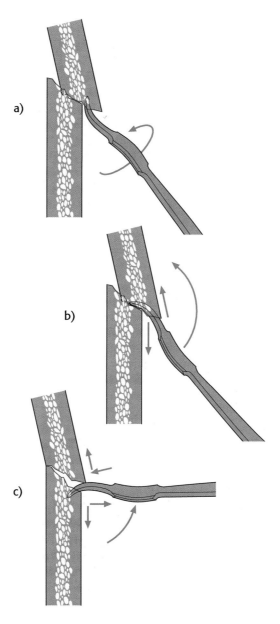

Fig. 3.1-11: In cortical bone the tip of the Hohmann retractor is placed between the two fragments. By turning and bending the retractor handle the fragments can be disengaged and reduced. Another turn is usually required to remove the Hohmann retractor.

a bending force (**Fig. 3.1-12**) (**Video AO20194f**). This maneuver usually produces a small zone of impaction on the thin cortex of the fragment pushed down.

Fracture reduction in one direction can be carried out by instruments designed to push or pull. Using the ball spike, fragments can be pushed firmly into the right position (**Video AO20194g**). The bone impactor, used from within, serves to disimpact compressed fragments of an articular

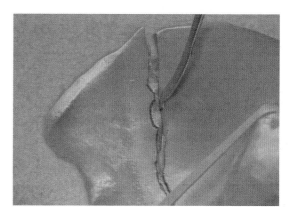

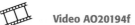
Video AO20194f

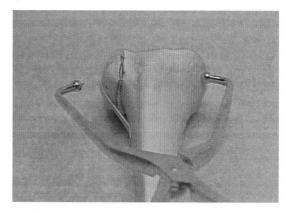
Video AO20194g

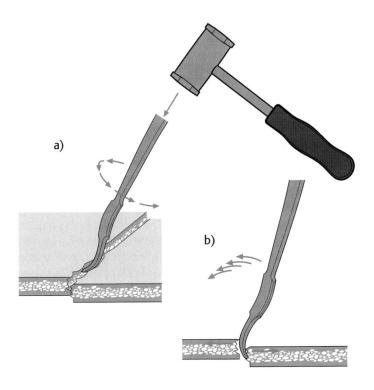

a)

b)

c)

Fig. 3.1-12: Hohmann retractor for reduction in cancellous bone. By placing the slightly curved tip of a Hohmann retractor between two overlapping fragments and then turning and tilting the retractor the fracture may be reduced and brought to interdigitate. A precondition is a solid layer of bone.

surface. The sharp hook (dental) or the regular bone hook can, with gentle traction, facilitate reduction of a fragment.

2.4 Implants used for reduction

Ideally an implant should contribute to the reduction as well as the stabilization of a fracture. Reduction may be obtained with an implant through interference with the bone. A simple example of this is the reduction achieved by an anatomically shaped intramedullary nail. As the nail crosses the fracture from one fragment to the other, reduction in the coronal and sagittal planes must occur.

In multifragment shaft fractures some lengthening can be obtained after distal interlocking by hammering the nail further distally. However, precise planning is needed with measure-

ment of the correct nail length on an x-ray of the entire opposite bone [1].

Fractures of any relatively straight portion of the diaphysis may be reduced by a plate which acts as a splint to restore alignment prior to fixation (**Video AO20194h**). By distracting the

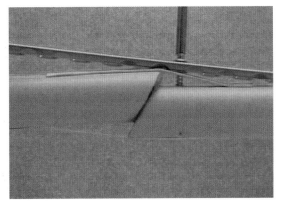

The ideal implant will both reduce and stabilize the fracture.

Video AO20194h

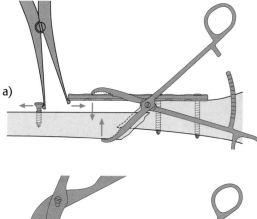

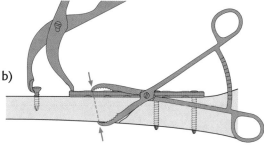

Fig. 3.1-13: Push-pull technique.
a) The laminar spreader, placed between the end of a plate and an independent screw, can be used to distract the fracture.
b) Using the same screw, interfragmentary compression is achieved with the small reduction forceps.

fracture the tension in the soft tissues is increased, which tends to realign the fragments to their original position. The push-pull technique with a laminar spreader and the reduction forceps is an elegant and regularly used way to distract and reduce a fracture, for example, of the forearm [1] (**Fig. 3.1-13**) (**Video AO20194i**).

Another simple and gentle reduction mechanism uses the plate in an antiglide function [11]. Applying a properly contoured plate to one fragment of an oblique metaphyseal fracture results in displacing the opposite fragment and automatically reducing it. This technique corrects small displacements and angulation while maintaining stability as the reduction occurs (**Fig. 3.1-14**) (**Video AO20194j**).

An angled blade plate, when correctly inserted in the epi-metaphyseal segment of the bone, will, by its shape, bring the diaphyseal segment into anatomical alignment. The blade of the plate is first inserted into the proximal or distal end-fragment. Then the shaft is reduced to the side-plate using the reduction forceps to hold the two together. Fine tuning of the reduction

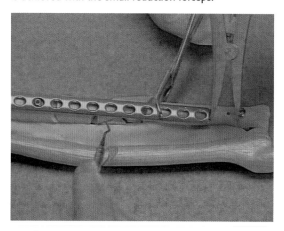

 Video AO20194i

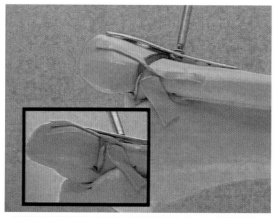

 Video AO20194j

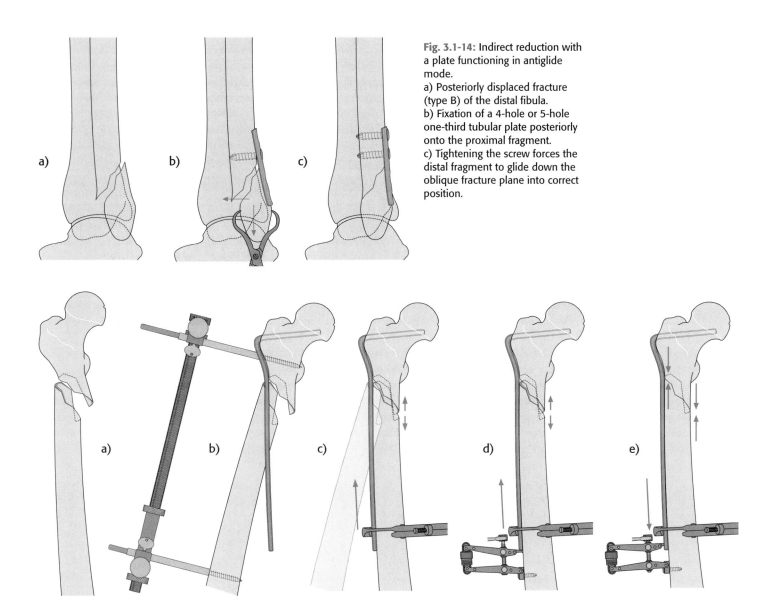

Fig. 3.1-14: Indirect reduction with a plate functioning in antiglide mode.
a) Posteriorly displaced fracture (type B) of the distal fibula.
b) Fixation of a 4-hole or 5-hole one-third tubular plate posteriorly onto the proximal fragment.
c) Tightening the screw forces the distal fragment to glide down the oblique fracture plane into correct position.

Fig. 3.1-15: Reduction with the aid of the condylar plate.
a) Displacement of the fracture with the proximal fragment in adduction and flexion.
b) Introduction of the condylar plate 95° and distraction of the fracture with the large distractor.
c) Provisional fixation with a reduction forceps distally.
d) Use of the tension device to distract the fracture and to allow complete reduction proximally.
e) Use of the tension device for interfragmentary compression.

is achieved by the push-pull technique using the articulated tension device [1, 2] (Fig. 3.1-15) (Video AO20194k). The same principles have recently been described for submuscular plate insertion, which is, however, technically much more demanding. After preparation of the blade seating canal, the plate is first inserted into the submuscular tunnel along the femoral shaft

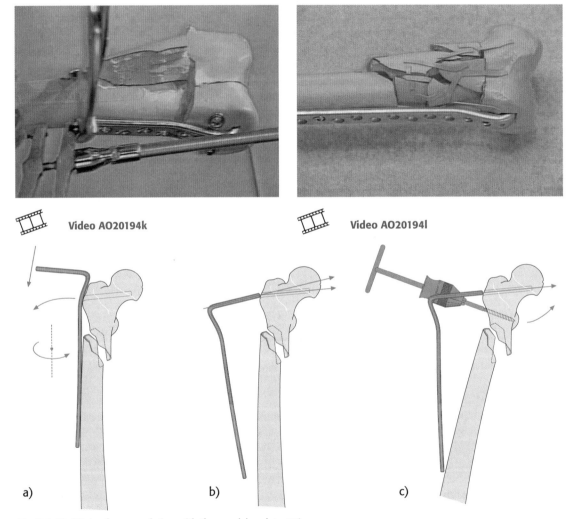

Video AO20194k

Video AO20194l

a)

b)

c)

Fig. 3.1-16: Minimal access plating with the condylar plate 95°.
a) Submuscular introduction of the long side plate (blade facing laterally) through a short proximal incision after preparation of the blade canal with the seating chisel.
b) After turning the condylar plate, the direction of the blade and the blade canal do not meet.
c) The proximal fragment must be brought into proper alignment to the blade using a Schanz screw as joystick.

with its blade pointing laterally. The plate is then turned through 180°, resulting in the blade now facing the bone. To insert the blade the metaphyseal fragment must now be manipulated with the aid of a joystick to align the blade canal to the blade (**Fig. 3.1-16**) (**Video AO20194l**). Length and axis are re-established with longitudinal traction (femoral distractor or push-pull technique).

2.4.1 Joystick reduction

The insertion of threaded K-wires or Schanz screws allows manipulation of bone fragments with or without a direct view. The technique is mainly used in articular fractures (distal radius, proximal humerus, acetabulum) [**3, 12**] (**Video AO20194m**).

2.4.2 Temporary cerclage

A temporary cerclage can be helpful in reducing a multifragmentary (mainly butterfly fragment) fracture in the diaphysis. The technique has the disadvantage of temporary circumferential denuding of the bone during the application of the wire [**2**], which is why only one wire should be used (**Video AO20194n**).

2.4.3 Kapandji reduction

With a K-wire introduced through the fracture line, the distal fragment of a distal radial fracture can be distracted and rotated similarly to the Hohmann technique. Definitive stabilization is achieved by inserting the K-wire into the opposite cortex of the radius.

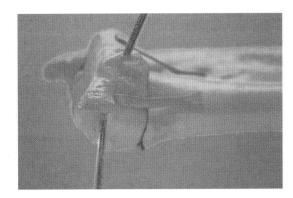

 Video AO20194m

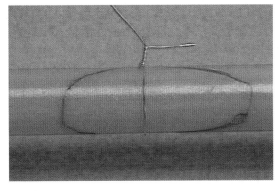

 Video AO20194n

2.4.4 External fixator

The external fixator can be used for indirect reduction, but gentle lengthening is more difficult than with the distractor. By applying traction across a joint, ligaments and soft tissues around the fracture area can assist in achieving reduction (ligamentotaxis, soft-tissue taxis) [**2**].

Intraoperative controlling of
reduction and fixation is
mandatory.

2.5 Assessment of reduction

Once reduction of a fracture is performed by either direct or indirect techniques, it must be checked. There are various ways to do so, including direct vision, palpation (digital or instrumental), clinical observation, x-ray or image intensifier, indirect vision using an arthroscope or an endoscope, or a computer-guided or computer-assisted system. Some of these techniques are more reliable than others; much, however, depends on their availability.

The small indentations or landmarks present in every fracture line must be observed if the fracture focus is visible (puzzle technique). When a fracture surface cannot be directly seen, but can be reached with a gentle fingertip, palpation may be helpful, for example, of the quadrilateral surface in the pelvis to control reduction of an acetabular fracture. This can also be performed with an appropriate instrument to evaluate the accuracy of reduction of an articular surface, for example, in a tibia plateau fracture.

Clinical judgement of reduction and rotational alignment may be difficult and unreliable. It is, however, frequently needed especially in closed intramedually nailing. Several methods are described in **chapter 3.3.1**.

When they are available, intraoperative assessment of the fracture reduction and fixation must be done by fluoroscopy or x-rays in two planes. In articular fractures the use of arthroscopy has been described to assist or check reduction (e.g., tibia plateau). However, this technique needs considerable experience and rigid asepsis.

2.5.1 Computer-assisted reduction control

Newest developments include the use of computer-guided systems for the placement of instruments and implants or localization of bone fragments in the 3-D space. Such systems are based on direct intraoperative imaging with an image intensifier or on a preoperative CT scan. Anatomical landmarks on the proximal and distal side of a fracture area can serve for the calculation of residual displacement (translational or rotational) using specific mathematical algorithms. In the future, at least semi-automated reduction of long bone fractures can be envisaged [13].

3 Bibliography

1. **Mast J, Jakob R, Ganz R** (1989) *Planning and Reduction Technique in Fracture Surgery.* 1st ed. Berlin Heidelberg New York: Springer-Verlag.

2. **Müller ME, Allgöwer M, Schneider R, et al.** (1990) *Manual of Internal Fixation.* 3rd ed. Berlin Heidelberg New York: Springer-Verlag.

3. **Schatzker J, Tile M** (1987) *The Rationale of Operative Fracture Care.* 1st ed. Berlin Heidelberg New York: Springer-Verlag.

4. **Brookes M** (1971) *The Blood Supply of Bone. An Approach to Bone Biology.* London: Butterworth.

5. **Kelly PJ** (1968) Anatomy, physiology, and pathology of the blood supply of bones. *J Bone Joint Surg [Am]*; 50 (4):766–783.

6. **Rhinelander FW** (1974) Tibial blood supply in relation to fracture healing. *Clin Orthop*; 105 (0):34–81.

7. **Trias A, Fery A** (1979) Cortical circulation of long bones. *J Bone Joint Surg [Am]*; 61 (7):1052–1059.

8. **Trueta J** (1974) Blood supply and the rate of healing of tibial fractures. *Clin Orthop*; 105 (0):11–26.

9. **Whiteside LA, Ogata K, Lesker P, et al.** (1978) The acute effects of periosteal stripping and medullary reaming on regional bone blood flow. *Clin Orthop*; (131):266–272.

10. **Gautier E, Perren SM, Ganz R** (1992) Principles of internal fixation. *Curr Orthop*; 6:220–232.

11. **Weber BG** (1981) *Special Techniques in Internal Fixation.* Berlin Heidelberg New York: Springer-Verlag.

12. **Heim U, Pfeiffer KM** (1988) *Internal Fixation of Small Fractures.* 3rd ed. Berlin Heidelberg New York: Springer-Verlag.

13. **Nolte L, Visarius H** (1998) Personal communication. *Maurice E. Müller Institute for Biomechanics.*

4 Updates

Updates and additional references for this chapter are available online at:
http://www.aopublishing.org/PFxM/31.htm

3.2.1 Lag screw

*Stephan M. Perren, Robert Frigg,
Markus Hehli, Slobodan Tepic*

1 General aspects

A screw is a very efficient tool for fixation of a fracture by interfragmentary compression or for fixing a splinting device such as a plate, nail, or fixator to bone. To exploit its possibilities to the full, it is recommended that the special characteristics of the screw are carefully studied and kept in mind during application. Biological advantages must be weighed against mechanical ones. First, we shall focus on the mechanical properties in general [1]. The biological aspects, which are even more important, are dealt with in the individual applications.

The axial force produced by a screw results from rotating the screw clockwise so that the inclined surfaces of its threads glide along a corresponding surface of the bone. The inclination of the thread must be small enough to provide "self-locking" of the screw, i.e., to prevent the screw from turning and becoming loose (**Fig. 3.2.1-1**). On the other hand, it must be large enough to allow full insertion with an acceptably low number of revolutions, something which also provides more familiar feedback to the surgeon's hand [2].

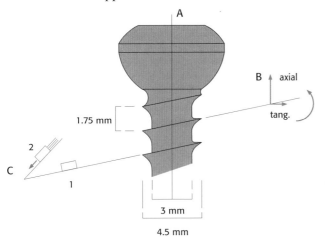

Fig. 3.2.1-1: Schematic drawing of a standard cortical bone screw, as used in diaphyseal bone.
(A) The undersurface of the screw head is spherical, allowing a congruent fit to be maintained while tilting the screw, e.g., within a plate hole. The thread is asymmetrical. The dimensions shown are designed to offer a good relation between axial force and torque applied (B) and these dimensions result in an inclination of the thread which is self-locking (C). The screw corresponds to the ISO standard 5835.

Two force components are active, namely one along the circumference of the thread, and one along the axis of the screw. The first results from the torque of tightening, the second produces axial tension. Of the torque applied during tightening, only about 40% is used for transformation into axial force; 50% is used to overcome friction at the screw head interface, and about 10% to overcome friction of the thread. This explains why, for instance, during bench test-ing, a plate screw can be tightened to nearly twice the torque that an isolated screw will tolerate. The relation between torque applied and axial force induced is about 6.7 kg/kg·cm for a standard 4.5 mm cortex screw [3].

The compression applied by a screw affects a comparatively small area of the bone by which it is surrounded. Therefore, **a single screw compressing an oblique fracture does not very effectively counteract rotation of the bone fragments around the axis of that screw.** The leverage of the compression induced around the screw is small. Similarly, a single screw applied to a flat surface is not very resistant to torque between two osteotomy fragments. Such situations require a second screw well apart from the first one. The leverage then corresponds to the distance between the screws plus twice the leverage of the single screw (**Fig. 3.2.1-2**).

A single interfragmentary lag screw does not prevent rotation between two fragments.

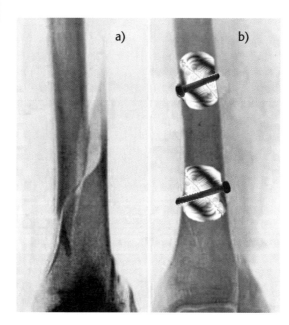

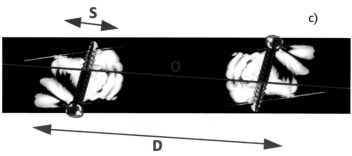

Fig. 3.2.1-2:
Different effects of using one or two lag screws for stabilization against torque in pure lag screw fixation.
a) Model of a spiral fracture in a diaphysis.
b) Fixation of the fracture using two lag screws. From a photoelastic experiment the extent of interfragmentary compression around a lag screw is demonstrated. The photoelastic pictures are superposed on the x-ray to give a rough idea of the distribution of compression.
c) In this figure the area of compression around a lag screw, as obtained from a photo-elastic experiment, has been inserted into a schmatic drawing of a long oblique osteotomy to explain the different effect of one lag screw alone compared to the effect of two well spaced lag screws.
  S Lever arm of a single lag screw.
  D Lever arm of double lag screws.
  O Osteotomy. Instead of a spiral fracture a shallow oblique osteotomy is shown. The same principles apply for both types of fractures.
This schematic diagram shows that whenever lag screws alone are used, there should be at least two well spaced screws.

1.1 Types of bone screws

There are two basic types of bone screws within the AO system: the cortex and the cancellous bone screws. The cancellous bone screws have a larger outer diameter, a deeper thread, and a larger pitch than the cortex screws and have their applications in metaphyseal or epiphyseal bone. The cortex screws are designed for the diaphysis.

Other screws

In recent developments of Schanz screws, the threads are shallower (i.e., the thread less deep) in order to provide less sharp edges and have a larger core diameter. This provides better buttressing against forces acting perpendicular to the long axis of the screw [4]. When applied in a technically correct way, self-cutting threads provide a good purchase.

Newly designed screws for diaphyseal application of internal fixators (PC-Fix and LISS) may be self-drilling, self-cutting, and unicortical and the screw head locks in the plate hole. They are "locked screws", as their inclination in relation to the "plate" body is fixed. Locked screws seem to provide better anchorage [5]. They can also function as a fixed angle device, which is an advantage in metaphyseal fractures and if a minimally invasive technique is used [6, 7] (see **chapters 3.3.2** and **3.4**).

1.2 Shaft screws

The functioning of a lag screw can be best understood by looking at a screw which has a short thread and a shaft, the diameter of which may be either that of the core or of the thread. The smooth shaft usually has a diameter corresponding to the inner core of the thread. When applied to a tubular (diaphyseal) bone, the thread anchors within the far *(trans)* cortex and in the near *(cis)* cortex the head provides a buttress against axial tension (**Fig. 3.2.1-3**), whereas the shaft does not produce any axial force.

1.3 Mode of application of a fully threaded lag screw

A fully threaded screw can be used as a lag screw, provided the thread is kept from engaging within the cortex close to the screw head *(cis* cortex). This is done by drilling, within the *cis* cortex, a clearance or gliding hole of a diameter slightly larger than the outer diameter

There are two basic types of screws: cortex screws and cancellous bone screws.

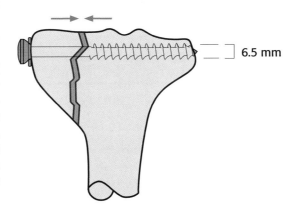

6.5 mm

Fig. 3.2.1-3: Compression of an epi-metaphyseal fracture using a shaft screw.
The thread pulls the opposite bone fragment towards the head of the screw. The shaft of the screw does not transmit any great axial force between the shaft and the surrounding bone. The length of the screw shaft must be chosen so that the threaded part of the screw lies fully within the opposite bone fragment. To prevent the screw head from sinking into the thin cortex, a washer is used.

To act as a lag screw the cortex screw requires a gliding hole in the near *(cis)* and a threaded hole in the far *(trans)* cortex.

of the screw thread. **Thus, the cortex lag screw is applied with a smaller pilot or threaded hole in the *trans* cortex and a larger clearance or gliding hole within the *cis* cortex (Fig. 3.2.1-4a) (Video AO00099a).** When an inclined screw thread produces axial

force, one component of the force tends to shift the screw head along the bone surface towards the fracture. Under such conditions the use of a lag screw with a shaft corresponding to the outer diameter of the thread (so-called shaft screws) may be advisable (**Fig. 3.2.1-4b**). Otherwise, the screw thread may engage within the gliding hole and some efficiency may be lost [8]. In diaphyseal bone, shaft screws or fully threaded screws are used because partially threaded cancellous bone screws are difficult to remove after healing (reverse cutting of the thread!).

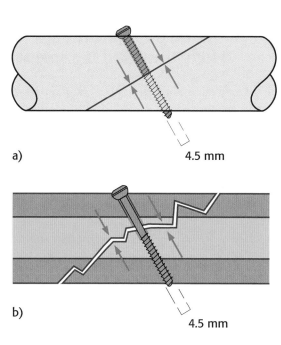

a)   4.5 mm

b)   4.5 mm

Fig. 3.2.1-4: Lag screw effect using a fully threaded screw.
a) By overdrilling the bone thread in the near fragment to the size of the outer diameter of the screw thread, the threaded part of the bone screw is enabled to glide in relation to the bone. When this technique is used for an inclined screw whose head rests on a surface parallel to the long axis of the bone (e.g., in DCP or LC-DCP), then one component of the axial screw force acts along the long axis of the bone. It tends to shift the screw head towards the fracture. The screw thread within the gliding hole may then engage and compression is lost to a varying degree.
b) This has led to the development of a cortex screw with a shaft corresponding to the outer diameter of the thread—the shaft screw.

1.4 Screw-tightening and torque-limiting screwdrivers

When an experienced surgeon tightens the screws to the degree which he considers as optimal and compatible with screw and/or bone strength, he achieves, on average, 86% of the thread-stripping torque [2]. In view of the fact that the screws produce very high amounts

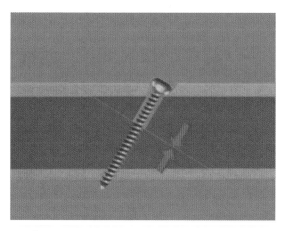

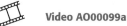 **Video AO00099a**

of axial force, it does not make sense to tighten the screws to the uppermost limit. Furthermore, when the holding force of a screw is fully utilized by static preload, there is limited holding force left to counter additional functional load. **The new self-locking screws of the PC-Fix and the LISS [5] lock upon tightening in the plate hole, and thus protect the screw and the bone.** For these new techniques a torque-limiting screwdriver will help to prevent the screw heads from jamming in the conical holes, whether threaded or not. In other applications where the bone density and thickness change from one area to another, torque-limiting screwdrivers are of little help.

Self-locking screws (LISS and PC-Fix) protect bone and screw from stripping.

1.5 Amount and maintenance of compression

Tests with expert surgeons [2] have shown that 4.5 mm screws are routinely tightened to a torque resulting in roughly 2,000–3,000 N of axial compression. *In vivo* measurements of compression applied to living bone demonstrated that the initially applied compression slowly decreases over months [9] which means that, in general, compression outlasts the time required for the fracture to heal.

In vivo, **loosening of well-placed screws is induced by micromotion at the interface between thread and bone** (Fig. 3.2.1-5) [10]. Such loosening, due to bone resorption, is seen with small rather than high axial forces. In most cases loosening is not a problem resulting from mechanical overload or hypothetical pressure necrosis, but rather from poor technique. When, however, excessive forces result in destruction of the threads in bone, the overall stability will also be irreversibly lost. Under stable conditions of rigid fixation, bone resorption at the interface will not be observed.

Loosening of screws is induced by micromotion.

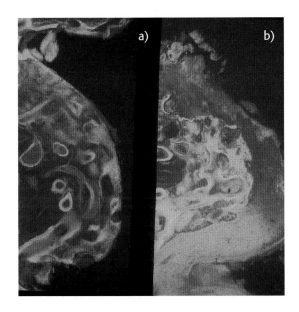

Fig. 3.2.1-5: Biological loosening of a bone screw.
a) Shows the biological reaction to a screw which does not move perpendicularly to the long axis of the screw. There is close contact between bone and adjacent screw. Bone remodeling proves that the absence of screw loosening is not due to a possible lack of biological reaction.
b) Shows the appearance of the "thread" where the screw had been undergoing movements within a range of micrometers. Bone has been resorbed, and instead, we now find fibrous tissue that no longer provides holding power.

1.6 Modes of failure

Screws can fail because of axial pull out, bending forces, or both. While screws usually resist axial pull out rather well, most conventional screws are fairly weak in bending due to their small core diameter. Based on the understanding that the core diameter of a screw may be increased without unduly forfeiting the pull out force, the resistance to bending may be increased threefold by only a 30% increase of the core size from, for example, 3.0–4.0 mm in diameter.

1.7 Special considerations of screw insertion

The following rather simplistic statements merit some attention in respect to practical use of screws. In the earlier days we considered the optimal torque and the maximum possible torque to be synonymous, i.e., as close to failure as possible. Based on our more recent knowledge, we can no longer hold this view. **Generally, a screw should not be tightened to the limits of strength or ductility, but to about 2/3 of these limits, to allow resistance to any additional functional loading.** Here, again, the principle of safe application should guide the hand of the surgeon who should strive for "best" axial compression, although, for reasons already given, this is not the same as the highest axial force.

In conventional plating, the inclination of the screws in relation to the long axis of the plate can be selected to provide optimal lag screw effect (**Video AO00099b**), or to bypass either an area of comminution or a fracture line in the cortex remote from the plate. The purchase of the screw in the remote cortex then locks the inclination of the screw. When unicortical screws are considered, the required angular stability must be provided by the special design of the screw head-to-plate locking process. A tightly fitting "Morse cone" or a conical thread provides this locking. We use the

> A screw should not be tightened to the limits of its strength, but to only about 2/3 of this, to allow additional functional loading.

general term of "locked screw" for this type of construction. Locked screws are easier to apply and less traumatizing, but their application is limited to procedures with less emphasis on lag screw compression. Furthermore, locked screws are increasingly being used to replace the DCS or the angled blade plate in minimally invasive techniques.

2　Clinical applications of lag screw

2.1 Positioning of the screw in respect to the fracture plane

Lag screws produce their best efficiency when the screw is perpendicularly oriented in relation to the fracture surface. As the fracture plane of, for example, a spiral fracture is subject not only

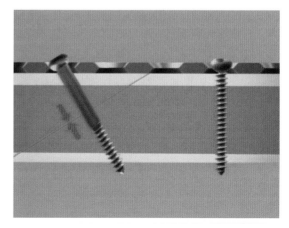

 Video AO00099b

to the compression by the screw but also to compression along the long axis of the bone, the ideal inclination is somewhat more perpendicular to the long axis of the bone (**Fig. 3.2.1-6**). This may cause the fracture to slide and so, to be on the safe side, the perpendicular position in relation to the fracture plane is in most cases simple to achieve and provides nearly optimal function of the lag screw. This inclination is, therefore, recommended. When several lag screws are used in a long spiral fracture in order to improve stability, the positioning of the screws must follow the spiral plane of the fracture. Such a procedure will cause considerable stripping of soft tissues and periosteum from the bone, which results in measurable damage to the periosteal circulation. Therefore, biology must be considered when applying lag screws. The clinical application of lag screws should go in line with our efforts to achieve indirect reduction of the fracture and minimal denudation of bone.

2.2 Lag screws in metaphyseal and epiphyseal regions

Articular and juxta-articular fractures usually need anatomical reduction and absolute stability in order to obtain perfect congruity of the joint. In this region, lag screw fixation is the predominant procedure. Large (6.5 mm) and small (4.0 mm) cancellous bone screws, as well as cannulated screws are used. To prevent the screw head from sinking into the bone, a washer is often needed (see **Fig. 3.2.1-3**) (**Video AO00097a**). For postoperative functional treatment in the ma-

To obtain anatomical reduction and absolute stability, interfragmentary lag screws are mandatory in articular fractures.

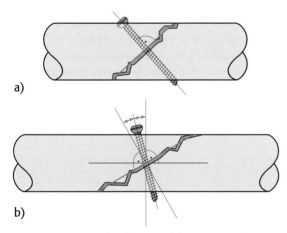

Fig. 3.2.1-6: Optimal inclination of the screw in relation to a simple fracture plane.
a) Shows a lag screw oriented perpendicular to the fracture plane. This is an ideal inclination in the absence of forces along the bone axis.
b) Shows an inclination half way between the perpendiculars to the fracture plane and to the long axis of the bone. This is an inclination which is better suited to resisting compressive functional load along the bone long axis.

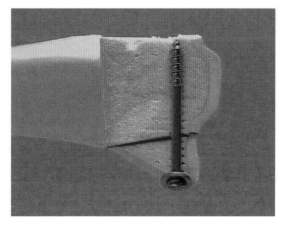

 Video AO00097a

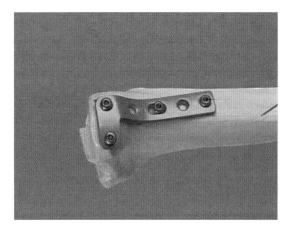

Video AO00097b

jority of these fractures, the combination of lag screw technique and buttressing by a plate is the method of choice (**Video AO00097b**).

2.3 Self-tapping screws

Self-tapping screws may be used for applications where the screw is applied only once. Self-tapping screws of modern design of [11] offer not only the advantage of simpler handling but also provide an optimal fit between the cut and the thread. This is normally the case for most plate screws, but lag screws are re-inserted, sometimes repeatedly, when reduction is optimized. In this situation a self-tapping screw might tend, in theory, to cut a new thread at each insertion, thereby reducing or losing its purchase in bone. **For clinical application it seems advisable, therefore, to revert to a conventional lag screw with tapping of the thread.** Another limitation regarding the use of self-tapping screws stems from the fact

Self-tapping screws are not recommended for use as lag screws.

that the cutting flutes of self-tapping screws are usually short. They may become clogged during insertion into a thick and dense cortical bone and this may damage the osseous thread. Here also the solution is to use a conventional pre-tapped application. Furthermore, a self-tapping screw may fail upon removal, when the cutting flutes are filled with ingrown new bone, or if the friction between screw and bone surfaces is very high. To avoid problems, the surgeon may try to loosen the screw, prior to removal, by first tightening it, thereby shearing off the ingrown bone from the cutting flutes. The design of the flutes of self-cutting screws must respond to these special demands.

3 Are screws forgiving?

Today, we tend to design implants in a way that offers high security for a wide variety of general applications. This requires an implant that tolerates intermittent peak (over-)load without irreversible loss of contact. While today's plates, nails, and external or internal fixators give way and spring back into their former shape, screw fixation is less tolerant in situations of peak load. Under overload, the bony thread strips and the screw permanently loses its holding power. This behavior must be considered in pure lag screw fixation and in combinations between screws and flexible devices such as nails and fixators. The lag screw, therefore, finds its application mainly in conventional fixation with interfragmentary compression and may have limited application for, and in certain situations even be incompatible with, biological internal fixation.

4 New trends in screw application: internal fixator with locked screws

The new technology of using the so-called internal fixators—PC-Fix and LISS—for biological internal fixation takes advantage of short, unicortical screws (see **chapter 3.4**). The unicortical screw offers the advantage of very simple handling as it allows safe application by self-drilling and self-tapping. The head of this screw is locked within the body of the fixator (plate) (**Fig. 3.2.1-7**) in a position perpendicular to the long axis of the fixator (**Fig. 3.2.1-8a/b**). The steep conical design of the interface, and/or

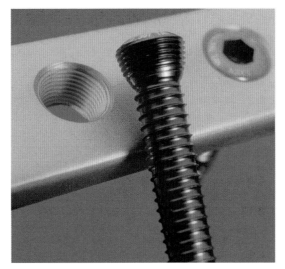

Fig. 3.2.1-7: The threaded screw head locks within the body of the fixator (plate).

Fig. 3.2.1-8:
Conventional and locked screws.
a) Shows the design and force components of a conventional screw as used for the DCP and LC-DCP. The screw acts by producing friction between the plate undersurface and the bone surface due to compression of the interface.

b) Locked screws as used in newer implants like the PC-Fix and the LISS. These are usually unicortical and work more like bolts than screws; the axial force produced by the screw is minimal. The screw provides fixation based on the fact that the screw head is locked in a position perpendicular to the "plate" body. Such systems act more like fixators than plates.

a)

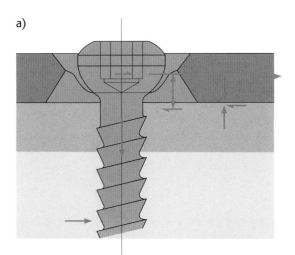

b)

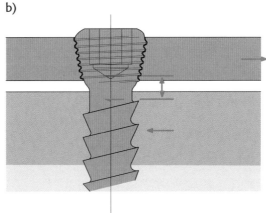

the newer conical thread, stop tightening well before the thread within bone sustains critical loads (**Video AO90063**). Clinical studies using the PC-Fix have shown that short unicortical screws do not require variable inclination and can be used safely in diaphyseal bone without stripping the bone thread [12, 13]. An essential advantage of locking the screws within the fixator is that of limiting the torque applied to the screw thread at insertion. Thus, the screw is not plastically deformed within its thread, allowing the safe use of implant materials of low ductility, such as titanium. While Banovetz et al. [14] reported an unusually high incidence of titanium screw failures in conventional applications, Haas [13] did not observe one single failure of titanium screws in a series of 387 PC-Fix insertions with an average of five to six screws per implant and a 96% follow-up rate. Unicortical screws should be used in diaphyseal, but preferably not in metaphyseal bone. In the metaphysis, the lack of a bony thick cortex, and a very short grip of the screw

in the bone, due to a generally imperfect fit between the undersurface of the "plate" body and the bone, result in too small an anchorage for this application. Locked screws may also be used as long screws, thereby eliminating the need for fixed angle blade plates in the metaphyseal area.

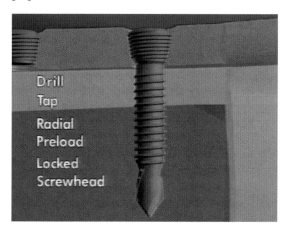

 Video AO90063

5 Bibliography

1. **Perren SM, Cordey J, Baumgart F, et al.** (1992) Technical and biomechanical aspects of screws used for bone surgery. *International Journal of Orthopaedic Trauma;* 2:31–48.

2. **Cordey J, Rahn BA, Perren SM** (1980) *Human Torque Control in the use of Bone Screws.* In: Uhthoff HK, editor. Current Concepts of Internal Fixation of Fractures. Berlin Heidelberg New York: Springer-Verlag: 235–243.

3. **Von Arx C** (1975) *Die Schubübertragung durch Reibung bei Plattenosteosynthese.* Diss. Basel: In AO Bulletin; 1–34, 1975.

4. **Schavan R** (1994) *Mechanische Testung von Schanzschen Schrauben.* Fachhochschule Aachen. (Thesis).

5. **Tepic S, Perren S** (1995) The biomechanics of the PC-Fix internal fixator. *Injury;* 26 (Suppl 2):5–10.

6. **Krettek C, Schandelmaier P, Miclau T, et al.** (1997) Minimally invasive percutaneous plate osteosynthesis (MIPPO) using the DCS in proximal and distal femur fractures. *Injury;* 28 (Suppl 1):20–31.

7. **Krettek CGE** (1998) Minimally invasive plate osteosynthesis (MIPO). *Injury;* 29 (Suppl 3).

8. **Klaue K** (1982) *The Dynamic Compression Unit (DCU) for stable internal fixation of bone fracture.* Diss. Basel.

9. **Blümlein H, Cordey J, Schneider U, et al.** (1997) Langzeitmessungen der Axialkraft von Knochenschrauben in vivo. *Med Orthop Tech;* 1:17–19.

10. **Ganz R, Perren SM, Ruter A** (1975) [Mechanical induction of bone resorption]. *Fortschr Kiefer Gesichtschir;* 19:45–48.

11. **Baumgart FW, Cordey J, Morikawa K, et al.** (1993) AO/ASIF self-tapping screws (STS). *Injury;* 24 (Suppl 1):1–17.

12. **Fernandez Dell'Oca AA, Tepic S, Frigg R, et al.** (In press) Treating forearm fractures using an internal fixator: a prospective study. *Clinical Orthopaedics and Related Research.*

13. **Haas NP, Hauke C, Schütz M, et al.** (In prep.) The principles of the internal fixator applied to diaphyseal fractures of the forearm using the Point Contact Fixator (PC-Fix): results of 387 fractures of a prospective multicentric study. *J Orthop Trauma.*

14. **Banovetz JM, Sharp R, Probe RA, et al.** (1996) Titanium plate fixation: a review of implant failures. *J Orthop Trauma;* 10 (6):389–394.

6 Updates

Updates and additional references for this chapter are available online at:
http://www.aopublishing.org/PFxM/321.htm

3.2.2 Plates

Bernd Wittner & Ulrich Holz

1 Introduction

In previous years, the technique of absolute stability leading to direct bone healing was usually recommended and employed in the management of operative fracture treatment [1]. Today, this approach is being challenged by less invasive, so-called biological, methods of fracture fixation [2]. **Nevertheless, osteosynthesis with plates providing rigid fixation still has a firm place in fracture treatment. Fractures with joint involvement are best fixed by absolutely rigid internal fixation, usually including plates. In these fractures, anatomical reduction is essential and abundant callus formation is not desired.** Provided intramedullary nailing techniques are not preferred, transverse and short oblique fractures of the shaft of long bones are still good indications for plating, be it for anatomical (forearm), local (contaminated wound), technical (short distal or proximal fragment), or general reasons (see **chapter 3.3.1**). In the case of local infections and in multiply injured patients with chest trauma, plate osteosynthesis competes with external fixation (see **chapters 3.3.3** and **3.4**).

While the development of callus is desirable in less stable fixation, its appearance after rigid fixation may be of concern, as it points to some degree of instability that ultimately may lead to implant fatigue and failure (see **chapter 1.2**). After stable osteosynthesis, fracture healing, especially in the region directly underneath a standard plate, probably takes longer than following other techniques. A plate placed in direct contact with and pressed to the bone surface can lead to a long-standing disturbance of the blood flow to the underlying cortex. The process of osteonal remodeling and revascularization is slow and can be observed as a porous condition of the cortical bone mirroring the footprints of the plate (see **chapter 1.2**). This disturbance of the cortical blood supply can be decreased by minimizing stripping of the periosteum, as a plate can be placed on top of it. Gentle use of small pointed hooks and pointed reduction clamps is recommended for reduction and, whenever possible, indirect reduction techniques, as described in **chapter 3.3.2**, should be applied to reduce the insult to bone and soft parts. Due to its reduced area of contact to the bone, the LC-DCP appears to preserve the blood supply better than the "old" DCP (see below), an effect which is even more evident with the PC-Fix or LISS (see **chapter 3.4**). In former times

Rigid fixation with plates and screws has a firm place in fracture treatment.

Articular fractures require anatomical reduction and stable fixation.

The potential compromise of cortical blood supply is a major draw back of conventional plating.

plates were said to perform so-called "stress protection", a term no longer used as the before-mentioned theory of a disturbed vascularity seems more plausible. "Refractures" after plate removal [3] may equally be explained by slower remodeling of the cortex underlying a plate.

As compared to osteosynthesis designed to heal by callus formation (biological fixation), the classical plating technique, providing rigid fixation, requires strict adherence to the principles of interfragmentary compression. Errors of technique and misapplied principles may lead to complications such as delayed healing, implant failure, and non-union.

2 Plate designs

AO has developed many different plates, most of which may be used for rigid internal fixation, as well as for biological plating with relative stability.

Most plates can be used for rigid as well as biological fracture fixation.

2.1 Dynamic compression plate (DCP) 3.5 and 4.5

The dynamic compression plate (DCP) was introduced in 1969 [4]. At the time, it represented a further development of the "coapteur" of Danis [5] and the modified plate of Bagby and Janes [6]. The DCP featured a new hole design allowing for axial compression by eccentric screw insertion. The plate functions in different modes: compression, neutralization, tension band, or as buttress.

The DCP design is available in three sizes for large and small bones:

1. The broad DCP 4.5 for fractures of the femur and, exceptionally, the humerus.
2. The narrow DCP 4.5 for fractures of the tibia and humerus.
3. The DCP 3.5 for the fractures of the forearm, fibula, pelvis, and clavicle.

The screw holes in the DCP are best described as a portion of an inclined and angled cylinder. Like a ball, the screw head slides down the inclined shoulder of the cylinder (**Fig. 3.2.2-1**). In practice, when the screw is inserted and

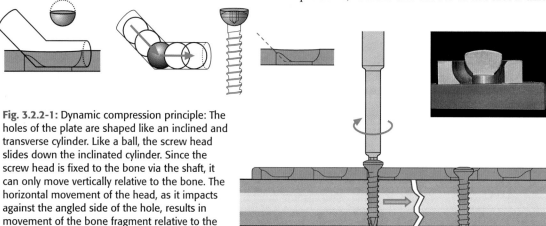

Fig. 3.2.2-1: Dynamic compression principle: The holes of the plate are shaped like an inclined and transverse cylinder. Like a ball, the screw head slides down the inclinated cylinder. Since the screw head is fixed to the bone via the shaft, it can only move vertically relative to the bone. The horizontal movement of the head, as it impacts against the angled side of the hole, results in movement of the bone fragment relative to the plate, and leads to compression of the fracture.

tightened, this results in a movement of the bone fragment relative to the plate, and consequently, compression of the fracture. The design of the screw holes allows for a displacement of up to 1.0 mm. After the insertion of one compression screw, additional compression using one more eccentric screw is possible before the first screw is "locked" (**Fig. 3.2.2-2**). For axial compression over a distance greater than 2.0 mm, the use of the articulated tension device is recommended (see **Fig. 3.2.2-19** and **Fig. 3.2.2-21**). The oval shape of the holes allows a 25° inclination of the screws in the longitudinal plane and up to 7° inclination in the transverse plane (**Fig. 3.2.2-3**).

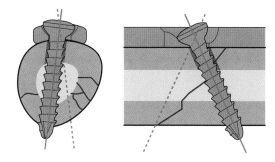

Fig. 3.2.2-3: The shape of the holes of the DCP allows inclination of the screws in transvers direction of ±7° and in longitudinal direction of 25°.

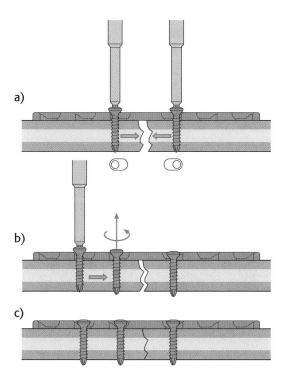

a)

b)

c)

Fig. 3.2.2-2: After insertion of one compressing screw it is only possible to insert one other screw with compressing function, otherwise the first screw locks. When the second screw is tightened, the first has to be loosened to allow the plate to slide on the bone, after which it is retightened.

2.1.1 Technique of application

The DCP 4.5 is used with 4.5 mm cortex screws, 4.5 mm shaft screws, and 6.5 mm cancellous bone screws. The DCP 3.5 is used with 3.5 mm cortex screws, 3.5 mm shaft screws, and 4.0 mm cancellous bone screws. There are two DCP drill guides, one with an eccentric (load) hole and a gold collar, the other with a concentric (neutral) hole and a green collar, for each size (4.5 or 3.5) plate/screws (**Fig. 3.2.2-4a/b**). Depending upon the intended function of the plate, the eccentric or neutral drill guide is chosen.

If the screw is to be inserted in neutral (green) position, the hole is, in fact, 0.1 mm off-center, which theoretically adds some compression even in neutral position.

The golden load drill guide produces a hole 1.0 mm off-center and away from the fracture, so that when the screw is tightened, the bone is displaced relative to the plate, applying compression to the fracture site (**Video AO00097a**).

If the plate is intended to function as a buttress (see below), the universal drill guide (or sleeve) may be used, placing the screw to the opposite end of the hole. This prevents any gliding of the plate relative to the bone (**Fig. 3.2.2-4c**).

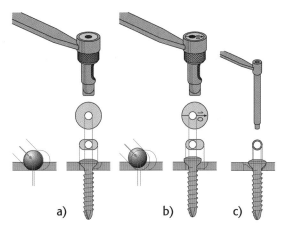

a) b) c)

Fig. 3.2.2-4: The application of the drill guides depends on the function the screw should have:
a) Neutral position (green end of the guide).
b) Compression (yellow end of the guide).
c) Buttressing (universal drill guide).

The LC-DCP design reduces the area of contact between plate and bone and thereby interferes less with bone biology.

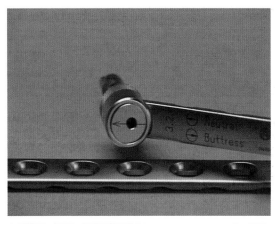

 Video AO00097a

2.2 Limited contact dynamic compression plate (LC-DCP) 3.5 and 4.5

(**Fig. 3.2.2-5**)

2.2.1 Design changes

The limited contact dynamic compression plate (LC-DCP) represents a further development of the DCP. Several elements of the design have been changed, and the plate is available both in stainless steel and in pure titanium. Titanium exhibits outstanding tissue tolerance (see **chapter 1.3**).

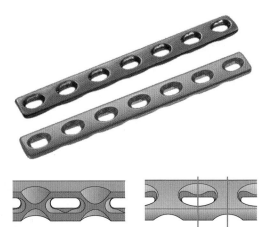

Fig. 3.2.2-5: The LC-DCP with its structured undersurface for limited contact between plate and bone and an even distribution of the holes throughout the plate.

By virtue of the changes in its design compared to the DCP, the area of the plate-bone contact (the plate "footprint") of the LC-DCP is greatly reduced. The capillary network of the periosteum is thereby less compromised, leading to a relative improvement of cortical perfusion, which reduces the porotic changes underneath the plate (see **chapter 1.3**).

The geometry of the plate, with its "structured" undersurface, results in an even distribution of stiffness, making contouring easier, and minimizing the tendency to "kink" at the holes when bent (**Fig. 3.2.2-6**). In bridging mode (**chapter 3.3.2**), this distribution of stiffness results in a gentle elastic deformation of the entire plate without stress concentration at one of the screw holes, as occurs in the DCP.

The plate holes have a symmetrical form, so that the self-tensioning principle is possible in each direction. This allows for compression at several levels, for example, in a segmental fracture.

The plate holes are evenly distributed over the entire length of the plate (see **Fig. 3.2.2-5**), which adds to the versatility of application.

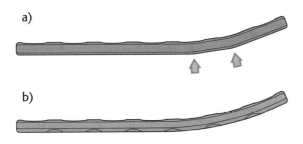

Fig. 3.2.2-6: In the DCP (a) the area at the plate holes is less stiff than the area between them. During bending, the plate tends to bend only in the areas of the hole. The LC-DCP (b) has an even stiffness without the risk of buckling at the screw holes.

In cross-section the plate has a trapezoidal shape. The bony ridges which form along the edges of the plate tend to be thicker and flatter, rendering them less prone to damage during plate removal (**Fig. 3.2.2-7**).

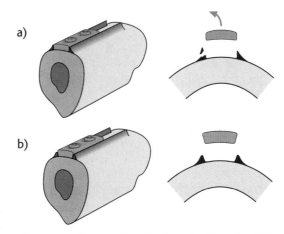

Fig. 3.2.2-7: Cross-section after bone healing using DCP (a) and LC-DCP (b); note the trapezoidal "footprint" of the LC-DCP.

2.2.2 Technique of application

As in the case of the DCP, the screws can be inserted in different modes: compression, neutral, and buttress. To facilitate insertion, there are two LC-DCP drill guides designed for each of the plates 3.5 and 4.5 (**Fig. 3.2.2-8a**), and the LC-DCP universal drill guide (**Fig. 3.2.2-8b**).

This new LC-DCP universal spring-loaded drill guide permits placement of the drill in neutral or eccentric position relative to the plate hole. If the inner drill sleeve is extended (normal) and placed against the end of the plate hole, an eccentric drill hole will result (**Fig. 3.2.2-9a**).

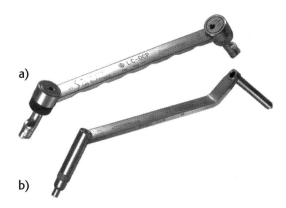

Fig. 3.2.2-8:
a) LC-DCP drill guide.
b) LC-DCP universal drill guide.

However, if the spring-loaded guide is pressed against the bone, the inner tube retracts, and the rounded end of the outer tube glides down the slope of the hole to the neutral position (**Fig. 3.2.2-9b**) (**Video AO00097b**).

2.3 Tubular plates (4.5/3.5/2.7)

(**Fig. 3.2.2-10**)

The one-third tubular plate exists only in the 3.5 version—its counterpart, in the 4.5 system, is the semi-tubular plate, which is less used than in the past. The one-third tubular plate is available in either titanium or stainless steel. As it is only 1.0 mm thick, its ability to confer stability is somewhat limited. However, it may be useful in areas with minimal soft-tissue covering, such as the lateral malleolus, the olecranon, and the distal end of the ulna. Each hole is surrounded by a small collar (**Fig. 3.2.2-10a'**) to prevent the spherical screwheads from penetrating the plate and producing cracks in the near cortex (**Fig. 3.2.2-10b/c**). The oval shape of each hole allows a certain degree of eccentric screw placement to produce fracture compression (**Fig. 3.2.2-10d**).

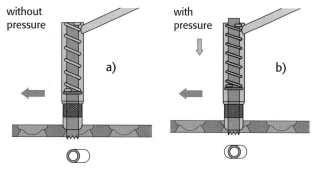

without pressure

with pressure

a)

b)

Fig. 3.2.2-9: Application of the LC-DCP universal drill guide:
a) Eccentric position.
b) Neutral position.

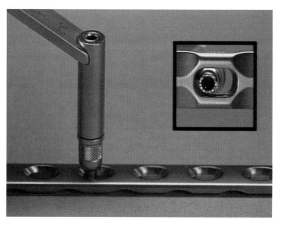

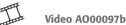
Video AO00097b

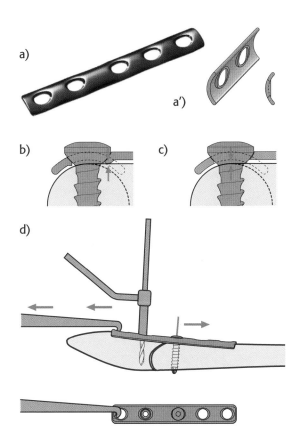

Fig. 3.2.2-10:
a) One-third tubular plate.
a′) The collar around the hole of the one-third tubular plate prevents the screw head from protruding and secures the plate/bone contact.
b) Without a collar, the screw head protrudes through the plate, preventing good fixation.
c) Thanks to the collar the plate-screw junction is improved.
d) The oval shape of each hole allows a certain degree of eccentric screw placement to produce fracture compression, which can be augmented by pulling at one end of the plate.

2.4 Reconstruction plate 3.5 and 4.5

(**Fig. 3.2.2-11**)

Reconstruction plates are characterized by deep notches between the holes that allow accurate contouring on the flat as well as standard bending (**section 3**). The plate is considered not to be as strong as the compression plates described before, and may be further weakened by heavy contouring—sharp bends in any direction should be avoided. The holes are oval, to allow for dynamic compression.

These plates are especially useful in fractures of bones with complex 3-D geometry, as encountered in the pelvis and the acetabulum, the distal humerus, and the clavicle. Special instruments are available for the contouring of these plates (**Fig. 3.2.2-11b**).

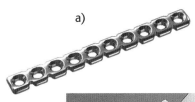

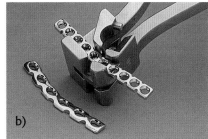

Fig. 3.2.2-11:
a) Reconstruction plate.
b) The special bending pliers for the reconstruction plates: Bending irons are available to twist the plate .

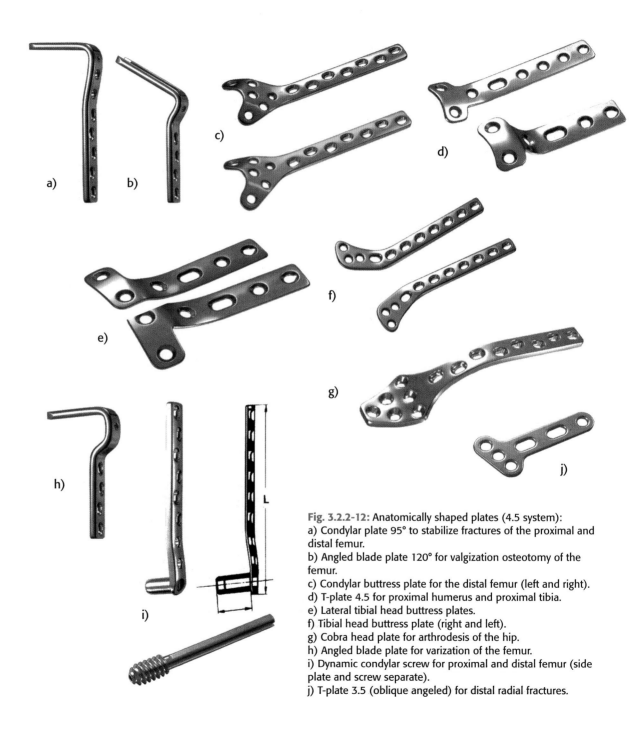

Fig. 3.2.2-12: Anatomically shaped plates (4.5 system):
a) Condylar plate 95° to stabilize fractures of the proximal and distal femur.
b) Angled blade plate 120° for valgization osteotomy of the femur.
c) Condylar buttress plate for the distal femur (left and right).
d) T-plate 4.5 for proximal humerus and proximal tibia.
e) Lateral tibial head buttress plates.
f) Tibial head buttress plate (right and left).
g) Cobra head plate for arthrodesis of the hip.
h) Angled blade plate for varization of the femur.
i) Dynamic condylar screw for proximal and distal femur (side plate and screw separate).
j) T-plate 3.5 (oblique angeled) for distal radial fractures.

2.5 Special plates

Several special plates for specific locations have been developed. They are shaped anatomically, corresponding to the site where they are to be applied. In some of these plates dynamic compression is possible. Application of these plates is described in the relevant chapters (**Fig. 3.2.2-12**).

3 Classical principles of rigid internal fixation with plates

Absolute stability of plated fractures depends on interfragmentary compression, which can be established by lag screws, axial compression by plate, or both. **Static compression between two fragments is maintained over several weeks [7] and does not enhance bone resorption or necrosis (Fig. 3.2.2-13). Interfragmentary compression leads to increased**

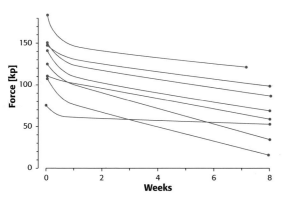

Fig. 3.2.2-13: Compression applied to cortical bone *in vivo*. The initial value of compression force decreases very slowly. This pattern of change in compression proved that pressure necrosis with surface resorption in the compressed area does not occur.

stability through friction, but has no direct influence on bone biology or fracture healing (**chapter 1.2**).

In order to achieve absolute stability, the compression over the whole cross-section of a fracture must be sufficiently high to neutralize all forces (bending, distraction, shear, and rotation).

There are four ways to obtain interfragmentary compression with a plate:

- Compression with the tension device.
- Compression with the dynamic compression principle (DCP/LC-DCP).
- Compression by contouring (over-bending) the plate.
- Additional lag screws through plate holes.

Interfragmentary compression provides stability through friction, but has no direct influence on bone bridging or fracture healing.

3.1 Rigid fixation by lag screw and neutralization (protection) plate

(**Fig. 3.2.2-14**)

The traditional and quite effective way to rigidly fix a simple diaphyseal fracture is to use lag screws (**chapter 3.2.1**) combined with a neutralization (protection) plate. In metaepiphyseal split fractures, lag screw fixation often needs to be combined with a buttress plate to protect the screws from shearing forces. A lag screw cor-

Static compression does not enhance bone resorption or necrosis.

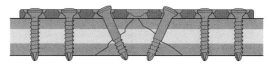

Fig. 3.2.2-14: Lag screw osteosynthesis with neutralization plate. Interfragmentary compression is achieved by lag screws. The function of the plate is to neutralize bending forces. Lag screws applied through the plate are preferable and do not require additional exposure.

rectly inserted in good bone generates forces up to 3,000 N. Since the same effect cannot be brought about by any of the methods listed below, lag screws should be used whenever the fracture pattern permits it (**Fig. 3.2.2-15**).

A lag screw can be placed either free standing or through the plate. To avoid any additional soft-tissue stripping, placement through the plate is to be preferred (**Video AO00097c**). The recommendations for positioning a lag screw as mentioned in **chapter 3.2.1** must be kept in mind. In the case of a wedge fragment opposite to the plate, the fragment should be reduced with the aid of pointed hooks or a pointed reduction clamp. Definitive fixation with a lag screw is best done—whenever possible—through the plate (**Fig. 3.2.2-16**).

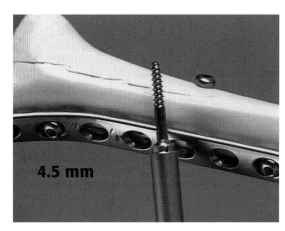

4.5 mm

Video AO00097c

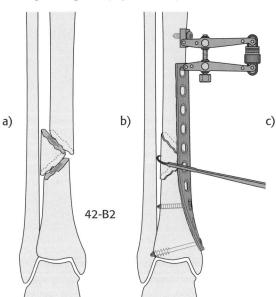

a)

b)

c)

42-B2

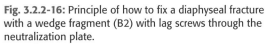

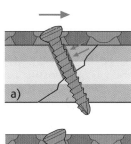

a)

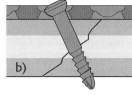

b)

Fig. 3.2.2-15: Cortex lag screw (a) and shaft screw (b) for compression of a fracture. The shaft screw exerts higher compression.

Fig. 3.2.2-16: Principle of how to fix a diaphyseal fracture with a wedge fragment (B2) with lag screws through the neutralization plate.
a) Wedge fracture (B2).
b) The plate, after contouring, is fixed with two screws to the distal main fragment, while the tension device is applied proximally. The wedge fragment is gently reduced with a small hook.
c) Final aspect of synthesis: the two middle screws introduced through the plate are lagging the wedge. No soft-tissue stripping required.

3.2 Compression with the tension device

In transverse or short oblique fractures of the diaphysis, placement of a lag screw is not always possible. The majority of these fractures are, anyhow, best treated by intramedullary fixation, except in the forearm. If nailing is not possible or not indicated, a compression plate should be used. The removable tension device was developed (**Fig. 3.2.2-16/17/18**) to achieve adequate compression (over 100 kp). Its use is also recommended for fractures of the femur or the humeral shaft, in osteotomies (see **chapter 6.4**) or when the gap to be closed exceeds 1–2 mm. Most plates have a notch at either end, which fits the hook of the tension device. Before use, the two branches of tension device should be opened completely. After fixation of the plate to one main fragment, the fracture is reduced and held in position with a reduction forceps. The tension device is now connected to the plate and fixed with a short cortical screw in the opposite main fragment. For application of forces in excess of 100–120 kp or in osteoporotic bone, a bicortical fixation is recommended. The wrench with universal joint is used for tightening.

In oblique fractures, to prevent displacement, the tension must be applied in such a way that the spike of the mobile fragment is pressed into the anxilla formed by the plate and the other main fragment to which it has been fixed (see **Fig. 3.2.2-18**). **Biomechanical studies**

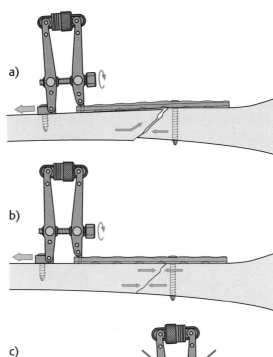

a)

b)

c)

Simple fracture patterns are still best reduced anatomically and rigidly fixed by a "classical" plate.

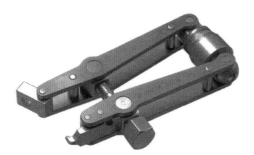

Fig. 3.2.2-17: Articulating tension device. Depending on the position of the hook, the device can be used for distraction or compression.

Fig. 3.2.2-18: a/b) In oblique fractures the tension device must be applied in such a way that the loose fragment locks in the anxilla if compression is produced. c) demonstrates the wrong position.

A lag screw placed through a plate hole greatly increases the stability.

If compression cannot be obtained through an interfragmentary lag screw, overbending of the plate is recommended.

have shown that the bending and rotational stability of such fractures is greatly increased if a lag screw through the plate and across the fracture is added once axial compression has been established (**Video AO00099a**).

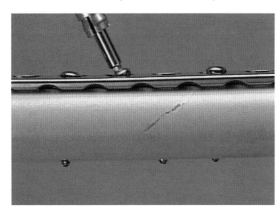

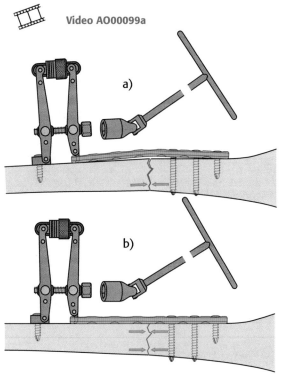

Video AO00099a

3.3 Compression by overbending

Due to the eccentric position of a straight plate on a straight bone, compressive forces are greater directly underneath the plate and less at the opposite cortex, where a small gap due to distraction can be observed (**Fig. 3.2.2-19**). This may induce micromovements. If the placement of an additional lag screw is not possible, prebending of the plate is essential (**Fig. 3.2.2-20**).

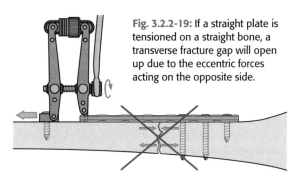

Fig. 3.2.2-19: If a straight plate is tensioned on a straight bone, a transverse fracture gap will open up due to the eccentric forces acting on the opposite side.

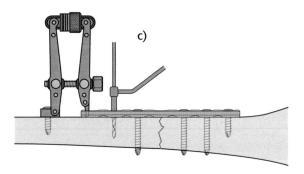

Fig. 3.2.2-20: If the plate is slightly pre-bent prior to the application (a), the gap in the opposite cortex will disappear as compression is built up (b), so that finally the whole fracture is firmly closed and compressed (c).

By applying tension, the overbent plate is straightened, which leads to compression of the opposite cortex, thereby adding to stability. There are special instruments available for pre-bending or contouring plates (**Fig. 3.2.2-21**).

3.4 Compression with the DCP or LC-DCP (dynamic compression principle)

Axial compression can also be generated with the DCP (see above). However, the compression force achievable is lower than with the tension device, while pre-bending of the plate is also necessary to obtain an even distribution of the compressive forces.

3.5 Contouring of plates

Straight plates often need to be contoured prior to application, to fit the anatomy of the bone. If this is not done, the reduction will be lost, especially if no lag screws are placed across the fracture. Even the anatomically shaped plates (see **section 2**) may require fine contouring before application. This is best done with the hand-held bending pliers or the bending press (see **Fig. 3.2.2-21**) as well as bending irons. If complex 3-D contouring is required, special flexible templates are available, which can be modeled to the bone surface (**Video AO00097d**). Repeated bending back and forth should, however, be avoided, because this weakens the plate.

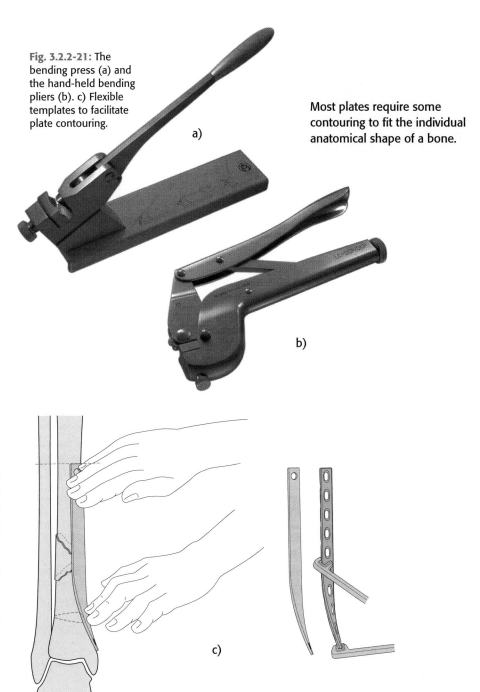

Fig. 3.2.2-21: The bending press (a) and the hand-held bending pliers (b). c) Flexible templates to facilitate plate contouring.

Most plates require some contouring to fit the individual anatomical shape of a bone.

a)

b)

c)

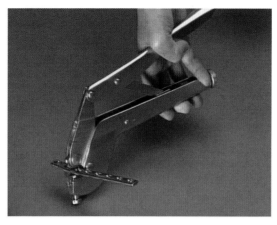

Video AO00097d

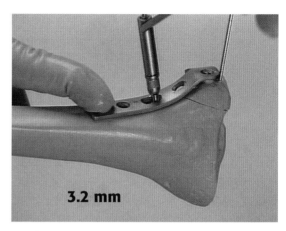

3.2 mm

Video AO00099b

4 Different functions of plates

The function assigned to a plate does not depend on its design.

Besides the plate functions already mentioned—neutralizing (protecting) or compressing—one and the same plate may also be used for other functions, such as buttressing, bridging, or to act as a tension band.

4.1 Buttress plate

In a metaphyseal/epiphyseal shear or split fracture, fixation with lag screws alone may not be sufficient. A lag screw should therefore be combined with a plate with buttress or antiglide function (**Video AO00099b**). In plates with DCP holes, the screws should be inserted in the buttress position (**Fig. 3.2.2-22**).

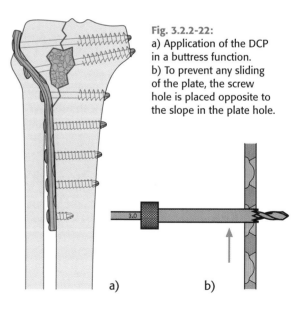

Fig. 3.2.2-22:
a) Application of the DCP in a buttress function.
b) To prevent any sliding of the plate, the screw hole is placed opposite to the slope in the plate hole.

a)   b)

4.2 Tension band plate

(see **chapter 3.2.3**)

The following four criteria must be fulfilled for a plate to act as a tension band:
1. The fractured bone must be eccentrically loaded, e.g., femur.
2. The plate must be placed on the tension side.
3. The plate must be able to withstand the tensile forces.
4. The bone must be able to withstand the compressive force which results from the conversion of distraction forces by the plate. There must be a bony buttress opposite to the plate to prevent cyclic bending.

A good example of a physiologically eccentrically loaded bone is the femur (**Fig. 3.2.2-23**). If a plate is placed on the lateral (tension) side of a transverse fracture, the distraction forces are converted to compressive forces across the

A plate under tension is much stronger than under bending forces.

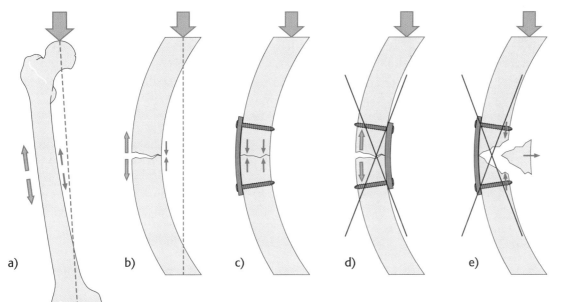

Fig. 3.2.2-23: Tension band principle at the femur.
The intact femur (a) is an eccentrically loaded bone with distraction or tensile forces laterally and compression on the medial side. In case of a fracture (b) the lateral fracture gap will open, whereas the medial will be compressed. If a plate is placed alongside the linea aspera of the femur (c), it will be under tension when loaded, thereby compressing the fracture gap, provided there is bony contact medially. If the plate is placed to the compression side (d), it is not able to prevent opening of the lateral gap (instability). If the medial cortex is not intact (e), the tension band principle cannot work, because of lack of buttress (see **chapter 3.2.3**).

whole fracture interface, provided the medial cortex is intact. If the same plate is placed medially, it cannot counteract the distractive forces, and the fixation will fail, especially under load.

4.3 Bridge plate

(see **chapter 3.3.2**)

In order to respect the biology of a complex multifragmentary fracture and to minimize any additional soft-tissue injury, presently a so-called bridge plate is advocated, which is fixed to the two main fragments only, leaving the fracture zone untouched. If feasible, bridge plates should be applied through minimal exposure in order to maintain length, correct axial alignment, and correct rotation. If the vascularity to bone and surrounding soft parts has not been disturbed too much, the physiological response to such a relatively flexible construction is rapid callus formation bridging the fragments, as happens in non-operative treatment or after gentle intramedullary nailing.

Bridge plates are indicated in complex diaphyseal fracture patterns.

5 Bibliography

1. **Müller ME, Allgöwer M, Schneider R, et al.** (1977) *Manual der Osteosynthese – AO-Technik.* 2nd ed. Berlin Heidelberg New York: Springer-Verlag.
2. **Miclau T, Martin RE** (1997) The evolution of modern plate osteosynthesis. *Injury;* 28 (Suppl 1):3–6.
3. **Kessler SB, Schweiberer L** (1988) Refrakturen nach operativer Frakturenbehandlung. *Hefte zur Unfallheilkunde;* 194:29–43.
4. **Perren SM, Russenberger M, Steinemann S, et al.** (1969) A dynamic compression plate. *Acta Orthop Scand Suppl;* 125:31–41.
5. **Danis R** (1949) *Théorie et practique de l'ostéosynthèse.* Paris: Masson.
6. **Bagby GW, Janes JM** (1957) An impacting bone plate. *Staff meeting: Mayo Clinic;* 32:55–57.
7. **Perren SM, Huggler A, Russenberger M, et al.** (1969) Cortical bone healing. The reaction of cortical bone to compression. *Acta Othop Scand;* 125 (Suppl):31–41.

6 Updates

Updates and additional references for this chapter are available online at:
http://www.aopublishing.org/PFxM/322.htm

3.2.3 Tension band principle

Christoph Josten & Gert Muhr

1 Biomechanical principles

Early concepts of load transfer within bone were developed and described by Frederic Pauwels [1]. He observed that a curved, tubular structure under axial load always has a compression side as well as a tension side. Using the eccentrically loaded femur as a model Pauwels, in the classical "load strain diagrams", schematically demonstrated the compression and tension forces present within that bone while it was under axial stress (**Fig. 3.2.3-1**).

From these observations the principle of the tension band evolved, which describes how **tensile forces are converted into compression forces** by applying a device eccentrically or to the convex side of a curved tube or bone (**Fig. 3.2.3-2**).

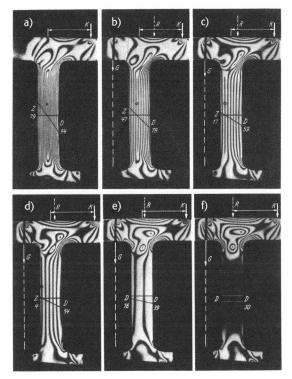

The tension band converts tensile forces into compression forces.

Fig. 3.2.3-1: To illustrate the effectiveness of the tension band principle, Pauwels used photo-elastic models. Eccentric loading produces a stress-strain differential within the material. These differentials can be equalized by a tension band applied to the tension side. It acts as a counterweight to eccentrically applied compression.
a) Eccentric force (K) is applied at a distance from the neutral axis (0), producing a tensile force of 79 kp/cm² (Z) and a compression force of 94 kp/cm² (D).
b) A weak tension band (G) is applied to the tension side (left column), producing a resultant force (R) more closely aligned with the neutral axis of the material. The tensile force Z is reduced to 47 kp/cm² while the compression force (D) is decreased to 79 kp/cm².
c–f) The application of a progressively stronger tension band (G) produces and intensifies the shift of forces toward the neutral axis. The resultant force (R) is shifted toward neutral force 0 until the tension-optical lines become collinear as seen in (f). There is now an equally acting compressive force of 30 kp/cm² [1].

The stresses (compression/ tensile forces) are given here in units of kp/cm², in order to match the labels in the original figure by Pauwels. To obtain the corresponding numbers in SI units N/cm², multiply by 9.81.

Since a fractured bone, if it is to unite, requires mechanical stability, as obtained, for example by compression, and reacts adversely under motion or repeated tension/distraction, it appears essential to neutralize such forces for the duration of the healing process [2].

This is especially important in articular fractures, which require early motion for a good functional outcome.

In those fractures where muscle pull during motion tends to distract the fragments, for example, fractures of the patella or olecranon, the application of a tension band will neutralize these forces and even convert them into compression when the joint is flexed (**Fig. 3.2.3-3**). Similarly, a bony fragment can be avulsed at the insertion of a tendon or ligament, for example, the greater tuberosity of the humerus, the greater trochanter of the femur, or the medial malleolus. Here too a tension band can firmly reattach the avulsed fragment allowing immediate motion of the involved joint.

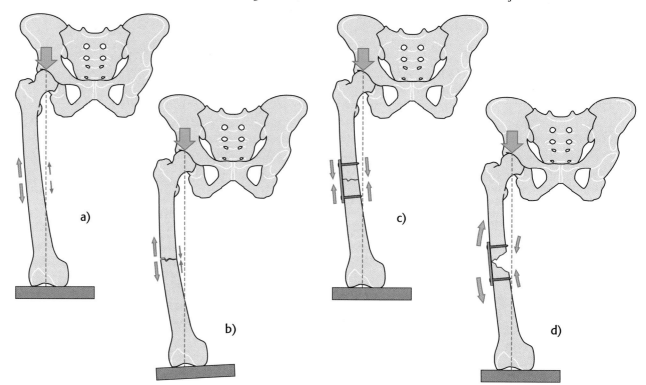

Fig. 3.2.3-2: When applied to the tension side of the bone a plate acts as a dynamic tension band.
a) The mechanical axis of the bone is not necessarily within the center of the bone.
b) Under vertical pressure the curved femur creates a tension force laterally and a compression force medially.
c) A plate positioned on the side of tensile forces neutralizes them at the fracture site provided there is cortical contact opposite to this plate.
d) In case of a cortical defect, the plate will undergo bending stresses and eventually fail due to fatigue.

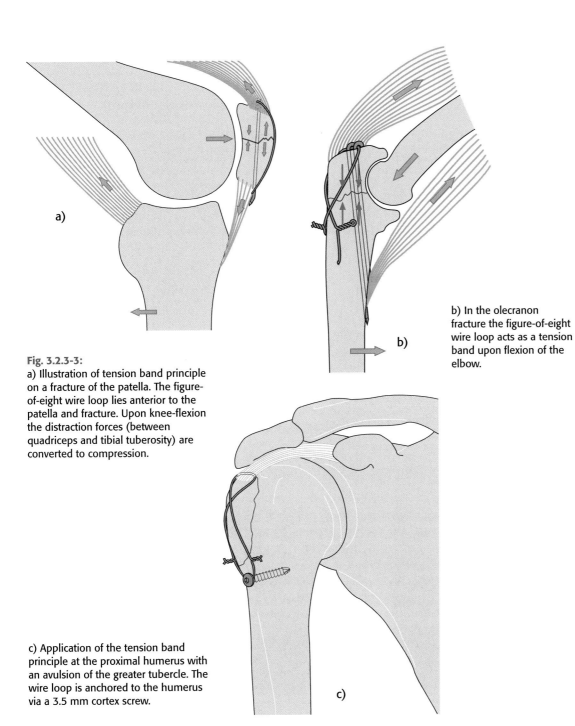

a)

b)

Fig. 3.2.3-3:

a) Illustration of tension band principle on a fracture of the patella. The figure-of-eight wire loop lies anterior to the patella and fracture. Upon knee-flexion the distraction forces (between quadriceps and tibial tuberosity) are converted to compression.

b) In the olecranon fracture the figure-of-eight wire loop acts as a tension band upon flexion of the elbow.

c) Application of the tension band principle at the proximal humerus with an avulsion of the greater tubercle. The wire loop is anchored to the humerus via a 3.5 mm cortex screw.

c)

In the diaphysis angular deformity (convexity) indicates the tension side.

2 Concepts of application

Historically a circumferential wire loop—so-called cerclage—was originally described by Berger in 1892. Multiple modifications of the technique have been presented since [3–5], while others introduced the combination of wiring with screw or K-wire fixation [6–8]. K-wires or lag screws stabilize the fragments against rotational forces and may serve as anchorage for the tension band material.

The types of articular fractures with avulsed fragments that typically profit from fixation according to the tension band principle have already been mentioned. However, there are situations where this principle can also be applied in diaphyseal fractures, for example, the femoral shaft, or in delayed unions or non-unions where the presence of **angular deformity indicates the tension side of the bone**. Any internal or external implant must be applied to the tension side to neutralize these forces. Bony union will then occur quite consistently. This demonstrates that not only loops of wires, cables, resorbable and non-resorbable suture materials, but also a plate or an external fixator can fulfill the function of a tension band (**Fig. 3.2.3-4**).

A tension band that produces compression at the time of application, for example, at the medial malleolus, is called a static tension band as the forces at the fracture site remain fairly constant during movement of the ankle.

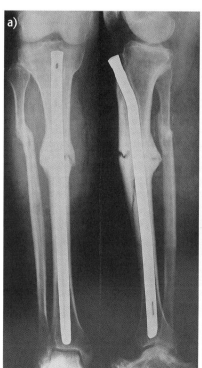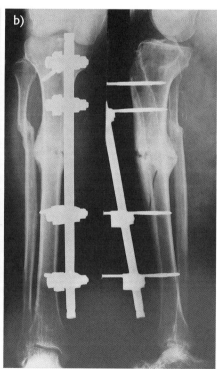

Fig. 3.2.3-4:
Clinical example of an external fixator acting as a tension band.
a) Symptomatic non-union after intramedullary nailing–note the hypertrophic area on the dorsal side of the tibia and the gap anteriorly.
b) After removal of the nail, a unilateral external fixator in the sagittal plane was applied and full weight bearing encouraged. The non-union consolidated within 8 weeks, while the patient was immediately asymptomatic.

However, if the compression forces increase with motion, for example, in the patella with knee flexion, the tension band is called dynamic.

3 Operative technique

Fractures subject to distraction are at risk of displacement if movement occurs, for example, patella with knee-flexion or greater tuberosity during contraction of the supraspinatus muscle. By applying a figure-of-eight or simple loop to the front of the patella with good purchase in the patellar and quadriceps tendons respectively, an excellent tension band mechanism is created which compresses the fracture under dynamic load (**Video AO51049**). The 1.0 or 1.2 mm wire must be anchored as close to the bone as possible. It can either be directed through the insertion of the tendon with a large gauge needle or run around longitudinal K-wires (see **Fig. 3.2.3-3a**) (see also **chapter 4.7**). The tension band loop can also be placed through a 2 mm drill hole in the neighboring bone, for example,

at the proximal ulna in olecranon fractures (see **Fig. 3.2.3-3b**) or around a screw head in the proximal humerus (see **Fig. 3.2.3-3c**).

As already mentioned, a plate or external fixator which is expected to function according to the tension band principle must be applied to the tension side of the bone or the convex side of a deformity or non-union (see **Fig. 3.2.3-4**). The following prerequisites are essential:

a) Bone or a fracture pattern that is able to withstand compression.

b) An intact cortical buttress on the opposite side of the tension band element.

c) Solid fixation that withstands tensile forces.

4 Pitfalls and complications

The most common complication is failure of the implant. A wire put under pure tension is very strong. However, if bending forces are added, it will break by fatigue quite rapidly. As this also holds true for plates, it appears essential that in the diaphysis the tension side of the bone is known and the opposite cortex is able to withstand compression forces (see **Fig. 3.2.3-2**). In the presence of a contralateral defect only the plate is load-bearing and repeated bending stresses invariably will lead to plate breakage by fatigue. A bone graft might be the answer to help to build up in due time a buttress in the cortex opposite to the plate.

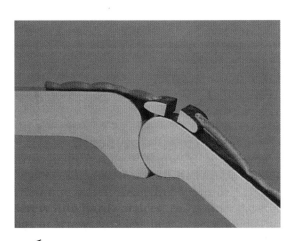

 Video AO51049

5 Bibliography

1. **Pauwels F** (1980) *Biomechanics of the Locomotor Apparatus*. Berlin Heidelberg New York: Springer-Verlag.

2. **Chandler WR** (1996) Fractures in adults. In: Rockwood CA, Green DP, Buchholz RW, editors. *Principles of internal fixation*. Philadelphia New York: Lippincott-Raven.

3. **Payr E** (1917) Zur Behandlung der Kniegelenksteife nach langdauernder Ruhigstellung. *Zentralbl Chir;* 44:809–816.

4. **Magnuson PB** (1936) *Fractures*. 2nd ed. Philadelphia: J.B. Lippincott.

5. **Anderson LD** (1971) In: Crenshaw AH, editor. *Campbell's Operative Orthopedics*. 5th ed. St Louis: C. V. Mosby.

6. **Müller ME, Allgöwer M, Schneider R, et al.** (1992) *Manual of Internal Fixation*. 3rd ed. Berlin Heidelberg New York: Springer-Verlag.

7. **DePalma AF** (1959) *The Management of Fractures and Dislocations*. Philadelphia: W. B. Saunders.

8. **Smillie IS** (1970) *Injuries of the Knee Joint*. Edinburgh: E & S Livingstone.

6 Updates

Updates and additional references for this chapter are available online at:
http://www.aopublishing.org/PFxM/323.htm

3.3.1 Intramedullary nailing

Christian Krettek

1 Types of intramedullary nailing

1.1 Classical Küntscher nail (tight fitting, unlocked)

Intramedullary nailing of long bone shaft fractures is generally accepted as a standard treatment. Use of the conventional "Küntscher nail" [1] with its longitudinal slot was restricted to relatively simple midshaft diaphyseal fractures because the stabilization was dependent on the contact between the elastic implant and the stiff bone (nailing principle). Reaming the medullary cavity increases the area of contact between the nail and bone and, therefore, extends the indication to fractures which are more complex or more proximal and distal in the shaft. Reaming also improves the mechanical properties of the bone-implant interface by allowing the use of larger diameter implants. However, the reaming process itself has some inherent biological disadvantages, especially when performed excessively. These are: a considerable rise in intramedullary pressure, temperature increase causing devitalized cortical layers, and bone necrosis. In the past, these disadvantages limited the use of reamed nails to fractures with minor soft-tissue injuries only.

1.2 Universal nail (tight fitting, locked)

The addition of **interlocking screws to the nail, as originally introduced by Grosse and Kempf [2], enhanced the mechanical properties of the intramedullary implant and widened the range of indications** to even more proximal and distal fractures, as well as to more complex and unstable patterns. However, if the fracture is more distal, more proximal, or more complex, its fixation mainly depends on the interlocking screws, and much less on the principle of friction. The length of the bone-implant construct is still effectively maintained, because the locking screws prevent

Nailing of diaphyseal fractures is a standard form of treatment.

Interlocking increases stability of fixation and widens the indications for nailing.

shortening. However, the longitudinal slot in the tubular nail results in decreased rotational stiffness which can lead to rotational instability, especially with smaller diameter nails [3].

1.3 Nailing without reaming or locking

A solid nail is less susceptible to infection than a tubular nail.

Several groups in Europe and North America have treated shaft fractures with significant soft-tissue injuries using intramedullary nails which were inserted without reaming, and which were, therefore, loose fitting. Since these implants (Ender nail, Lottes' nail, and Rush pins) were thin and could not be locked proximally or distally, longitudinal and rotational instability resulted, especially in complex fractures. Despite the "low" infection rates, a major disadvantage was the frequent need for additional external stabilizers, such as plaster casts, which are undesirable for other reasons.

1.4 Nailing without reaming, with locking ("unreamed solid nail")

Damage to cortical blood supply after reaming is reversible.

There was a manifest need for a small diameter solid nail that could be locked. While the absence of a slot considerably increases the torsional stiffness of the implant, it also carries a reduced capacity to adapt to the shape of the bone. If the insertion site is not optimally chosen or the shape and radius of the intramedullary canal diverge from those of the nail geometry, a proper "fit" may be a problem. With a smaller outer diameter (i.e., 9 mm) in the femur, the material strength of the nail must be reinforced to keep the risk of implant failure as low as

possible. Both of these demands (low stiffness and high fatigue strength) were met by a change of material from stainless steel to the titanium alloy Ti-6Al-7Nb. The higher strength of the nail allows the use of larger locking bolts of 4.2/4.9 mm diameter (initially 3.2/3.9 mm). The solid cross section of the nail does not add much to its mechanical bending properties but it does have biological advantages. **Results of animal experiments indicate that the susceptibility to infection is lower for the solid nail compared with the tubular nail with its inner dead space [4].** On the other hand, a hollow or cannulated system allows for the use of a guide wire, which makes nail insertion easier.

2 Pathophysiology of intramedullary nailing

2.1 Nailing with reaming

2.1.1 Local changes

Reaming the medullary cavity causes damage to the internal cortical blood supply, which, in animal experiments, was shown to be reversible within 8–12 weeks [5]. This reduced blood supply during the early weeks after trauma and reaming might account for the increased risk of infection, especially in open tibial fractures. Because of infection rates as high as 21% [6], the use of reamed intramedullary nails in open fractures, even on a delayed basis, was not recommended. Although new bone formation has been observed around reaming dust, and some viable bone cells have been identified in reaming products, the often cited osteo-inductive effect of such material remains controversial.

Since the femur has a good soft-tissue envelope, femoral shaft fractures are more often closed than open and treatment by intramedullary nailing is, therefore, more straightforward and less risky than for the tibia. The infection rates for grade I and grade II open fractures of the femur following reamed intramedullary nailing are 1–2%, whereas for open fractures with extensive soft-tissue injury (grade III) the infection rates range between 4–5% [7].

2.1.2 General changes

General changes, apart from several other effects of reaming, have to be considered. These include pulmonary embolization, temperature-related changes of the coagulation system and humoral, neural, and inflammatory reactions among others. The development of post-traumatic pulmonary failure (including ARDS) following early femoral nailing in the multiply injured patient is associated with the reaming process (see **chapter 5.3**). The passage of thrombi into the pulmonary circulation after reaming has been demonstrated in studies focusing on this topic [8, 9]. **Intramedullary nailing appears to be a particular insult to the patient's pulmonary system, especially in cases of polytrauma, since the lungs are very sensitive to any additional stress in the period immediately following trauma.**

The results of ongoing multicenter studies with large numbers of patients will hopefully help to indicate the actual risk of pulmonary complications. However, the advantages of unreamed nails are already emerging [10]. Any device introduced into the medullary canal (guide wire, reamer, nail) acts as a piston and forces the contents of the medullary cavity either through the fracture gap into the adjacent tissue or into the venous system. Wenda et al. [9], measuring intramedullary pressures intraoperatively, found values between 420–1,510 mm Hg with reaming procedures, as compared with 40–70 mm Hg in cases where solid nails were used without reaming. In addition, intraoperative transesophageal echocardiography showed solid emboli in the reamed group, which were not observed in the unreamed group.

In contrast to the reaming procedure, where the introduction of the reamer into the canal is repeated many times (up to twelve times for a 14 mm nail), the thinner solid nail without reaming is gently pushed into the diaphysis only once.

Nevertheless, there is a continuing controversy between those who recommend reamed nailing for all patients with severe trauma and those with concerns about its role in pulmonary impairment in multiply injured patients (see **chapter 5.3**).

2.2 Nailing without reaming

Smaller diameter implants are used in nail insertion without reaming. The benefits are less heat production and less disturbance of the endosteal blood supply. Although the insertion of thinner implants certainly disturbs the blood supply, it is to a lesser extent [11]. There is also considerably less bone necrosis, which appears to be one of the risk factors for the development of postoperative infection.

The susceptibility to experimentally induced infection has recently been studied, comparing solid with tubular nails in an animal model. The statistically significant results showed higher

Intramedullary nailing in severe trauma may cause respiratory distress.

susceptibility to infection in the group treated by tubular nails when compared to the solid nail group [12]. The dead space within the tubular nail is probably the main reason for the difference. The influence of nail diameter on blood perfusion and mechanical parameters was also studied in a dog model. Following segmental osteotomy of the tibia, it was shown that a loose-fitting nail did not affect cortical perfusion as much as a tight-fitting nail and it allowed more complete cortical revascularization at 11 weeks post-nailing. On the other hand, stiffness and load to failure were not found to be different [13]. These findings, therefore, have implications for the treatment of tibial shaft fractures with severe soft-tissue injury, in which the blood supply is significantly compromised [13].

3 General techniques

3.1 Preoperative planning and management

3.1.1 Patient positioning

The fracture table or a standard radiolucent operating table, with or without the use of the femoral distractor, are alternatives for patient positioning for femoral nailing. The use of a fracture table will maintain a defined reduction throughout the procedure, which might be helpful in the placement of reamed nails. However, positioning on the fracture table can put skin and neurovascular structures at risk and the setup process is time-consuming. Recent studies, without use of a fracture table, showed significantly shorter operation and anesthesia time compared to when either a

fracture table or femoral distractor was used [14]. Much depends, however, on personal experience and preference as well as on the OR-environment. With the unreamed nail, maintenance of accurate reduction is only necessary for the short period of time required to pass the nail from the proximal fragment into the distal main fragment. In reamed nailing, however, preservation of fracture reduction is required for every passage of the reamer and finally of the nail as well. Multiply injured patients with ipsilateral and/or bilateral tibial and/or femoral fractures can be treated on a regular table without the need to change either the position of the patient or the drapes. This appears to be safer and quicker [15]. A simple external fixator frame, or one constructed from the tubular external fixator and four tube-to-tube clamps, supports the injured leg, while padding the hollow of the knee helps to obtain gross reduction of the fracture in the tibia [16].

3.1.2 Sequence of stabilization in multiple extremity fractures

The recommended order for the treatment of closed fractures is: 1) femur; 2) tibia; 3) pelvis or spine; 4) upper limb. To follow this sequence, alternative methods were developed for the treatment of concomitant ipsilateral and/or bilateral fractures of the lower limb [15]. In multiple fractures of the lower limb, standardized stabilization protocols have been helpful for the sequence and method of stabilization according to the patient's condition (good, questionable, and critical). More recent techniques for intramedullary stabilization are no longer based on a fracture table but show a preference instead for the temporary use of a distractor [14, 17] (Table 3.3.1-1). This allows a single positioning and draping procedure for multiple fractures and semi-parallel fracture stabilization.

3.1.3 Correct implant selection

Preoperative selection of nail length

Templates are commonly recommended for the preoperative planning of intramedullary nailing. The accuracy of templates, however, is dependent upon the x-ray magnification. Unfortunately, there is currently no accepted standard for long bones, and magnification ranges from 10–20%. In a recent study, 200 randomly selected x-rays of femurs and tibias following fracture stabilization with an intra-

medullary nail were analyzed. The mean magnification factor in the femur was 1.09 and in the tibia 1.07 [18]. It was concluded that the templates currently used are highly unreliable for selecting correct nail length. Therefore, implant selection should be based on a x-ray of the intact contralateral bone or on intraoperative clinical or image intensifier-based measurements [15].

Intraoperative nail length selection with the use of radiolucent rulers or by clinical means

Intraoperative nail length measurement with a radiolucent ruler under C-arm control is an accurate method. If the proximal and distal ends of the bone are centered in the x-ray beam and the ruler is placed parallel to the diaphysis,

Table 3.3.1-1: Protocol [15] for the management of ipsilateral femoral and tibial fractures (floating knee) for patients in good, questionable, and critical condition.

Proposals for management of ipsilateral femoral and tibial fractures			
Step	**Patient condition stable**		**Patient condition questionable**	**Patient condition critical ISS > 40**
1	standard radiolucent table or fracture table, whole extremity draped			
2	**a) Femur** UFN retrograde	**a) Femur** distractor	**a) Femur** distractor	**a) Femur** external fixator
2	**b) Tibia** UTN	**b) Tibia** UTN	**b) Tibia** UTN	**b) Tibia** external fixator (standard or pinless)
3		**c) Femur** UFN antegrade	**c) Re-evaluation of the patient: if stable:** UFN femur **if unstable:** leave femoral distractor, ICU	
4			**d) Femur** UFN	**c) Tibia** UTN **d) Femur** UFN

Fig. 3.3.1-1:
Intraoperative determination of nail length with the use of the image intensifier.
a)–c) Highlights of potential sources of error. Note that these errors can occur in various combinations to produce different patterns of error.

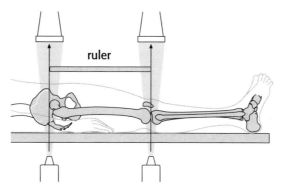

a) Correct position of patient, C-arm, and ruler parallel to the femur.

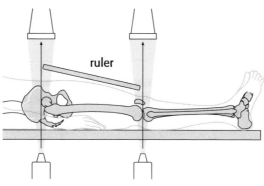

b) "Not parallel" ruler position results in too short a measurement.

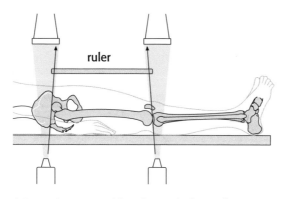

c) Excentric C-arm position also results in too short a measurement.

projection-induced misjudgment of implant length is minimized (**Fig. 3.3.1-1**).

An alternative nail length selection can be easily and accurately performed clinically. Landmarks are drawn on the skin using a sterile pen and measured by a ruler.

The proximal landmark in the femur is the tip of the greater trochanter, which is identified by touch and marked on the skin after the approach has been performed. The distal landmarks are the lateral knee joint space and/or the superior edge of the patella. In simple fracture patterns, one shot of the reduced fracture site (shortening?) with the image intensifier allows correct measurement and choice of a nail of appropriate size.

Proximal landmarks for the tibia are both the medial and lateral knee joint spaces; the distal point is the anterior part of the ankle joint with a dorsiflexed foot (**Video 3.3.1-1**).

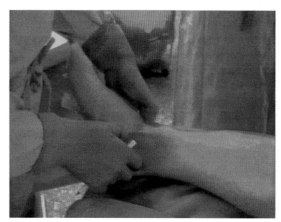

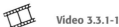 **Video 3.3.1-1**

Nail diameter

The radiolucent ruler also permits measurement of the implant diameter (**Video 3.3.1-2**). A technical trick for the selection of the cavity diameter during nailing is the use of the reamer head as a probe.

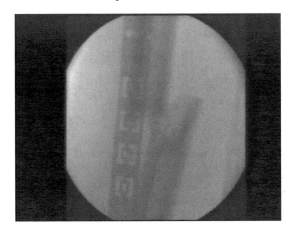

 Video 3.3.1-2

3.2 Insertion techniques

3.2.1 Surgical approach and preparation of the starting point

Several textbooks, including the AO Manual, recommend relatively long incisions for nail insertion. In intramedullary nailing without reaming, the approach can be much smaller for three reasons:
- The position of the starting hole is not identified by direct vision.
- A wide access to protect the soft tissues from the reamers is not needed.

- Clinical observation has shown that usually only the most proximal portion of these approaches is used. Stab incision techniques have been developed for the femur [15] and the tibia [16]. In both bones care must be taken to place the approaches in line with the axis of the medullary cavity and not too close to the chosen starting point on the bone (**Fig. 3.3.1-2**, **Fig. 3.3.1-3**).

These smaller approaches decrease blood loss [19] and reduce the risk of heterotopic ossification[20] at the tip of the trochanter.

3.2.2 Preparation of the starting point in antegrade femoral nailing

A correct starting point is crucial in intramedullary nailing. In the femur, flexion and adduction of the hip joint facilitate the approach for antegrade nailing. This measure decreases the length of the incision, especially in obese patients. The greater trochanter, lateral femoral condyle, and, if possible, the femoral shaft, are palpated and, if necessary, identified with a marker. A slightly curved line is drawn in a proximal direction corresponding to the curvature of the femur. A stab-incision about 3–5 cm long is made approximately 10 cm above the tip and towards the greater trochanter (**Fig. 3.3.1-3**). This allows insertion of a palpating finger alongside the implant (**Video 3.3.1-3**). Incisions should not be placed too posteriorly, since abductor muscle weakness has been recorded after nailing.

The guide wire is rarely perfectly positioned in both planes on the first attempt, especially in the femur. In these cases, a correct second pin is in-

A correct starting point is crucial in intramedullary nailing.

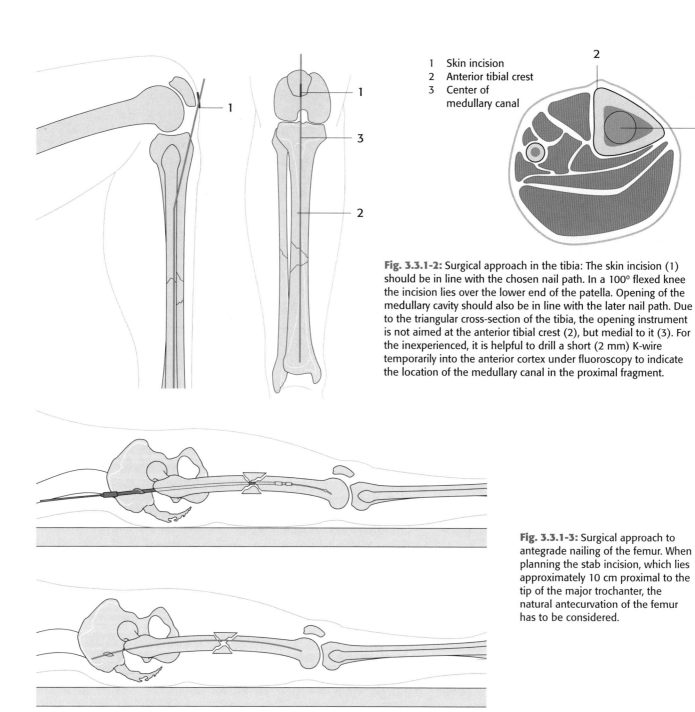

1 Skin incision
2 Anterior tibial crest
3 Center of
   medullary canal

Fig. 3.3.1-2: Surgical approach in the tibia: The skin incision (1) should be in line with the chosen nail path. In a 100° flexed knee the incision lies over the lower end of the patella. Opening of the medullary cavity should also be in line with the later nail path. Due to the triangular cross-section of the tibia, the opening instrument is not aimed at the anterior tibial crest (2), but medial to it (3). For the inexperienced, it is helpful to drill a short (2 mm) K-wire temporarily into the anterior cortex under fluoroscopy to indicate the location of the medullary canal in the proximal fragment.

Fig. 3.3.1-3: Surgical approach to antegrade nailing of the femur. When planning the stab incision, which lies approximately 10 cm proximal to the tip of the major trochanter, the natural antecurvation of the femur has to be considered.

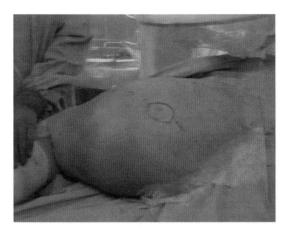

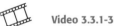
Video 3.3.1-3

serted using the initial wire as a reference. Once the starting point and direction are perfect, the malpositioned wire is removed (**Fig. 3.3.1-4**). A sleeve protects the soft tissues from the 13.0 mm cannulated drill bit that prepares the entry point.

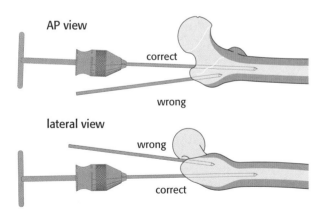

AP view

correct

wrong

lateral view

wrong

correct

Fig. 3.3.1-4: Technique for selection of starting point by entering the medullary cavity with the 3.2 mm guide wire and universal chuck with T-handle. The position of the guide wire is assessed in two planes by the image intensifier. If the position is not accurate, it must be corrected, as this may be decisive for the entire nailing procedure. The first wire is left in place as a reference for the second wire.

3.2.3 Preparation of the starting point in retrograde femoral nailing

For retrograde nailing of the femur, the knee is flexed approximately 30°. A guide wire is lined up with the midline of the medullary cavity of the distal femoral shaft using an image intensifier. The stab incision is placed in this line and a K-wire with a protection sleeve is pushed through the ligamentum patellae into the distal femur. Its position is also checked in a lateral view. Care must be taken that the origin of the posterior cruciate ligament (PCL) is not injured. The important landmark in the lateral view is the "Blumensaat's line", a radiodense line representing the cortical bone of the roof of the intercondylar notch of the femur.

3.2.4 Antegrade tibial nailing

In the tibia, a 15–20 mm stab incision using a large blade is made in line with the medullary cavity. The incision passes through skin and the patellar tendon at the inferior pole of the patella. The knee is flexed as much as possible (**Fig. 3.3.1-2**). The proximal anterior edge of the tibia can be easily identified by palpation with the sharp tip of the guide pin.

The 4.0 mm centering pin, mounted on an universal chuck with T-handle, is pushed through the thin cortex in the direction of the center of the medullary canal. The position may be checked with image intensification. The protection sleeve for the cannulated cutter is placed through the stab incision and through the patellar ligament directly onto the bone. The cannulated cutter ("cheese cutter") for the medullary canal cuts out a cylinder of cortico-cancellous bone, which may be used as bone

When using short incisions for "minimal" approaches careful planning with identification of the landmarks is essential.

The choice of the correct entry point is crucial for the whole procedure.

Never ream with an inflated tourniquet on the limb.

Closed reduction of fractures is more difficult in the femur than in the tibia.

Design of reamers and reamer shaft influences intramedullary pressure and temperature.

graft. For proximal fractures and in order to prevent malalignment, it is essential to place the starting point exactly in line with the center of the medullary cavity.

3.2.5 Floating knee: retrograde femoral nailing and antegrade tibial nailing

In the case of retrograde femoral and antegrade tibial nailing, both nail insertions can be performed through the same skin incision. In this situation the surgeon must ensure that the incision is proximal enough to allow insertion of the retrograde nail (close to the patella).

3.2.6 Technique of reaming

For fresh fractures, power reamers are more convenient and faster than hand reamers. However, for more difficult situations, (i.e., pseudarthrosis with sclerosis of the medullary cavity) specially designed hand reamers are safer and more effective. Besides the problems of pressure rise and heat production by reaming, the influence of reamer design (cutting flutes, geometry and diameter of the reamer shaft, sharpness of reamers, etc.) was analyzed. It was shown that **blunt reamers, small flutes, high axial forces, and large diameters of the reamer shaft cause increased pressure and temperature [21]**. It was shown by Pape [8] that the risk of pulmonary embolization depends to some extent on different reamer constructions.

The efficacy of a distal venting hole is strongly dependent on its diameter and a proposed flushing technique of the medullary canal is not yet widely in use, but it may decrease the risk of complications. **Never ream**

with an inflated tourniquet as the normal circulation is an effective "cooling system".

3.3 Reduction techniques

3.3.1 Considerations for the reduction maneuvers in antegrade femoral nailing

For several reasons, **femoral fractures are usually more difficult to reduce than tibial fractures:**
- A thicker soft-tissue envelope and less direct access to bone.
- A somewhat hidden starting point.
- The presence of the iliotibial tract, which tends to shorten the fracture if the leg is adducted.

The demands of each step in femoral nailing may create a conflict with the others.

3.3.2 Reduction of tibial fractures

The most effective and gentle instruments for reducing fresh tibial fractures are our hands. In contrast to the femur, large parts of the tibia, especially the anterior crest, are easily palpated. Since most fractures are simple A and B types in the midshaft or distal diaphysis, they are quite suitable for simple manual reduction during implant insertion. Temporary over-correction of the fracture zone during nail passage is sometimes advantageous and helpful in oblique fractures. With the tip of the un-reamed nail, the distal fragment can be "felt" during manipulation. Once the nail has engaged in the medullary canal of the distal main fragment, this can be recognized immediately by the increase in stiffness.

Positioning of leg in antegrade femoral nailing

Steps	Problem	Solution
1. Starting point and nail insertion in proximal main fragment.	In neutral position, soft tissues and iliac crest prevent easy access.	AD-duction and flexion of the proximal femur or entire leg.
2. Passing the nail into the distal main fragment.	In adducted position, the iliotibial tract is under tension and shortens the fracture.	AB-duction or neutral position of the distal main fragment with the proximal main fragment in neutral position.

3.3.3 Reduction aids

While reduction of fresh fractures for closed intramedullary nailing is rarely a problem, most situations of delayed nailing require additional tools to overcome shortening and to control axial alignment.

The simplest "towel-sling" and "beanbag" techniques are easy, non-invasive, and cheap ways to manipulate the main fragments. However, they are rather imprecise and not suitable for adjusting the length. In the tibia, pointed reduction clamps are best used, since they can be applied percutaneously or through an open wound, without additional soft-tissue trauma.

The use of temporarily inserted Schanz screws is an effective way to get direct contact with the bone. This is especially helpful in femoral or delayed tibial fractures [15, 16]. Three principles have to be respected:
- Screw placement as close to the fracture as possible.
- Unicortical insertion in the proximal fragment.
- Connection with universal chuck with T-handle for easier manipulation.

There are two planes in which reduction has to be controlled: frontal, or AP, and sagittal, or lateral. Use of the image intensifier can be reduced by fixing universal chucks with T-handle to the Schanz screws and analyzing their position relative to each other. Furthermore, tactile control of the main fragments may also decrease the need for a C-arm (**Fig. 3.3.1-5**).

Reduction for closed nailing in fresh fractures is rarely a problem; for delayed nailing additional tools may be needed.

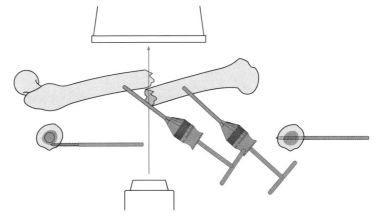

Fig. 3.3.1-5: The use of Schanz screws for reduction. In the proximal fragment the Schanz screws are placed in one cortex, in the distal fragment in both. With two universal chucks with T-handle the fragments are manipulated under C-arm control (AP view). The orientation in the sagittal plane is obtained by "feeling" the fragments touching each other.

In cases of delayed nailing with shortening of the limb, the use of the large distractor may be essential for restitution of length and axis [17]. Care has to be taken, since the single Schanz screw tends to bend and rotate under strain. If a distractor is not available, a tube-to-tube construct and a distraction tool can be used for the same purpose (**Fig. 3.3.1-6**).

Nailing of fractures in the metaphysis is associated with a higher rate of malalignment. A strong muscle pull [22] and, often, a wide medullary canal can lead to post-fixation instability, even with locking [16]. Blocking screws, placed adjacent to the nail, have been proposed as a possible solution to prevent lateral or medial translation in both the tibia [16] and the femur [15]. These screws, also called Poller screws, decrease the width of the metaphyseal medullary canal, forcing the nail to the center of the bone, thereby also increasing the mechanical stiffness of the bone-implant-construct. Poller screws can be used for: 1) alignment, 2) stabilization, and 3) manipulation. The screw is placed perpendicular to the direction in which the implant might displace (**Fig. 3.3.1-7**).

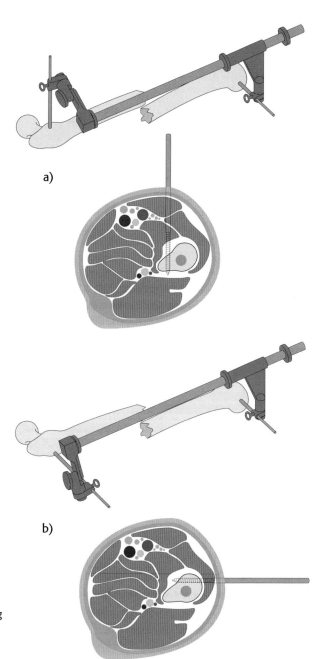

a)

b)

Fig. 3.3.1-6: The use of a distractor for reduction.
a) Standard application of the large distractor. Proximally, the AP Schanz screw is inserted just proximal to the lesser trochanter and medial to the nail path and lateral to the medial cortex. In the cross-section (insert) the "safe" relation of this Schanz screw to the neurovascular structures can be appreciated.
b) Alternative application, with both Schanz screws coming from lateral. The proximal Schanz screw usually interferes with the insertion handle of the nail, so that the distractor has to be removed before the nail is fully introduced.

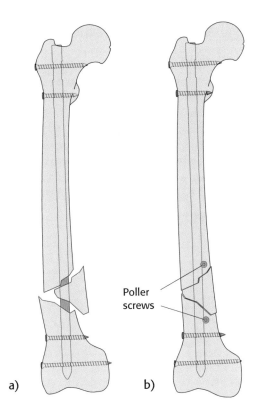
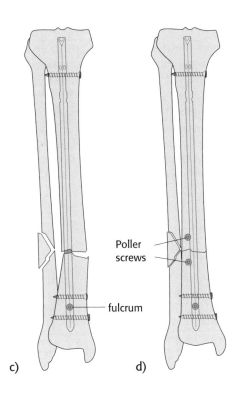

a) b) c) d)

Fig. 3.3.1-7: With the aid of Poller screws, undesirable nail positions, as well as malalignments, can be prevented or corrected while simultaneously stability is increased.
a) Example of a distal femur fracture: Due to the large discrepancy between medullary canal and nail diameter, the nail may slide a few millimeters along the locking bolts, which results in varus deformity and instability.
b) Placement of one (distal) or two (distal and proximal) Poller screws prevents malalignment and increases stability.
c) Example of a distal tibia fracture: Despite the presence of an AP screw, displacement in the frontal plane can occur in cases of short distal fragments or poor bone stock. The AP screw acts as a fulcrum in these cases.
d) Closed reduction and either unilateral or bilateral support with Poller screws placed bicortically in the sagittal direction prevents angulation in the frontal plane.

Poller screws

Poller screws

fulcrum

In oblique metaphyseal fractures of the distal tibia or femur the Poller screw may help with stabilizing, because shear forces are transformed into compression forces (**Video 3.3.1-4**).

The Poller screw may help to prevent displacement in situations where a previously malplaced nail tends to slip again into the old nail path. Similarly, it can also be used in situations where the antegrade starting point, for example, in the tibia, was originally badly chosen, forcing the proximal bone fragment into malalignment. In this situation, the nail has to be removed temporarily and the Poller screw placed to block the incorrect path, while the nail is reinserted (**Fig. 3.3.1-8**).

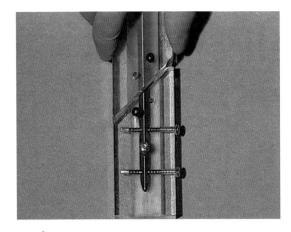

Video 3.3.1-4

Use of an extra wide tourniquet as a reduction tool for closed tibial fractures is also possible. Inflation of the circumferential aircushion and simultaneous longitudinal traction bring about smooth reduction and temporary stabilization. In addition, the tourniquet can be combined with the distractor [23]. However, this technique carries certain risks in cases of fractures with severe soft-tissue injury. The application time should be as short as possible and reaming must never be done with the tourniquet inflated.

3.3.4 Sequence of locking

Nails may produce fracture distraction upon insertion by pushing the distal fragment. This causes a sharp rise in compartment pressure and may delay fracture healing. In a statically locked diastasis, the weight-bearing load is directly transmitted to the locking screws, which will eventually fail. Axial deformities are also more likely to develop, especially in distal metaphyseal fractures. In contrast to the pre-

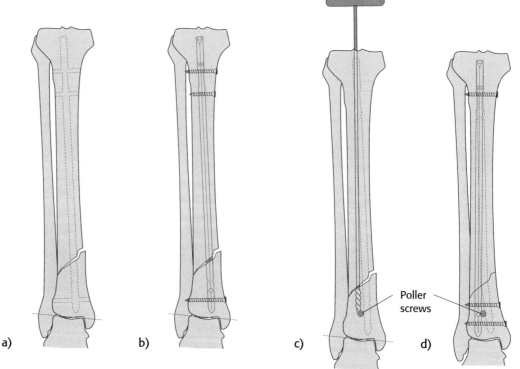

a)   b)   c)   d)

Poller screws

Fig. 3.3.1-8: Poller screws as reduction tool.
a) Schematic drawing of a clinical case: After nail removal a refracture occurred which healed in valgus malalignment.
b) Since the original nail path is sclerotic, the new nail follows the pre-existing path with the same malalignment.
c) This problem can be solved with a Poller screw as a reduction tool: The nail is temporarily removed. The Poller screw is placed in the old nail path, to block it, while a new path is prepared with a hand reamer.
d) Once the new nail path has been prepared, the Poller screw remains in place and the new nail is reinserted and locked.

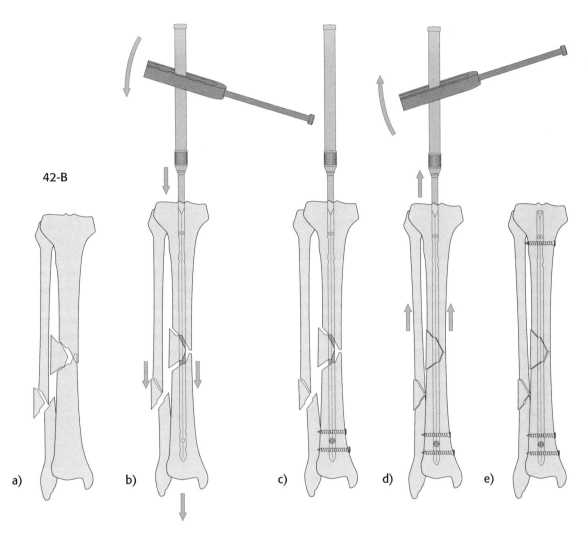

42-B

a)   b)   c)   d)   e)

vious manuals and teaching videos, we now recommend locking of the distal end as a first step [16]. This gives the opportunity to apply the "backstroke technique", which adapts and compresses the fracture fragments after distal locking (**Fig. 3.3.1-9**). If the nail length has been correctly chosen, there should be no problem; otherwise the nail may protrude proximally by a few millimeters.

Fig. 3.3.1-9:
Backstroke technique for correction of fragment diastasis.
a/b) Insertion of an unreamed nail frequently results in fracture distraction, which may worsen a compartment syndrome and delay healing.
c) Distal locking first with three locking bolts (increasing strength).
d) Careful backstrokes under fluoroscopic control until main fragments are reduced or the planned length is achieved.
e) Proximal locking, dynamic or static, according to fracture pattern and fracture location. If the nail is proud proximally, a shorter one should be chosen.

3.3.5 Intraoperative techniques for the control of alignment

Length

Doing the distal locking first brings the additional advantage that the distal fragment is fixed to the nail. Any further reduction maneuvers can be performed with the insertion handle. After distal locking of all C fractures and certain A1 and B1 fractures, the reduction, especially length, should be radiologically assessed.

In femoral fractures the upper margin of the femoral head is brought into line with the measuring device under image intensification (see **Fig. 3.3.1-1**). This has the length of the contralateral femur marked on it with a clip (femoral head—lateral femoral condyle). Subsequently, the knee joint is viewed and any length discrepancy can be measured between the lateral femoral condyle and the position of the clip. By using a ram with handle, limb length can be continuously adjusted in both directions (**Fig. 3.3.1-10**). The length of the tibia is much easier to evaluate than that of the femur and clinical means are usually sufficient.

Frontal-sagittal plane

In simple midshaft fractures of the femur and tibia, frontal and sagittal plane alignment is usually not a problem. While CCD angles can be measured and checked by fluoroscopy, the evaluation of the correct weight-bearing axis is usually more difficult, especially in complex, multifragmented, or metaphyseal fractures.

The recently described "cable-technique" greatly facilitates intraoperative assessment of axis in the frontal plane. With the patella facing anteriorly, the centers of the femoral head and of the ankle joint are marked under fluoroscopy either on the skin or the surgical sheets. The long cable of electrocautery is then spanned between these two points with the image intensifier centered on the knee joint. Varus/valgus alignment can now be determined using the projection of the cable (**Fig. 3.3.1-11**). The sagittal alignment is determined using a lateral fluoroscopic image.

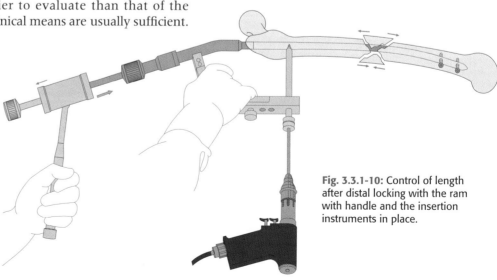

Fig. 3.3.1-10: Control of length after distal locking with the ram with handle and the insertion instruments in place.

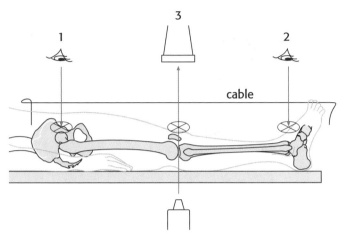

Fig. 3.3.1-11: Cable technique for checking alignment in the frontal plane: The knee is fully extended and the patella must face anteriorly. Step 1) With the image intensifier beam strictly vertical, the center of the femoral head is centered on the screen. A pen then marks the center of the femoral head on the patient's skin. Step 2) In a similar way the center of the ankle joint is marked. An assistant now spans the cable of the electrocautery between these two landmarks. Step 3) When the knee joint is viewed the cable should run centrally. Any deviation of the projected cautery cable from the center of the joint indicates the axial deviation in the frontal plane.

Rotation

There are several methods for intraoperative assessment of the rotation of nailed fractures of the femur and the tibia:

Clinical judgment is not very precise and depends on the position of the patient and the leg during surgery. Preoperatively, the rotation of the intact limb is established with the knee and the hip flexed at 90°. Intraoperatively, after nailing and temporary locking of the fractured bone, the rotation is checked again. To do this correctly the insertion handle has to be removed.

In the tibia, rotation should be checked with the knee in flexion and the foot dorsiflexed. However, as well as comparing the position of the feet, the range and symmetry of foot rotation has also to be taken into account.

Several signs have recently been described for x-ray assessment of femoral rotation. These include the shape of the lesser trochanter, the cortical step sign, and the sign of the diameter difference [15].

The x-ray contour of the lesser trochanter in relation to the proximal femoral shaft depends on the rotation of the bone. Preoperatively, the shape of the lesser trochanter of the uninjured

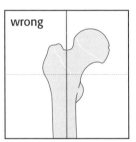 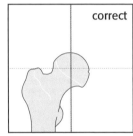 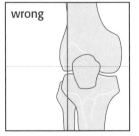 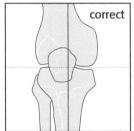 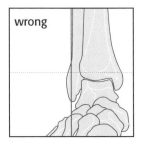 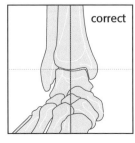

wrong | correct (×3)

Cable technique, lesser trochanter sign, cortical step sign, and cortical thickness are all useful to assess the correctness of reduction.

limb with the patella facing anteriorly is analyzed and stored in the fluoroscope. Before proximal locking, with the patella facing anteriorly, the proximal fragment may be rotated around the nail, using a Schanz screw, until the shape of the lesser trochanter appears to be symmetrical with the stored image of the uninjured side. In the case of an external malrotation, the lesser trochanter is smaller because it is partially hidden by the femoral shaft. With internal malrotation, however, the lesser trochanter looks bigger [15] (**Fig. 3.3.1-12** and **Video 3.3.1-5**).

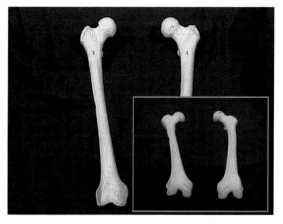

Video 3.3.1-5

Fig. 3.3.1-12: Intraoperative radiological assessment of rotation with comparison of the shape of the lesser trochanter with the contralateral side (lesser trochanter shape sign).
a) Before positioning the patient, the shape of the lesser trochanter of the intact opposite side (patella facing anteriorly) is stored in the image intensifier.
b) After distal locking and the patella facing anteriorly, the proximal fragment is rotated until the shape of the lesser trochanter matches the one of the intact side already stored.
c) In cases of external malrotation the lesser trochanter is smaller and partially hidden behind the proximal femoral shaft.
d) In cases of internal malrotation the lesser trochanter appears enlarged.

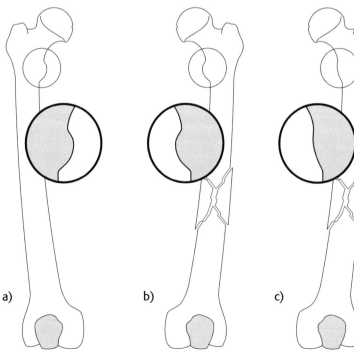
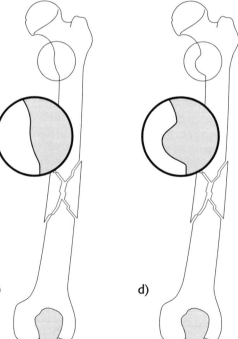

a)   b)   c)   d)

In transverse or short oblique fractures the correct rotation may be judged by the thickness of the cortices of the proximal and distal main fragments (cortical step sign). This is less sensitive, however, than the sign of the lesser trochanter [15] (**Fig. 3.3.1-13**).

The sign of bone diameter is positive at levels where the bone diameter is oval, rather than round. In cases of malrotation, the transverse diameters of proximal and distal fragments are projected with different diameters. Again, this sign also is much less sensitive[15] (**Fig. 3.3.1-13**).

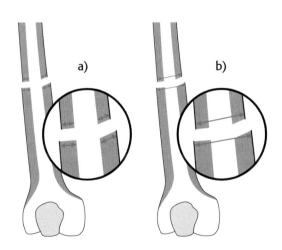

a)   b)

Fig. 3.3.1-13: Radiological signs of malrotation depending on the cortical thickness and the bone diameter.
a) Cortical step sign: In the presence of a considerable rotational deformity, this can be diagnosed by the different thickness of the cortices.
b) Diameter difference sign: This sign is positive at levels where the bone cross-section is oval rather than round. With malrotation, the diameters of proximal and distal main fragments appear to be of different sizes.

3.3.6 Reduction techniques for delayed cases and non-unions

In delayed cases, and depending on the time interval, we are faced with the following problems:

- Axial deformation (shortening, angulation, and/or translation).
- Connective tissue ingrowth and early callus formation making reduction difficult.
- Sclerosis at the fracture site with sealed medullary cavity and osteoporosis of the main fragments.

These conditions make intramedullary nailing difficult, because instruments (reamer) and nails are easily deflected and tend to penetrate the cortex in the wrong direction. While angular deformities can be corrected by the use of a distractor, an offset due to fragment translation is much more difficult to overcome.

In these situations, the use of Poller screws, as already described in **section 3.3.4**, helps to guide instruments and implants in the desired direction. Alternatively, plates may be used.

3.3.7 Techniques for prevention of malalignment

Selection of the correct starting point in the proximal fragment and a central nail position in the distal fragment are the most important points to observe in order to avoid varus-valgus and antecurvatum deformities.

In malunions and non-unions nailing may be difficult. Alternatively plates can be used.

In the case of a proximal or distal metaphyseal fracture, the relatively loose contact between locking screws and nail may lead to malalignment, but this can be used to correct malalignment as well. An increase in the stability of the bone-implant construct can be obtained with the temporary addition of external fixation devices, (pinless or standard), Poller screws, or plates (see **Fig. 3.3.1-8**).

In unreamed nailing the use of locking bolts is mandatory.

3.4 Fixation techniques/ interlocking

3.4.1 Interlocking screws

While locking is advisable in reamed nailing, it is mandatory in unreamed nailing, since the nails used here are thinner. Stable fracture patterns are locked in a dynamic mode, which allows for axial compression, but prevents rotational instability. Distal interlocking may be done with the free-hand technique, using a radiolucent drive and fluoroscopy. Proximal interlocking is performed through the guide attached to the insertion handle.

Distally, at least two (femur) or three (tibia) interlocking screws are recommended for the following reasons:

As there is no tight fit between the locking screws and nail, "toggling" may occur. This can lead to instability and malalignment, especially in the frontal plane. The insertion of two (femur) or three (tibia) distal screws, which are usually not quite parallel, reduces the toggling.

Breakage of locking bolts is dependent on implant material, design, surface finishing, and cross sectional area as well as on the amount of load applied and the number of cycles. With smaller diameter nails (unreamed systems), the locking bolts are of smaller diameter, which may result in more screw breakage. This is, however, clinically not relevant in the vast majority of cases. Since the distal interlocking screws are usually the weakest part in the nailing system, we recommend using the full range of locking options, especially in the distal tibia [25].

3.4.2 Technique for distal interlocking without fluoroscopy (DAD)

Radiation exposure during nailing procedures continues to be a controversial issue. Every attempt should be made to develop aiming devices that are precise, reliable, and easy to apply without fluoroscopy.

Recently, a radiation-independent proximally mounted distal aiming device (DAD) has been developed for solid intramedullary nails, which do not undergo any significant torque upon insertion. The DAD is based on an aiming arm which is readjusted to the deformed nail through a distal working channel and an asymmetric spacer. In a prospective randomized study using human leg specimens, the DAD and the radiolucent drill guide were compared in the hands of inexperienced surgeons measuring the radiation and operating time. In the DAD group, fluoroscopy time was significantly shorter, while failure rates were equal in both groups. However, the operating time was longer with DAD (**Fig. 3.3.1-14** and **Video 3.3.1-6**).

Locking protocol tibia

Segment	Fracture type	Proximal locking pattern
3–5	All A3 Well-adapted B2-3, C2 fractures	Dynamic hole
3–5	All A1-2, B1 Insufficiently adapted B2-3, C2 All C1 and C3 fractures	Static + dynamic hole
1–2	All A, B, and C fractures	Static + dynamic + oblique hole

Table 3.3.1-2: Location refers to the most proximal extension of the fracture in the proximal half of the tibia, and to the distal aspect of the fracture in the distal half of the tibia.

Distally, all three locking options are used. Proximal in the first and second fifth, always use three screws. Fractures in segment 3–5 are locked according to fracture type.

In the tibia distal locking must always comprise all three possibilities.

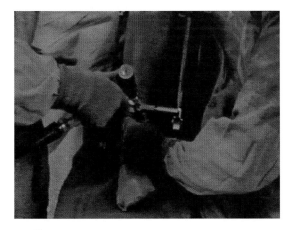

Video 3.3.1-6

3.4.3   Dynamization

In the femur, dynamization of statically locked nails is rarely necessary. In the tibia, it may be recommended (in combination with bone graft) **for certain fracture patterns** with a high risk of delayed fracture healing [**24**]. The best time seems to be 2–3 months after initial surgery; the removal of one or both locking bolts proximally can be done on an outpatient basis.

Dynamization is rarely necessary in the femur, while in the tibia it may be recommended for certain fracture patterns.

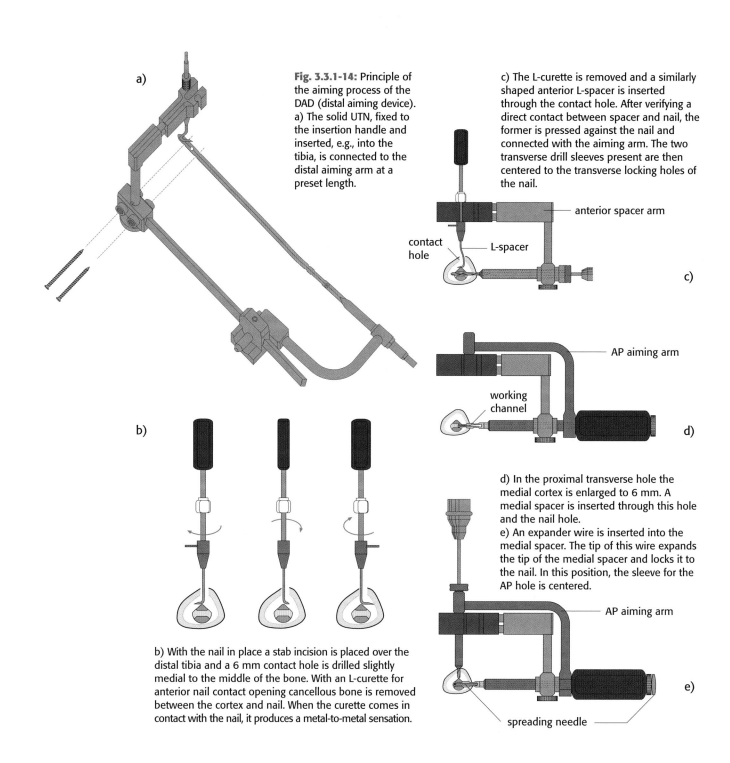

a)

Fig. 3.3.1-14: Principle of the aiming process of the DAD (distal aiming device).
a) The solid UTN, fixed to the insertion handle and inserted, e.g., into the tibia, is connected to the distal aiming arm at a preset length.

c) The L-curette is removed and a similarly shaped anterior L-spacer is inserted through the contact hole. After verifying a direct contact between spacer and nail, the former is pressed against the nail and connected with the aiming arm. The two transverse drill sleeves present are then centered to the transverse locking holes of the nail.

anterior spacer arm

contact hole

L-spacer

c)

AP aiming arm

working channel

d)

d) In the proximal transverse hole the medial cortex is enlarged to 6 mm. A medial spacer is inserted through this hole and the nail hole.
e) An expander wire is inserted into the medial spacer. The tip of this wire expands the tip of the medial spacer and locks it to the nail. In this position, the sleeve for the AP hole is centered.

AP aiming arm

b)

b) With the nail in place a stab incision is placed over the distal tibia and a 6 mm contact hole is drilled slightly medial to the middle of the bone. With an L-curette for anterior nail contact opening cancellous bone is removed between the cortex and nail. When the curette comes in contact with the nail, it produces a metal-to-metal sensation.

spreading needle

e)

4 Contraindications

The development of new nails designed for different indications has greatly expanded the spectrum of nailing in terms of fracture location, fracture pattern, soft-tissue damage, and concomitant injuries. **There are, however, still several biological and mechanical concerns or contraindications for nailing,** which include:

- Infection at the entry site, within the medullary canal, at pin sites, or sepsis.
- Femoral fracture(s) in the multiply injured patient with pulmonary trauma, where temporary stabilization by external fixation or plating is advocated.
- Metaphyseal fractures where fixation of locking bolts may be insufficient to control malalignment.

5 Bibliography

1. **Küntscher G** (1962) *Praxis der Marknagelung.* Stuttgart: Schattauer.

2. **Kempf I, Grosse A, Beck G** (1985) Closed locked intramedullary nailing. Its application to comminuted fractures of the femur. *J Bone Joint Surg [Am];* 67 (5):709–720.

3. **Krettek C, Miclau T, Blauth M, et al.** (1997) Recurrent rotational deformity of the femur after static locking of intramedullary nails: case reports. *J Bone Joint Surg [Br];* 79 (1):4–8.

4. **Melcher GA, Claudi B, Schlegel U, et al.** (1994) Influence of type of medullary nail on the development of local infection. An experimental study of solid and slotted nails in rabbits. *J Bone Joint Surg [Br];* 76 (6):955–959.

5. **Schemitsch EH, Kowalski MJ, Swiontkowski MF, et al.** (1994) Cortical bone blood flow in reamed and unreamed locked intramedullary nailing: a fractured tibia model in sheep. *J Orthop Trauma;* 8 (5):373–382.

6. **Wiss DA, Stetson WB** (1995) Unstable fractures of the tibia treated with a reamed intramedullary interlocking nail. *Clin Orthop;* (315):56–63.

7. **Brumback RJ, Ellison PS, Jr., Poka A, et al.** (1989) Intramedullary nailing of open fractures of the femoral shaft. *J Bone Joint Surg [Am];* 71 (9):1324–1331.

8. **Pape HC, Krettek C, Maschek H, et al.** (1996) Fatal pulmonary embolization after reaming of the femoral medullary cavity in sclerosing osteomyelitis: a case report. *J Orthop Trauma;* 10 (6):429–432.

9. **Wenda K, Ritter G, Degreif J, et al.** (1988) [Pathogenesis of pulmonary complications following intramedullary nailing osteosyntheses]. *Unfallchirurg;* 91 (9):432–435.

10. **Pape HC, Regel G, Dwenger A, et al.** (1993) Influences of different methods of intramedullary femoral nailing on lung function in patients with multiple trauma. *J Trauma;* 35 (5):709–716.

11. **Klein MP, Rahn BA, Frigg R, et al.** (1990) Reaming versus non-reaming in medullary nailing: interference with cortical circulation of the canine tibia. *Arch Orthop Trauma Surg;* 109 (6):314–316.

12. **Melcher GA, Metzdorf A, Schlegel U, et al.** (1995) Influence of reaming versus non-reaming in intramedullary nailing on local infection rate: experimental investigation in rabbits. *J Trauma;* 39 (6):1123–1128.

In spite of many new nail designs, there remain valid contradictions for nailing of long bone fractures.

13. **Hupel TM, Aksenov SA, Schemitsch EH** (1998) Cortical bone blood flow in loose and tight fitting locked unreamed intramedullary nailing: a canine segmental tibia fracture model. *J Orthop Trauma;* 12 (2):127–135.

14. **McFerran MA, Johnson KD** (1992) Intramedullary nailing of acute femoral shaft fractures without a fracture table: technique of using a femoral distractor. *J Orthop Trauma;* 6 (3):271–278.

15. **Krettek C, Rudolf J, Schandelmaier P, et al.** (1996) Unreamed intramedullary nailing of femoral shaft fractures: operative technique and early clinical experience with the standard locking option. *Injury;* 27 (Suppl 4):233–254.

16. **Krettek C, Schandelmaier P, Tscherne H** (1995) Non-reamed interlocking nailing of closed tibial fractures with severe soft-tissue injury. *Clin Orthop;* (315):34–47.

17. **Baumgaertel F, Dahlen C, Stiletto R, et al.** (1994) Technique of using the AO femoral distractor for femoral intramedullary nailing. *J Orthop Trauma;* 8 (4):315–321.

18. **Krettek C, Blauth M, Miclau T, et al.** (1996) Accuracy of intramedullary templates in femoral and tibial radiographs. *J Bone Joint Surg [Br];* 78 (6):963–964.

19. **Tornetta P, III, Tiburzi D** (1997) The treatment of femoral shaft fractures using intramedullary interlocked nails with and without intramedullary reaming: a preliminary report. *J Orthop Trauma;* 11 (2):89–92.

20. **Furlong AJ, Giannoudis PV, Smith RM** (1997) Heterotopic ossification: a comparison between reamed and unreamed femoral nailing. *Injury;* 28 (Suppl 1):9–14.

21. **Müller C, Frigg R, Pfister U** (1993) Effect of flexible drive diameter and reamer design on the increase of pressure in the medullary cavity during reaming. *Injury;* 24 (Suppl 3):40–47.

22. **Freedman EL, Johnson EE** (1995) Radiographic analysis of tibial fracture malalignment following intramedullary nailing. *Clin Orthop;* (315):25–33.

23. **Ryf C, Melcher GA, Rüedi T** (1993) Pneumatic tournique as a repositioning aid in closed intramedullary nailing. *Unfallchirurg;* 98:617–619.

24. **Bone LB, Kassman S, Stegemann P, et al.** (1994) Prospective study of union rate of open tibial fractures treated with locked, unreamed intramedullary nails. *J Orthop Trauma;* 8 (1):45–49.

25. **Hajek PD, Bicknell HR, Jr., Bronson WE, et al.** (1993) The use of one compared with two distal screws in the treatment of femoral shaft fractures with interlocking intramedullary nailing. A clinical and biomechanical analysis. *J Bone Joint Surg [Am];* 75 (4):519–525.

6 Updates

Updates and additional references for this chapter are available online at:
http://www.aopublishing.org/PFxM/331.htm

220

3.3.2

3.3.2 Bridge plating

Fred Baumgaertel

1 Introduction

In general, plate fixation of fractures represents a form of stabilization with load bearing and load sharing properties. Functional treatment of the limb for preservation of muscle strength, coordination, and joint mobility depends on the stability provided by the plate-bone construct. Fracture consolidation is to be expected if the mechanics of fixation and the biology of the fracture are compatible and mutually beneficial.

Biological or bridge plating uses the plate as an extramedullary splint fixed to the two main fragments, while the complex fracture zone is virtually left untouched, or rather bridged, by the plate. **This concept combines adequate mechanical stability offered by the plate with uncompromised natural fracture biology to achieve rapid interfragmentary callus formation and fracture consolidation.** Bridge plating techniques are applicable to all long bone fractures where complex fragmentation is present and which are not suitable for intramedullary nailing (**Fig. 3.3.2-1**).

With "classical" direct open fracture reduction and rigid plate fixation, the viability not only of soft tissues but also of the fragments may be jeopardized. This risk occurs to a lesser degree in simple than in multifragmentary fractures. Indeed, it is the concern to maintain the vascularity at the fracture site which creates such a strong indication for the use of bridging techniques in fracture patterns with significant fragmentation.

In type C fractures of the diaphysis (see **chapter 1.4**), the endosteal blood supply of fragments is, as a rule, interrupted. Preservation of bone vitality relies predominantly on periosteal vascularity, which is also responsible for fracture healing. In the absence of mechanical continuity between the two main fragments, maintenance of stability becomes a function of the bridging plate. Wide exposure, with periosteal stripping for precise fragment reduction, and fixation by interfragmentary compression and plating carry the risk of higher rates of bone-healing complications in type C fractures [1–7]. **Mechanistic thinking and technique, together with misapplication and misinterpretation of the principles of interfragmentary compression, are probably responsible for most failures.**

An attempt to reconstruct anatomically and rigidly fix a widely fragmented fracture area is to be considered a precarious undertaking and will most probably result in some sort of complications, followed by loss of stability and implant failure or, in the worst case, by infection.

In bridge plating the plate acts as an extramedullary splint.

Biological plating combines adequate stability with uncompromised biology.

Misinterpretation of principles and misapplied techniques are responsible for most failures.

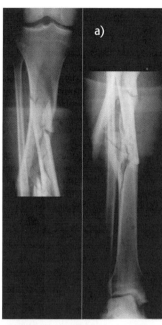
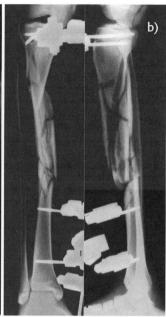

Fig. 3.3.2-1:
a) Complex fracture of tibia and fibula (42-C) not suitable for nailing with severely compromised soft tissues in a 41-year-old polytrauma patient (ISS = 48) after MVA.
b) As emergency fixation a conventional unilateral external fixator was applied. In the same session, the opposite femur was plated and the femoral neck fixed with screws while the other tibia was nailed.

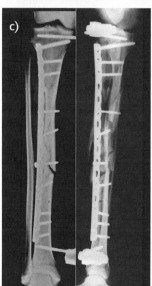
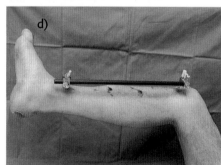
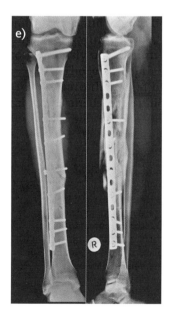

c) With the external fixator in place to hold alignment, 3 weeks after the injury, a contoured 16-hole LC-DCP was pushed through a short incision from the tibial plateau along the lateral side of the tibia and fixed with percutaneously applied 4.5 mm cortex screws, some as lag screws. To provide a medial support, the external fixator was retained with one pin in each main fragment.
d) Clinical aspect 8 weeks after the accident.
e) X-ray follow-up at 29 weeks.

However, in type C fractures of the metaphyses, including articular fractures (see **chapter 2.3**) with various degrees of fragmentation, anatomical reconstruction and rigid fixation of the joint surface is paramount, while the metaphyseal bone, given its good healing qualities, will withstand a higher degree of iatrogenic damage from manipulation than will the diaphysis. The endangered area is not the metaphysis but its junction with the more compact bone of the diaphysis. These regions of transition remain under continuous bending loads and show a distinct tendency to delay or failure of fracture healing. In any bone deprived of the possibility of developing adequate callus, fracture fixation is likely to fail. In the past, therefore, liberal use of bone grafting was advocated and indeed, if biology is ignored, bone grafting had to assume the role of problem solver.

The current plating concepts embrace the principle of placing biology before mechanics. This development has led to a more flexible and individual approach to internal fixation, based on the nature and severity or the personality of a fracture.

Simple type A diaphyseal fractures require a high degree of mechanical stability, which can be obtained quite well by compression plating or intramedullary nailing. In type C fractures involving not only two main fragments but numerous intermediate pieces, the fixation device must allow for some micromovements between the different fragments, thereby stimulating the healing process, for example, callus formation. **Tissue strain within minimal ranges enhances bone healing by producing callus** [8]. If, for example, a complex, multifragmentary fracture, rather than being anatomically reduced, is splinted, for example, in a cast, the movement between intermediate but viable fragments will be minimal, while the system as a whole will tolerate a significant amount of deformation. This allows tissue differentiation to progress and callus formation between intermediate fragments occurs rapidly, even in the presence of considerable fragment diastases. Prerequisites for the success of bone healing under such conditions are optimal preservation of fragment vascularity and a favorable mechanical and cellular environment for the production of callus. Bone fragments, once they have been stripped of their soft-tissue attachments (periosteum, muscles, etc.), will not be incorporated into the early callus formation.

The surgeon attempting operative stabilization of a complex multifragmentary fracture must therefore be able to reduce the fracture without interfering with the blood supply and, at the same time, apply a fixation device that provides adequate fixation while also stimulating callus healing.

2 Indirect reduction techniques

(see **chapter 3.1**)

Biological or bridge plating is usually applied following some form of indirect reduction.

The goal of indirect reduction is to achieve preliminary alignment of a fractured bone, either before any attempt at internal fixation is made or in conjunction with a fixation device [9–12]. The mechanical principle underlying indirect reduction is distraction and applies to diaphyseal as well as to metaphyseal bone. The muscular envelope surrounding the diaphysis of most long bones provides a logical rationale for indirect reduction, since a controlled pull on

The current plating concepts embrace the principle of placing biology before mechanics.

Biological plating requires indirect fracture reduction.

Tissue strain within minimal ranges enhances callus formation.

the muscle and periosteal attachments of any single fragment tends to align it in the desired direction. Furthermore, a muscle envelope under distraction exerts concentric pressure on the shaft, easing fragments into place. This also holds true for metaphyseal and epiphyseal bone, although the distraction required to align fragments is transferred not so much via muscular attachments as through capsular tissues, ligaments and, less often, tendons. This phenomenon, regularly seen as part of conservative fracture management, is described by the term **"ligamentotaxis"**, coined by Vidal [13]. Similarly, traction applied by a traction table to an entire limb produces indirect reduction at a fracture focus. However, the use of an implant or large distractor (**Video AO20163**) to a single bone controls reduction more effectively and permits subtle adjustments as well. If feasible, indirect reduction techniques with distractor or external fixator and plate can be combined (**Fig. 3.3.2-1d**). Other tools for indirect reduction, plates in conjunction with the articulated tension device, or bone spreaders are described in **chapter 3.1** (**Fig. 3.3.2-2**) (**Video AO20194a**).

Ligamentotaxis = traction via ligaments and capsule.

3 Implant considerations

In biological or bridge plating, the surgeon must study the fracture morphology, carefully plan reduction, and finally choose a plate appropriate to the anatomical location and extent of the fracture. In general, **most plates are suitable to be used either for conventional or bridge plating.** In case an angled blade plate is used, it is first placed submuscularly and then inserted into the metaphyseal fragment prior to reduction. Subsequently, reduction is obtained with the help of the plate as a reduction aid as described in **chapter 3.1** (**Fig. 3.3.2-3**) (**Video AO20194b**).

Most plates can be used either for conventional or bridge plating.

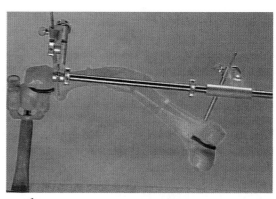
Video AO20163

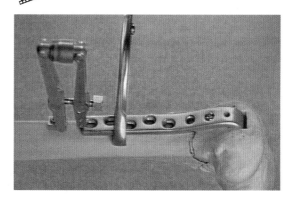
Video AO20194a

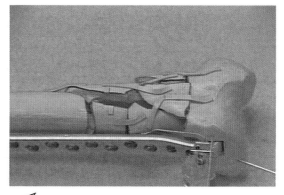
Video AO20194b

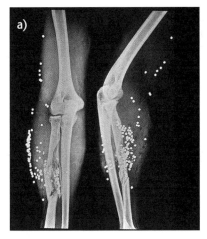
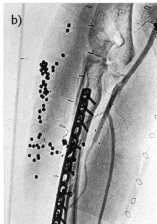
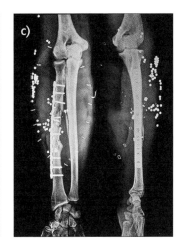
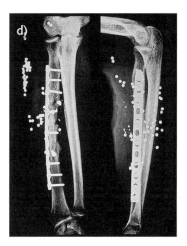

Fig. 3.3.2-2:
a) 24-year-old man with shotgun injury, right forearm. Grade III open comminuted radial shaft C1 fracture with radial artery disruption and compartment syndrome.
b) Intraoperative arteriography after fasciotomy, arterial repair with saphenous vein interposition and stabilization of the radial shaft by a long LC-DCP 3.5 through a Henry approach.
c) Postoperative x-ray showing the bridging plate on the radial shaft to correct length, axis, and rotation. Three major fragments are held by additional lag screws. Functional aftercare.
d) Follow-up x-ray after 3 months with adequate indirect bone healing.

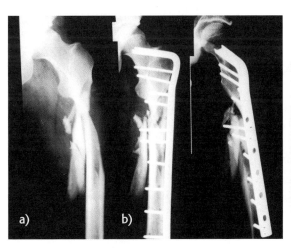
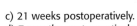
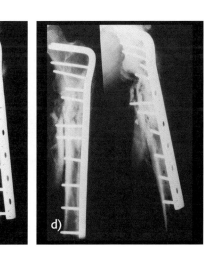
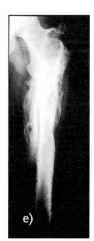

Fig. 3.3.2-3: Subtrochanteric C1.1 fracture.
a) Indirect reduction with plate and bridging of fracture zone. Large intermediate fragment deliberately left unreduced. No bone graft.
b) Postoperative x-ray.
c) 21 weeks postoperatively.
d) 7 months postoperatively with gradual filling of bone defect.
e) At 24 months and after implant removal. Complete reconstitution of cortical continuity, massive stable callus.

The common denominator in all bridge plating is the use of the plate as a splint on the outside of a bone, in the same way as a nail which splints the bone from within. Splintage of complex fractures has been a principle for a number of surgeons over many years, but has only recently become accepted as a recommendable concept and a principle to be taught. The wave plate (**Fig. 3.3.2-4**), with its central curved segment, provides three theoretical advantages for the treatment of fractures:

a) by reducing interference with the vascular supply to the fracture site by avoiding bone contact,

b) by providing excellent access for the application of a bone graft at the fracture site,

c) by altering the load to pure tension forces on the plate.

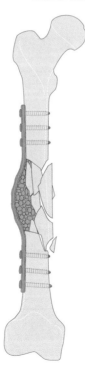

In practice, either end of a bridge plate is solidly fixed to the main fragment by three to four screws. Strength of fixation to each main fragment should be balanced. Long plates bridging an extensive zone of fragmentation with only short fixation on either end of the bone will undergo considerable defor-

Fig. 3.3.2-4: Wave plate allowing for grafting of lateral defect.

mation forces. As bending stresses are distributed over a long segment of the plate, the stress per unit area is correspondingly low, which reduces the risk of plate failure. In short fractures, repetitive bending stresses will be concentrated and centered on a short segment or screw hole of the plate, which will thereby break more easily due to fatigue (**Fig. 3.3.2-5**). The risk of mechanical failure can be considerably reduced if longer plates are used despite

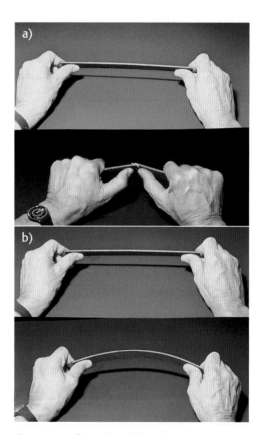

Fig. 3.3.2-5: Illustration of "stress concentration" (a) and "stress distribution" (b) on the model of a strip of plywood.

short zones of comminution, so that stresses are deliberately distributed over a proportionately longer section of the plate. This is accomplished by fixing the plate end well away from the fracture. The entire construct becomes "elastic", and even simple fracture patterns can be successfully bridged [14, 15]. Furthermore, the bridging concept using plates has been supported by new developments in plate design, such as the LC-DCP, PC-Fix, and LISS (see **chapters 3.2.2** and **3.4**). **These new implants are designed to minimize the area of contact between plate and bone, and they also display an even distribution of strength throughout the plate, thereby eliminating stress raisers at a screw hole.**

4 Soft-tissue considerations

As already stated, biological plating serves to preserve the vascularity around the fracture area, resulting in more rapid and abundant callus formation as observed in nailing or in non-operative fracture treatment. However, the success in using this operative approach depends very much on how the surgeon handles the soft tissues and on how well the anatomical characteristics of any given fracture have been taken into consideration during the planning of surgery.

Ideally, the muscle envelope over the fracture site, for example, the vastus lateralis muscle in the femur, is elevated from its insertion to the intermuscular septum by blunt dissection. The periosteum is left untouched and the perforator vessels are not ligated, while the plate is pushed through a tunnel between remaining muscle fibers and the bone. The exposure can safely be extended to control plate position and fracture alignment at either end of the long bridging plates where close contact between bone and plate is necessary. This technique enables the surgeon to avoid long incisions by restricting the exposure to the area of the bone required for plate fixation [16–18]. Thus, **plating becomes a semi-closed technique.** This principle can, however, not be applied to every long bone. Tunneling is not feasible in the humerus because of the different tendinous muscle insertions anteriorly and the course of the radial nerve posteriorly. Similar considerations apply to the radius. In the tibia a plate can be introduced subcutaneously on the medial side. There should, however, not be too much tension on the delicate skin cover [19]. For placement lateral to the tibial crest, somewhat more dissection with a sharp elevator is necessary. Screws are easily introduced through stab incisions.

Other areas of interest for minimal access plating include the distal femur or the proximal tibia [16]. Both locations, however, have distinct anatomical characteristics requiring precision not only in positioning, but also in contouring the plate. The surgeon may find it necessary to combine open reconstruction of the articular components with submuscular positioning of the plate on the adjacent shaft of the bone, where plate contouring is unproblematic. **If difficulties occur, a conventional approach is advisable** which still allows careful handling of the soft-tissue cover and minimal exposure of the bone itself. Even when using biological techniques, the surgeon must always be mindful of whatever soft-tissue damage was caused by the initial trauma. This consideration seems to preclude the use of standard instruments usually helpful in making an exposure. Hohmann retractors and reduction tools such as Verbrugge clamps should not be used. We recommend

Plating becomes a semi-closed technique.

Use LC-DCP, PC-Fix, or LISS for bridge plating.

If difficulties are anticipated, a conventional approach is advisable.

pointed reduction forceps, ball spikes, picks, and awls as instruments for bone manipulation and Langenbeck retractors for the soft tissues.

In grade III open fractures or closed injuries with considerable soft-tissue contusion, bridge plating is not the first choice for fixing a multifragmentary fracture in the emergency situation. Here, we prefer external fixation or the use of an unreamed nail (see **chapters 3.3.3**, **3.3.1** and **5.1**). The management of such difficult fractures is most demanding and requires much experience, as well as careful planning of all the many options and tactical steps.

5 Experimental verification

Biological techniques are supported by good clinical studies.

Numerous clinical studies have demonstrated excellent results when applying the biological or bridging technique of plating [10, 16, 18, 20–24].

In addition, animal experiments were performed to study the effect of biological plating in multifragment subtrochanteric fracture in sheep in order to compare anatomical reduction with various forms of indirect reduction followed by bridge plating [25]. Compared to the open, anatomically reduced group, the indirect reduction group healed with greater bone mass and higher breaking resistance, resulting in a decrease in the failure rate due to other causes.

6 Summary

Whenever the indication for plating of complex, multifragmentary fractures has been established, indirect reduction techniques in combination with bridge plating have proved, experimentally and clinically, to optimize the overall results. The classical former concept of direct anatomical reduction and rigid fixation by interfragmentary compression should therefore be reserved for simple type A and B fractures that are not considered for intramedullary nailing. With newly developed implants (PC-Fix and LISS), the trend to minimal access surgery continues, so that submuscular tunneling and plate introduction will be facilitated with other reduction tools and instruments for endoscopic viewing. A prerequisite for successful biological plating is, however, a sound knowledge supported by practical experience in the art of conventional compression plating.

7 Bibliography

1. **Lies A, Scheuer I** (1981) Die mediale Abstützung — Bedeutung und Möglichkeiten der Wiederherstellung bei Osteosynthesen. *Hefte Unfallheilkd;* 153:243–248.

2. **Loomer RL, Meek R, De Sommer F** (1980) Plating of femoral shaft fractures: the Vancouver experience. *J Trauma;* 20 (12):1038–1042.

3. **Lüscher JN, Rüedi T, Allgöwer M** (1979) Erfahrungen mit der Plattenosteosynthese bei 131 Femurschafttrümmerfrakturen. *Helv Chir Acta;* 45:39–42.

4. **Magerl F, Wyss A, Brunner C, et al.** (1979) Plate osteosynthesis of femoral shaft fractures in adults. A follow-up study. *Clin Orthop;* (138):62–73.

5. **Merchan EC, Maestu PR, Blanco RP** (1992) Blade-plating of closed displaced supracondylar fractures of the distal femur with the AO system. *J Trauma;* 32 (2):174–178.

6. **Tscherne H, Trentz O** (1977) [Technique of internal fixation and results in comminuted and multifragment fractures of the femoral shaft (collective study by the German Section of AO International) (author's transl)]. *Unfallheilkunde;* 80 (5):221–230.

7. **Wagner R, Weckbach A** (1994) [Complications of plate osteosynthesis of the femur shaft. An analysis of 199 femoral fractures]. *Unfallchirurg;* 97 (3):139–143.

8. **Perren SM** (1991) The concept of biological plating using the limited contact-dynamic compression plate (LC-DCP). Scientific background, design and application. *Injury;* 22 (Suppl 1):1–41.

9. **Bolhofner BR, Carmen B, Clifford P** (1996) The results of open reduction and internal fixation of distal femur fractures using a biologic (indirect) reduction technique. *J Orthop Trauma;* 10 (6):372–377.

10. **Baumgaertel F, Gotzen L** (1994) [The "biological" plate osteosynthesis in multifragment fractures of the para-articular femur. A prospective study]. *Unfallchirurg;* 97 (2):78–84.

11. **Baumgaertel F, Perren SM, Rahn B** (1994) [Animal experiment studies of "biological" plate osteosynthesis of multifragment fractures of the femur]. *Unfallchirurg;* 97 (1):19–27.

12. **Tepic S, Remiger AR, Morikawa K, et al.** (1997) Strength recovery in fractured sheep tibia treated with a plate or an internal fixator: an experimental study with a two-year follow-up. *J Orthop Trauma;* 11 (1):14–23.

13. **Vidal J** (1979) External Fixation: Current State of the Art. In: Brooker HS, Edward CC, editors. *Treatment of articular fractures by "ligamentotaxis" with external fixation.* Baltimore: Williams & Walkins.

14. **Schmidtmann U, Knopp W, Wolff C, et al.** (1997) [Results of elastic plate osteosynthesis of simple femoral shaft fractures in polytraumatized patients. An alternative procedure]. *Unfallchirurg;* 100 (12):949–956.

15. **Stürmer KM** (1996) [Elastic plate osteosynthesis, biomechanics, indications and technique in comparison with rigid osteosynthesis]. *Unfallchirurg;* 99 (11):816–817.

16. **Krettek C, Schandelmaier P, Miclau T, et al.** (1997) Transarticular joint reconstruction and indirect plate osteosynthesis for complex distal supracondylar femoral fractures. *Injury;* 28 (Suppl 1):A31–A41.

17. **Krettek C, Schandelmaier P, Miclau T, et al.** (1997) Minimally invasive percutaneous plate osteosynthesis (MIPPO) using the DCS in proximal and distal femoral fractures. *Injury;* 28 (Suppl 1):A20–A30.

18. **Wenda K, Runkel M, Degreif J, et al.** (1997) Minimally invasive plate fixation in femoral shaft fractures. *Injury;* 28 (Suppl 1):A13–A19.

19. **Helfet DL, Shonnard PY, Levine D, et al.** (1997) Minimally invasive plate osteosynthesis of distal fractures of the tibia. *Injury;* 28 (Suppl 1):A42–A48.

20. **Gerber C, Mast JW, Ganz R** (1990) Biological internal fixation of fractures [published erratum appears in Arch Orthop Trauma Surg 1991; 110 (4):226]. *Arch Orthop Trauma Surg;* 109 (6):295–303.

21. **Kinast C, Bolhofner BR, Mast JW, et al.** (1989) Subtrochanteric fractures of the femur. Results of treatment with the 95 degrees condylar blade-plate [see comments]. *Clin Orthop;* (238):122–130.

22. **Heitemeyer U, Hierholzer G** (1985) [Bridging osteosynthesis in closed compound fractures of the femur shaft]. *Aktuelle Traumatol;* 15 (5):205–209.

23. **Kleining R, Hax PM** (1981) Die interne Überbrückungsosteosynthese ohne Reposition des Stückbruchbereiches als Alternative zur internen Fragment-fixation von Stückbrüchen nach anatomischer Reposition. *Hefte Unfallheilkd;* 153:213–223.

24. **Thielemann FW, Blersch E, Holz U** (1988) [Plate osteosynthesis of femoral shaft fracture with reference to biological aspects]. *Unfallchirurg;* 91 (9):389–394.

25. **Heitemeyer U, Kepmer F, Hierholzer G, et al.** (1987) Severely comminuted femoral shaft fractures: treatment by bridging- plate osteosynthesis. *Arch Orthop Trauma Surg;* 106 (5):327–330.

8 Updates

Updates and additional references for this chapter are available online at:
http://www.aopublishing.org/PFxM/332.htm

3.3.3 External fixation

Alberto Fernandez Dell'Oca

1 Introduction

An external fixator is a device placed outside the skin which stabilizes the bone fragments through wires or pins connected to one or more longitudinal bars/tubes. When wires are used they must be under tension. This requires rings or half rings.

One of the main characteristics of external fixators is skin penetration creating so-called pin tracks. Most of the disadvantages of external fixation are related to pin-track complications [1].

Advantages

- Less damage to blood supply of bone.
- Minimal interference with soft-tissue cover [2].
- Useful for stabilizing open fractures (see **chapter 5.1**).
- Rigidity of fixation adjustable without surgery [3].
- Good option in situations with risk of infection.
- Requires less experience and surgical skill than standard ORIF.
- Quite safe to use in cases of bone infection.

Disadvantages

- Pin and wires penetrating the soft tissues.
- Restricted joint motion.
- Pin-track complications in long-lasting external fixation.
- Cumbersome and not always well tolerated.
- Limited stiffness in certain locations (e.g., femur fracture in adults).

Thanks to its position "outside" the soft parts, the external fixator is a safe device for stabilizing all sorts of different fractures.

2 Biomechanical aspects

2.1 Components of standard external fixators

(**Fig. 3.3.3-1**)

The main components of external fixator systems are:
- Pins (Schanz screws/Steinmann pins).
- Stainless steel tubes or carbon fibre rods.

- A variety of clamps to fasten pins/wires to tubes/rods.
- Clamps to connect tubes/rods to tubes/rods.

There is a variety of pins/wires available:
- Steinmann pins for bilateral frames.
- Schanz screws, either self-drilling or requiring pre-drilling.
- Schanz screws with small diameter tips for use in small bones.
- 2.0 and 1.8 mm K-wires (±olives) for ring fixator.
- Threaded K-wires for the small external fixator [4].

The two main systems are the standard tubular/rod external fixator and the small external fixator.

Only few components are needed for the standard external fixator.

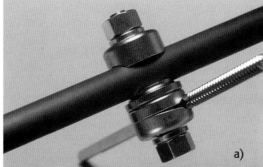

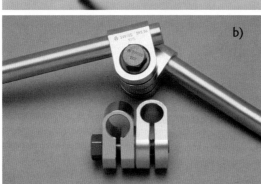

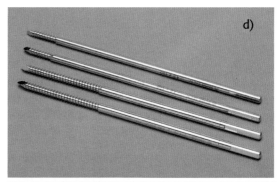

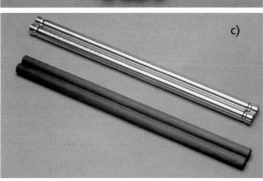

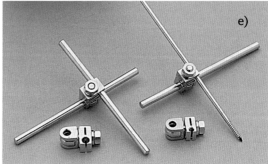

Fig. 3.3.3-1:
Components of tubular and small external fixators:
a) Adjustable open clamp.
b) Tube-to-tube clamp.
c) Stainless steel tubes, carbon fibre rods.
d) Different pins, Schanz screws.
e) Small external fixator.

The standard tubular system is employed for treatment of fractures in large bones, for arthrodesis, and for bone lengthening and transport systems. The small external fixator is used mainly for fractures of the distal radius and forearm as well as for fractures in children and adolescents.

Thanks to its modular concept, the external fixator with its different components can be employed in many different configurations and constructs, which allows a unique versatility (see **section 4**).

2.2   Stiffness of the frame

Stiffness of the frame depends upon the following factors:

- Distance of pins/Schanz screws
  - from the fracture line: the closer the better (x),
  - within each main fragment, the further apart the better (y).
- Distance of longitudinal connecting tube/ bar from bone: the closer the better (z).
- Number of bars/tubes: two are better than one.
- Configuration: unilateral/V-shaped/bilateral or triangular frame (**Fig. 3.3.3-2**).
- Combination of limited internal fixation (lag screw) with external fixation.

Insufficiently stable external fixation may delay fracture healing and lead to pin loosening. However, **too much stiffness or rigidity of the external fixator construct may also delay fracture healing,** especially in open fractures.

In the management of such fractures it may be necessary to "dynamize" an initially quite stable configuration or add stability in case of pin loosening [**5–10**].

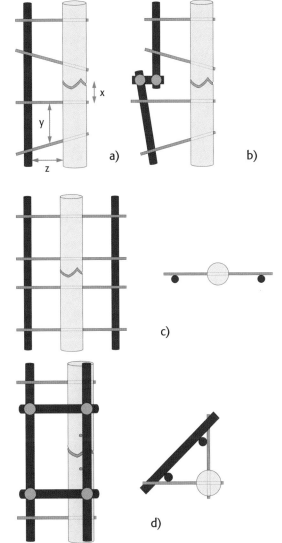

Fig. 3.3.3-2: Different constructions of external fixators:
a) Unilateral uniplanar single tube fixator.
b) Modular construct with 3 tubes: a useful configuration with wide applications.
c) Bilateral frame: now seldom used.
d) Unilateral biplanar frame.

Fixation which is insufficiently stable is either too elastic or too rigid and can delay fracture healing.

2.3 Types of external fixators

(Fig. 3.3.3-2)
- Pin fixators:
  - unilateral,
  - V-shaped,
  - bilateral frame,
  - triangular.
- Ring (wire fixators).
- Hybrid fixators (wire and pin).
- Pinless external fixator.
- Mefisto.

2.3.1 Hybrid external fixator

(Fig. 3.3.3-3)
The hybrid external fixator is a construct used in fractures close to a joint. It is called "hybrid" because it combines wire fixation (3/4 ring fixator) with pin fixation (unilateral fixator in the diaphysis). It requires K-wires for the half-ring and conventional Schanz screws for the shaft. There are K-wires with an olive which allows for fragment adaptation by applying some compression (**Video AO20166Ba**).

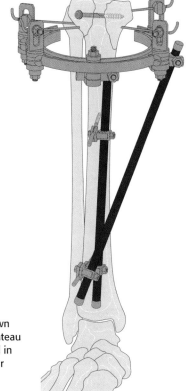

Fig. 3.3.3-3:
Hybrid fixator shown here on a tibial plateau fracture, but useful in other juxta-articular tibial fractures.

Advantages
- Minimally invasive alignment of simple articular fractures.
- Better anchorage of thin wires than of conventional pins in cancellous bone.
- Free postoperative joint motion.
- Can be combined with lag screws.

Disadvantages
- Risk of articular infection. The proximity of K-wire pin tracks to a joint may be hazardous [11].
- Radiopaque ring may obstruct x-ray assessment of the reduction in standard views.

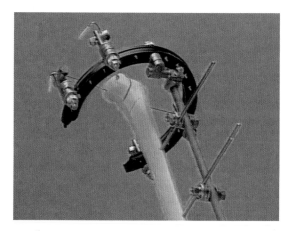

Video AO20166Ba

Hybrid ring fixators have been mainly used in type A and B fractures of the proximal and distal tibia, either free-standing or to protect a lag screw internal fixation [11].

It is not easy to insert a hybrid fixator correctly in an articular fracture, nor is it a quick procedure. It may therefore be done as a second step, for example, in polytraumatized patients or open fractures after initial joint-bridging fixation.

2.3.2 Pinless fixator

(**Fig. 3.3.3-4**)

The main goal of the pinless fixator design was to avoid penetration of the medullary canal, thereby reducing the risk of deep infection in case of secondary intramedullary nailing.

The sharp points of the forceps-like fixator are applied to the bone by a rocking motion and should only penetrate the cortex superficially. Forceps of varying sizes and shapes are available to adapt to the triangular cross-section of the tibia at different levels (**Video AO20166Bb**).

Once the forceps are well anchored in the bone, the fracture is reduced and the four forceps are connected by a simple bar or as a tube-to-tube arrangement.

> Hybrid and pinless fixators are mostly used for temporary fracture stabilization in case of critical soft-tissue conditions.

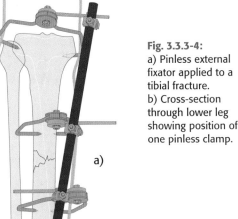

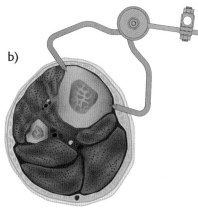

Fig. 3.3.3-4:
a) Pinless external fixator applied to a tibial fracture.
b) Cross-section through lower leg showing position of one pinless clamp.

a)

b)

Video AO20166Bb

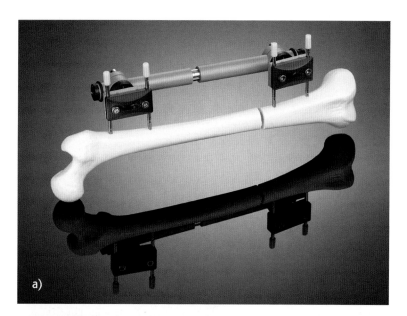

a)

b)

2.3.3 Mefisto

The Mefisto is a recently introduced external fixator. It was designed for fracture treatment (**Fig. 3.3.3-5a**) and for limb lengthening and bone transport (**Fig. 3.3.3-5b**). Thanks to the modular configuration it proved also to be a very useful tool for the management of fractures.

3 Surgical technique

3.1 Pin insertion technique

In order to avoid tendon penetration or injuries to nerves, vessels, and muscles, the surgeon must be familiar with the anatomy of the different cross-sections of the lower leg and make use of the recommended pin placement sites [**11, 12**] (**Fig. 3.3.3-6** "safe pin sites").

Fig. 3.3.3-5:
a) Mefisto (monolateral external fixation system for trauma and orthopedics): Carbon fiber tube with double pin clamps.
b) Aluminum central body with T-configuration.

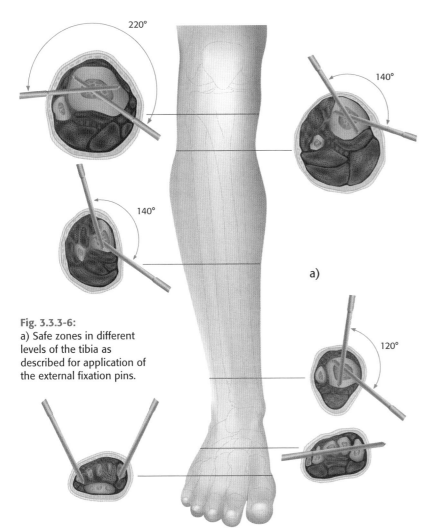

Fig. 3.3.3-6:
a) Safe zones in different levels of the tibia as described for application of the external fixation pins.

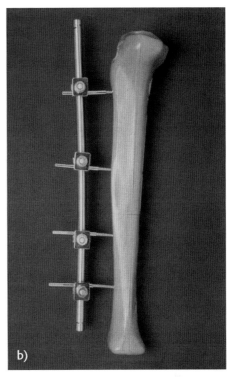

b) Standard unilateral external fixator on bone model.

3.1.1 Diaphyses

It is important to avoid heat damage to the bone when inserting a pin or Schanz screw into hard cortices. The sharper the drill bits or screws, the less heat is generated. The temperature rises as insertion speed increases [1].

Burning the bone can be a serious problem and may result in early loosening due to ring sequestrum formation. A correctly inserted pin or screw should catch the opposite cortex but not protrude too far past it. Correct depth insertion may be achieved by feeling the opposite cortex (probably the best way), using measuring gauges (fairly difficult), or by intraoperative x-ray (which may be misleading).

To avoid heat damage, the holes for Schanz screws and Steinmann pins must be predrilled.

There is no way to build a solid frame over poorly inserted pins.

Joint involvement of any pin must be avoided.

If the inserted Schanz screw points to the opposite cortex without reaching it, it may be short or the image misleading. If the control x-ray shows an empty hole in the opposite cortex, the screw has not been inserted far enough (**Fig. 3.3.3-7**).

There is no way to build a solid frame over poorly inserted pins.

3.1.2 Metaphyses

In metaphyseal bone heat generation is not such a problem. Since it is easy to miss the predrilled hole, the use of self-drilling screws may be safer. **Joint involvement must, however, be avoided** because of the danger of pin-track infection which could progress into the joint.

When inserting a pin or Schanz screw it is important:

- not to injure nerves or vessels,
- not to place them into the joint,
- to avoid the fracture line,
- not to "burn" the bone,
- to insert a screw of the correct length,
- to use self-drilling screws in metaphyseal bone.

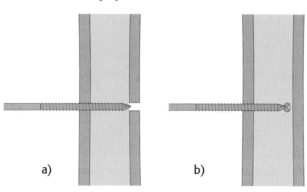

a)   b)

Fig. 3.3.3-7: Deceptive x-ray appearances: short pin not reaching opposite cortex showing empty screwhole.
a) AP, b) oblique view. This will result in instability.

3.2 Frame construction

Depending on what is easier and on local priorities, the fixator is applied after reduction (reduction first) or the fixator is used as a reduction tool (fixator first). For the latter technique a modular frame (**Fig. 3.3.3-8**) construction is required.

A pair of pins is inserted into each main fragment and joined by a short tube or rod. The two tubes or rods are then connected by a short third tube and two special tube-to-tube clamps. This construct allows the surgeon to manipulate and reduce the fracture and to hold it after reduction [13] (**Video AO20166Bc**).

Advantages

Free pin placement allowing the surgeon:

- to spread both pins, increasing frame stiffness,
- to position pins according to the fracture pattern or soft-tissue injury,
- to avoid injury to nerves or vessels.

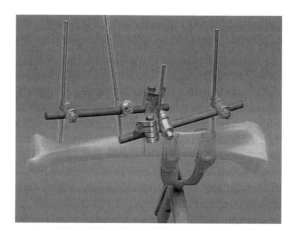

 Video AO20166Bc

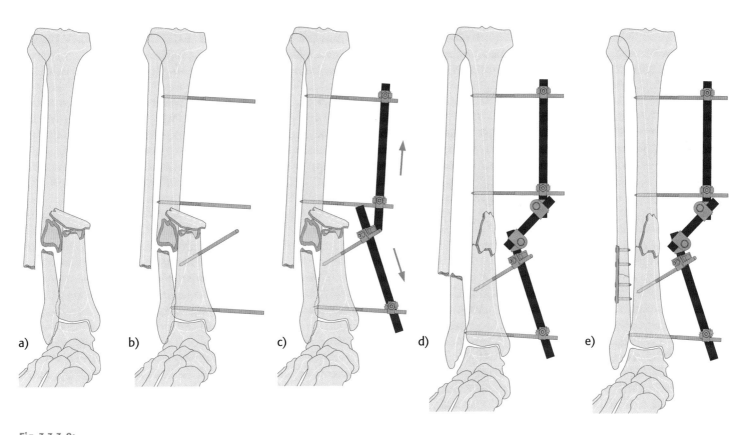

Fig. 3.3.3-8:
a) Schema illustrating the "fixator first" protocol for a complex open fracture.
b) In each main fragment two pins are inserted according to the soft-tissue conditions.
c) Fixed to a bar by universal clamps two "handles" are obtained for reduction.
d) After reduction the two bars are united by a third tube and two tube-to-tube clamps.
e) The fibula has been plated adding stability.

The application of the external fixator "first" means reduced x-ray time. This type of fixator can even be applied without x-ray facility or image intensification in the OR, since minor improvements of reduction and axial alignment can be made later on without the need of anesthesia or more surgery.

Every large long bone can be fixed with this technique using few components and only three tubes. This is useful when there are only limited resources, in situations of catastrophe, or in a patient with multiple injuries or fractures.

Tube-to-tube clamps have a better grip on stainless steel tubes than on carbon fiber rods; the latter should therefore be double-stacked (**Fig. 3.3.3-9**).

External fixation is the gold standard in open fractures, avoiding additional damage to an already compromised limb.

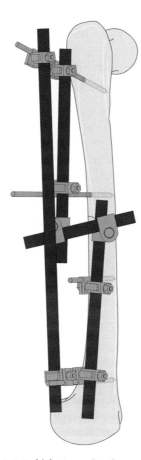

Fig. 3.3.3-9: In high-stress situations carbon fiber rods, (CFR) for modular frames should be double-stacked (holding power of tube-tube clamps on CFR is not so high as it is on stainless steel tubes). Example on a femur.

4 Indications for external fixation

4.1 Open fractures

External fixation is only one possibility for skeletal stabilization in open fractures. It is, however, a very useful device for managing such injuries and still the gold standard, with the following relevant advantages:

It offers the possibility of **atraumatic insertion, avoiding additional damage to the soft tissues and bone vascularity already compromised by the injury.**

It is advisable to apply the fixator using the modular technique as already mentioned (**Fig. 3.3.3-8**), thus avoiding the use of bone forceps, retractors, etc.

Furthermore, it does not compromise any secondary procedure and is rapidly applied in the emergency situation, even in the hemodynamically unstable patient [2].

In long oblique spiral fractures, a pointed reduction clamp, gently applied percutaneously to the bone, may be used to improve and hold the reduction temporarily while the fixator is aligned and tightened.

Lag screws are to be used only exceptionally when dealing with open fractures (**Fig. 3.3.3-10**). They may be required in very long oblique spiral fractures or in the presence of a large well-vascularized third fragment, which lends itself to fixation.

In the tibial fracture, the pinless fixator (see **Fig. 3.3.3-4**) may be a valuable alternative. Its main advantages are that the medullary canal is not opened or penetrated since the clamps (forceps) are anchored in the cortex only. This allows for safe, secondary intramedullary nailing. Fixation with the pinless system is, however, somewhat less stable.

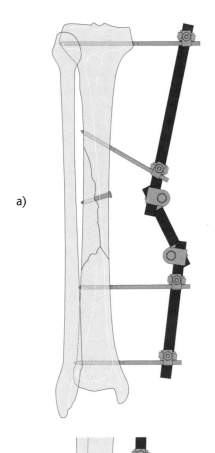

4.2 Closed fractures

In closed fractures, external fixation is rarely indicated, except in severe polytrauma (ISS > 40), severe closed contusions or degloving, for temporary joint bridging, as well as in children.

4.3 Polytrauma

In severe polytrauma (ISS > 40) (see **chapter 5.3**), **external fixation may be the most adequate way to initially stabilize multiple fractures;** being minimally invasive it should not add any additional surgical insult to the patient. External fixation can deal with almost every long bone fracture except the proximal femur or humerus. The main advantages of this approach lies in the rapid achievement of stability, which helps in pain control, decreases bleeding, and facilitates nursing care.

In polytrauma, ISS > 40, external fixation is the safest means to stabilize multiple long bone fractures temporarily.

4.4 Children's fractures

In children, whether following polytrauma or not, there may be good indications for external fixation, especially in the lower limb or in case of open fractures. One must avoid going through the growth plate with a pin, whereas relatively small implants (small external fixator) may be sufficiently rigid even on the tibia or humerus.

Pediatric fractures are good indications for external fixation.

Fig. 3.3.3-10: The modular frame used in association with lag screw employed:
a) to hold a large vital butterfly bone fragment,
b) to restore joint surface.

4.5 Special indications— articular fractures/joint bridging

Perfect joint reconstruction and a stable fixation with interfragmentary compression allowing early pain-free motion are the treatment goals for articular fractures. This goal can be reached by ORIF or in simpler fracture patterns by a combination of interfragmentary lag screw fixation with an external or hybrid fixator. These two options are recommended in cases of open or closed fractures with severe soft-tissue compromise (**Fig. 3.3.3-11**).

Furthermore, the external fixator can be applied in a joint-bridging fashion, usually as a temporary measure in order to protect the delicate soft-tissue cover in unstable or complex articular fracture, or joint dislocations which do not allow a more definitive internal fixation.

Except for the shoulder, any major joint can be bridged in this way [14].

Bridging external fixation of the wrist in complex or open distal radius fractures is a standard procedure (see **chapter 4.3.3**) [15]. In this situation the external fixator is used first to reduce the fracture indirectly by distraction (ligamentotaxis) and then to hold the fragments in place. Care has to be taken, however, not to overdistract the wrist joint or to maintain distraction for a prolonged period of time (maximum 3–4 weeks) [15, 16].

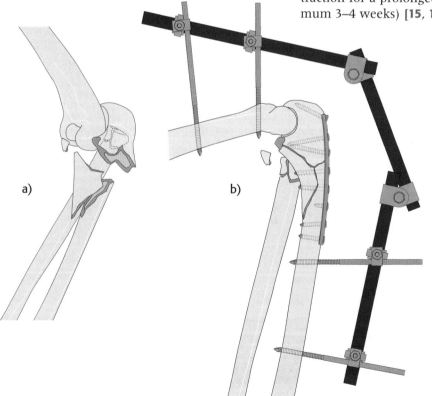

a)

b)

Fig. 3.3.3-11: A bridging frame used to protect a potentially unstable elbow.
a) Complex proximal forearm fracture. (Note the displaced radial head and the floating coronoid process.)
b) The ulna has been plated and the still unstable elbow is bridged with a temporary external fixator.

In open tibial shaft fractures, bridging external fixation is frequently applied to the first metatarsal in order to hold the foot and ankle in neutral position (see **Fig. 3.3.3-10b**).

As joint-bridging external fixation is usually only a temporary measure, careful planning of pin placement is essential in order not to compromise or interfere with definitive internal fixation 1–2 weeks later. In case of large soft-tissue defects, consultation with a plastic surgeon is recommended to avoid compromising the access for later reconstructive procedures.

5 Postoperative treatment

5.1 Pin-track care

Pin-track care starts with correct pin insertion. Undue soft-tissue tension around the pins must be released during surgery. Correct care of the pin-track sites is important for reducing the risk of pin-track complications [1]. Daily cleansing and desinfection with Betadine paste is recommended.

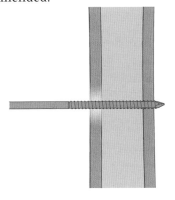

Fig. 3.3.3-12: X-ray appearance of bone resorption around a loose pin.

In case of persistant pin-track infection the pin has usually lost its firm hold in the bone. On x-ray a seam of bone resorption can be observed and mechanically the pin appears "loose". Only change of the pin to a new site can solve the problem (**Fig. 3.3.3-12**).

5.2 Change to internal fixation

The advantages of the external fixator as an emergency device in open fractures and polytrauma patients are well established. For the definitive treatment of a fracture with external fixation, there are, however, major drawbacks, such as the bulk of the device, its discomfort, the need for daily pin care, and the possible limitation of joint movement. The patient's wish to change to an internal stabilization is therefore understandable.

5.3 Timing of the procedure

Intramedullary nailing, preferably without reaming, is considered safe if performed within the first 2 weeks after external fixation, provided the pin sites are clean without signs of infection. If the change to intramedullary nailing is decided later than 2 weeks or in case of pin-site infection, it is advisable to remove the external fixator, curette the pin tracks, and place the limb in a plaster cast until all signs of infection are gone. An alternative may be to replace the standard external fixator by a pinless device.

Where plating is planned, the fixator may be kept a week or two longer prior to change; however, here too the pin tracks should be clean!

Joint-bridging external fixation has to be planned carefully in order not to compromise later ORIF.

Pin-track care starts with correct pin insertion.

A change to internal fixation (intramedullary nail or plate) should occur not later than 2 weeks after external fixation.

6 Special applications

6.1 Arthrodesis

One of the first applications of external fixation was for ankle fusion by applying compression through a bilateral frame. This principle is also used for knee and elbow fusion, especially in case of infection [17].

6.2 Infection

(see **chapter 6.1**)

In acute or chronic infection, external fixation may be the ultimate way of stabilizing an infected fracture or non-union, as the pins can usually be inserted away from the infected focus. Techniques and guidelines are essentially the same as for fresh fractures.

6.3 Limb lengthening/ bone transport

(see **chapters 6.3** and **6.4**)

The technique of distraction osteogenesis was introduced by Ilizarov with the ring fixator [18]. The same technique can also be applied using the tubular external fixator and the Mefisto, with the limitation, however, that angular and rotational corrections cannot be performed simultaneously.

6.4 Corrective osteotomies

(see **chapter 6.4**)

External fixation for osteotomies should only be used in case of poor or compromised soft-tissue cover, or in combination with bone transport; in other circumstances there are better ways and techniques, in particular, plating.

7 Bibliography

1. **Green S** (1982) Complications of external fixation. In: Uhthoff HK, editor. *Current Concepts of External Fixation of Fractures*. Berlin Heidelberg New York: Springer-Verlag.

2. **Burny F** (1979) Elastic external fixation of tibia fractures: a study of 1421 cases. In: Brooker A, Edwards C, editors. *External Fixation: The Current State of the Art*. London: Williams & Wilkins: 55–73.

3. **Canadell J, Forriol F** (1993) *Fijacion Externa Monolateral*. Pamplona: Eurograf.

4. **Perren S** (1990) Basic aspects of internal fixation. In: Müller ME, Allgöwer M, Schneider R, editors. *Manual of Internal Fixation*. Berlin Heidelberg New York: Springer-Verlag: 1–112.

5. **Mooney V, Claudi B** (1982) How stable should external fixation be? In: Uhthoff HK, editor. *Current Concepts of External Fixation of Fractures*. Berlin Heidelberg New York: Springer-Verlag: 21–26.

6. **Mears D** (1983) Nonunions, infected nonunions and arthrodeses. In: Mears D, editor. External Skeletal Fixation: 93–160. Baltimore London: Williams & Wilkins.

7. **Edwards C** (1982) The timing of external fixation. In: Uhthoff HK, editor. *Current Concepts of External Fixation of Fractures.* Berlin Heidelberg New York: Springer-Verlag: 27–42.

8. **Mears D** (1983) Fracture healing: pathophysiology and biomechanics. In: Mears D, editor. *External Skeletal Fixation.* Baltimore London: Williams & Wilkins: 42–92.

9. **De Bastiani G, Aldegheri R, Renzi Brivio L** (1984) The treatment of fractures with a dynamic axial fixator. *J Bone Joint Surg [Br];* 66 (4):538–545.

10. **Lazo-Zbikowski J, Aguilar F, Mozo F, et al.** (1986) Biocompression external fixation. Sliding external osteosynthesis. *Clin Orthop;* (206):169–184.

11. **Fernandez A, Masliah R** (1991) *Modular External Fixation in Emergency.* Montevideo: Intergraf.

12. **Behrens F, Searls K** (1982) Unilateral external fixation: experience with the ASIF "tubular" frame. In: Uhthoff HK, editor. *Current Concepts of External Fixation of Fractures.* Berlin Heidelberg New York: Springer-Verlag: 177–183.

13. **Fernandez A** (1992) External fixation using simple pin fixators. *Injury;* 23 (Suppl 4):1–54.

14. **Vidal J, Buscayret C, Coones H** (1979) Treatment of articular fractures by "ligamentotaxis" with external fixation. In: Brooker A, Edwards E, editors. *External Fixation: The Current State of the Art.* London: Williams & Wilkins: 75–82.

15. **Jakob R, Fernandez D** (1982) The treatment of wrist fractures with the small AO external fixation device. In: Uhthoff HK, editor. *Current Concepts of External Fixation of Fractures.* Berlin Heidelberg New York: Springer-Verlag: 307–314.

16. **Fernandez D, Jupiter JB** (1996) *Fractures of the Distal Radius.* Berlin Heidelberg New York: Springer-Verlag.

17. **Mears D** (1983) Clinical techniques in the lower extremity. In: Mears D, editor. *External Skeletal Fixation.* Baltimore London: Williams & Wilkins: 210–338.

18. **Ilizarov GA** (1971) [Basic principles of transosseous compression and distraction osteosynthesis]. *Ortop Travmatol Protez;* 32 (11):7–15.

8 Updates

Updates and additional references for this chapter are available online at:
http://www.aopublishing.org/PFxM/333.htm

3.4 Newer technologies

*Alberto Fernandez Dell'Oca, Pietro Regazzoni,
Christoph Sommer, Michael Schütz*

1 Introduction

In the preceding chapters the conventional techniques of intramedullary nailing, plating, and the use of the tension band, as well as external fixation have been described, all of them having specific indications and a firm position in the growing field of operative fracture fixation.

The introduction some 10 years ago of the combination of biological bridge plating with indirect reduction techniques was considered by some to be an important and welcome evolution, but by others [2, 5, 6] as a revolution against rigid AO principles.

It had become evident that in the cortex directly underneath a plate, and to a lesser extent in the vicinity of an intramedullary nail, considerable structural changes occur. These changes were first attributed to so-called stress protection by a metallic implant much more rigid than bone. Further research [1, 3] gave rise to the theory that disturbed blood flow within the cortical bone was responsible for the intense remodeling processes that could be observed underneath every plate that was pressed against bone by screws (see **chapter 1.2**).

Reducing the area of contact between plate and bone, as achieved by the LC-DCP design, significantly reduced the vascular changes caused by pressure on the cortex. However, the LC-DCP also has to be pressed against the bone in order to create the friction needed to fulfill its function. **In order to abolish the ill effects of any plate to bone contact, a completely different approach had to be chosen.** With the introduction of screws or bolts that rigidly lock into the plate hole when driven home, the plate is no longer pressed against the underlying bone [4]. Furthermore, the use of unicortical self-tapping screws seemed, in *in vitro* experiments, equally as effective as external fixation in obtaining a stable construct [4]. In a way similar in principle to the external fixator (see **chapter 3.3.3**) **this new and quite different technique of applying a plate has been termed the internal fixator system, as the implant functions more like a fixator than a plate, while the whole construct is covered by soft tissues and skin.**

Such devices, since they are designed to avoid the ill effects of conventional plating, might be expected to offer a higher resistance to infection and other complications.

To prevent the pressure of a plate against bone a completely new system was chosen: the internal fixator.

This new device functions as a subcutaneous or submuscular fixator.

2 PC-Fix (point contact fixator)

The first implant designed to fulfill the new requirements was the small PC-Fix for forearm bones.

PC-Fix has been tested in more than 1,000 fractures with very promising results.

The first implant designed to fulfill the new requirements was the small PC-Fix for forearm bones. The PC-Fix is a narrow plate-like implant with a specially designed undersurface having only small points that come into contact with bone (**Video AO90072a**). The screws are self-

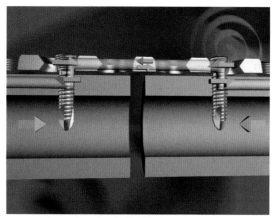

Video AO90072a

tapping and unicortical and are available in one length only. The screw head locks firmly in the plate hole with a fine thread (**Video AO20168b**).

As in biological plating, long implants with few screws are applied to fractures which have already been adequately reduced and axially aligned, because the plate as such cannot be used as a reduction tool, or to obtain inter-fragmentary compression. For surgeons accustomed to conventional plating, this is a major change, acceptance of which may require a little time. The PC-Fix plate can, if necessary, be gently contoured to meet the shape of the bone (**Video AO20168c**). So far, this new fixator system has been tested in several clinical studies in **over 1,000 fractures, mostly of the forearm, with very promising results.** Once the procedure has been learned, the healing rate is consistently high and reliable (**Fig. 3.4-1**).

A larger PC-Fix version for other long bones (tibia and humerus) is under development.

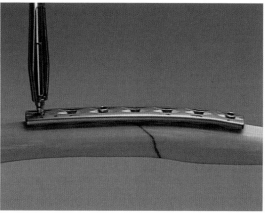

 Video AO20168b

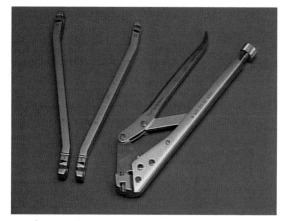

 Video AO20168c

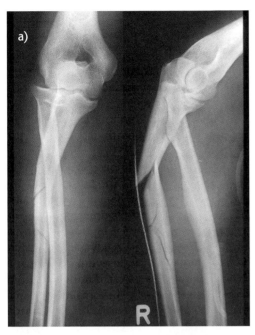

3 LISS (less invasive stabilization system)

While the PC-Fix has limited applications in the metaphyseal and epiphyseal areas, the LISS (**Fig. 3.4-2**) was conceived for precisely these regions—initially for the distal femur and later for the proximal tibia. Its shape conforms to the anatomical contours of the specific area of the bone so separate implants are required for the

Fig. 3.4-1: Clinical example of PC-Fix:
a) Complex Monteggia-type fracture of the ulna with associated radial head fracture-dislocation in a 40-year-old male.
b) Reconstruction of ulna with a 12-hole PC-Fix and one independent lag screw. The radial head reduced spontaneously and was left untouched. Functional aftercare.
c) One year follow-up with well-healed fracture and excellent elbow function.
The undisplaced radial head fracture healed without incident.

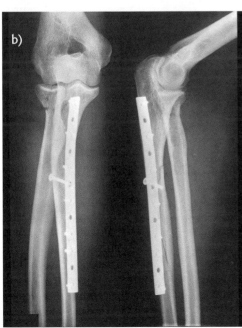

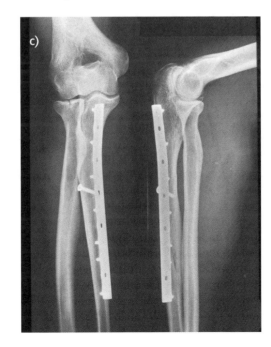

right and left sides. Additional contouring is not required as the "plate" fixator does not necessarily need to touch the bone. In addition to the locked unicortical screws, this implant is designed and instrumented for application via a minimally invasive submuscular approach [7, 8] (**Video AO90063**) (see **chapter 4.6.3**).

As with the PC-Fix, the fracture must be adequately reduced and aligned prior to the application of the LISS. This is especially true for the articular components of the distal femur or proximal tibia which must be anatomically reconstructed and held by plate-independent lag screws. The LISS can accommodate long, fully threaded self-tapping screws that are locked in plate holes when driven home, thereby providing the attributes of a fixed-angle device.

The insertion handle for submuscular insertion of the long plate also serves simultaneously as a drill guide for precise screw placement through separate small incisions (**Fig.3.4-2d**).

LISS was designed for the distal femur and proximal tibia, to be inserted à la MIPO (minimal invasive plate osteosynthesis).

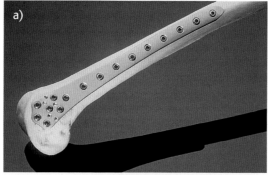

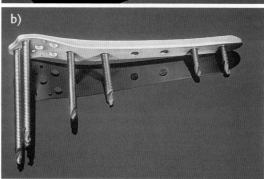

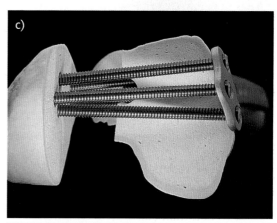

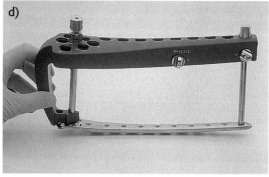

Fig. 3.4-2: Less invasive stabilization system.
a) LISS fixator applied to lateral aspect of distal femur.
b) The self-tapping bolts (long in metaphysis and epiphysis, short in diaphysis) are locked in the plate when driven home, thereby providing angular stability.
c) Arrangement and direction of bolts in the metaphysis and epiphysis.

d) To be introduced with minimal exposure underneath the lateral vastus muscle, the fixator plate is mounted on a handle which acts as a guide to the percutaneous placement of the bolts.

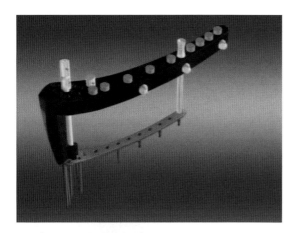

 Video AO90063

In summary, the new internal fixator systems LISS and PC-Fix

- constitute a completely new, but promising alternative to conventional plating,
- preserve vascularity of bone in an optimal way,
- should have a better resistance to infection than conventional plates,
- are designed to be inserted in a minimally invasive fashion (LISS only),
- provide a fixed-angle plate screw device consisting of two components for easy application in complex fractures,
- are, because of their self-tapping, unicortical screws, easily and rapidly applied to a reduced fracture.

4 LCP (locking compression plate)

A further refinement of internal fixator systems (see **chapter 3.2.1**, **section 4**), with screw heads locking firmly into the plate hole, has now been devised. This is a new plate hole configuration which brings to this most valuable innovation the advantages of conventional plating, for example, placement of a lag screw across the plate for certain fracture configurations. This is achieved through a new design, the "combination" plate hole which can accommodate either a conventional screw or the new "locking head screw (LHS)" which has a conical threaded head (**Fig. 3.4-3**). The LHS comes in two forms. the self-tapping LHS has self-tapping grooves and is designed for use in sites such as the metaphysis where exact measurement of screw length is required. It can be bicortical or monocortical and predrilling is needed. The self-drilling and self-tapping LHS is of the same design but with the addition of a drilling tip of conventional design; it is for monocortical use only (see **Fig. 3.4-4**). The standard screw can be applied in the usual fashion. Alternatively, the combination design enables the new screw to be locked in any hole along the plate, so providing angular stability (**Video AO90072a**).

The new combination hole has two parts:

1. The first part has the design of the standard DC/LC-DCP compression hole (dynamic compression unit: DCU) which accepts a conventional screw allowing axial compression or the placement of an angled lag screw through the plate.
2. The other part is conical, and threaded, to accept the locking head screw.

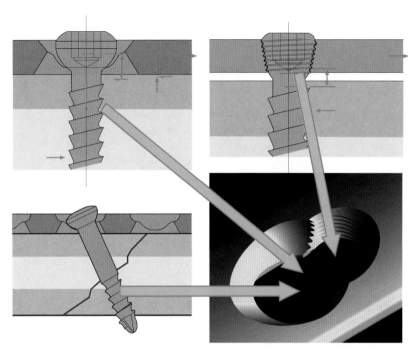

Fig. 3.4-3: LCP combination hole combining three proven elements. It mainly consists of two parts:
1) One half of the hole has the design of the standard DC/LC-DCP (dynamic compression unit: DCU) for conventional screws (incl. lag screws).
2) The other half is conical and threaded to accept the matching thread of the new locking head screw providing angular stability.

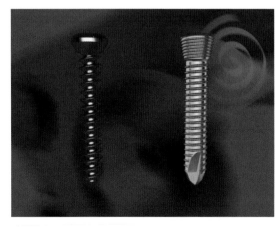

 Video AO90072a

Currently, all standard Synthes plates of the 3.5 and 4.5 systems (DCP, LC-DCP, L-plates, and T-plates, as well as reconstruction plates) are available in versions with the new combination hole, but without any change in the overall plate dimensions.

Depending on the desired function the locking compression plate (LCP) can be applied in three different ways:

1. As a conventional dynamic compression plate: With the use of an eccentric drill guide, axial compression can be obtained or a lag screw can be placed through a plate hole. This classical type of rigid fixation is still applicable in simple type A and B1 fractures in the meta-epiphyseal area, where anatomical reduction may be required and can easily be achieved without wide exposure.

2. As a "pure" internal fixator according to PC-Fix and LISS principles (**Fig. 3.4-4**): Here locked screws exclusively are used. The complex type C fracture zone is bridged—without being exposed—by a long plate. This allows rapid indirect fracture healing with external callus formation. While the fractured bone must be appropriately aligned before the LCP is applied, little or no contouring is needed. Due to the locking mechanism the fragments are not pulled towards the plate. This facilitates percutaneous plate insertion and the use of unicortical screws (**Video AO90072b**).

Furthermore, the fixed angle principle appears to be very effective in stabilizing fractures in osteoporotic bone because the resistance to pull-out is much greater than for the standard screw.

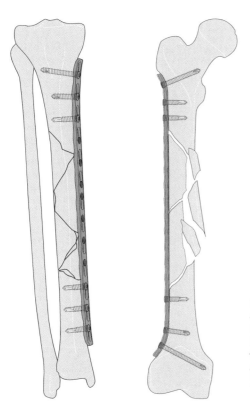

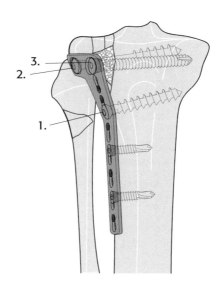

Fig. 3.4-4: LCP applied as pure internal fixator in a bridging function in a complex type C fracture using the different types of locking head scews.

Fig. 3.4-5: LCP application in a combined fashion using the lag screw principle for the reconstruction of the articular components, and the locking head screw to provide angular stability.

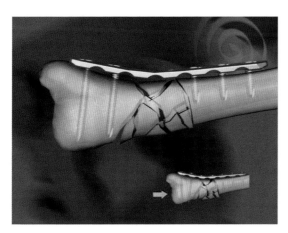

 Video AO90072b

3. In combined fashion where both techniques are employed; using conventional lag screws as well as locked screws. In articular fractures requiring an anatomical reduction and fixation by interfragmentary compression lag screws may be essential for the reconstruction of any articular components (**Fig. 3.4-5**). At the same time the locking head screw provides angluar stability, helping to prevent secondary displacement in case of metaphyseal comminution or other bony deficiency.

Fig. 3.4-6: An example for how to use a lag screw in combination with the internal fixator principle to approximate a fragment to an already applied percutaneous plate.

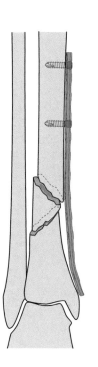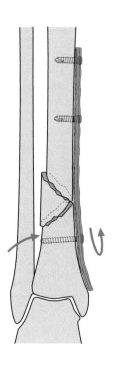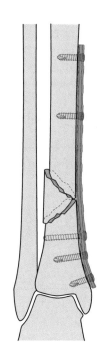

Similarly when a long bridge plate is applied with locking screws, a conventional lag screw may be used to approximate a grossly displaced large fragment in order to improve stability and alignment (**Fig. 3.4-6**).

In summary, the existing benefits of the new internal fixator principles are enhanced by the combination hole concept in the following respects:

- Improvement in angular stability due to locking head screws (even if unicortical) which do not tend to loosen.
- Accurate plate contouring not required.
- Less damage to the periosteum and its blood supply.
- More options and greater versatility in fracture management.

However, these new techniques demand very careful preoperative planning, especially in the sequence of applying the different types of screws, since this process requires a clear understanding of the principles governing each technique.

5 Bibliography

1. **Perren SM** (1991) Basic aspects of internal fixation. In: Müller ME, Allgöwer M, Schneider R, et al., editors. *Manual of Internal Fixation.* Berlin Heidelberg New York: Springer Verlag: 1–112.
2. **Schatzker J** (1995) Changes in the AO/ASIF principles and methods. *Injury;* 26 (Suppl 2):51–56.

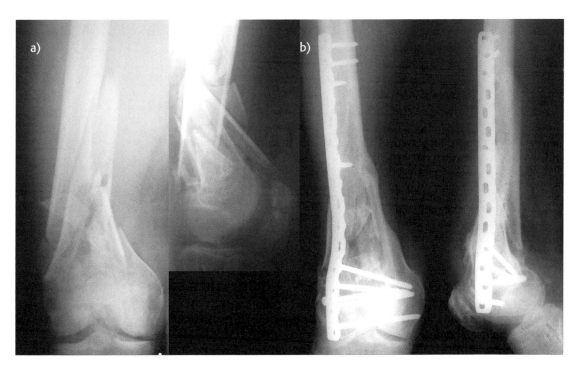

Fig 3.4-7: a) 37-year-old male with distal femur fracture 33-C2. Use of a straight, large LCP 4.5 to reconstruct and stabilize the femur. Percutaneous insertion of the bridging plate after reconstruction of the articular component with lag screws.
b) Follow-up x-rays after 6 months with sound fracture healing in correct axial alignment.

3. **Perren SM, Buchanan J** (1995) Basic concepts relevant to the design and development of the point contact fixator (PC-Fix). *Injury*; 26 (Suppl 2):1–4.

4. **Tepic S, Perren SM** (1995) The biomechanics of the PC-Fix internal fixator. *Injury*; 26 (Suppl 2):5–10.

5. **Ganz R, Mast J, Weber BG, et al.** (1991) Clinical aspects of biological plating. *Injury*; 22 (Suppl 1):4–5.

6. **Mast J** (1991) Preoperative planning and principles of reduction. In: Müller ME, Allgöwer M, Schneider R, et al., editors. *Manual of Internal Fixation.* Berlin Heidelberg New York: Springer-Verlag: 159–178.

7. **Krettek C** (1997) Concepts of minimally invasive plate osteosynthesis. *Injury*; 28 (Suppl 1):1–6.

8. **Krettek C, Schandelmaier P, Miclau T, et al.** (1997) Minimally invasive percutaneous plate osteosynthesis (MIPPO) using the DCS in proximal and distal femoral fractures. *Injury*; 28 (Suppl 1):20–30.

6 Updates

Updates and additional references for this chapter are available online at:
http://www.aopublishing.org/PFxM/34.htm

4.1 Scapula and clavicle

Christoph W. Geel

1 Scapular fractures

In 1805 Desault produced what was probably the first ever report on scapular fractures. Since then only a small number of studies have been published, thus confirming the rarity of these fractures, accompanied as they are by a high incidence of associated ipsilateral chest injuries [1–4].

Closed management has been the rule for the vast majority of these fractures. More recent studies, however, have raised some questions about this approach to their management.

1.1 Assessment of fractures and soft tissues

Shoulder contusions and skin marks are telltale signs. The most common fracture type, representing about 35% of all scapular fractures, occurs in the body of the scapula. Fractures of the scapular neck are second in frequency. Injuries to the scapular spine, glenoid, and acromion are about equal in incidence. A high proportion of these particular injuries show complex multiple fracture patterns.

Blunt trauma frequently results in combination fractures of the clavicle and the scapula, but there is also a 25% incidence of injury to the ipsilateral chest wall. The overall incidence of pulmonary injuries from this high-energy complex trauma is 37%, mostly hemopneumothorax and lung contusion.

An incidence of 8% of skull fractures and 12% cervical spine injuries has been documented [4, 5]. Clearly, in many cases, the scapular fracture per se is not to be considered an "isolated injury" but as the centerpiece of a regional injury.

Scapular fractures are classified (**Fig. 4.1-1**) on the basis of their anatomy [6–9]. We can **distinguish between stable and unstable extra-articular and intra-articular fracture** patterns. Stable extra-articular fractures comprise injuries of the scapular body and processes, and can be simple or fragmented. Fractures of the scapular neck, in spite of some displacement, usually appear to be stable and so fall into this category.

Unstable extra-articular fractures of the scapular neck are typically associated with a displaced fracture of the midshaft of the ipsilateral clavicle (see **Fig. 4.1-5a**). This combination may make the entire shoulder girdle unstable and gives it a tendency to rotate caudally due to

Closed management has been the rule for the vast majority of scapular fractures.

Distinguish between stable and unstable extra-articular and intra-articular fractures.

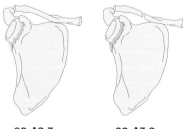

09-A2.3   09-A3.2

Fig. 4.1-1: OTA Classification

the weight of the arm. The severe force necessary to cause such a complex injury often results in a fracture of the upper three to four ipsilateral ribs and may also damage the neurovascular bundle including the brachial plexus [10].

Such a fracture combination deserves the label "floating shoulder".

Intra-articular fractures are much less common and mostly present with a transverse fracture line through the entire glenoid.

Glenoid rim fractures are in general associated with a dislocation of the shoulder and have to be considered as an integral part of posttraumatic shoulder instability [11].

1.1.1 Indications

The unconstrained structure of the shoulder and associated joints results in unique axial and rotational mobility. At less than 90° of abduction the deltoid muscle force generates a shear vector in the glenoid fossa. This force is neutralized by the rotator cuff muscle, which creates a stabilizing compressive force across the glenoid. If there is a change in the glenoid axis caused by fracture displacement, the lever arm of the rotator cuff muscles is altered, converting the compressive force into a shear or sliding force. The situation worsens markedly at about 45° or more of glenoid varus tilt. In addition, fracture of the scapular spine may cause rotator cuff dysfunction because the entire scapula collapses with shortening of the leverage of the rotator cuff muscles.

It is evident that severely **displaced and unstable fractures of the scapular neck** with greater than 40° angulation in either the transverse or coronal plane or greater than 1 cm displacement are **indications for operative management**. In addition, the instability of

Indications for operative management are displaced and unstable fractures of the scapular neck.

the scapular neck is augmented by the displaced ipsilateral fracture in the clavicle, which is the ultimate stabilizer of the shoulder girdle. Fractures of the acromion and the coracoid process, if displaced greater than 5–8 mm, are indications for surgery.

Glenoid rim fractures and intra-articular glenoid fractures resulting in a remaining shoulder instability are indications for surgery. Intra-articular displacement of 3–5 mm is considered enough to warrant operative reduction and stabilization.

1.2 Surgical anatomy

Attempt at surgical exposures, anteriorly or posteriorly, through limited approaches, will only prove frustrating and are not recommended.

Structures at risk in the posterior approach are the axillary nerve as well as the humeral circumflex artery and the suprascapular nerve at the level of the scapular neck.

1.3 Preoperative planning

Accurate radiographic assessment and preoperative planning are essential factors for successful surgical treatment of scapular fractures. The chest x-ray, which should be taken in all multiple trauma cases, is used as a first screening.

A true anterior/posterior x-ray and a lateral scapular view to assess displacement of the glenoid in the coronal plane, as well as a transaxillary axial view, are essential minimum studies. In those cases with suspected fractures of the glenoid in combination with, or without, ipsilateral rib fractures, a CT scan and reconstruction views provide the needed information as to the best surgical approach, as well as to determine the amount of displacement and the size of the fragments. In addition, the ipsilateral chest, its volume (pneumothorax?), as well as the chest wall with rib fractures are documented.

1.3.1 Positioning and approaches

Anterior approach: Details see **chapter 4.2.1**, **Fig. 4.2.1-3** and **Fig. 4.2.1-5**.

Anterior glenoid fragments and anterior glenoid rim fractures are approached through a standard Bankart dissection using the delto-pectoral incision. The axillary nerve on the undersurface of the deltoid as well as the neuro-vascular bundle medially are at risk. The patient is positioned in a beach chair position (see **chapter 4.2.1**, **Fig. 4.2.1-4**) with the arm draped free. Alternatively, the patient may be positioned supine with a radiolucent roll under the spine to allow the involved arm to extend. It is very helpful if a complete radiolucent operating table is used to facilitate intraoperative radiographic imaging. In a large or muscular patient the coracoid process or the conjoint tendon of the short head of the biceps muscle and coraco-brachialis muscle must be taken down in order to have satisfactory exposure of the medial extent of the neck of the glenoid.

Posterior approach: Lateral decubitus positioning is preferable because of possible ipsilateral chest wall injuries.

Posteriorly the extensile approach runs from the tip of the acromion along the inferior margin of the scapular spine to the medial scapular border, down which it curves to the inferior angle of the scapula (**Fig. 4.1-2a**).

The posteromedial angle of the deltoid is sharply dissected from the spine and base of the acromion, leaving a small tissue border at the spine to facilitate reattachment. The deltoid is then folded very cautiously laterally because the axillary nerve and the circumflex artery are attached to its lateral border. The interface between infraspinatus and teres minor offers an approach to the lateral margin and border of the scapula. With this approach, the inferior aspect of the base of the scapular spine, the base of the acromion, the lateral scapula border and the scapular neck are seen. If necessary, a small arthrotomy can be carried out to look at the posterior part of the glenoid (**Fig. 4.1-2b**).

1.4 Surgical treatment—tricks and hints

1.4.1 Fractures of the glenoid rim

Isolated fractures of the anterior and/or inferior glenoid rim are usually associated with shoulder dislocations. Larger rim fragments should be provisionally stabilized with a K-wire and fixed with one or two 4.0 mm cancellous bone screws. The inclination of the glenoid fossa serves as a guide to the positioning of the K-wires, whether these are preliminary prior to screw fixation, or definitive for the siting of 4.0 mm or 4.5 mm cannulated screws. The soft tissue of the labrum is frequently disrupted and small washers may be helpful in reattaching it.

1.4.2 Fractures of the glenoid fossa

Undisplaced fractures are usually managed without surgery and show good functional results. Only unstable and displaced fractures of the glenoid need to be reduced and stabilized. For these fractures, which are mostly transverse through the glenoid, lag screw fixation with 4.0 mm cancellous bone, or cannulated screws

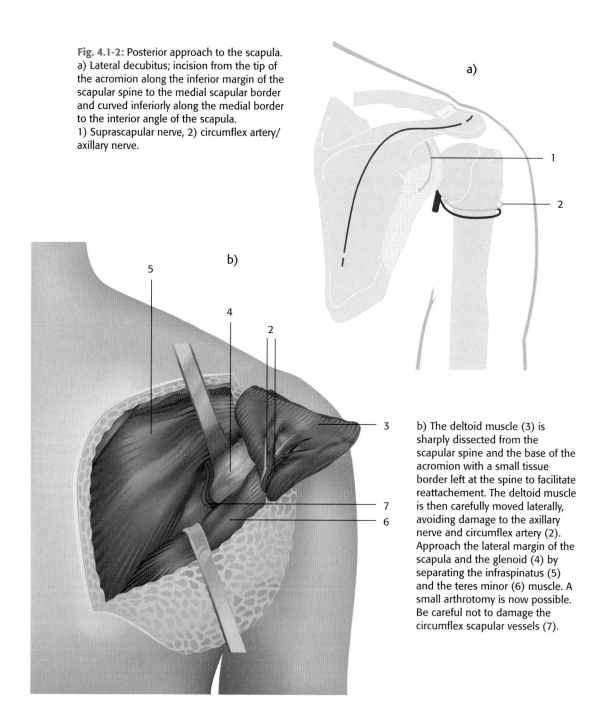

Fig. 4.1-2: Posterior approach to the scapula. a) Lateral decubitus; incision from the tip of the acromion along the inferior margin of the scapular spine to the medial scapular border and curved inferiorly along the medial border to the interior angle of the scapula.
1) Suprascapular nerve, 2) circumflex artery/ axillary nerve.

b) The deltoid muscle (3) is sharply dissected from the scapular spine and the base of the acromion with a small tissue border left at the spine to facilitate reattachement. The deltoid muscle is then carefully moved laterally, avoiding damage to the axillary nerve and circumflex artery (2). Approach the lateral margin of the scapula and the glenoid (4) by separating the infraspinatus (5) and the teres minor (6) muscle. A small arthrotomy is now possible. Be careful not to damage the circumflex scapular vessels (7).

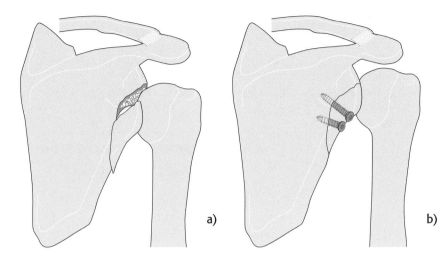

Fig. 4.1-3:
a) Transglenoid fracture with marked dislocation of the fragment.
b) Reduction through partially open joint capsule, temporarily fixation with a K-wire and fixation with two lag screws.

provides enough stabilization for active range of motion postoperatively (**Fig. 4.1-3**). If the fragment size is large, a one-third tubular plate at the inferior lateral border, fixed with 3.5 mm cortex screws, is recommended.

1.4.3   Fractures of the neck of the scapula

Isolated fracture of the scapular neck

Some minimally displaced fractures without involvement of the ipsilateral shoulder girdle or ipsilateral chest wall are treated with early functional aftercare.

The inserting triceps muscle attachment at the infraglenoid tubercle may pull the glenoid distally and tilt it laterally (**Fig. 4.1-4**).

Depending on the fragment size and the fracture pattern the implant choice lies between independent lag screws (see **Fig. 4.1-3b**) and a buttress plate. With the posterior approach, the individual lag screws can be driven into the

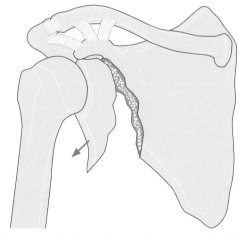

Fig. 4.1-4: Isolated scapular neck fracture lateral to the coracoid. The fragment is displaced by the force of the triceps muscle traction.

tubercle from behind. Larger fragments should be buttressed posteriorly with a one-third tubular plate, pressing the articular fragment against the proximal lateral border of the scapula. Combining the plate with a 3.5 mm cortex lag screw increases the stability of the fixation.

Combination fractures with scapular neck fractures

When a fracture of the clavicle and/or rib fractures combined with a displaced scapular neck fracture occur on the same side, the shoulder girdle becomes unstable (see **Fig. 4.1-5a**). The weight of the arm drags the shoulder, as well as the chest wall, distally and anteriorly, which may compromise the chest volume. How much the scapular neck is displaced and how unstable it is depends on the integrity of the coracoclavicular and acromioclavicular ligaments. Associated injuries of the brachial plexus are very common in those circumstances.

The **first step to restore the stability is to fix the clavicle,** which is the only attachment of the shoulder girdle to the sternum.

First step to restore stability: fix the clavicle.

The clavicular fracture is fixed with a DCP 3.5, LC-DCP 3.5, or reconstruction plate 3.5. This usually reduces the neck fracture, at least partially; additional fixation of the scapular neck fracture is rarely required (**Fig. 4.1-5**).

1.4.4 Fractures of the acromion and coracoid process

Operative treatment is only indicated for markedly displaced fractures and painful nonunions. A lateral fracture of the acromion may be stabilized with K-wires and a tension band. Small fragments may be excised and a detached deltoid muscle is reattached in a transosseous fashion.

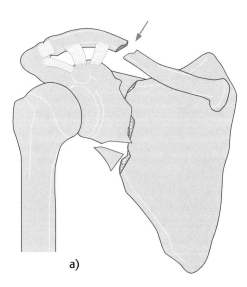
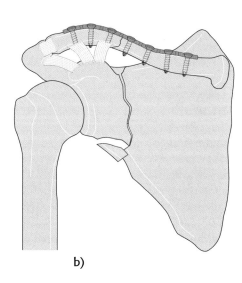

a)

b)

Fig. 4.1-5:
a) The combination of fractures of the clavicle and the scapular neck renders the entire shoulder girdle unstable. The lateral fragment of the scapula rotates due to the weight of the arm.

b) To restore stability it is usually sufficient to fix the clavicle with a 3.5 mm plate.

For fractures of the coracoid process surgery is indicated only if there is marked coraco-clavicular displacement or if the neurovascular bundle is compromised.

Internal fixation is, however, used after osteotomy of the coracoid in order to gain access to the anterior part of the shoulder joint. Inter-fragmentary screw compression is satisfactory using a screw of suitable size for the patient's bone. This may be supplemented with a tension band wire [12].

1.5 Postoperative treatment

Temporary immobilization in a Gilchrist or Desault sling is recommended for 3–4 post-operative days and then active assisted functional after treatment is instituted. After the third postoperative week, a complete program of rotator cuff strengthening with resistive exercises is mandatory for a good result.

1.6 Results

The outcome is in part determined by the initial damage to the cartilage of the glenohumeral joint caused by the high impact and, in part, by the quality of the reduction.

Hardegger and Simpson reported 79% good to excellent results in 37 operated patients. Others report good results in 75% of operated intra-articular glenoid fractures [2, 9, 10, 13].

2 Clavicular fractures and dislocations of adjacent joints

Falls on the outstretched hand and direct trauma are the likeliest causes of fractures of the clavicle. With an intact sternoclavicular joint, the force of the entire shoulder and the scapula, directed posteriorly, creates the fracture of the clavicle over the fulcrum of the first rib. With this mechanism in mind, it becomes obvious that the neurovascular bundle is at risk and needs to be evaluated carefully.

The OTA compendium lists diaphyseal fracture (06) as simple, wedge, and complex (**Fig. 4.1-6**).

Clavicular fractures in children, adolescents, and adults will heal with a minimum of treatment in the vast majority of the cases. Treatment with figure-of-eight strapping relieves most of the discomfort and pain, and allows early motion.

There is some controversy in the literature regarding the non-union rates, which range between 0.1% up to 23% [14, 15].

The treatment goal is the restoration of normal function in the shoulder girdle and, therefore, immobilization should be kept to an absolute minimum.

2.1 Assessment of fractures and soft tissues

The few **indications for primary operative fixation of clavicular fractures** include the open fracture, impending perforation of the skin by a sharp irreducible fragment, and an **associated injury to the subclavian artery and brachial plexus, as well as an ipsilateral scapular neck fracture** resulting in instability

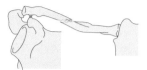

06-A1

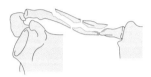

06-C1

Fig. 4.1-6: OTA Classification

Indications for primary operative fixation of clavicular fractures:
- associated injury to the subclavian artery and brachial plexus,
- an ipsilateral scapular neck fracture,
- painful non-union.

[12]. Relative indications are a clavicular fracture in a multiply injured patient, if it seems likely to help in mobilization, and bilateral fractures.

The third **indication is painful non-union** of the clavicle, with or without compromise of the neurovascular bundle due to abundant callus formation. Efforts must be made beforehand to distinguish between pain from a plexus injury and pain from the non-union site [14].

Grossly displaced lateral clavicular fractures may require operative treatment since the rates of painful non-union are significant in this group.

In very rare cases where surgical access to the subclavian artery has to be facilitated by an osteotomy of the clavicle, plating of the osteotomy can be considered in preference to clavicular resection which, though frequently recommended, can result in an unstable shoulder girdle [15].

2.2 Surgical anatomy

The close proximity of the brachial plexus and the subclavian vessels makes the use of oscillating drill bits recommendable to reduce the risk of perforating and injuring those structures. The saber cut incision in closed injuries gives the best cosmetic result in a skin area that tends to form hypertrophic scarring. The exposure is sufficient if the medial and lateral fragments are alternately exposed and only one window at a time is used. Incisions parallel to the clavicle should only be used in open fractures where the laceration can be incorporated in the incision following the Langer's lines, as well as in cases needing access to the subclavian artery and brachial plexus. The plate can be placed anteriorly or superiorly, depending upon the fracture pattern and the position of the wedge fragment. Anterior placement of the plate eliminates the

Complex fractures require longer plates.

risk of a vascular injury and allows the use of longer screws but poses some threat to the brachial plexus. Straight plates are more easily contoured!

2.3 Preoperative planning

The chest x-ray serves as a screening tool. Specific views of the clavicle in straight AP direction are augmented with oblique views. Scapular Y-views are helpful in determing the relationship between acromion/coracoid and the scapula.

To evaluate acromioclavicular joint dislocation AP and lordotic views of the clavicle are used. The degree of instability is best documented by gentle palpation of the acromioclavicular joint while supporting the arm at the elbow and lifting it up and down. The use of weights to displace the dislocation may be painful and should be avoided.

2.4 Surgical treatment— tricks and hints

Spiral or short oblique fractures are easily reduced and temporarily stabilized with pointed reduction forceps. A 7-hole or 8-hole LC-DCP 3.5 or a reconstruction plate 3.5 can be used to stabilize the fracture (**Fig. 4.1-7**). If possible, an independent lag screw should be inserted to stabilize a wedge fragment.

More **complex fractures require longer plates**, although, contouring may become difficult. In complex multifragmentary fractures the plate is best used as a bridge spanning the fragments, which is far more successful than dissecting each fragment. Cancellous bone grafting is only performed for bone defects or devitalized bone.

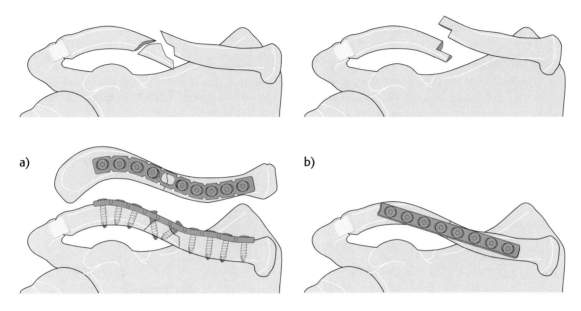

Fig. 4.1-7: Midshaft fractures of the clavicle.
a) Wedge fracture fixed with a 10-hole reconstruction plate 3.5 on top. Two lag screws are placed through the plate.

b) Anterior placement of a LC-DCP 3.5 for better purchase of the screws.

2.4.1 Fracture of the lateral clavicle

(**Fig. 4.1-8**)

Provisional reduction is secured by a trans-acromial K-wire. The definitive fixation is accomplished with a figure-of-eight tension band wire combined with two—preferably threaded—K-wires (**Fig. 4.1-9**). To avoid articular disc injury, this fixation should not encroach upon the acromioclavicular joint. As an alternative, a one-third tubular plate or small fragment T-plate can be used according to the size of the fragments. In multifragmentary fractures a reconstruction plate 3.5 is a valid alternative.

An alternative is the technique with a screw through the plate into the base of the coracoid as described by Bosworth [16, 17] (**Fig. 4.1-10**).

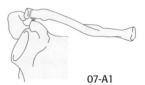
07-A1

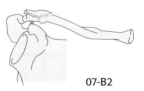
07-B2

Fig. 4.1-8: OTA Classification

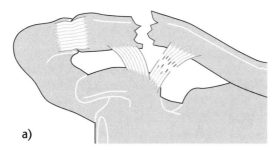

a)

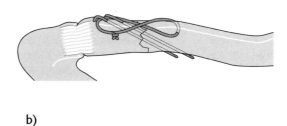

b)

Fig. 4.1-9:
a) Lateral clavicular fracture with partial disrupture of the coracoclavicular ligament.

b) Fixation with two K-wires brought in through the cranial aspect of the lateral fracture fragment. The fracture is anchored by a figure-of-eight cerclage through a 2 mm drill hole.

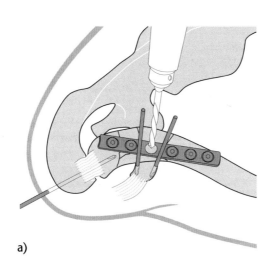

a)

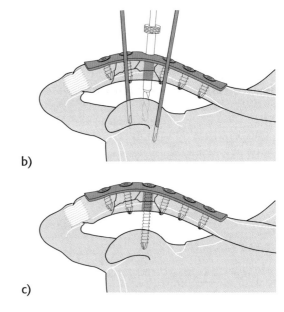

b)

c)

Fig. 4.1-10:
a) Temporary fixation of the acromioclavicular joint, localization of the coracoid with K-wires, and fixation of the plate omitting the screw opposite the coracoid.

b) A 3.5 mm gliding hole is drilled through the LC-DCP 3.5 and the coracoid perforated by a 2.5 mm drill bit.
c) A 3.5 mm cortex screw is placed in the coracoid and the temporary K-wires are removed.

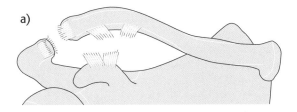
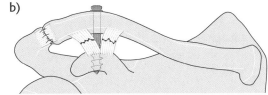

Fig. 4.1-11: Acromioclavicular dislocation type Tossy III.
a) Through a sabre cut incision, the remnants of the coracoclavicular ligament are identified and—if feasible—prepared for suture.
b) After temporary fixation of the reduced acromioclavicular joint with a K-wire, a 3.2 mm hole is drilled centrally through the clavicle into the coracoid. Both

cortices of the clavicle are overdrilled and a 6.5 mm cancellous bone screw is placed with a washer. The shaft of the screw should only be in loose contact with the clavicle to allow for some movement of the shoulder girdle. Suture of the acromioclavicular joint capsule and removal of the transfixing K-wire.

2.4.2 Acromioclavicular joint dislocation

Complete disruption of the acromioclavicular joint (Tossy III), especially if irreducible, is indication for operative care [18].

Many techniques have been proposed in the treatment of acromioclavicular joint separation [18, 19]. We describe two possibilities:

Indirect purchase on the acromioclavicular joint with coracoclavicular fixation using screws, wire loops, or sutures (**Fig. 4.1-11**). These procedures may be combined with débridement of the acromioclavicular joint and repair of the coracoclavicular ligaments. Saber cut incision gives the best exposure. Transosseous sutures may be placed between the avulsed ligaments and holes in the lateral end of the clavicle. After identification of the coracoid with two temporary K-wires, a 3.2 mm drill bit is used to drill a hole through the clavicle into the coracoid. Both cortices of the clavicle are then overdrilled with a 4.5 mm drill and a 6.5 mm cancellous bone screw with 16 mm thread, and a washer

is inserted. The overdrilling of both cortices of the clavicle allows it to rotate without loosening of the screw in the coracoid anchor. Tying the sutures of the acromioclavicular reconstruction completes the procedure. Screw removal is planned after 8–10 weeks postoperatively.

Alternatively, the acromioclavicular joint is exposed in a similar fashion as for the coracoclavicular screw and the joint debrided. Following reduction it is stabilized with a 2 mm K-wire inserted from the outer lateral aspect of the acromion across the joint and into the clavicle. It is important that this wire impale the cortex of the clavicle to prevent migration. Instead of a K-wire, a 3.5 mm cancellous bone screw or a 4.5 mm cannulated cortex screw may be used. This screw is inserted through a gliding hole in the acromion and into the medullary canal of the clavicle. It will normally exit from the cortex of the clavicle due to the curve of the bone. After stabilization of the joint, a tension band of either wire or non-absorbable suture is placed through a drill hole in the clavicle and runs under the deltoid attachment to the acromion and the wire or screw head. The patient is not allowed to use the extremity in abduction to prevent breakage of the wire or screw but may use the extremity for other activities. At 3 months the wire or screw is removed and full activity is commenced.

2.4.3 Sternoclavicular joint dislocation

Sternoclavicular dislocations in patients of 20 years or younger may constitute a Salter Type I or II physeal injury, as the medial clavicle ossifies late. The diagnosis is based on physical and radiographic findings with apical lordotic views. Only the CT scan allows an accurate characterization of these lesions. Sternoclavicular joint dislocations, whether anterior or posterior, can be complete or incomplete. Anterior dislocations have generally little long-term functional impact but remain unstable when reduced.

Posterior dislocations are more serious due to the adjacent mediastinal and cervical structures. Dysphagia or dyspnea have been reported [20].

Surgical treatment—tricks and hints

Symptomatic posterior dislocations are reduced with a towel clip or pointed bone-holding forceps applied percutaneously. Once reduced those dislocations are stable.

Dislocations that cannot be managed with closed reduction techniques receive surgery. Techniques to stabilize these dislocations remain debatable and range from transosseous sutures to excisional arthroplasty.

Functional aftercare is as described for fractures of the clavicle.

2.4.4 Clavicular non-unions

The main indications for secondary operations on the clavicle are the painful non-unions of the middle third as well as post-traumatic shortening with deformity. The major goals of surgery are pain relief and improvement of shoulder function. Any plexus injuries must be thoroughly examined and evaluated beforehand [14].

Preoperative planning

Careful preoperative planning is required with possible inclusion of a CT scan to rule out malalignment in the acromioclavicular and sternoclavicular joints. Reference to preoperative x-rays of the healthy opposite side is helpful to avoid further deformities. Bone grafts should only be needed in atrophic non-unions.

Surgical treatment—tricks and hints

Osteotomy of clavicular non-union is only performed during reconstructive surgery of ipsilateral brachial plexus injures. Due to the fibrotic scar tissue and callus formation around the clavicle, contouring the plate is more difficult than in the acute situation. The remaining fragments must be opposed without force and without rotational malalignment, to reduce the risk of posttraumatic arthritis in the adjacent joints. The anatomic length of the clavicle should be accurately restored to reduce secondary weakening of the rotator cuff strength.

A stable construct with a DCP 3.5 or LC-DCP 3.5 is recommended.

For an atrophic clavicular non-union, a cancellous bone graft is added with or without decortication.

Postoperative treatment

Operated midshaft fractures, as well as lateral clavicular fractures should be stable enough to undergo active range of motion after operation, following pendulum exercises for the first two weeks out of the sling. Full function should be restored at 4–6 weeks postoperatively. Heavy labor and contact sports should be possible at 3–5 months postoperatively.

2.4.5 Results

The operative fixation of non-united clavicular fractures should have a rate of 80–95% good to excellent results overall. A hypertrophied scar may ensue in spite of the care exercised in the incision planning and wound closure.

3 Pitfalls and complications in ORIF of scapula and clavicle

K-wires bridging the acromioclavicular joint have a tendency to migrate and can cause problems, even when the threaded version is used. Early removal of those K-wires after fracture healing is recommended as a further precaution against secondary migration.

Meticulous evaluation of the soft tissue surrounding the clavicle with careful choice of the incision site as well as handling of the soft tissue during surgery (windows) can reduce the risks of infection, which are reported to be as high as 10% [21].

Intra-articular placement of screws in the glenoid fossa can be prevented when preliminary K-wires are placed in the joint to help in determing the axis of the glenoid cavity. Intra-operative C-arm views in at least two planes or intra-articular inspection is mandatory to rule out any intra-articular instrumentation.

4 Bibliography

1. **Goss TP** (1992) Fractures of the glenoid cavity. *J Bone Joint Surg [Am]*; 74 (2):299–305.
2. **Ada JR, Miller ME** (1991) Scapular fractures: analysis of 113 cases. *Clin Orthop*; (269):174–180.
3. **Bauer G, Fleischmann W, Dussler E** (1995) Displaced scapular fractures: indication and long-term results of open reduction and internal fixation. *Arch Orthop Trauma Surg*; 114 (4):215–219.
4. **Thompson DA, Flynn TC, Miller PW, et al.** (1985) The significance of scapular fractures. *J Trauma*; 25 (10):974–977.
5. **Simpson NS, Jupiter JB** (1995) Complex fracture patterns of the upper extremity. *Clin Orthop*; (318):43–53.
6. **Vecsei V, Dann K** (1990) [Surgical management of shoulderblade fractures]. *Aktuelle Traumatol*; 20 (6):277–282.
7. **Euler E, Habermeyer P, Kohler W, et al.** (1992) [Scapula fractures—classification and differential therapy]. *Orthopade*; 21 (2):158–162.
8. **Ideberg R, Grevsten S, Larsson A, et al.** (1995) Epidemiology of scapular fractures. Incidence and classification of 338 fractures. *Acta Orthop Scand*; 66 (5):395–397.
9. **Hardegger FH, Simpson LA, Weber A, et al.** (1984) The operative treatment of scapular fractures. *J Bone Joint Surg [Br]*; 66 (5):725–731.

10. **Rickli D, Regazzoni P, Renner N** (1995) The unstable shoulder girdle: early functional treatment utilizing open reduction and internal fixation. *J Orthop Trauma*; 9 (2):93–97.

11. **Kligman M, Roffman M** (1997) Posterior approach for glenoid fracture. *J Trauma*; 42 (4):733–735.

12. **Goss TP** (1996) The scapula: coracoid, acromial, and avulsion fractures. *Am J Orthop*; 25 (2):106–115.

13. **Guttentag IJ, Rechtine GR** (1988) Fractures of the scapula. A review of the literature. *Orthop Rev*; 17 (2):147–158.

14. **Jupiter JB, Leffert RD** (1987) Non-union of the clavicle. Associated complications and surgical management. *J Bone Joint Surg [Am]*; 69 (5):753–760.

15. **Echtermeyer V, Zwipp H, Oestern HJ** (1984) [Errors and dangers in the treatment of fractures and pseudarthroses of the clavicle]. *Langenbecks Arch Chir*; 364:351–354.

16. **Bosworth BM** (1941) Acromioclavicular separation: a new method of repair. *Surg Gynecol Obstet*; 73:866–871.

17. **Ballmer FT, Gerber C** (1991) Coracoclavicular screw fixation for unstable fractures of the distal clavicle. A report of five cases. *J Bone Joint Surg [Br]*; 73 (2):291–294.

18. **Tossy JD, Mead NC, Sigmond HM** (1963) Acromioclavicular separations: useful and practical classification for treatment. *Clin Orthop*; 28:111–119.

19. **Winkler H, Schlamp D, Wentzensen A** (1994) [Treatment of acromioclavicular joint dislocation by tension band and ligament suture]. *Aktuelle Traumatol*; 24 (4):133–139.

20. **Lewonowski K, Bassett GS** (1992) Complete posterior sternoclavicular epiphyseal separation. A case report and review of the literature. *Clin Orthop*; (281):84–88.

21. **Böstman O, Manninen M, Pihlajamaki H** (1997) Complications of plate fixation in fresh displaced midclavicular fractures. *J Trauma*; 43 (5):778–783.

5 Updates

Updates and additional references for this chapter are available online at:
http://www.aopublishing.org/PFxM/41.htm

4.2.1 Humerus: proximal

Rudolf Szyszkowitz

1 Assessment of fractures

1.1 X-rays and classification

After the patient's clinical status has been established and stabilized, **at least two x-rays of the glenohumeral joint taken at right angles to each other are mandatory to identify the fracture type.** Even better, especially for preoperative planning of B and C fractures, are the three x-rays of the "trauma-series" (**Fig. 4.2.1-1**). Furthermore, x-rays in external and internal rotation of the humerus can be important if tuberosity

fractures are suspected. CT is useful, if these standardized x-rays do not allow clear evaluation of the main fracture features, as well as of articular damage, displacement of fragments, and soft-tissue involvement (e.g., long biceps tendon). It must be possible to determine whether the fracture runs through the anatomical or surgical neck, and this leads on to classification (**Fig. 4.2.1-2**), surgical decision-making, and a view of the prognosis.

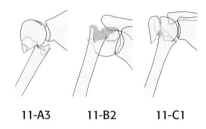

11-A3   11-B2   11-C1

Fig. 4.2.1-2: Müller AO Classification

At least two x-rays of the shoulder joint are required.

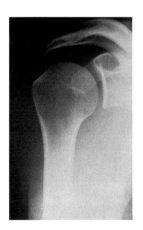

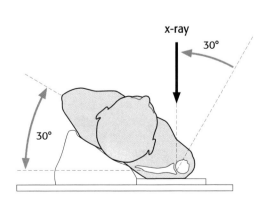

Fig. 4.2.1-1a:
"Trauma-series x-rays": For the AP-view of the shoulder the patient must be placed with the posterior aspect of the affected side against the x-ray plate and the opposite side of the trunk elevated at least 30°.

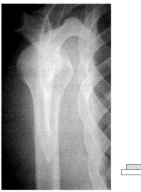 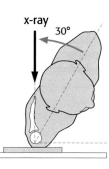

Fig. 4.2.1-1b: The lateral/anterior aspect of the affected shoulder is placed against the x-ray plate. The x-ray beam is then directed posteriorly along the spine of the scapula at an angle of 90° to the direction of the AP.

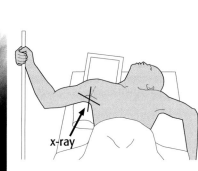

Fig. 4.2.1-1c: For an axillary view the patient is supine with the x-ray plate placed above the shoulder. Abduction of about 30° is needed; this is painful but usually tolerated by the patient.

1.2 Objective indications for surgery

The goal is to restore function.

Conservative treatment is to be preferred for elderly patients and only minimally displaced fractures.

Indications for surgical intervention are governed by general and local concomitant injuries, the type and stability of the fracture, and the patient's age and general state, as well as the quality of the bone (osteoporosis). Stability and displacement are often interdependent. The greater the damage to the adjacent soft tissues and the periosteum, the more likely the need for internal fixation and early functional post-operative treatment. However, in nearly 80% of cases the fracture fragments are held together by muscles, tendons, the attachment of the rotator cuff, and the periosteum, **so treatment—especially in elderly patients—is usually conservative**. In only 20% may reduction and operative fixation be necessary. This group consists mainly of younger patients with fractures in which the tuberosities are displaced more than 5 mm, shaft fragments displaced more than 2 cm, or where head fragment displacement is greater than 40°.

1.3 Subjective indications for surgery

Patient expectations are likely to play an increasingly important part in future decision-making. **In young individuals the goal will be to restore pre-injury levels of function**. Some elderly patients, even when aged over 70, wish to resume such sporting activities as swimming, sailing, cross country skiing, or golf; others, however, require merely to be able to go back to their everyday lives.

2   Surgical anatomy

It is crucial to differentiate between fractures of the anatomical and surgical neck, because the blood supply to the main head fragment after anatomical neck fractures is usually disrupted and AVN is likely to occur. Surgical neck fractures, by contrast, are relatively benign, as the blood supply to the head is usually preserved.

The tendon of the long head of the biceps plays an important role in orientation between the greater and lesser tuberosities. Moreover, in displaced proximal humeral fractures or epiphysiolysis, it can be trapped between bony fragments, making closed reduction impossible. Finally, a few millimeters posterior and parallel to the tendon runs the lateral ascending branch of the anterior circumflex humeral artery (**Fig. 4.2.1-3**). This carries the most important blood supply for the upper part of the humeral head **and damage to it may lead to avascular necrosis** to this part of the head [**1**, **2**]. The

anterior and posterior circumflex humeral arteries anastomose on the lateral side of the surgical neck. Should these vessels be ruptured, the medial aspect of the capsule is the most important remaining blood supply, especially to the lower part of the head, and if a larger medial spike of the head-fragment is present [**3**]. If the head fragment has no soft-tissue connections, AVN develops followed by collapse and deformity, usually within 5 years.

The acromion, along with the coracoacromial ligament and the coracoid process, forms an arch under which the humeral head passes and rotates. Upwards, downwards, or sideways movement of the humeral head is constrained by this arch and the subscapularis, supraspinatus, infraspinatus, and teres minor muscles. These are attached to the tuberosities and, together with the other surrounding muscles, maintain dynamic glenohumeral function. Because of this and to avoid impingement, **it is most important to reduce and to fix the tuberosities with their muscle insertions as closely as possible to their original anatomical sites.**

Vascular damage especially to the lateral ascending branch of the anterior circumflex artery may lead to AVN.

Good function depends on reduction and fixation of the two tuberosities.

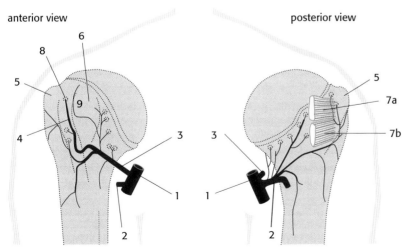

anterior view   posterior view

Fig. 4.2.1-3:
1   Axillary artery
2   Posterior circumflex artery
3   Anterior circumflex artery
4   Anterolateral branch of the anterior circumflex artery
5   Greater tuberosity
6   Lesser tuberosity (anterior)
7   Tendon insertions:
    a   infraspinatus
    b   teres minor
8   Constant site of entry of the anterolateral branch into bone
9   Intertubercular groove

3 Preoperative planning

For every osteosynthesis a preoperative drawing should be carried out: The more complicated the fracture, the greater the need for a detailed plan (see **chapter 2.4**).

3.1 Closed reduction

If general anesthesia is possible, the patient is placed supine on a radiolucent table or in a "beach-chair" position with the affected arm supported on an armrest and free-draped for mobility (**Fig. 4.2.1-4**). Before draping, however, **closed manipulation should be tried** under image intensification. In acute fractures, including about 20% of type B3 and type C3 fracture dislocations, reduction quite often succeeds. If not, after sterile draping there is a second chance using joysticks (small Schanz pins), K-wires, or hooks, so that even after severe initial displacement, near-anatomical reduction—more often in young patients—can be achieved. This means that the possibility of **minimally invasive osteosynthesis** (especially by means of cannulated screws) **should be kept in mind and preoperatively planned.**

> Often closed reduction and percutaneous K-wire fixation will be successful.

3.2 Approaches

If closed reduction cannot be achieved, assisted percutaneous reduction by means of a joystick or hook, or open reduction will be necessary in order to get a good alignment as well as fixation for functional after-treatment.

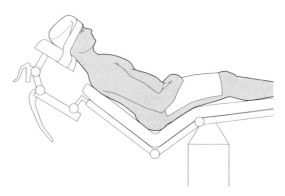

Fig. 4.2.1-4: Beach-chair position with the right shoulder resting on a translucent part of the operating table; the entire shoulder is checked first with the image intensifier before draping.

3.2.1 Deltopectoral approach

The standard approach for reduction and internal fixation of fractures of the proximal humerus is between the deltoid and the pectoral muscles (**Fig. 4.2.1-5**). The cephalic vein can normally be identified proximally with its main connections on the lateral side. The fascia is incised medial to the vein and with slight abduction of the arm, the fracture and the humeral head can be palpated after blunt separation of the deltoid muscle from the bursa, soft tissues, and hematoma around the fracture. After washing out the hematoma, the long biceps tendon can usually be identified under internal and external rotation and will lead to the greater and lesser tuberosities. These, even if they are fractured, have some connections to the adjacent tissues and to their attached muscles. Distally on the shaft, especially in comminuted fractures, the insertion of both the deltoid and the pectoralis muscle may have to be incised to some extent, especially for reduction or to put a plate on the lateral aspect of the humeral shaft. The plate should lie dorsal to the long biceps tendon and the lateral ascending branch of the anterior circumflex humeral artery (**Fig. 4.2.1-3**). The position of this artery should be kept in mind; ligation or coagulation should be avoided along with damage to the axillary nerve.

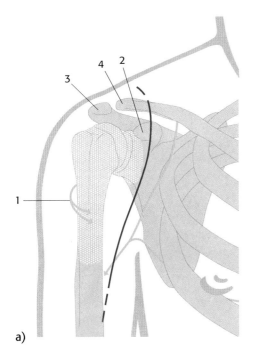

a)

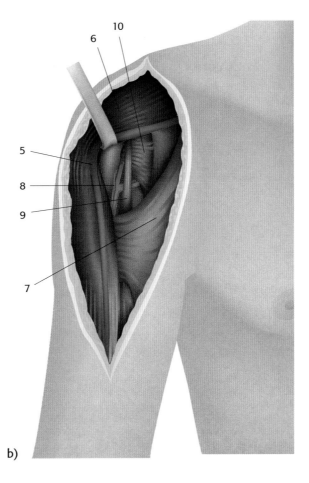

b)

In ORIF, keep fragment exposure to a minimum.

Fig. 4.2.1-5: Deltopectoral approach:

a) The skin incision starts from the coracoid process and runs slightly convex towards the medial side, as far as the insertion of the deltoid muscle on the lateral humeral shaft. 1) Axillary nerve, 2) coracoid process, 3) acromion, 4) lateral end of clavicle.

b) Retraction of the deltoid muscle to the lateral side looking for the humeral head. 5) Cephalic vein, 6) deltoid muscle, 7) pectoralis major muscle, 8) anterior circumflex humeral artery, 9) conjoint tendon of the subscapularis muscle (10).

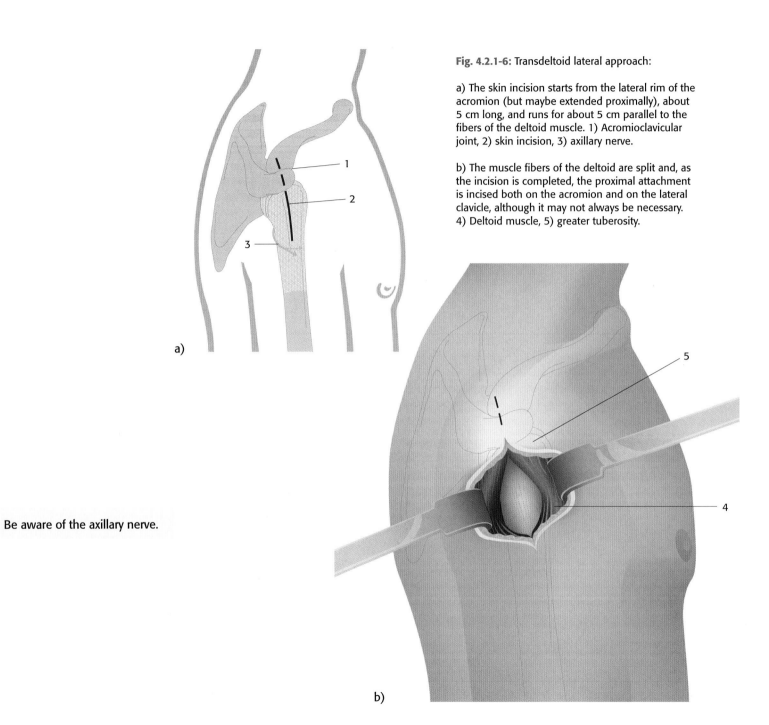

Fig. 4.2.1-6: Transdeltoid lateral approach:

a) The skin incision starts from the lateral rim of the acromion (but maybe extended proximally), about 5 cm long, and runs for about 5 cm parallel to the fibers of the deltoid muscle. 1) Acromioclavicular joint, 2) skin incision, 3) axillary nerve.

b) The muscle fibers of the deltoid are split and, as the incision is completed, the proximal attachment is incised both on the acromion and on the lateral clavicle, although it may not always be necessary. 4) Deltoid muscle, 5) greater tuberosity.

Be aware of the axillary nerve.

3.2.2 Transdeltoid lateral approach

This approach is used for lesions and fractures of the tuberosities and injuries of the rotator cuff (**Fig. 4.2.1-6**). Blunt dissection is used to part the fibers of the deltoid muscle. Rarely, this needs to be detached from the acromion and/or lateral clavicle but must be refixed at closure. Care must be taken not to proceed too far distally because of the axillary nerve and a "safety-suture" should be placed at a distance of 5 cm. During internal and external rotation the fragments can usually be palpated, reduced, and stabilized, as described under **A1 fractures**.

3.3 Instruments and implants for osteosynthesis

We try to **employ as few implants as possible** and plan to have cannulated screws of different diameters and lengths as well as resorbable and non-resorbable atraumatic sutures and 1 mm wire available. Plates are mainly used for surgical neck fractures—where the risk of AVN is smaller—and especially in subcapital fractures with a metaphyseal comminution zone. The aim is to bridge this area and to gain adequate stability for functional after-treatment. T-plates come in different lengths and are fixed by 4.5 mm cortex screws and by 6.5 mm cancellous bone screws, both partially and fully threaded. Cloverleaf plates, which accept small fragment 3.5 mm screws, should also be available. For subcapital fractures, intramedullary nails may sometimes be preferable. Finally, a right-angle plate is available (on request) which is inserted over a K-wire and allows placement of screws into the head or the medial cortex. This plate is especially useful in delayed union and non-unions and is sometimes used together with small fragment screws.

If bone grafting is anticipated, especially after impaction at the fracture site or after comminution, the contralateral iliac crest is prepared, so that bone grafts or even a little cancellous block can be harvested to gain more stability after reduction of the head fragment and to promote earlier bony consolidation [4]. In addition, the use of bone cement might be considered in severe porosis or in pathological fractures to provide a good anchorage for screws.

Bone grafting must be planned (iliac crest) ahead of time.

3.4 Prosthetic replacement

During preoperative planning, cemented prosthetic replacement, especially in complex C fractures, should also be considered, since reconstruction of multiple fragment fractures may not be possible particularly in osteoporotic bone. Reconstruction might also not be advisable in elderly patients with little or no soft-tissue connections to the main head fragment. Under these conditions results are better after primary than after secondary head replacement. This is mainly because functional treatment can only be allowed with stable fixation or after prosthetic replacement [3, 5–7].

Proximal humeral fractures require only a minimum of implants—4.0 mm screws, K-wires, tension band wires, or strong (resorbable) sutures.

4 Surgical treatment

4.1 Extra-articular unifocal A fractures (Fig. 4.2.1-7)

4.1.1 A1 fractures

Unifocal fractures of the greater tuberosity should be treated by sling immobilization in the following circumstances:

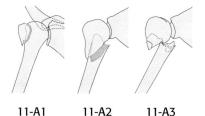

11-A1   11-A2   11-A3

Fig. 4.2.1-7: Müller AO Classification

- if, in younger patients, they are undisplaced or not more than 5 mm displaced,
- if, in older patients (60 and above), they are not more than 10 mm displaced,
- if the angulation of the fragments is less than about 40° (A1.1).

Displacement of tuberosity fragments is best verified with x-rays in internal and external humeral rotation.

When fragments are further displaced, especially the superior part of the greater tuberosity (A1.2), they may intrude between the head and the acromion, due to the pull of the supraspinatus muscle. Such fragments need to be reduced, held temporarily with K-wires running through to the medial side, and then fixed with a cannulated screw (**Fig. 4.2.1-8a/b**). The screw should find a good bite in the cancellous bone.

If open reduction using the deltopectoral approach becomes necessary, a tension-absorbing suture or tension band wire can also be used, alone or as an addition (**Fig. 4.2.1-8c**). After perforation of the cuff close to its bony insertion by means of an atraumatic curved needle carrying a size 1 or 2 resorbable suture, the fragment is reduced and held in place with a figure-of-eight loop which is tightened around a screw head or through a 2.0 mm drill hole in the lateral cortex.

For years we have used only resorbable atraumatic sutures [4] instead of wires [8] with good results. Wires tend to cut through the bone and may break. Patients notice this on the x-ray and may feel disturbed.

If there is an associated glenohumeral dislocation (A1.3), careful closed reduction should be attempted first. In case of significant displacement of the greater or lesser tuberosity, as described above, closed reduction under image intensifier followed by percutaneous fixation is preferable.

Displaced tuberosity fragments are best fixed with a tension band or cannulated screws.

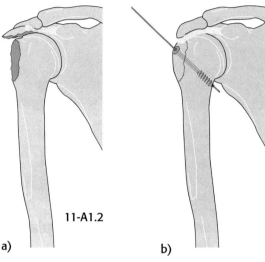

11-A1.2

a)

b)

Fig. 4.2.1-8: Displaced greater tuberosity fracture (A1.2). Reduction and fixation with 4.5 mm cannulated cancellous bone screw following provisional K-wire fixation.

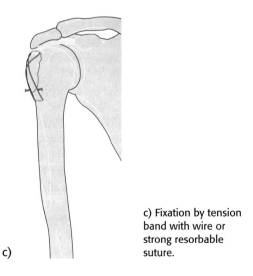

c)

c) Fixation by tension band with wire or strong resorbable suture.

If this proves impossible, open fixation should be achieved as described for the A1.2 fractures.

4.1.2 A2 fractures

Surgical neck or subcapital fractures without major displacement (A2.1: less than 10 mm and angulation below 30° to 45°) will, depending on the patient's age, etc., be treated by sling immobilization until the pain is gone. Afterwards, passive motion, followed by active motion, will be carefully encouraged. If the fracture is impacted with an acceptable amount of varus or valgus malalignment (A2.2 and A2.3) in relation to the patient's age, functional treatment can also be allowed after a few days.

4.1.3 A3 fractures

In these unstable fractures, even when they are impacted or can be reduced closed, redisplacement occurs, leading to prolonged pain, immobilization, and stiffness.

If they can be reduced, maintenance of the reduction is most often attempted by percutaneous pinning under general anesthesia [3, 9, 10]. Alternatively, instead of simple pinning, we favor the use of 7.0 or 4.5 mm cannulated screws following optimal placing of, usually, three 1.6 mm K-wires. These screws are inserted with power after the lateral cortex has been opened with a 4.5 mm drill bit (3.2 mm in younger patients). Two from the lateral cortex

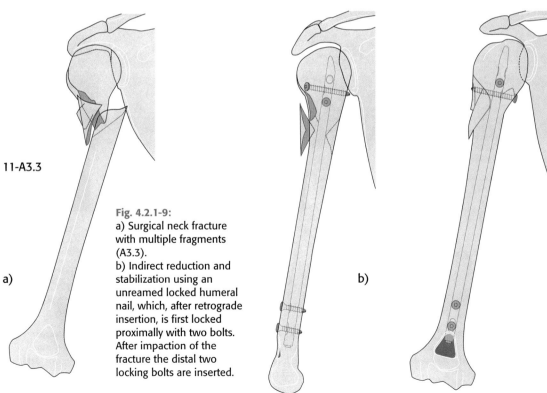

11-A3.3

Fig. 4.2.1-9:
a) Surgical neck fracture with multiple fragments (A3.3).
b) Indirect reduction and stabilization using an unreamed locked humeral nail, which, after retrograde insertion, is first locked proximally with two bolts. After impaction of the fracture the distal two locking bolts are inserted.

a)

b)

and perhaps one from anteriorly are driven towards the center of the head.

One or two K-wires may also be inserted from the greater tuberosity into the medial shaft cortex and usually one or two long cannulated cancellous bone screws are inserted to impact the fracture. After removal of the K-wires, passive motion under image intensification will confirm whether the fixation is stable enough for postoperative functional treatment.

An alternative method of fixation after closed reduction is the use of intramedullary pins or nails, usually by retrograde insertion from about 3 cm proximal to the olecranon tip. **Unreamed interlocking nails provide satisfactory stability, even in A3.3 fractures** with metaphyseal comminution (**Fig. 4.2.1-9**). In severe

open, comminuted, and contaminated fractures an external fixator can be applied.

Inability to reduce the fracture by closed means is usually due to interposition of the long biceps tendon, buttonholing through a split muscle or interposed fragments. Under these conditions a delto-pectoral approach is performed and the situation is corrected. Valgus impaction of up to 10° can be accepted and for stable fixation lag screws and/or plates may be used. Most often a 3-hole or 4-hole T-plate is inserted (**Fig. 4.2.1-10**). If the anchorage of the screws is not reliable, bone cement may be put into the drill holes. The reduction, screw length, screw position, and stability should be checked by image intensifier before the wound is closed. Even pathological fractures can be reliably stabilized in this way.

> In case of inability to reduce the fracture, tendon interposition must be assumed.

> Unstable subcapital fractures (incl. A3.3) may be stabilized using unreamed nails or T-plates.

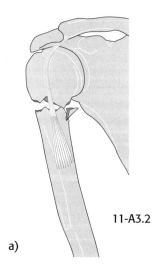
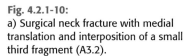
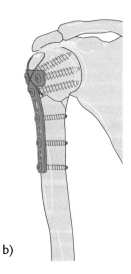
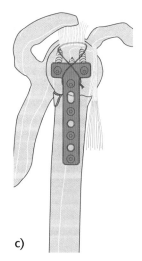

11-A3.2

a)   b)   c)

Fig. 4.2.1-10:
a) Surgical neck fracture with medial translation and interposition of a small third fragment (A3.2).

Correct T-plate fixation AP (b) and lateral (c) after anatomical reduction of the main fragments. Three fully threaded 6.5 mm cancellous bone screws are applied into the head fragment, and 4.5 mm cortex screws into the distal fragment.

In multifragmentary fractures at the surgical neck area or fractures extending further into the shaft, longer T-plates bridging the medial comminution zone will be used. Under these conditions removal of the anterior part of the deltoid insertion has to be accepted; it should be sutured back.

4.2 Bifocal B fractures

(**Fig. 4.2.1-11**)

4.2.1 B1 fractures

These bifocal fractures with little or no displacement display metaphyseal impaction, which can be lateral, medial, or posterior. **Displaced tuberosity fractures must be reduced and fixed** as described for A1 fractures. The impacted metaphyseal fracture is usually stable and treated by conservative means, if the malposition is acceptable.

4.2.2 B2 fractures

These are unstable at the surgical neck and if they are combined with a **rotary displacement of the head fragment** (B2.2), due to the muscle pull on the intact tuberosity, reduction will be required (**Fig. 4.2.1-12a/b**). If this cannot be done closed, percutaneous reduction under image intensifier using a small hook or threaded K-wire as a joystick will be needed (**Fig. 4.2.1-12c/d**). Stabilization by means of cannulated cancellous bone screws is the treatment of choice [5] (**Fig. 4.2.1-12e/f**). Washers are advisable for osteoporotic fragments.

For open reduction the delto-pectoral approach will be used. Tension-absorbing sutures or wires around the tuberosity fragments are anchored to screw heads or in plate holes (**Video AO20080**). In multifragmentary fractures (B2.3) plates will be used routinely, although in the type B fractures it is most important not to damage the residual blood supply to the head.

Hemiarthroplasty in these three-part fractures remains a salvage procedure when stable fixation cannot be achieved.

4.2.3 B3 fractures

Closed reduction is possible in only about 20% of bifocal fracture dislocations, even under full relaxation. If necessary, a joystick and/or hook should be tried, under sterile conditions and using the image intensifier. However, in 80% of cases, open reduction of the dislocated head fragment is necessary, employing the techniques described for B2 fractures. Good results, even

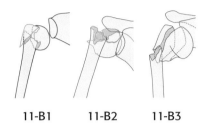

11-B1   11-B2   11-B3

Fig. 4.2.1-11: Müller AO Classification

Reduce and fix displaced tuberosity fragments.

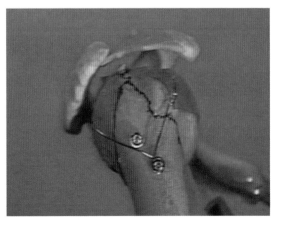

In B2 fractures the head fragment may be rotated.

Video AO20080

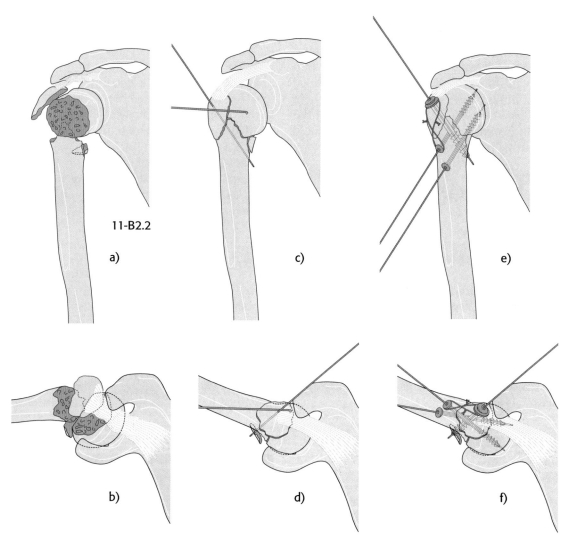

11-B2.2

a)

c)

e)

b)

d)

f)

Fig. 4.2.1-12: Bifocal B2.2 fracture:
a) AP-view: Rotation of the head fragment caused by the sub-scapularis muscle with complete avulsion of the greater tuberosity.
b) Axial view showing 60° angulation deformity.

c) Closed reduction by longitudinal traction, external rotation of the head fragment by means of a hook and stabilization of the greater tuberosity fragment by means of a K-wire.
d) Axial view showing reduction with 15° anterior angulation.

e) Percutaneous K-wire and cannulated screw fixation using 4 mm cannulated cancellous bone screws for the head fragment and one 7.0 mm cannulated cancellous bone screw with washer for the greater tuberosity fragment.
f) Axial view: Fixation in place with angular deformity corrected.

in posterior fracture dislocation with avulsion of both tuberosities (B3.3) can be achieved [5, 11]. **A head endoprosthesis should be restricted to elderly patients only** [12]. Humeral head impaction fractures (Hill-Sachs-lesions) are caused by the glenoid during dislocation and may be treated by elevation and bone grafting to restore the anatomy and to prevent recurrent displacement.

4.3 Articular C fractures

(Fig. 4.2.1-13)

4.3.1 C1 fractures

In this type of fracture of the anatomical neck, there is less than 40° tilting of the head fragment and less than 1 cm shifting of the tuberosity fragment. However, even in minimally displaced neck fractures, without fracture of one of the tuberosities, **the risk of avascular necrosis of the humeral head is more than 50%**, depending on the connection of the head fragment to the capsule on the antero- and postero-medial sides. Often the head is displaced no more than a few millimeters medially on the shaft fragment and is impacted so that its articular surface looks upwards ("ice-cream cone type") [4, 13]. With **the blood supply already at risk**, only closed reduction and **minimal internal fixation** through very limited approaches should be performed. However, in slightly displaced four-part fractures treated by open reduction and minimal internal fixation surprisingly good results, without head necrosis during the first two years, have been described [5, 12, 14]. Prosthetic replacement for these fractures should

therefore be avoided. The technique of closed manipulation and minimally invasive internal fixation is similar to that described for type B fractures (**Fig. 4.2.1-12**). The open fixation technique will be described in the section on **C2.2** and **C3.2** fractures.

In elderly patients varus impaction may be accepted. The fragments, mainly from the tuberosity, may be pulled distally and laterally and fixed with tension-absorbing sutures.

4.3.2 C2 fractures

These fractures are the "real" four-part fractures with more than 40° of angulation of the head fragment and more than 1 cm displacement of at least one tuberosity fragment [6]. If the medial capsule is disrupted, there is usually a displacement of more than 1 cm on the medial side between the head and the shaft fragment—and the joint surface of the head fragment is directed towards the lateral and/or posterior side (**Fig. 4.2.1-14a**).

Using percutaneous reduction and screw fixation, some authors [12] achieved near-anatomical reduction and very good end results in a high percentage of patients with three-part and four-part fractures.

If open reduction is necessary, the deltopectoral approach is used. Many authors prefer osteosynthesis with compression screws and tension-absorbing bands or sutures (**Fig. 4.2.1-14b–d**), but without plates, to reduce the risk of AVN [4, 5, 7, 8, 12–18].

In elderly patients, after impaction of cancellous bone or major displacement, with tilting of the head fragment, a defect persists after reduction, which must be filled with cancellous bone grafts—or substitutes—to gain more stability. Screws placed in the head fragment

Endoprosthesis in elderly patients or unreconstructable fractures only.

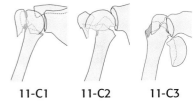

11-C1   11-C2   11-C3

Fig. 4.2.1-13: Müller AO Classification

Risk of avascular necrosis is > 50% in C1 fractures.

Minimal ORIF is recommended when blood supply is at risk.

Fig. 4.2.1-14: Articular four-part C2.2 fracture in a 20-year-old male.

In case of bone defects or impaction use bone grafts.

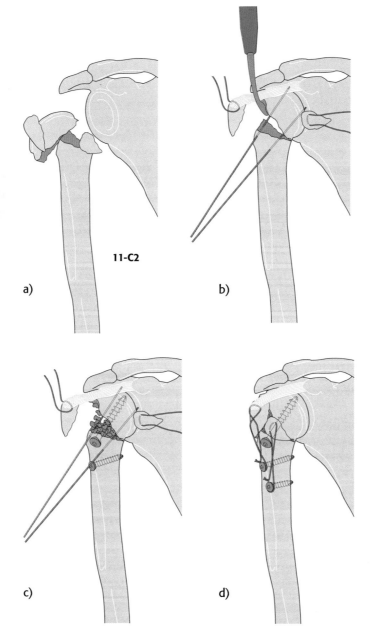

11-C2

a)

b)

c)

d)

a) AP-view: Considerable displacement of head fragment. Large greater tuberosity fragment overlying the head fragment.
b) During open reduction, the head fragment is elevated and placed in correct relationship to the glenoid fossa. Reduction is held with K-wires. The greater and lesser tuberosity fragments are retracted laterally and medially respectively by pulling on resorbable sutures or wires.

c) The K-wires and one 4.5 mm cancellous bone screw hold the position while the defect is partly filled up with cancellous bone graft and the first (proximal) 3.5 mm cortex screw is inserted.
d) The greater tuberosity fragment is reduced and the tension-absorbing suture is tightened around the head of the cortex screw. The lesser tuberosity fragment is also reduced and similarly held by another tension-absorbing figure-of-eight suture tightened around the head of a second more distal 3.5 mm cortex screw.

function more as positioning than compression screws; we have used 7.3 mm self-tapping cancellous bone screws in this situation [12]. In addition, impaction techniques, extra screws, and tension-absorbing sutures and staples or other fixation aids may have a place (**Fig. 4.2.1-14b**).

4.3.3 C3 fractures

For anatomical neck fracture-dislocations (C3.1), many surgeons prefer primary hemiarthroplasty [3, 6], some only if they cannot reconstruct the head fracture or—in elderly patients—if no soft-tissue connections to the head fragment were found during the attempt at open reduction. **Even if these fractures are internally fixed, and later head necrosis is diagnosed on x-ray or MRI, function is often astonishingly good** [5, 7, 12]. The results of secondary endoprosthetic replacement, if necessary, are also satisfying.

If prosthetic replacement is carried out, tuberosity fragments should be accurately reduced to the shaft and held as rigidly as possible, using non-resorbable sutures or wires. The stem should be cemented to ensure rotational stability and to guarantee adequate height of the head. Otherwise, secondary prosthesis migration, displacement, and resorption of the tuberosity fragments, generally with poor clinical results, will occur more often during the later years [6, 18].

5 Postoperative treatment

The shoulder is perhaps the most challenging joint to rehabilitate both postoperatively and after conservative treatment. Early passive motion according to pain tolerance can usually be started after the first postoperative day—even following major reconstruction or prosthetic replacement. The program of **rehabilitation has to be adjusted to the ability and expectations of the patient and the quality and stability of the repair.** Poor purchase of screws in osteoporotic bone, concern about soft-tissue healing (e.g., tendons or ligaments) or other special conditions (e.g., percutaneous cannulated screw fixation without tension-absorbing sutures) may enforce delay in beginning passive motion, usually to be performed by a physiotherapist.

The full exercise program progresses to protected active and then self-assisted exercises. The stretching and strengthening phases follow. The ultimate goal is to regain strength and full function.

Postoperative physiotherapy must be carefully supervised. Mild pain and some restriction of movement at the shoulder joint should not, however, interfere with daily activities. The more severe the initial displacement of the fracture and the older the patient, the greater will be the likelihood of some remaining stiffness. Progress of physiotherapy and callus formation should be monitored regularly. If necessary, closed mobilization of the joint, even under general anesthesia, may be indicated; however, the danger of additional loosening, or of fractures later on, especially in elderly patients, should be kept in mind. Arthroscopy and even open release and manipulation may be considered under certain circumstances, especially in younger individuals.

The patient and stability of repair govern rehabilitation.

In spite of partial AVN, function remains often satisfactory.

6 Pitfalls and complications

Both B and C fractures frequently result in some AVN.

6.1 Positioning of implants

Incorrect placement of implants and displacements of fragments and/or implants can all occur, especially in osteoporotic bone. Not only do screws in the head need to be of optimal length but also in the metaphyseal shaft area they tend to loosen and to migrate. Muscular activity and passive external forces, working on a long lever arm, are often underestimated. Therefore, checking optimal bone and implant position intraoperatively under image intensifier should be the routine. If the hold in subchondral bone or cortex is found to be inadequate, a larger size screw or bone cement should be used prophylactically.

The range of motion to be allowed postoperatively has to be decided intraoperatively under direct view and image intensifier. The stability of the bone-implant construct must be established together with the absence of any resistance or obstruction to the range and directions in which passive movement is to be permitted.

The nerve most frequently at risk is the axillary.

6.2 Malunion and non-union

Malunions and non-unions are rare. If they are causing significant symptoms, such as major discomfort and the loss of function, open correction and internal fixation will benefit reliable patients whose bone and soft tissues are of suitable quality (see chapter 6.2).

Brachial plexus may be damaged by dislocations and fracture dislocations.

6.3 Avascular necrosis

AVN of the humeral head is relatively frequent in B and especially in C fractures and is due to the particular arrangement of its blood supply. This must be known and understood by the surgeon, with the aim of preserving as many vessels and soft-tissue attachments as possible. Accordingly, the use of plates and excessive numbers of sutures and tension-absorbing bands is to be avoided where possible [3, 6].

Avascular necrosis is not in itself a clinical problem. However, it may end up in partial or total collapse of the humeral head with incongruency. This may result in malfunction and pain, although the x-ray appearance frequently does not correlate with the clinical picture [5, 12, 13, 15, 16, 18].

In elderly patients with a life expectancy of not more than 10–20 years, primary prosthetic replacement, if performed as a primary procedure, seems to have a better prognosis in C2.3 fractures and C3 fractures and will avoid the need for a second operation.

6.4 Nerve lesions

The axillary nerve is the one most often damaged both during the accident and iatrogenically—even by closed manipulation and percutaneous fixation. During open reduction the danger occurs especially during soft-tissue retraction using Hohmann retractors or hooks. The musculocutaneous nerve can be damaged in a similar way and especially if an osteotomy of the coracoid process was performed—which is usually not necessary. The adjacent brachial plexus is at risk in dislocations and fracture dislocations. Care must be taken while

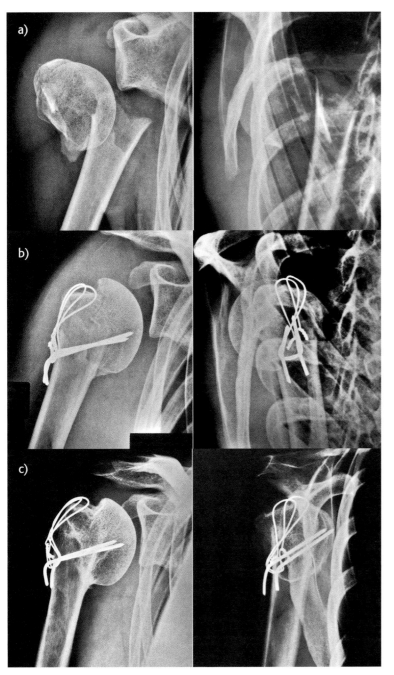

Fig. 4.2.1-15: 26-year-old female, skiing injury.
a) Fracture dislocation of articular fracture (11-C3), AP and axial view.

b) After reduction with two K-wires and two tension band wires. Active postoperative mobilization, AP and axial view.

c) One year follow-up with good range of motion, AP and axial view. In this case, cannulated screws would be an acceptable alternative to K-wires.

6.5 Infection

Aggressive management of deep infection is always required.

positioning the patient before and during the operation so as not to stretch the plexus or damage its blood supply by indirect or direct manipulations.

Percutaneous K-wires may cause irritation and infection along their tracks.

If deep infection occurs, it should be handled aggressively (see **chapter 6.1**). It will be necessary to wash out and debride soft tissues and occasionally necrotic fragments. On rare occasions, and usually only after a second or third look, has the whole head fragment to be removed. This leaves the possibility that later when the infection has settled, prosthetic replacement may be indicated.

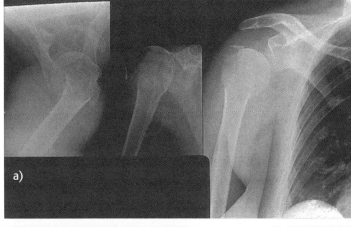

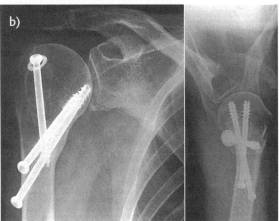
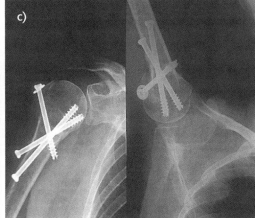

Fig. 4.2.1-16:
a) B1.3 fracture of proximal humerus in a middle aged woman.
b) Postoperative x-rays after reconstruction and fixation with three large cannulated screws.
c) 6 months follow-up, good function.

7 Bibliography

1. **Plaschy S, Leutenegger A, Rüedi TP** (1995) Humeruskopf C-Brüche beim jungen Patienten: Kann die Kopfnekrose vermieden werden? *Unfallchirurg*; 92:63-68.

2. **Cornell CN, Levine D, Pagnani MJ** (1994) Internal fixation of proximal humerus fractures using the screw tension band technique. *J Orthop Trauma*; 8 (1):23–27.

3. **Gerber C, Schneeberger AG, Vin H** (1990) The arterial vascularization of the humeral head. *J Bone Joint Surg [Am]*; 72 (10):1486–1494.

4. **Szyszkowitz R, Seggl W, Schleifer P, et al.** (1993) Proximal humeral fractures. Management techniques and expected results. *Clin Orthop*; (292):13–25.

5. **Jakob RP, Miniaci A, Anson PS, et al.** (1991) Four-part valgus impacted fractures of the proximal humerus. *J Bone Joint Surg [Br]*; 73 (2):295–298.

6. **Jaberg H, Warner JJ, Jakob RP** (1992) Percutaneous stabilization of unstable fractures of the humerus. *J Bone Joint Surg [Am]*; 74 (4):508–515.

7. **Speck M, Regazzoni P** (1997) [4-fragment fractures of the proximal humerus. Alternative strategies for surgical treatment]. *Unfallchirurg*; 100 (5):349–353.

8. **Ochsner PE, Ilchmann T** (1991) [Tension band osteosynthesis with absorbable cords in proximal comminuted fractures of the humerus]. *Unfallchirurg*; 94 (10):508–510.

9. **Schippinger G, Szyszkowitz R, Seibert FJ** (1997) Current concepts in the treatment of proximal humeral fractures. *Curr Orthop*; 11:203–214.

10. **Szyszkowitz R, Schippinger G** (1999) Die Frakturen des proximalen Humerus. *Unfallchirurg*; 102 (6):422–428.

11. **Bigliani LU** (1996) Fractures of the proximal humerus. In: Rockwood CA, Green DP, Buchholz RW, et al., editors. *Fractures in Adults*. 4th ed. Philadelphia: Lippincott-Raven: 1055–1109.

12. **Resch H, Povacz P, Fröhlich R, et al.** (1997) Percutaneous fixation of three- and four-part fractures of the proximal humerus. *J Bone Joint Surg [Br]*; 79 (2):295–300.

13. **Neer CS, II** (1990) Fractures. Shoulder Reconstruction. Philadelphia: W. B. Saunders Co.: 363–364.

14. **Kuner EH, Siebler G** (1987) [Dislocation fractures of the proximal humerus—results following surgical treatment. A follow-up study of 167 cases]. *Unfallchirurg*; 13 (2):64–71.

15. **Kasperczyk WJ, Engel M, Tscherne H** (1993) [4-fragment fracture of the proximal upper arm]. *Unfallchirurg*; 96 (8):422–426.

16. **Böhler J** (1962) Perkutane Osteosynthese mit dem Röntgenbildverstärker. *Wien Klin Wchnschr*; 74:482–485.

17. **Münst P, Kuner EH** (1992) [Osteosynthesis in dislocated fractures of the humerus head. *Orthopade*; 21 (2):121–130.

18. **Siebler G, Walz H, Kuner EH** (1989) [Minimal osteosynthesis of fractures of the head of the humerus. Indications, technic, results]. *Unfallchirurg*; 92 (4):169–174.

8 Updates

Updates and additional references for this chapter are available online at:
http://www.aopublishing.org/PFxM/421.htm

4.2.2 Humerus: shaft

Pol M. Rommens, Donald P. Endrizzi,
Jochen Blum, Raymond R. White

1 Assessment of fractures and soft tissues

1.1 General remarks

Humeral shaft fractures make up approximately 1% of all fractures. Typically they are the result of direct trauma. They also occur in those sports where rotational forces are great, particularly baseball or arm wrestling [1]. Fractures of the proximal humerus can lead to axillary nerve damage. Fractures of the middle and distal thirds of the shaft can give rise to injuries of the radial nerve. Vascular injury is associated with humeral shaft fractures in a small percentage of cases.

The upper arm should be examined for swelling, ecchymosis, and deformity. The entire limb is carefully examined for vascular and neurological changes. Evaluation of the function of the radial nerve is especially crucial prior to any reduction [2].

X-rays are obtained in two planes. If the fracture extends into the shoulder or elbow, oblique x-rays are helpful. Evaluation of the patient with emphasis on associated injuries and concurrent disease is critical in treatment selection.

1.2 Indications (general)

For conservative management of humeral shaft fractures numerous methods have been described, including casting, splinting, Velpeau immobilization, and others. Currently, **functional bracing is probably the most widely accepted** treatment. Good to excellent results have been reported [3, 4]. Moderate angulation (less than 20° anterior and 30° varus angulation), rotation, and shortening (less than 3 cm) are well tolerated.

There are absolute or relative indications for surgical stabilization (**Table 4.2.2-1**). The patient's age, fracture pattern, associated injuries or disease, and ability to comply with treatment must all be considered.

Plate fixation can be used for almost all humeral fractures, especially in the **proximal or the distal shaft**, particularly if there is a concomitant joint fracture.

Plating enables the surgeon to reduce and hold the critical articular or juxta-articular components. Although plating can be technically demanding and requires considerable surgical experience, the results are predictably good and there is little associated shoulder or elbow stiffness [5–9]. Plating is also best for holding cor-

For conservative management of humeral shaft fractures numerous methods have been described—functional bracing is probably the most widely accepted.

Plate fixation can be used for almost all humeral fractures, while intramedullary nailing is gaining in significance.

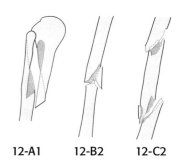

12-A1   12-B2   12-C2

Fig. 4.2.2-1: Müller AO Classification

Table 4.2.2-1: Indications for osteosynthesis.

Absolute indications

- Multiple trauma
- Open fractures
- Bilateral humeral fractures
- Pathological fractures
- Floating elbow
- Vascular injury
- Radial nerve palsy after closed reduction
- Non-union

Relative indications

- Long spiral fractures
- Transverse fractures
- Brachial plexus injuries
- Primary nerve palsy
- Inability to maintain reduction
- Neurologic deficits, Parkinson's disease
- Non-compliance due to alcohol or drug abuse
- Obesity

rected malunions and remains a standard regime for non-unions of the humerus.

Intramedullary nailing is growing in significance as a means of managing humeral fractures. This is due to disappointing experiences in conservative treatment of some fracture types or combinations, or the technical difficulties of plate osteosynthesis in some situations [10]. With smaller, more flexible humeral nails inserted either antegrade or retrograde in an unreamed locked fashion, nailing can be performed more safely (**Fig. 4.2.2-2**). The fracture must be localized between the surgical neck and the transition between shaft and distal metaphysis. Every fracture type, as well as pseudarthroses and pathological fractures, can be nailed [11]. Done properly, nailing permits good fracture alignment and adequate stability. Postoperative rehabilitation is short, uneventful healing the rule, and functional results are excellent [12, 13].

External fixation is mainly used in treating humeral shaft fractures with extensive soft-tissue injury, bone loss, or infection such as occurs in gunshot wounds or accidents with agricultural machinery.

2 Surgical anatomy

The humeral shaft extends from the surgical neck proximally to the condyles distally. It has a cylindrical shape proximally, is conical in its middle section, and in the distal third becomes more flattened in the coronal plane.

The humeral head is just proximal to, and in line with, the medullary canal. The humeral condyles are, however, not in line with the distal end of the canal. Proximally, the articular cartilage of the humerus is separated from greater and lesser tuberosities by the anatomical neck. Distally, a triangular dorsal surface is bounded by the medial and lateral supracondylar crests and the olecranon fossa.

The muscles are divided into flexor and extensor compartments. If the fracture is situated between the rotator cuff and the pectoralis major muscle, the humeral head will be abducted and internally rotated. If the fracture lies between the pectoralis muscle and the deltoid insertion, the proximal fragment will be adducted and the distal fragment laterally displaced. In fractures distal to the deltoid insertion, the proximal fragment will be abducted. In case of a fracture proximal to the brachioradialis and extensor muscles, the distal fragment will be rotated laterally.

The brachial artery and vein, as well as the median and ulnar nerves, traverse the anterior compartment in the medial bicipital groove.

The radial nerve runs through the triceps muscle, **occupying the radial groove in the midshaft area** and perforating the intermuscular septum further down. Here the nerve **becomes less mobile and is vulnerable** when displacement of fragments occurs. The axillary nerve and the posterior circumflex humeral artery originate posteriorly and wind round the surgical neck about 5–6 cm below the acromion.

The radial nerve crossing the humerus becomes most vulnerable at the intramuscular septum.

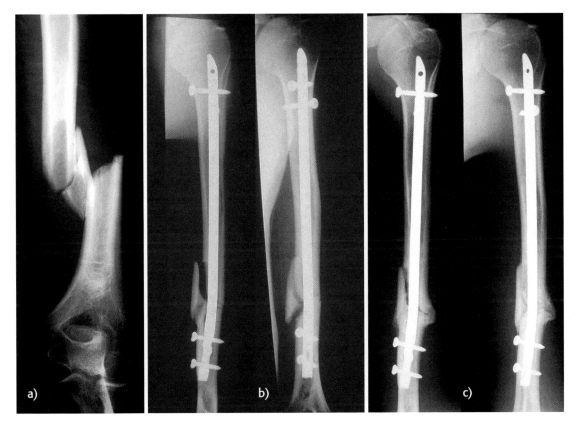

Fig. 4.2.2-2:
a) 26-year-old male with a 12-B2 fracture of the humeral shaft. Intact neurovascular function.
b) Good alignment after retrograde insertion of a solid nail (UHN) with static interlocking.
c) Good callus has bridged the main fragments as well as the wedge at 8 weeks postoperatively.

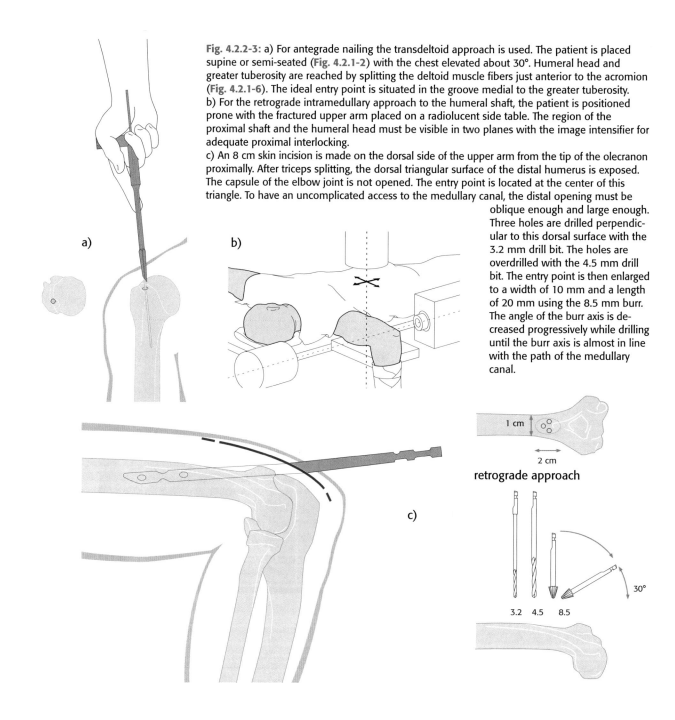

Fig. 4.2.2-3: a) For antegrade nailing the transdeltoid approach is used. The patient is placed supine or semi-seated (Fig. 4.2.1-2) with the chest elevated about 30°. Humeral head and greater tuberosity are reached by splitting the deltoid muscle fibers just anterior to the acromion (Fig. 4.2.1-6). The ideal entry point is situated in the groove medial to the greater tuberosity.
b) For the retrograde intramedullary approach to the humeral shaft, the patient is positioned prone with the fractured upper arm placed on a radiolucent side table. The region of the proximal shaft and the humeral head must be visible in two planes with the image intensifier for adequate proximal interlocking.
c) An 8 cm skin incision is made on the dorsal side of the upper arm from the tip of the olecranon proximally. After triceps splitting, the dorsal triangular surface of the distal humerus is exposed. The capsule of the elbow joint is not opened. The entry point is located at the center of this triangle. To have an uncomplicated access to the medullary canal, the distal opening must be oblique enough and large enough. Three holes are drilled perpendicular to this dorsal surface with the 3.2 mm drill bit. The holes are overdrilled with the 4.5 mm drill bit. The entry point is then enlarged to a width of 10 mm and a length of 20 mm using the 8.5 mm burr. The angle of the burr axis is decreased progressively while drilling until the burr axis is almost in line with the path of the medullary canal.

a)

b)

c)

1 cm

2 cm

retrograde approach

3.2   4.5   8.5

30°

3   Preoperative planning

3.1   Positioning and approaches

Access to the humeral shaft for plating may be by either anterolateral or dorsal approaches. The proximal transdeltoid and the distal dorsal approaches are employed for nailing.

For the antegrade approach the patient is placed supine or semi-seated with the chest elevated about 30°. For the dorsal approach, the patient lies prone on the table with the fractured side near to its edge and the head facing away. The fractured upper arm rests on a radiolucent side table with the forearm hanging down (**Fig. 4.2.2-3b**) [14, 15].

3.1.1   Transdeltoid approach

This is the approach used for antegrade nailing (**Fig. 4.2.2-3a**).

3.1.2   Anterolateral approach

Plating of proximal humeral shaft fractures may be performed through the anterolateral approach. This can be extended down the shaft for middle-third fractures. Care must be taken if this approach is used in distal-third fractures as the radial nerve hugs the lateral cortex and may be trapped under the distal corner of the plate (**Fig. 4.2.2-4** and **Fig. 4.2.2-5**).

3.1.3   Dorsal approach (Henry)

This is most commonly used for fractures of the distal half of the humerus (**Fig. 4.2.2-6** and **Fig. 4.2.2-7**). However, it is easily extended for more proximal fractures once the radial nerve is identified. Access for nailing requires an incision about 8 cm in length over the distal portion (**Fig. 4.2.2-3b/c**) (**Video AO40080a**).

3.2   Reduction techniques and tools

Reduction for plating should be atraumatic. It is achieved by careful traction to restore length, which is then maintained with pointed reduction forceps in oblique or spiral fractures. Transverse

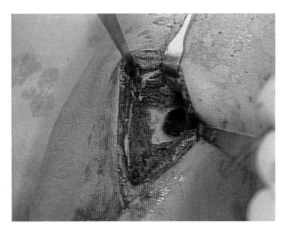

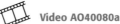 **Video AO40080a**

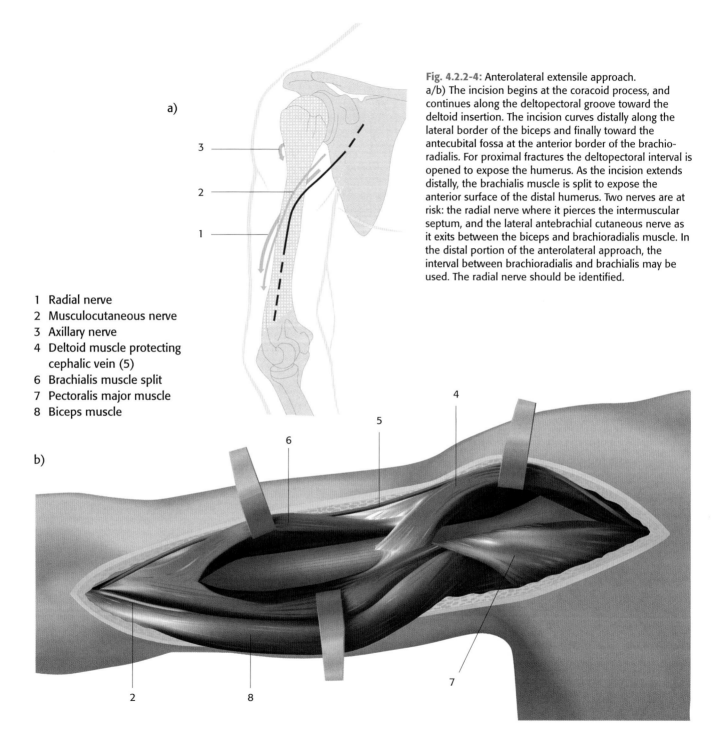

a)

3

2

1

1 Radial nerve
2 Musculocutaneous nerve
3 Axillary nerve
4 Deltoid muscle protecting
   cephalic vein (5)
6 Brachialis muscle split
7 Pectoralis major muscle
8 Biceps muscle

b)

Fig. 4.2.2-4: Anterolateral extensile approach.
a/b) The incision begins at the coracoid process, and
continues along the deltopectoral groove toward the
deltoid insertion. The incision curves distally along the
lateral border of the biceps and finally toward the
antecubital fossa at the anterior border of the brachioradialis. For proximal fractures the deltopectoral interval is
opened to expose the humerus. As the incision extends
distally, the brachialis muscle is split to expose the
anterior surface of the distal humerus. Two nerves are at
risk: the radial nerve where it pierces the intermuscular
septum, and the lateral antebrachial cutaneous nerve as
it exits between the biceps and brachioradialis muscle. In
the distal portion of the anterolateral approach, the
interval between brachioradialis and brachialis may be
used. The radial nerve should be identified.

6

5

4

7

2   8

fractures are best reduced using the plate. The plate is placed extraperiosteally.

In closed nailing, reduction is done with the nail partially inserted. Then, using it as a reduction tool, the opposing fragment is picked up and engaged. Additional external manipulation will help the process.

In case of open reduction, the usual tools can be used.

3.3 Choice of implant

In the past, the recommended implant for plating was the broad DCP 4.5. Today the narrow LC-DCP 4.5 is preferred (**Fig. 4.2.2-7**). This plate will fit well on either posterior or lateral surface. It is important that the screws should be inserted in an offset pattern rather than in parallel sequence, to reduce the risk of fatigue fractures through rotational load.

The solid humeral nail (UHN) is available in three diameters: 6.7, 7.5, and 9.5 mm. Its length varies from 190–325 mm. Both parameters must be determined before nail insertion. A radiographic ruler is available to measure length and diameter intraoperatively. The 7.5 mm nail is used as standard.

4 Surgical treatment—tricks and hints

In order to achieve adequate fixation of the plate, the screws should engage six to eight cortices (usually three to four holes) both above and below the fracture. The aim, wherever possible, should be interfragmentary compression, either by placing a lag screw through the

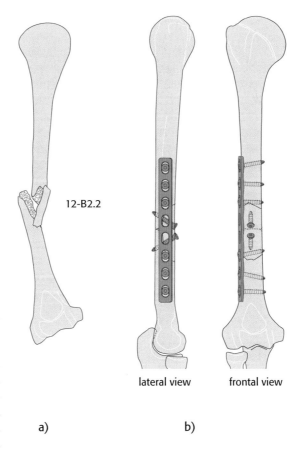

12-B2.2

lateral view   frontal view

a)   b)

Fig. 4.2.2-5:
a) Humeral fracture in the middle third of the right shaft, type 12-B2.2.
b) Anterolateral approach. ORIF with two independent lag screws and a narrow 8-hole LC-DCP 4.5 as protection plate.

a)

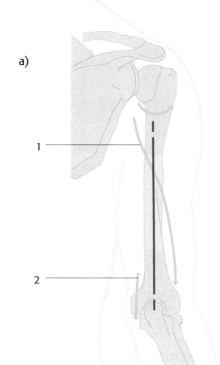

1 Radial nerve
2 Ulnar nerve
3 Lateral intermuscular
  septum

Fig. 4.2.2-6:
Dorsal approach for the distal third of the shaft.
a) The skin incision begins at the tip of the olecranon and runs in a straight line over the posterior midline of the arm proximally.
b) The triceps muscle is split bluntly between the long and the lateral heads. Distally, in the tendon, sharp dissection is necessary. The profunda brachii artery runs with the radial nerve in the spiral groove and is also at risk of injury. The radial nerve (1) must be identified. The ulnar nerve (2), though not generally seen, can be injured by careless retraction. Lateral intermuscular septum (3).

b)

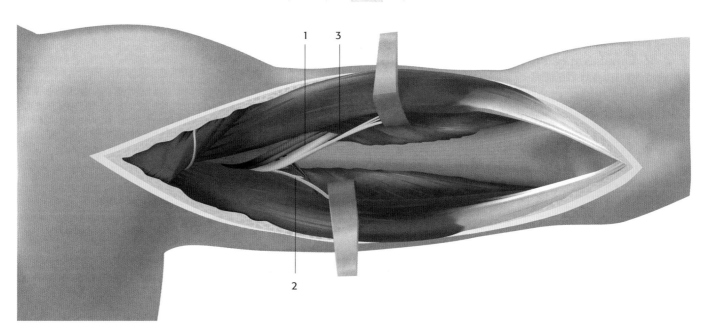

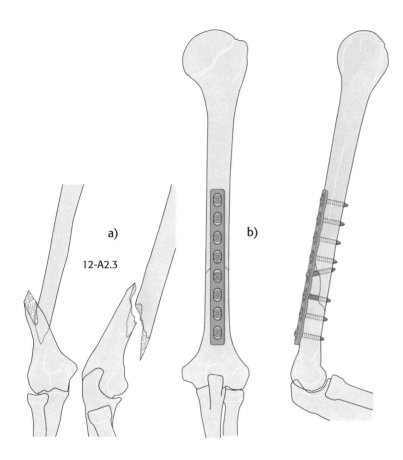

a)

b)

12-A2.3

Fig. 4.2.2-7:
a) Distal humeral shaft fracture, type 12-A2.3.
b) Dorsal approach for the distal third of the shaft. ORIF with a narrow 8-hole LC-DCP 4.5 as protection plate. The two screws crossing the fracture line are lag screws.

plate, or by applying axial load using the DC holes or the articulated tension device. No periosteal stripping should be done, either for plate fixation or screw placement. The use of a nerve stimulator during surgery can be helpful in finding the radial nerve [16]. However, it is much **safer to inspect the nerve** and make sure it is not under the plate, especially at the ends of the plate.

Two different modes of nail assembly are available for nailing. To add interfragmentary compression and to enhance rotational stability, a specific compression device is used in transverse or short oblique fractures. This device has

to be coupled from the start with the insertion handle and the nail. If no additional compression is to be applied, only the insertion handle is connected with the nail. Only minimal force is used for nail insertion.

With careful rotational movements without using a hammer, the nail is advanced by hand to the fracture gap and beyond, after fracture reduction (**Video AO40080b**). Proximal interlocking is done through the targeting device and distal interlocking is carried out freehand in anteroposterior direction.

Various interlocking combinations proximally and distally are possible. The authors

To be safe, inspect the redial nerve.

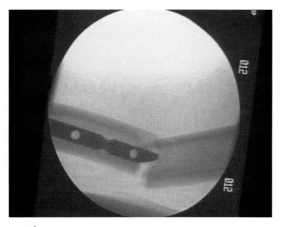

 Video AO40080b

Double interlocking is recommended proximally and distally.

advise double interlocking both proximally and distally (**Fig. 4.2.2-8**) [**15**].

Retrograde nailing (**Fig. 4.2.2-3a/b**): When the canal is very narrow, hand reamers are used to widen it. The nail is inserted without force, while its progress is monitored under image intensification. The nail tip should protrude just slightly into the humeral head. Only then are the locking bolts inserted by freehand technique into the proximal third of the diaphysis where the cortex is thick enough for a reliable hold.

Distally, dorsoventral interlocking is performed through the handle of the targeting device (**Video AO40080c**).

Pin placement in the humerus must respect the courses of nerves.

For external fixation, a unilateral, half-pin frame is sufficient for fracture stabilization (**Fig. 4.2.2-9**). Because the courses of nerves and vessels vary, limited open placement of the pins is recommended. A small incision is made and bluntly dissected to bone and the guide is placed through this [**17, 18**].

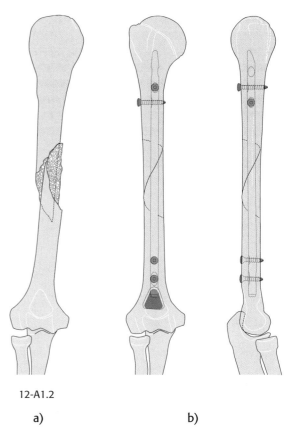

12-A1.2

a)   b)

Fig. 4.2.2-8:
a) Spiral fracture of the humerus type 12-A1.2.
b) Dorsal approach: Retrograde nailing with a 9.5 mm solid humeral nail (UHN) and two 3.9 mm locking bolts at the base and two perpendicular 3.9 mm locking bolts at the nail's tip for static interlocking without the compression device. Periosteal consolidation after 15 weeks.

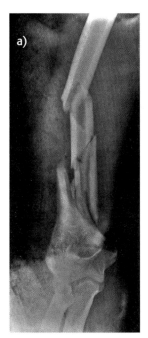

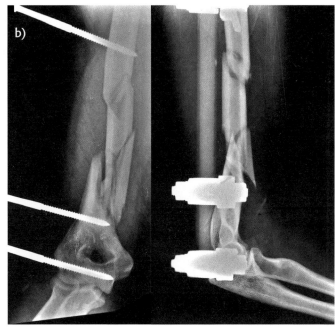

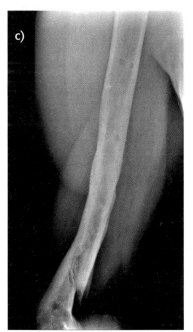

Fig. 4.2.2-9: External fixation.
a) Closed complex humeral shaft fracture (type 12-C3.1).
b) Unilateral external fixation. The most distal Schanz screw is placed distal to the olecranon fossa.
c) The one year follow-up shows complete consolidation.

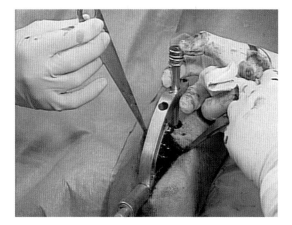

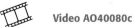 **Video AO40080c**

5 Postoperative treatment

Postoperative management after stable osteo-synthesis with plates is straightforward. Mobilization begins with active assisted elbow and shoulder range of motion (ROM) until the incision is healed. Active motion can then begin. Resistive exercises should be started only when evidence of bridging callus is visible on x-rays.

After nailing, a sling is seldom required. Shoulder and elbow exercises can start immediately, but rotational movements against resistance should be avoided until bridging periosteal callus formation is visible on x-rays.

It is possible to treat the humerus until union with the external fixator. When a fixator has been in place a short time, less than 4–5 days, conversion to plate or nail may be performed in a single step. If the pins have been in place for longer, primary exchange to internal fixation may not be safe. After removal of the fixator, a brace can be used as the clinical situation warrants and the soft tissues allow.

6 Pitfalls and complications

A complication in retrograde nailing is the creation of a supracondylar fracture.

Inadequate fixation, poor soft-tissue handling, and circumferential periosteal dissection may all contribute to the development of a non-union. In plating, the principles of careful soft-tissue management should be followed closely.

The most dramatic **complication in retro-grade nailing is the creation of a supra-condylar fracture**. Since a non-elastic implant has to be introduced through an eccentric portal into the intramedullary canal, the entry portal itself must be made large enough for the chosen nail. Moreover, the nail must always be introduced by hand and not with a hammer.

Another feared complication is radial nerve palsy. In cases of secondary nerve palsy, exploration of the nerve is required. To prevent axillary nerve damage, it is advisable to make small skin incisions and perform blunt dissection to the bone, followed by drilling and interlocking. Careful soft-tissue management prevents peri-articular ossification in the rotator cuff or on the dorsal side of the elbow joint.

7 Clinical results

7.1 Nailing

In a prospective multi-center study, 104 patients were healed with the UHN for humeral shaft fractures (**Table 4.2.2-2**). The average age was 56.2 years. There were seven patients with severe closed soft-tissue damage and six open fractures. Primary radial nerve palsy was present in seven (6.7%) cases. Surgeons evaluated the procedure as excellent or good in 90% and patients as excellent or good in 95% of cases (**Table 4.2.2-3**).

Plate fixation has consistent, good results when used for both open and closed fractures. Reviewing some published reports [7–9, 19], there are 214 humerus platings. There was a 98% union rate with primary bone grafting used only for complex fragmented fractures. Infection was less than 1% and iatrogenic radial nerve palsy was 3%. Over 97% of these patients achieved a fully functional result for their own needs, as they perceive them.

Table 4.2.2-2: Indications for nailing in 104 patients (prospective multi-center study).

Fracture type		Distribution	
Fresh fractures	84	Proximal third	24 (23%)
Pseudarthroses	11	Middle third	68 (66%)
Pathological	7	Distal third	12 (11%)
Refractures	2		

Table 4.2.2-3: Results of prospective series of 104 fractures fixed with UHN.

Postoperative joint function		
Antegrade nailing **41 cases**		**Retrograde nailing** **63 cases**
Shoulder		
35 (85%)	excellent	57 (90%)
4 (10%)	moderate	5 (8%)
2 (5%)	bad	1 (2%)
Elbow		
37 (90%)	excellent	56 (89%)
3 (7%)	moderate	5 (8%)
1 (3%)	bad	2 (3%)

8 Bibliography

1. **DiCicco JD, Mehlman CT, Urse JS** (1993) Fracture of the shaft of the humerus secondary to muscular violence. *J Orthop Trauma*; 7 (1):90–93.

2. **Pollock FH, Drake D, Bovill EG, et al.** (1981) Treatment of radial neuropathy associated with fractures of the humerus. *J Bone Joint Surg [Am]*; 63 (2):239–243.

3. **Sarmiento A, Kinman PB, Galvin EG, et al.** (1977) Functional bracing of fractures of the shaft of the humerus. *J Bone Joint Surg [Am]*; 59 (5):596–601.

4. **Zagorski JB, Latta LL, Zych GA, et al.** (1988) Diaphyseal fractures of the humerus. Treatment with prefabricated braces. *J Bone Joint Surg [Am]*; 70 (4):607–610.

5. **Gregory P, Sanders R** (1997) Compression plating versus intramedullary fixation of humeral shaft fractures. *J Am Acad Orthop Surg*; 5(4):215–223.

6. **Rodriguez-Merchan E** (1995) Compression plating versus hackenthal nailing in closed humeral shaft fractures failing nonoperative reduction. *J Orthop Trauma*; 9 (3):194–197.

7. **Bell MJ, Beauchamp CG, Kellam JK, et al.** (1985) The results of plating humeral shaft fractures in patients with multiple injuries. The Sunnybrook experience. *J Bone Joint Surg [Br]*; 67 (2):293–296.

8. **Dabezies EJ, Banta CJ, Murphy CP, et al.** (1992) Plate fixation of the humeral shaft for acute fractures, with and without radial nerve injuries. *J Orthop Trauma*; 6 (1):10–13.

9. **Vander Griend R, Tomasin J, Ward EF** (1986) Open reduction and internal fixation of humeral shaft fractures. Results using AO plating techniques. *J Bone Joint Surg [Am]*; 68 (3):430–433.

10. **Riemer B** (1996) Intramedullary nailing of the humerus. In: Browner B, editor. *The Science and Practice of Intramedullary Nailing.* Baltimore: Williams & Wilkins: 241–263.

11. **Redmond BJ, Biermann JS, Blasier RB** (1996) Interlocking intramedullary nailing of pathological fractures of the shaft of the humerus. *J Bone Joint Surg [Am]*; 78 (6):891–896.

12. **Blum J, Rommens PM, Janzing H** (1997) The unreamed humeral nail—a biological osteosynthesis of the upper arm. *Acta Chir Belg*; 97 (4):184–189.

13. **Blum J, Rommens PM, Janzing H, et al.** (1998) [Retrograde nailing of humerus shaft fractures with the unreamed humerus nail. An international multicenter study]. *Unfallchirurg*; 101 (5);342-352.

14. **Rommens PM, Verbruggen J, Broos PL** (1995) Retrograde locked nailing of humeral shaft fractures: a review of 39 patients. *J Bone Joint Surg [Br]*; 77 (1):84–89.

15. **Ingman AM, Waters DA** (1994) Locked intramedullary nailing of humeral shaft fractures. Implant design, surgical technique, and clinical results. *J Bone Joint Surg [Br]*; 76 (1):23–29.

16. **Jupiter JB** (1990) Complex non-union of the humeral diaphysis. Treatment with a medial approach, an anterior plate, and a vascularized fibular graft. *J Bone Joint Surg [Am]*; 72 (5):701–707.
17. **Smith DK, Cooney WP** (1990) External fixation of high-energy upper extremity injuries. *J Orthop Trauma*; 4 (1):7–18.
18. **Zinman C, Norman D, Hamoud K, et al.** (1997) External fixation for severe open fractures of the humerus caused by missiles. *J Orthop Trauma*; 11 (7):536–539.
19. **Heim D, Herkert F, Hess P, et al.** (1993) Surgical treatment of humeral shaft fractures—the Basel experience. *J Trauma*; 35 (2):226–232.

9 Updates

Updates and additional references for this chapter are available online at:
http://www.aopublishing.org/PFxM/422.htm

4.2.3 Humerus: distal

Brian J. Holdsworth

1 Introduction

Fractures of the distal end of the humerus can lead to difficult management decisions. There are fractures with a relatively good prognosis represented by extra-articular injuries and some of the partial articular injuries involving one or other of the condyles. The fractures with a bad prognosis are those that are complete articular as well as the multifragmented types of the supracondylar region.

Significant stiffness, pain, and deformity can be seen following improper treatment of the fractures in both the adult and the child. Prolonged immobilization usually leads to this stiffness, as would traction. In order to overcome this, stable reduction and fixation of the fractures are required so that active motion can be started early to produce the best possible result.

Other factors influence the outcome apart from the fracture. The age of the patient is significant for the risk of osteoporosis. The weakest link of any internal fixation construct is the attachment to the bone. If the patient has osteoporotic bone, it will be difficult to hold the fixation and thus achieve a stable construct and early motion.

The type of fracture is significant in that it involves the joint surface itself, and if the surface is fragmented, a poor result will also occur. Whether or not the fracture is open or closed, and the amount of soft tissue associated with this, will also influence the functional outcome. Other soft-tissue injuries, notably vascular injuries, are particularly important for the overall function of the extremity.

These factors may lead to changes in the decision making as to how one would best obtain stable internal fixation and postoperative motion, but do not negate the concept that a well reconstructed and stable joint fixation with early active motion will produce the best result.

2 Assessment of fractures and soft tissues

2.1 Classification

The pattern of elbow fractures can vary considerably and an understanding of the different types, leading to proper classification, is indispensable for correct decision making (**Fig. 4.2.3-1**). Certain important groups require comment.

Type A (extra-articular) avulsion fractures of the condyle(s) are usually associated with dislocation. Treatment of the dislocation takes precedence. Entrapment within the reduced joint of bony fragments, with or without nerve or soft-tissue attachments, must be avoided. The elbow must be stable after reduction.

Type B3: These may be multifragmentary and, in the elderly, very difficult to stabilize.

Type C1: This fracture is easy to fix, but uncommon. Hidden fracture lines should be carefully sought.

2.2 Neurovascular problems

Severe disruption of any nerve or vessel passing the elbow may occur with distal humeral fractures. Laceration of nerves is rare, but traction injuries or nerve entrapment may occur. Finger movements and sensation are tested with the arm gently supported. Enormous swelling may threaten the circulation but it may usually be maintained by simple elevation in extension while treatment is planned.

Severe pain and the inability to tolerate finger extension, whether active or passive, point to the presence of a compartment syndrome (see **chapter 1.5**). If the brachial artery has been divided, the excellent collateral circulation can sustain the forearm tissues. Simple ligation of the lacerated artery relaxes collateral spasm and micro-vascular repair may not be needed. Small penetrating wounds are common but, in civilian practice at least, major skin loss is rare. Prompt surgery reduces the risk of sepsis. Crushing injuries carry a risk of major skin necrosis from degloving, so incisions must be planned and placed with care. The elbow is intolerant of immobilization and delay while assessing tissue viability is not usually an option.

2.3 History of mechanism of injury

The amount of energy imparted to the tissues is estimated by a careful history. The strength of the patient's bone is crucial; in the elderly a simple fall may cause complex fractures. Osteoporosis makes fixation difficult, but it is still feasible [1]. The general medical history is also vital. Good results after fixation require cooperative patients willing to practice active postoperative movements. Problems can arise in patients with severe head injuries, dementia, alcoholism, or drug addiction. Non-operative treatment, despite some inevitable stiffness, may be preferable to failed internal fixation.

Heterotopic ossification may follow intracranial damage and is made more likely by delayed fixation and by passive stretching of the elbow.

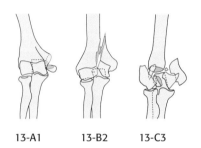

13-A1   13-B2   13-C3

Fig. 4.2.3-1: Müller AO Classification

Be aware of nerve injury!

2.4 Imaging

High-quality plain x-rays (AP, lateral ± oblique views) are needed. **Sedation or anesthesia will permit the use of gentle traction during x-ray.** This helps to clarify the fracture pattern and to assist in preparing the definitive preoperative drawings. Views of the normal side are helpful for planning. Hidden fragmentation is a hazard and is not always detected by less experienced surgeons. CT or MRI scanning has so far proved to be of limited use but, with better resolution techniques, 3-D reconstruction scans may prove helpful. **Fixation and approach vary with the type of fracture, hence accurate classification of the fracture is essential.**

3 Surgical anatomy

The lower humerus forms a strong bony triangle. The radial column has the capitellum on its front surface but its back is non-articular and may be used as a site for a plate. The bobbin-shaped trochlea is central rather than medial and the axis of rotation lies slightly in front of the humeral shaft.

The small anterior fossa accommodates the radial head in flexion, and for full movement the anterior and posterior fossae must be clear of metal. The collateral ligaments are essential for stability. The ulnar ligament lies close to the wall of the trochlea, where it is vulnerable to excessive dissection (**Fig. 4.2.3-2**).

4 Preoperative planning

Planning includes the entire surgical tactic (antibiotics, surgical approach, bone grafting, etc.), set out step by step (**Fig. 4.2.3-3**). If it is not possible to make an exact drawing of the planned fixation, the choice of procedure (or of surgeon) should be reviewed [2].

Traction views facilitate assessment and planning.

Careful planning according to fracture pattern.

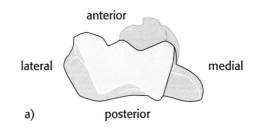

a)

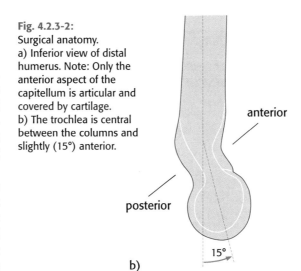

b)

Fig. 4.2.3-2:
Surgical anatomy.
a) Inferior view of distal humerus. Note: Only the anterior aspect of the capitellum is articular and covered by cartilage.
b) The trochlea is central between the columns and slightly (15°) anterior.

4.1 Positioning and approach

A tourniquet is rarely required.

For elbow fractures a prone position is best.

The lateral decubitus position is usual, as most fractures are type C2 or C3. For severe C3 fractures, in otherwise fit patients, the **fully prone position allows excellent access.** The arm rests on a padded bar of about 4 cm diameter allowing 120° flexion of the elbow (**Fig. 4.2.3-4**). A bone graft is rarely needed, but with C3 fractures it is wise to prepare a donor site.

In most cases a tourniquet, preferably sterile, is placed high on the arm and sealed at its lower edge to avoid chemical burns from skin preparation fluid. **A tourniquet is not essential but can make it easier to identify the ulnar nerve.** It may be omitted if the humerus is short or when the fracture extends far up the shaft and should in any event be released and, if possible, removed after a maximum of two hours.

All fractures are approached through a slightly curved posterior incision just radial to

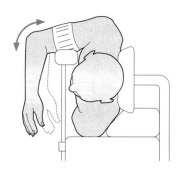

Fig. 4.2.3-4: a) Positioning of the patient in lateral decubitus with the upper arm supported by a padded post.

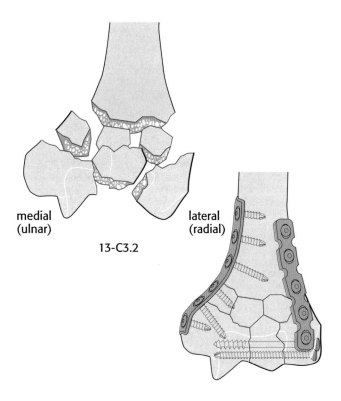

medial (ulnar)

lateral (radial)

13-C3.2

Fig. 4.2.3-3: Planning: The different fragments are outlined and reduced on paper using the intact opposite bone as the template. The plates (reconstruction plate 3.5, LC-DCP 3.5, or one-third tubular plate 3.5) are then drawn in appropriate length and position for placement on the bone.

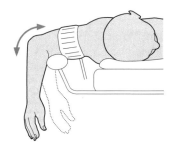

b) The patient lies prone with the arm on a radiolucent support, or (as illustrated) a padded post. Either gives maximum freedom to approach the elbow.

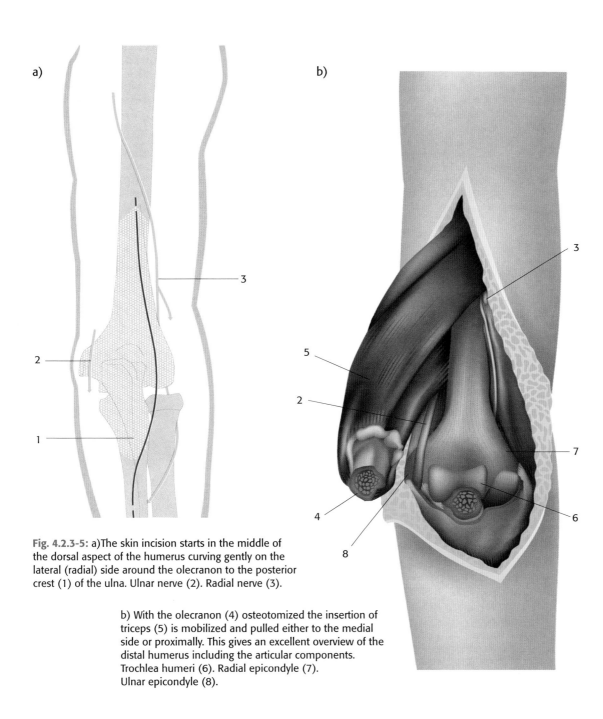

Fig. 4.2.3-5: a)The skin incision starts in the middle of the dorsal aspect of the humerus curving gently on the lateral (radial) side around the olecranon to the posterior crest (1) of the ulna. Ulnar nerve (2). Radial nerve (3).

b) With the olecranon (4) osteotomized the insertion of triceps (5) is mobilized and pulled either to the medial side or proximally. This gives an excellent overview of the distal humerus including the articular components. Trochlea humeri (6). Radial epicondyle (7). Ulnar epicondyle (8).

Olecranon osteotomy with reflection of triceps gives the best exposure of trochlea and capitellum.

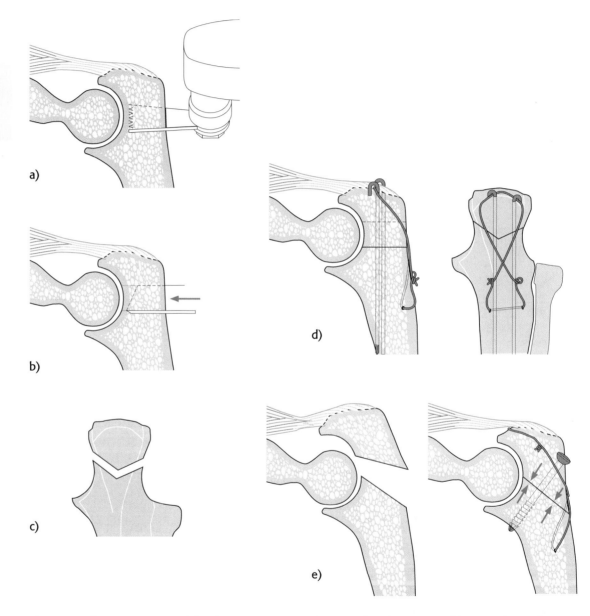

a)

b)

c)

d)

e)

Fig. 4.2.3-6: Chevron osteotomy of the olecranon: starting with a fine oscillating bone saw (a) and finishing by breaking the last few millimeters with an osteotome (b & c).

Reconstruction after surgery with two K-wires and figure-of-eight tension band wire (d) or tension band wire and 3.5 mm lag screw (e).

the olecranon. A **distally pointed chevron olecranon osteotomy best exposes the fracture** [3] (**Video AO20142Ba**) and allows stable fixation (**Fig. 4.2.3-5**, **Fig. 4.2.3-6**). The ulnar nerve is gently identified and may need to be isolated and elevated at the ulnar epicondyle.

4.2 Reduction techniques and tools

An experienced assistant helps to control the fragments during the **reduction phase, often the most demanding part of surgery**. There are situations when distraction with an external fixator may be helpful. Temporary K-wire fixation helps during this process but should never be relied on for definitive fixation. The plan should be consulted throughout surgery, to ensure that definitive placement of implants is not hampered by inappropriate siting of temporary fixation. Pointed reduction forceps, small and large, are most useful. Assembly of the trochlear fragments, in accordance with the standard technique, may well prove possible, but when any large fragment obviously fits well to the shaft, it is often preferable to reduce and fix it first, whether or not it forms part of the main joint surface. **A plastic model is useful to recall the complex shape of the lower humerus** (**Video AO20142Bb**).

4.3 Choice of implant

Within fracture types, a pattern of implant selection emerges as follows:

Type A: Fixation is rarely needed, as the principal injury is a dislocation. For larger fragments, 3.5 or 4.0 mm screws are more reliable than K-wires. Cannulated screws may greatly facilitate the procedure.

Type B: There is a need to be wary of possible trochlear involvement as revealed by a double capitellar outline on the lateral x-ray [4]. For simple isolated lateral column injuries, a single plate may be used or screws alone from back to front, but without penetrating the articular surface.

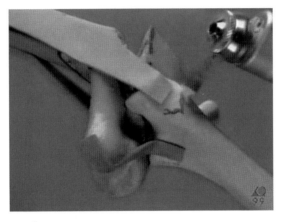

Video AO20142Ba

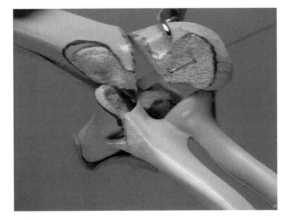
Video AO20142Bb

A distally pointed chevron olecranon osteotomy best exposes the fracture.

Reduction is usually the most demanding part of surgery.

Use bone model to recall shape of distal humerus.

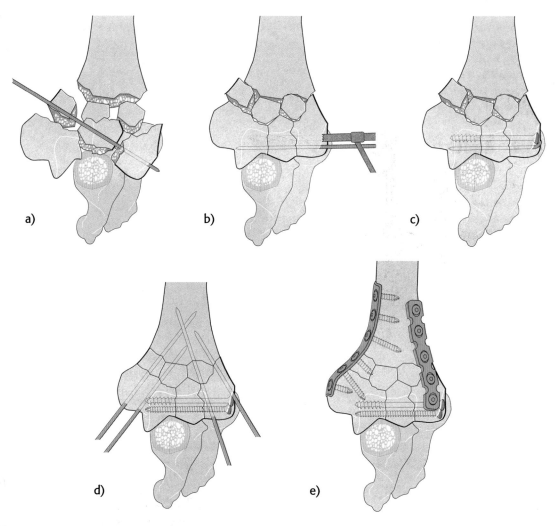

a)

b)

c)

d)

e)

Fig. 4.2.3-7:
Different steps in reconstructing a complex, multifragment distal humerus fracture.
a) Inside-out technique for the K-wire (1.6 mm) to reconstruct the trochlea and capitellum.
b) After reduction of three articular fragments, the K-wire is drilled in the reverse direction. It may be used as a guide for a 3.5 mm

cannulated screw or a screw may be placed parallel to it (c).
d) Once the articular components are firmly fixed as one block, this is then joined to the shaft of the humerus, again using temporary K-wires.
e) To join the articular block to the humerus we first place a precisely contoured reconstruction plate 3.5 on the postero-lateral side. It may

curve around the capitellum which has no cartilage cover posteriorly. On the medial side we prefer to place the plate on the crest of the bone (at right angles to the lateral plate), which increases stability. Again, a reconstruction plate may be used although the one-third tubular plate serves the same purpose and fits very well onto the crest.

Type C: Two plates are needed for adequate strength, which may be increased by placing them at right angles to each other. The forces generated in everyday exercise may disrupt unprotected screw fixation. For firm fixation, the lateral plate should reach down to the joint line. The complex shape of the restored lower humerus requires a full range of plate bending and twisting equipment.

A DCP 3.5 or reconstruction plate 3.5 must be used. The medial plate lies virtually along the supracondylar crest, though this is very narrow. It curves forward very little, if at all. One-third tubular plates may be used but are not recommended; reconstruction plates 3.5 are preferable. For the capitellum, fully threaded small fragment cancellous bone screws are introduced through the radial plate (**Fig. 4.2.3-7**). In the humerus, K-wires are used only for provisional fixation.

5 Surgical treatment— tricks and hints

Because adult elbows are intolerant of even a few days of immobilization and heterotopic ossification tends to follow operations delayed a week or more, the window of opportunity for fixation is quite narrow. In open fractures urgent débridement and stable internal fixation are essential. Major soft-tissue loss, rare in civilian trauma, requires immediate assistance from a plastic surgeon.

These fractures require classical stable internal fixation. "Minimalist" procedures will not allow early and enthusiastic movement, so, in adults, tenuous fixation by screws or wires alone is never appropriate.

Active movement starts within 24 hours. Children are more tolerant of joint immobilization and, for them, minimal fixation may be used [**5**].

For optimal fixation, a well-drawn plan should be followed throughout the operation, the aim, when feasible, being to place two, or preferably, three screws above and below the fracture in each plate. The fossae must be free of screw shafts. When possible, plates at right angles to each other create a girder-like structure, which strengthens the fixation (**Fig. 4.2.3-7**). The postero-lateral plate, which will function as a tension band during elbow flexion, is first provisionally applied. It is contoured according to the shape of the bone to restore the anterior tilt of the capitellum. It may reach down to the joint surface. Initial fixation around the triangle of the distal humerus should be provisional only. A slight malrotation of the trochlear fragments frequently prevents completion of the final corner of the triangle, requiring that the initial fixation be adjusted. Once the medial side plate is in place, the lateral plate can be definitively fixed. A long cortex screw, lagged to allow stable compression, passes transversely through the medial plate. However, if this screw is lagged in the presence of central comminution or a gap, it may result in articular incongruity. **Precise plate positioning is critical for optimal fixation.** Fragments should not be thrown away as even the smallest may give a clue to correct re-assembly. Small fragments may safely be left in place if the remainder of the fixation is stable. Bone grafts for articular defects are rarely needed (**Video AO20142Bc**).

Soft-tissue attachments are preserved as far as possible but even if fragments have become detached, they rarely cause any late problems if soundly fixed, unless gross contamination has

Correct plate positioning is critical for optimal fixation.

Articular fractures require classical ORIF with anatomical reconstruction and rigid internal fixation.

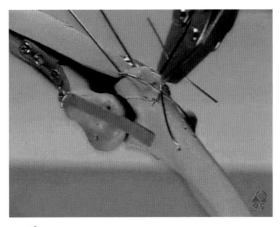

Video AO20142Bc

occurred in open fractures. Well-buried tension band wiring allows full excursion of the triceps in extension and reliably fixes the olecranon osteotomy. Some surgeons doubt that straight K-wires add much to olecranon stability and use two simple figure-of-eight wires. A large cancellous bone screw, even with a loop of wire, cannot function as a tension band and has an increased rate of non-union (**Fig. 4.2.3-6**) [6, 7].

Finally, the reconstructed elbow is put through a full range of movement, including rotation. Careful palpation is needed to exclude impinging screws or wires and to detect any movement between the fragments.

The ulnar nerve is usually replaced in its bed, even when near a plate, with its position precisely recorded in the operation note.

Before the patient is woken from anesthesia, on-table x-rays are carefully scrutinized (close-

up!). A casual glance will miss subtle problems.

With practice the great majority of fractures can be firmly fixed using the techniques described. However, for elderly patients with grossly fragmented soft bone and a very distal fracture pattern, total elbow replacement may be a good option [8].

This is not appropriate in younger fit adults or when the supracondylar ridges are badly disrupted. For very low fractures at epicondylar level, tension band wiring is a possibility.

Wound closure: Operative incisions are closed gently with fine sutures or staples, avoiding excess tension. A suction drain is used for 24 hours. Lacerations in open fractures are never closed at the first operation. Delayed primary closure at 72 hours is much safer. Small puncture wounds are left to heal and active exercises practiced as normal.

6 Postoperative treatment

After effective fixation, plaster of Paris should not be needed or used. Postoperative swelling is usual and tight bandages or plaster risk a compartment syndrome. Active movements start at 24 hours, when the drain is removed. Intermittent passive stretching by a second person is not allowed. However, continuous passive motion (CPM) seems safe but is not obligatory. A loosely applied sling is used for respite following frequent spells of active exercise. **Active assisted exercises are allowed, but resisted exercises are delayed for 4 weeks**.

Postoperatively active assisted exercises are best.

7 Pitfalls and complications

7.1 Stiffness

The most common error is not to achieve sound fixation. This often means splinting the arm for several weeks and is followed by extreme and usually persistent stiffness. Heterotopic ossification varies in severity [9]. The presence of a little collateral new bone on x-rays does not represent a clinical problem. Head injured patients are more vulnerable, especially when operation is delayed above 5 days. Radiotherapy has been suggested, but young adults have many years during which to develop unforeseeable complications [10].

7.2 Non-union

Inadequate fixation will not withstand the considerable forces generated by early active movement and so non-union may follow. It also results from breakage of implants, and use of one-third tubular plates is no longer recommended as a routine [11]. The exception may be on the ulnar side if a strong fixation has been achieved radially by a well-positioned and more robust plate.

7.3 Infection

This is relatively rare despite the thin soft-tissue cover, which is often punctured in the initial trauma. Prophylactic antibiotics are given and, in open fractures, continued for 48 hours at most or until the wound is dry. If the wound is becoming inflamed, early revision and débridement may prevent a disaster.

7.4 Ulnar neurapraxia

Tingling in the ulnar nerve distribution is common but rarely persists. **Traction on the retracted nerve must be avoided during the operation**. Occasional late ulnar palsy may need decompression, hence the need to record the exact position of the nerve relative to the metalwork. Prophylactic transposition is not recommended. It causes a longer period of initial neurapraxia and seems not to be necessary.

The ulnar nerve is a most vulnerable structure.

7.5 Failure of initially sound fixation

Loosening of olecranon wires, common in the elderly, is minimized by burying them deep to the triceps. Screw fixation in osteoporotic bone may fail. Early weight bearing on the arms is forbidden.

8 Results

Before stable fixation techniques were developed, a strong body of opinion was opposed to operative intervention. An average range of about 90° follows the "bag of bones" technique of fostering early movement ignoring the fracture [12]. It was believed that recovery to anything resembling normality was impossible and any discernible movement was hailed as a "good" result. Limited open reduction, inevitably requiring immobilization, combines the disadvantages of both closed and open treatment [13].

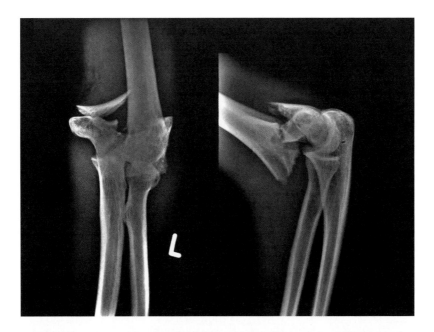

Fig. 4.2.3-8a: Fracture of distal humerus 13-C in an 18-year-old male.

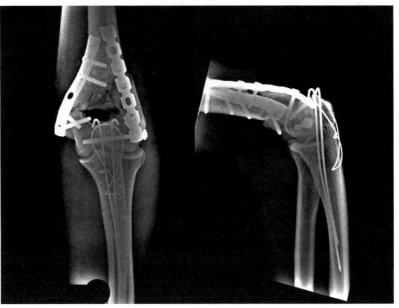

Fig. 4.2.3-8b: Postoperative view with stable internal fixation.

Comparisons between series are hampered by use of differing criteria for "good", "fair", etc. However, the Cassebaum rating has proved helpful [3]. This defines "excellent" as pain free with no more than 15° loss of flexion or extension, reducing to "good" at 40–120° and to "fair" when flexion was less than 110°.

Most recent series using these criteria found 75–80% of patients achieved at least a "good" rating [13–15]. Fractures of the distal humerus are very difficult and no one claims less than about 15% of poor results.

8.1 Conclusion

Planning is mandatory. If it is not possible to plan and draw the proposed fixation or a very close approximation to it, then the patient should be referred immediately to a surgeon more experienced in elbow problems.

Sound fixation and early active movement are essential. If this looks impossible to achieve, the operation should not be started.

With sound technique and cooperative patients, excellent or good results, measured by relatively strict functional criteria, should be achieved in about 80% of patients.

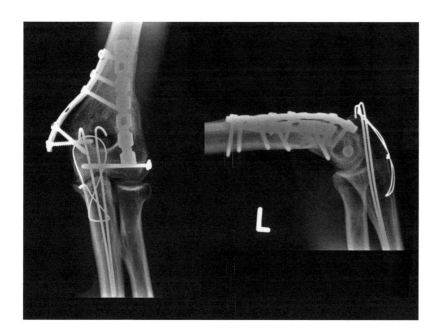

Fig. 4.2.3-8c: One-year follow-up with excellent functional result.

9 Bibliography

1. **John H, Rosso R, Neff U, et al.** (1994)
   Operative treatment of distal humeral
   fractures in the elderly.
   J Bone Joint Surg [Br]; 76 (5):793–796.
2. **Holdsworth BJ** (1989) Planning in
   fracture surgery. In: Bunker TD, Colton
   CL, Webb JK, editors. *Frontiers in Fracture
   Management.* London: Martin Dunitz: 1–15.
3. **Cassebaum WH** (1969) Open reduction
   of T & Y fractures of the lower end of the
   humerus. *J Trauma*; 9 (11):915–925.
4. **McKee MD, Jupiter JB, Bamberger HB**
   (1996) Coronal shear fractures of the
   distal end of the humerus.
   J Bone Joint Surg [Am]; 78 (1):49–54.
5. **Sodergard J, Sandelin J, Bostman O**
   (1992) Postoperative complications of
   distal humeral fractures. 27/96 adults
   followed up for 6 (2–10) years.
   Acta Orthop Scand; 63 (1):85–89.
6. **Gainor BJ, Moussa F, Schott T** (1995)
   Healing rate of transverse osteotomies of
   the olecranon used in reconstruction of
   distal humerus fractures.
   J South Orthop Assoc; 4 (4):263–268.
7. **Letsch R, Schmit-Neuerburg KP,
   Sturmer KM, et al.** (1989) Intra-
   articular fractures of the distal humerus.
   Surgical treatment and results.
   Clin Orthop; (241):238–244.
8. **Cobb TK, Morrey BF** (1997) Total
   elbow arthroplasty as primary treatment
   for distal humeral fractures in elderly
   patients. *J Bone Joint Surg [Am]*;
   79 (6):826–832.

9. **Summerfield SL, DiGiovanni C,
   Weiss AP** (1997) Heterotopic ossification
   of the elbow. *J Should Elbow Surg*;
   6 (3):321–331.
10. **Jupiter JB** (1994) Complex fractures of
    the distal part of the humerus and
    associated complications.
    J Bone Joint Surg [Am]; 76:1252–1263.
11. **Henley MB, Bone LB, Parker B** (1987)
    Operative management of intra-articular
    fractures of the distal humerus.
    J Orthop Trauma; 1 (1):24–35.
12. **Riseborough EJ, Radin EL** (1969)
    Intercondylar T fractures of the humerus in
    the adult. A comparison of operative and
    non-operative treatment in twenty-nine
    cases. *J Bone Joint Surg [Am]*; 51 (1):130–141.
13. **Rommens PM** (1996) Fractures of the
    distal third of the humerus. In: Flatow EC,
    editor. *Muskuloskeletal Trauma Series—
    Humerus.* 1st ed. Oxford: Butterworth
    Heinemann: 156–183.
14. **Holdsworth BJ, Mossad MM** (1990)
    Fractures of the adult distal humerus.
    Elbow function after internal fixation.
    J Bone Joint Surg [Br]; 72 (3):362–365.
15. **Jupiter JB, Neff U, Holzach P, et al.**
    (1985) Intercondylar fractures of the
    humerus. An operative approach.
    J Bone Joint Surg [Am]; 67 (2):226–239.

10 Updates

Updates and additional references for this chapter
are available online at:
http://www.aopublishing.org/PFxM/423.htm

4.3.1 Olecranon/radial head/ complex elbow injures

Jaime Quintero

1 General aspects of proximal forearm injuries

Proximal forearm fractures can lead to severe dysfunction, arising from posttraumatic instability, impingement, malunion, or non-union. These injuries may involve one or more of the three different articulations that constitute the elbow: the ulnotrochlear joint, the radiocapitellar joint, and the proximal radioulnar joint [1–6].

The structural anatomy of the elbow joint is considered in **Fig. 4.3.1-1**.

Osteochondral fractures or loose bodies are not uncommon, especially with radial head injuries associated with capitellar abrasions. Higher energy fractures may produce associated distal injuries, such as forearm and distal radial fractures and disruptions of the interosseous membrane or the distal radioulnar joint; these must be diagnosed, so an x-ray of the entire forearm is advisable.

In order to promote **early functional treatment, it is essential to achieve precise anatomical reconstruction of the different ring structures** [2]. **This requires not only reduction of the osseous components but also the restoration of the tension of the ligamentous and capsular avulsions.**

Occasionally, and in the absence of associated ligamentous instability, grossly comminuted fragments may be excised. In elderly people a comminuted olecranon may be treated by resection and reattachment of the triceps, provided no fractures of the coronoid process or avulsion of the anterior capsule are present. Similarly, the comminuted radial head, if not amenable to reconstruction, may be replaced by a prosthetic spacer, which will allow healing of the torn capsule or ligaments without compromising the function of the elbow or forearm [2, 6–8].

Classification of proximal forearm fractures is illustrated in **Fig. 4.3.1-2**.

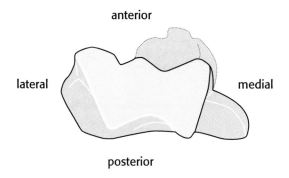

anterior

lateral   medial

posterior

Fig. 4.3.1-1: Distribution of articular cartilage on distal humerus viewed from below, see also **Fig. 4.2.3-2** on distal humerus fractures.

Early functional treatment calls for precise anatomic reconstruction of the different components: osseous, ligamentous, and avulsed fragments.

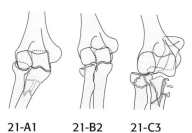

21-A1   21-B2   21-C3

Fig. 4.3.1-2: Müller AO Classification

2 Olecranon

Because its subcutaneous position makes it quite vulnerable to direct trauma, hyperextension, and torsion, fractures of the olecranon are among the most common of elbow injuries.

2.1 Assessment of fractures and soft tissues

The fracture usually represents a disruption of the triceps mechanism combined with a bending moment over the distal end of the trochlea, inducing the characteristic transverse and oblique B1 patterns. More direct forces generate comminution (fragmentation) and impaction of the central portion of the olecranon articular surface and, occasionally, avulsions of the coronoid process [5].

The patient has pain and usually is not able to use the elbow. The skin can be swollen, contused, or bruised. The lateral view clearly shows the fracture line, the amount of displacement and, usually, the degree of comminution (fragmentation), if present. A lateral tomogram is useful to clarify the degree of articular impaction. Complex fractures may be associated with an anterior dislocation of the forearm (transolecranon fracture-dislocation) or a posterior type II Monteggia lesion [4, 9].

Several classification systems have been described, **but what matters is that simple transverse or oblique fractures cannot be relied on to represent the typical stable pattern as they can be associated with elbow or forearm dislocations.** In the same way, multifragment fractures are likely to be more stable if confined to the trochlear notch, or grossly unstable if they involve the coronoid process or proximal ulna [8].

Even simple transverse or oblique fractures may be associated with dislocations.

2.2 Preoperative planning

2.2.1 Positioning and approaches

The patient should either be prone or in the lateral position with the elbow flexed over a side rest (see **Fig. 4.2.3-4**). The supine position with the forearm placed across the chest is an acceptable option (**Fig. 4.3.1-3**), especially with

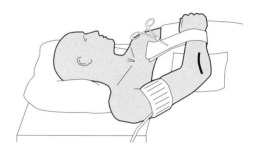

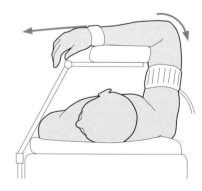

Fig. 4.3.1-3: Supine position of the patient. The elbow is placed onto the chest of the patient or on an armrest. Olecranon fractures are easily approached from the posterior aspect. The ulnar nerve is usually identified and protected during the operative fixation. If needed, separating some of the fibers of the anconeus muscle from the lateral side can adequately expose the joint and depressed fragments.

extended approaches to the lateral pillar or column. A sterile tourniquet is placed on the upper arm after skin preparation and draping.

The skin incision runs posteriorly from the supracondylar area to a point 4 or 5 cm distal to the fracture. It can be gently curved to the radial side to protect the ulnar nerve or to avoid skin bruises or lacerations. **Large skin flaps may not heal well and should be avoided** (see **Fig. 4.2.3-5**).

2.2.2 Reduction techniques and tools

A direct reduction technique, using hooks, pointed reduction forceps, or K-wires, is the method of choice for articular fractures (**Fig. 4.3.1-4**). Multifragmentary fractures may require an indirect reduction technique.

2.2.3 Choice of implants—tension band principle

Two K-wires (1.8 or 1.6 mm) as internal splints and a 1.0 mm stainless steel cerclage wire are the implants of choice for simple transverse and oblique fractures (**Video AO00072**). An additional lag screw should be used in selected oblique fractures to obtain uniform compression (**Fig. 4.3.1-5**). An interfragmentary cancellous bone lag screw with an additional cerclage wire is an alternative. A posterior plate (one-third tubular plate, LC-DCP 3.5, or reconstruction plate) is preferred for comminuted fractures (**Fig. 4.3.1-6**).

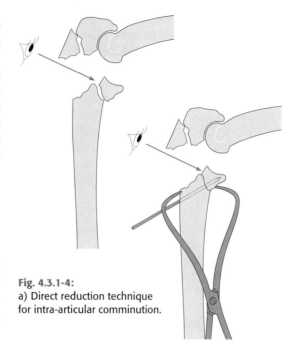

Large skin flaps may not heal well and should be avoided.

Fig. 4.3.1-4:
a) Direct reduction technique for intra-articular comminution.

b) Correct reduction of the coronoid process must be checked before its preliminary fixation with a K-wire.

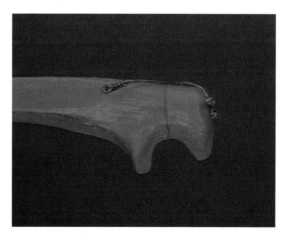

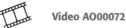 **Video AO00072**

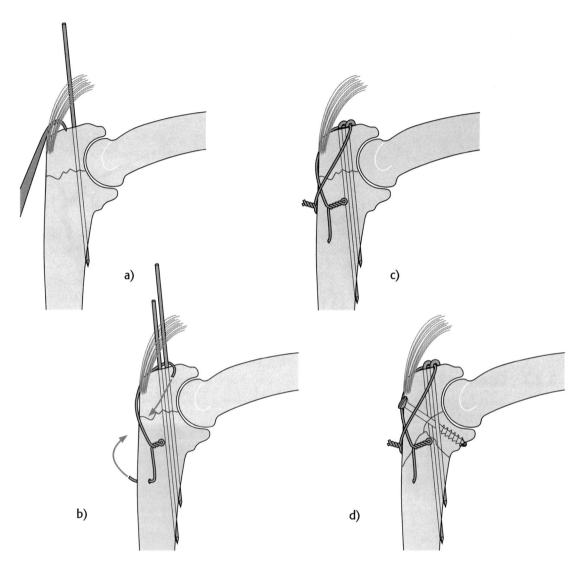

Fig. 4.3.1-5: a) Simple olecranon fractures are best reduced and held in place with a hook, followed by two 1.6 mm K-wires, which are introduced parallel to each other and which must penetrate the distal cortex.
b) A 1 mm stainless steel wire is passed through a 2.0 mm hole in the ulna and in a figure-of-eight through the triceps insertion at the olecranon.

c) The final aspect with the tension band wire in place.
d) In case of an oblique fracture that tends to shear off when the wire is tightened, a 4.0 mm lag screw may be used in place of the K-wires.

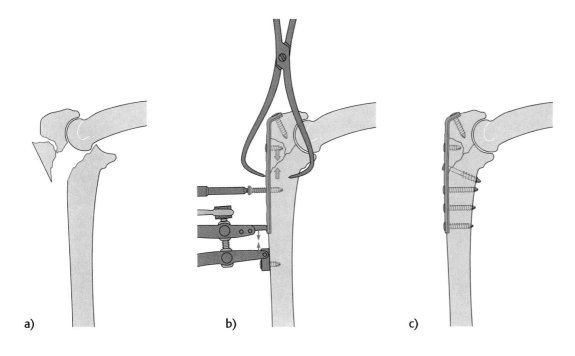

a)   b)   c)

Fig. 4.3.1-6:
a) In more complex olecranon fractures, the tension band principle with cerclage wire may not work. Therefore, a small plate (one-third tubular plate, DCP 3.5, LC-DCP 3.5, or reconstruction plate) is used.

b) These plates require considerable contouring to bend around the tip of the olecranon. The plate is first anchored to the olecranon by two screws and then the tensioning device is added distally to compress the fracture.
c) The final aspect of the fixation with an additional lag screw through the plate.

2.3   Surgical treatment— tricks and hints

Transverse and oblique fractures

Flexing the elbow and detaching some fibers of the anconeus muscle from the lateral aspect exposes the fracture and articular surface. After irrigation and cleaning of the joint, the fracture is reduced.

Direct reduction is achieved by extending the elbow and simultaneously reducing the fragments with a pointed clamp, anchoring its distal point on the diaphysis in a predrilled small hole. The method of choice is tension band fixation with two K-wires; for technique see **Fig. 4.3.1-5**.

For oblique fractures, prior to the tension band fixation, an additional lag screw may be inserted at a right angle to the fracture plane. For more distal fractures, or those associated with soft-tissue instability, a posterior plate is preferred.

Multifragmented fractures

In cases where a simple depressed fragment can be directly reduced and fixed with one or two K-wires, a regular tension band is then applied as described. For more complex comminuted fractures an indirect reduction is preferred. Definitive fixation is obtained using a DCP 3.5 or LC-DCP 3.5 contoured to the proximal ulna. The most proximal screws are directed to the medullary canal and placed at a 90° angle to the other screws, thereby creating an interlocking construct [9–11].

An alternative option requires a one-third tubular plate. This is cut through an end screwhole and bent to form a bifid hook, which engages into the proximal fragment where it can be additionally fixed with screws (**Fig. 4.3.1-7**).

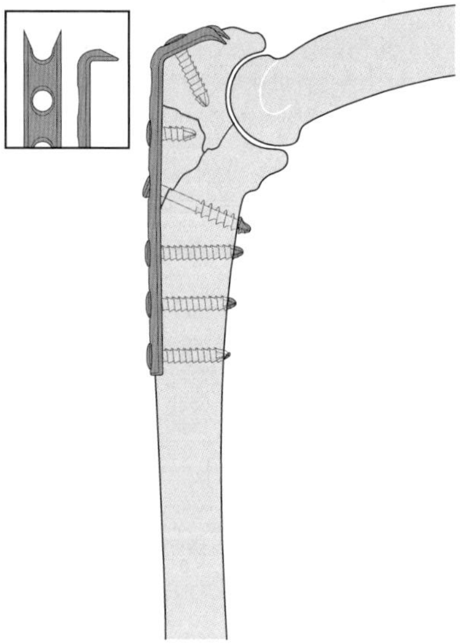

Active assisted exercises are started on the first post-operative day.

Fig. 4.3.1-7: Alternatively to **Fig. 4.3.1-6**, a one-third tubular plate may be shaped—or cut—to form two sharp hooks that engage into the tip of the olecranon for better purchase in case of quite small fragments.

If a distractor is not available, the plate is used as a lever to facilitate reduction to the diaphysis. Because the plate is thin and can fail under load, this fixation should be augmented with a tension band wire or a further one-third plate on top [12].

2.4 Postoperative treatment

A suction drain is placed and the elbow is wrapped in a bulky dressing. During the first 24–48 hours, a dorsal splint may promote comfort but is not essential. **Active assisted exercises are started the day after**, including gravity assisted elbow flexion with the patient lying supine. During the first weeks an active exercise program should be closely monitored by the treating surgeon in order to avoid elbow contractures. At 3–4 weeks resisted exercises can be started and the patient usually returns to work.

2.5 Pitfalls and complications

After the fracture has healed, prominent or protruding K-wires may cause pain and require removal, which is otherwise optional. Nonunions are rare and usually unite after repair with the methods already described [10, 13].

2.6 Results

Most olecranon fractures heal primarily. The majority of patients recover a functional range of motion, frequently with small losses of extension, usually with no associated disability.

3 Radial head

3.1 Assessment of fractures and soft tissues

Fractures of the radial head are caused by a fall on the outstretched hand, with the forearm slightly flexed and pronated. Fracture patterns range from simple and non-displaced to multifragmentary and severely impacted. Elbow dislocation and associated soft-tissue injuries are not uncommon, as are fractures of the distal radius.

The patient is usually in severe pain and cannot rotate the forearm. Because extension is also difficult and painful, an AP view is taken perpendicular to the forearm (**Fig. 4.3.1-8**) with, in addition, lateral and oblique radiocapitellar views. However, simple x-rays are often difficult to interpret and an accurate assessment of the fracture configuration and associated injuries may be possible only at the time of surgery. Additional imaging techniques (tomograms, CT scan, MRI) are seldom indicated [14].

Stable fractures which do not interfere with forearm rotation may be best treated by early motion.

Unstable fractures (**Fig. 4.3.1-9**) include those with displaced or loose fragments, associated fractures of the capitellum, olecranon or coronoid process, elbow dislocations, ligamentous avulsions, and distal wrist injuries. These unstable fracture configurations are best treated by operative fixation or radial head replacement [5–8, 15–19].

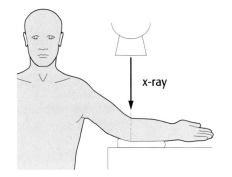

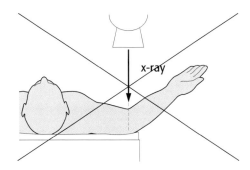

Fig. 4.3.1-8: For the AP x-ray of the radial head the direction of the beam must be perpendicular to the radial head, as the elbow can rarely be extended.

3.2 Preoperative planning

3.2.1 Positioning and approach

The patient is positioned supine on the table and the extremity is prepared from the axilla to the hand to allow rotation of the forearm and flexion and extension of the elbow during the operative fixation. The standard lateral approach is most commonly used (**Fig. 4.3.1-10**). Care must be taken to avoid the deep branch of the radial nerve, which runs anteriorly to the capsule and the radial head. To minimize the risk of

Stable fractures are best treated by early motion.

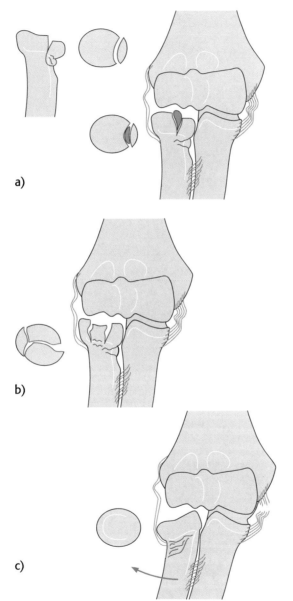

a)

b)

c)

Fig. 4.3.1-9:
Typical radial head fractures (21-A and 21-B).
a) Displaced shearing fractures B2, b) complex articular fracture with impaction B3, c) extra-articular tilt of radial head A2 often combined with ligamentous avulsion.

operative disruption of the lateral collateral ligament, the capsular incision should remain in front of the anterior margin of the anconeus muscle and parallel to the fascial limit of the extensor carpi ulnaris. The annular ligament, a true thickening of the capsule, is opened laterally or slightly anteriorly to allow full inspection of the fragments. In selected cases an osteotomy of the lateral epicondyle should provide an extensile approach [19, 20].

3.2.2 Reduction techniques

Direct reduction and temporary fixation are obtained with a dental hook and fine pointed forceps. Gentle rotation of the forearm allows inspection of the circumference of the radial head and neck. Provisional fixation is then performed with 1.0 mm K-wires (Fig. 4.3.1-11).

3.2.3 Choice of implant

Mini fragment screws can provide stable fixation when interfragmentary compression is applied, with 1.5 and 2.0 mm screws used as lag screws to fix marginal or wedge fragments. In impacted fractures the same screws can be used as positioning screws, i.e., not as lag screws, to avoid compression, which would narrow and distort the radial head. In fractures that are impacted, comminuted, or associated with a fracture of the radial neck, a mini T-plate or L-plate should be used to support the repair.

Fig. 4.3.1-10: Approach to the radial head.
a) The incision starts 2–3 cm proximal to the lateral epicondyle and curves dorsal to it across the joint parallel to the radius for 3–4 cm.

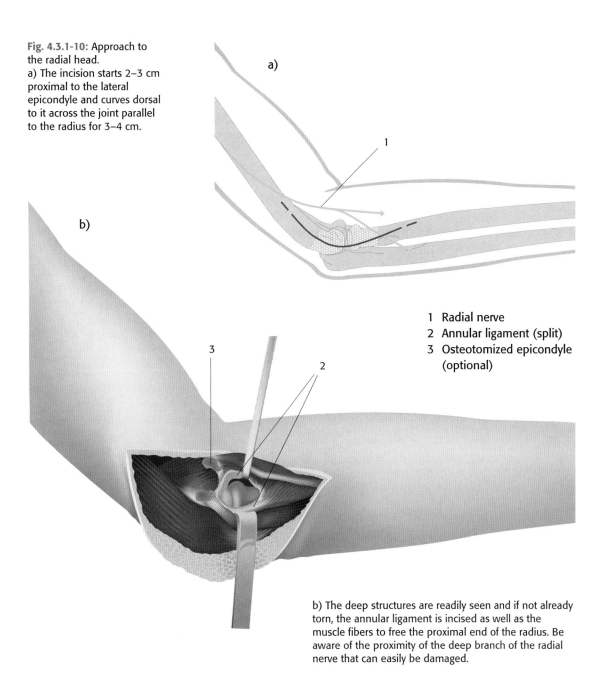

a)

b)

1   Radial nerve
2   Annular ligament (split)
3   Osteotomized epicondyle (optional)

b) The deep structures are readily seen and if not already torn, the annular ligament is incised as well as the muscle fibers to free the proximal end of the radius. Be aware of the proximity of the deep branch of the radial nerve that can easily be damaged.

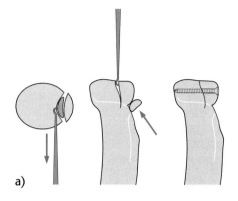

Fig. 4.3.1-11: a) The articular surface must be freed from interposed fragments and precisely reduced with K-wire fixation. Finally, one or two 1.5 mm or 2.0 mm cortex lag screws are inserted. The screw head should be slightly countersunk.

b) In case of comminution a bone graft (from the epicondyle) may be needed for the reconstruction as well as several small screws inserted in different directions.

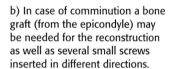
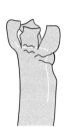
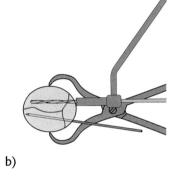
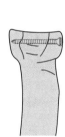

b)

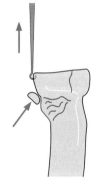

c) If the radial head is tilted more than 20°, it should be elevated and fixed. Again, a bone graft is required. For the fixation, a 1.5 or 2.0 mm screw may be sufficient. Otherwise an adaptation plate 1.5 or 2.0 or a T-plate 1.5 is applied.

c)

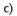
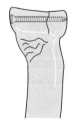
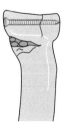
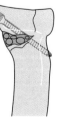
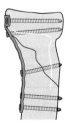

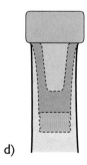

d)

d) Irreparable radial heads should be replaced by prostheses, especially if elbow stability is at stake.

3.3 Surgical treatment— tricks and hints

From the standpoint of **operative reconstruction,** four types of fracture patterns should be identified [20]: **wedge, impacted, multifragmentary, and neck fractures** (Fig. 4.3.1-11a–c).

- Wedge fractures: The fracture is easily reduced and fixed with one or two 2.0 mm lag screws. Small pieces of capitellar cartilage are frequently found entrapped in the fissure and should be removed. The screw heads should be countersunk to allow free forearm rotation.
- Impacted fractures: Impacted fragments can be found as depressions of the periphery or on the central surface. These are gently lifted using a dental hook or small elevator. If necessary, the remaining defects may be filled with small amounts of cancellous bone obtained from the lateral epicondyle. Provisional fixation is secured by means of 1.0 mm K-wires. Mini screws are used as position screws or a small mini plate may be added to support the reduction.
- Multifragmented fractures: The fragments are carefully reduced and provisionally fixed with K-wires. Two or three 2.0 mm screws are used to hold the reduced articular surface, as described. Usually one pillar of the radial head remains intact and some thin periosteal connections remain between the fragments. These should be preserved while reducing the fragments. Even in complex injuries there are sites where a small T-plate or L-plate can be contoured and adapted without impinging on the proximal radioulnar joint. Prosthetic replacement of the radial head represents a realistic option for badly comminuted fractures.
- Radial neck fractures: These fractures are uncommon in adults. Once the head is realigned, the resulting defect is filled with bone graft and supporting screws or a mini plate are placed to avoid displacement.

Following fixation of the radial head the annular ligament is repaired and stability of the elbow is checked through a full range of motion. In those cases associated with an elbow dislocation, repair of the lateral collateral ligament complex should follow. If instability persists, the medial complex should be explored and repaired.

3.4 Postoperative treatment

As described with olecranon fractures, a well-padded splint is placed with the elbow in extension to avoid edema. The day after surgery, active exercise is started by elevating the arm in a supine position and flexing the elbow by gravity. An active exercise program is then started. A posterior removable splint is worn for 3–4 weeks.

Wedge, impacted, multifragmentary, and neck fractures need operative reconstruction.

3.5 Pitfalls and complications

If intraoperative reconstruction of the head becomes impossible, replacement with a prosthesis is an option to restore stability and avoid secondary valgus and migration (Fig. 4.3.1-11d).

A recent report of 73 patients has shown a 13% rate of non-union and implant failure after open reduction and internal fixation of complex, multifragmented fractures. In these cases the reconstructed head functioned well as a spacer and late resection led to good results without compromising the function [21].

3.6 Results

Recent literature has shown excellent and good functional results of surgical reconstruction even in complex or multifragmented fractures. Some loss of full extension may be expected but without compromising the overall function [15–19, 21].

Implant removal has only been necessary if palpable screw heads cause pain or discomfort to the patient; it is seldom indicated.

4 Complex elbow injuries

4.1 Anterior or transolecranon fracture dislocation

This complex injury occurs when a high-energy direct blow is applied to the dorsal aspect of the forearm with the elbow in 90° flexion. It must be distinguished from anterior Monteggia lesions because both radius and ulna dislocate anteriorly leaving the proximal radioulnar joint intact. The proximal ulna is often multifragmented with a large coronoid fragment. Associated radial head fractures are uncommon. A posterior approach is performed and an indirect reduction of the ulna is accomplished as described for complex olecranon fractures. Fixation of the coronoid process with a screw will enhance stability. A dorsally placed pre-contoured LC-DCP 3.5 or alternatively a one-third tubular hook plate augmented with a tension band cerclage wire are the methods of fixation of choice [9, 12].

4.2 Posterior Monteggia fracture dislocation

(Fig. 4.3.1-12)

The mechanism of injury is similar to the posterior dislocation, but in this case a failure occurs through the proximal ulna resulting in a multifragmented fracture with a triangular or quadrangular fragment that can involve the coronoid process or be located more distally. Usually the radial head is fractured and dislocated postero-laterally [4].

Reconstruction of the proximal ulna with a posterior plate, as described above, will reduce the dislocation of the proximal radioulnar joint. Direct fixation of the coronoid process with a lag screw is achieved through the posterior approach. Occasionally, as distraction is applied, the fragment will reduce and become aligned to the montage. Reconstitution of the anterior ulnar cortex is essential to allow the plate to function as a tension band. Fixation of the head and reattachment of the lateral ligamentous complex will provide adequate stability to the lateral column.

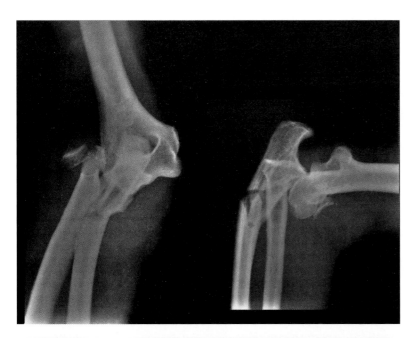

Fig. 4.3.1-12a/b:
Clinical example of a
reconstruction of a complex
radial/ulnar fracture 21-B3.
a) Complex elbow fracture
dislocation in a young woman
(dominant arm) with multifragment fracture of the
olecranon and split radial head.
No neurovascular deficit.

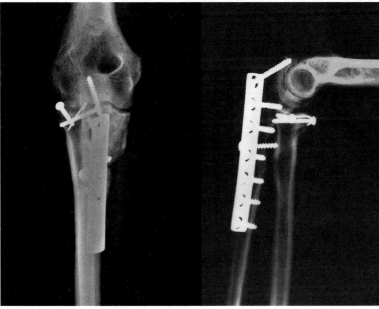

b) After emergency reconstruction of both olecranon (7-hole
DCP 3.5) and radial head
(two small fragment screws plus
K-wire), the patient is encouraged to move the elbow and
forearm immediately as pain
allows.

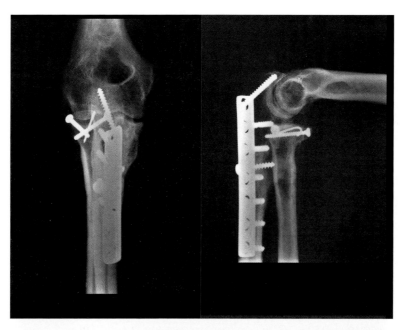

Fig. 4.3.1-12c/d:
c) 28 weeks postoperatively the fractures are well consolidated, the elbow joint stable with excellent function. Implant removal after one year.

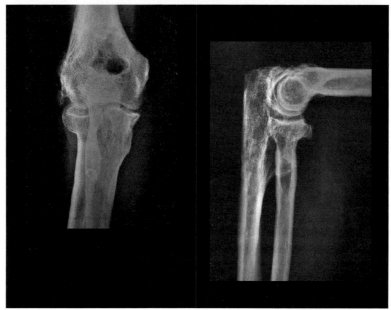

d) 14-years follow-up of the same still asymptomatic elbow with minimal signs of arthrosis and only slight limitation of function.

4.3 Bipolar fracture dislocation

This complex injury involves a fracture dislocation of the elbow associated with a distal fracture dislocation of the radius or disruption of the distal radioulnar joint. A segmental or "floating" radial diaphysis is present and this, associated with the disruption of both proximal and distal radioulnar joints, can lead to severe disability. The same fixation tactics recommended for Monteggia and Galeazzi lesions are applicable in the bipolar fracture dislocation [22].

5 Bibliography

1. **Teasdall R, Savoie FH, Hughes JL** (1993) Comminuted fractures of the proximal radius and ulna. *Clin Orthop*; (292):37–47.

2. **Ring D, Jupiter JB** (1998) Fracture dislocation of the elbow. *J Bone Joint Surg [Am]*; 80 (4):566–580.

3. **Modabber MR, Jupiter JB** (1995) Reconstruction for post-traumatic conditions of the elbow joint. *J Bone Joint Surg [Am]*; 77 (9):1431–1446.

4. **Jupiter JB, Leibovic SJ, Ribbans W, et al.** (1991) The posterior Monteggia lesion. *J Orthop Trauma*; 5 (4):395–402.

5. **Heim U** (1998) [Combined fractures of the radius and the ulna at the elbow level in the adult. Analysis of 120 cases after more than 1 year]. *Rev Chir Orthop Reparatrice Appar Mot*; 84 (2):142–153.

6. **Heim U** (1994) Kombinierte Verletzungen von Radius und Ulna im proximalen Unterarmsegment. *Unfallchirurg*; 241:62–79.

7. **Knight DJ, Rymaszewski LA, Amis AA, et al.** (1993) Primary replacement of the fractured radial head with a metal prosthesis. *J Bone Joint Surg [Br]*; 75 (4):572–576.

8. **Jupiter JB** (1994) Internal fixation for fractures about the elbow. *Operative Techniques in Orthopaedics*; 4 (1):31–48.

9. **Simpson NS, Goodman LA, Jupiter JB** (1996) Contoured LCDC plating of the proximal ulna. *Injury*; 27 (6):411–417.

10. **Healy W** (1991) Tension band plating for nonunion of proximal ulna and olecranon. *Techniques in Orthopaedics*; 6 (2):51–54.

11. **Webb LX** (1991) Use of a hook plate technique in the management of proximal ulna fractures. *Techniques in Orthopaedics*; 6 (2):45–50.

12. **Gerber C, Stokar P, Ganz R** (1991) The technique of open reduction and tension band augmented plate fixation of comminuted fractures of the olecranon. *Techniques in Orthopaedics*; 6 (2):41–44.

13. **Papagelopoulos PJ, Morrey BF** (1994) Treatment of nonunion of olecranon fractures. *J Bone Joint Surg [Br]*; 76 (4):627–635.

14. **Quintero J** (1994) Fractura de la cúpula radial. In: Malagón V, Soto D, editors. *Tratado de Ortopedia y Fracturas*. Bogotá: Celsus: 1497–1507.

15. **Ebraheim NA, Skie MC, Zeiss J, et al.** (1992) Internal fixation of radial neck fracture in a fracture dislocation of the elbow. A case report. *Clin Orthop*; (276):187–191.

16. **Khalfayan EE, Culp RW, Alexander AH**
(1992) Mason type II radial head
fractures: operative versus nonoperative
treatment. *J Orthop Trauma*; 6 (3):283–289.

17. **King GJ, Evans DC, Kellam JF** (1991)
Open reduction and internal fixation of
radial head fractures. *J Ortrhop Trauma*;
5 (1):21–28.

18. **Morales LC, Quintero J, Bustillo E**
(1989) Osteosíntesis estable en fracturas
conminutas de la cúpula radial. *Rev Colom
Ortop Traumatol*; 3 (1):1497–1507.

19. **Heim U** (1992) [Surgical treatment of
radial head fracture]. *Z Unfallchir
Versicherungsmed*; 85 (1):3–11.

20. **Heim U** (1988) The elbow. In: Heim U,
Pfeiffer KM, editors. *Internal Fixation of
Small Fractures*. Berlin Heidelberg New
York: Springer-Verlag: 107–137.

21. **Ring D, Kharrazi FD, Jupiter JB, et al.**
(1998) Non-union following ORIF of
radial head fractures. *Am Soc Surg Hand*.

22. **Jupiter JB, Kour AK, Richards RR,
et al.** (1994) The floating radius in
bipolar fracture-dislocation of the
forearm. *J Orthop Trauma*; 8 (2):99–106.

6 Updates

Updates and additional references for this chapter
are available online at:
http://www.aopublishing.org/PFxM/431.htm

4.3.2 Forearm shaft fractures

Dominik Heim

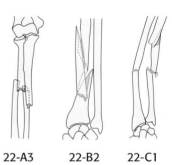

22-A3   22-B2   22-C1

Fig. 4.3.2-1: Müller AO Classification

1 Assessment of fractures

In the AO documentation (1980–1996) 10–14% of all fractures recorded occurred in the forearm. **Because the relationships of the radius and ulna are so important for the range of wrist and elbow movement, treatment in adults is generally surgical.**

1.1 Goals of treatment

- Restoration of length, axial alignment, and rotation so as to guarantee full pronation and supination.
- Fixation sufficient to allow free post-operative movement of adjacent joints.

1.2 General considerations

Indications for surgery:
- Combined fracture of radius and ulna.
- Displaced, isolated fracture of either bone (rotational deformity). A simple, non-displaced shaft fracture may, as an exception, be treated by non-operative means.
- Monteggia and Galeazzi fractures.
- All open fractures.

Imaging: Conventional x-rays of the forearm in two planes are usually sufficient. They must include the elbow and wrist in order to exclude associated articular fractures or specific fracture types, such as Monteggia or Galeazzi fractures. **Further imaging by CT scan or by MRI is seldom required**.

   Timing of surgery: As with most diaphyseal fractures of the human skeleton, forearm fractures are best operated on within 6–8 hours of the accident, including open fractures. Delayed fixation seems to increase the risk of radioulnar synostosis [1–2].

Treatment of forearm shaft fractures is mainly surgical.

CT scans or MRI are seldom required.

2 Surgical anatomy

The anatomy of the forearm is quite complex and preoperative planning is advised. Drawings are made using the techniques already described in **chapter 2.4**.

Both-bone fractures are best approached through separate incisions.

3 Preoperative planning

3.1 Positioning and approaches

The patient is usually placed supine with the affected limb supported on an arm rest. The use of a tourniquet is practical but should not be a routine without careful consideration of each individual case; it should be placed as high as possible on the arm in case the incision needs to be extended proximally.

If bone grafting is anticipated, one iliac crest is prepared. If during the operation only a small amount is needed, the radial condyle of the humerus is another possiblity.

Approaches

Several approaches may be used to fix shaft fractures of the forearm:

1 Entire shaft of the ulna: a single straight incision with the plate on the dorso-lateral aspect of the ulna.
2 Distal and middle shaft of the radius: a lateral approach with the plate on the dorsolateral aspect of the radius, or a palmar Henry incision.

3 Proximal shaft of the radius: the palmar approach according to Henry [3] with the plate on the ventral aspect of the radius.
4 Radius and ulna: a separate incision for each bone, preserving a broad skin bridge between the two incisions. **Attempting to fix both bones through a single approach increases the risk of nerve injury and radio-ulnar synostosis [1, 4].**

Approach to the ulna

Landmarks: Olecranon, styloid process of ulna (**Fig. 4.3.2-2a**).

The skin incision runs parallel to the ulnar crest (**Fig. 4.3.2-2b**). Access to the shaft is gained between the extensor carpi ulnaris and the flexor carpi ulnaris muscles. For dorsal plate positioning, the extensor is detached from the bone. In the very distal part of the incision, care is needed not to damage the dorsal branch of the ulnar nerve.

Dorsolateral approach to the radius

Landmarks: Lateral epicondyle of the humerus, styloid process of radius (**Fig. 4.3.2-3a**).

The skin is incised between the two landmarks. Access to the radial shaft runs in the septum between the extensor carpi radialis brevis and the extensor digitorum muscles.

These two muscle groups are split along the septum, commencing just proximal to the muscle belly of the abductor pollicis longus, which is easily recognized in the distal part of the incision. It might be necessary to mobilize this muscle in order to slip the plate underneath

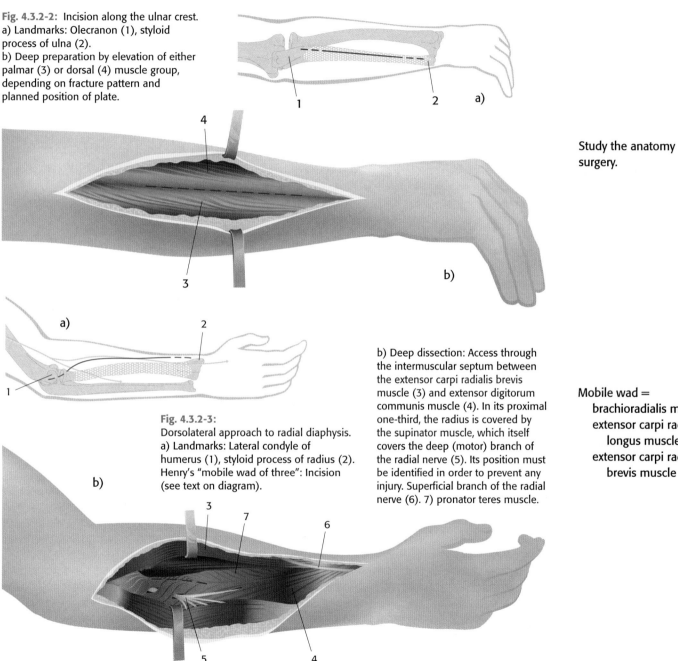

Fig. 4.3.2-2: Incision along the ulnar crest.
a) Landmarks: Olecranon (1), styloid process of ulna (2).
b) Deep preparation by elevation of either palmar (3) or dorsal (4) muscle group, depending on fracture pattern and planned position of plate.

Study the anatomy prior to surgery.

Fig. 4.3.2-3:
Dorsolateral approach to radial diaphysis.
a) Landmarks: Lateral condyle of humerus (1), styloid process of radius (2). Henry's "mobile wad of three": Incision (see text on diagram).

b) Deep dissection: Access through the intermuscular septum between the extensor carpi radialis brevis muscle (3) and extensor digitorum communis muscle (4). In its proximal one-third, the radius is covered by the supinator muscle, which itself covers the deep (motor) branch of the radial nerve (5). Its position must be identified in order to prevent any injury. Superficial branch of the radial nerve (6). 7) pronator teres muscle.

Mobile wad =
brachioradialis muscle
extensor carpi radialis longus muscle
extensor carpi radialis brevis muscle

in more distal shaft fractures of the radius (**Fig. 4.3.2-3b**, **Video AO22022**). The superficial branch of the radial nerve, which appears in the distal part of the incision along the brachioradialis muscle crossing the abductor pollicis longus in the subcutaneous layer, is vulnerable here.

During proximal exposure of the radial shaft, there could be damage to the deep branch of the radial nerve (posterior interosseous nerve), which runs through the supinator muscle at right angles to its fibers. The nerve can be felt as a bulge within the muscle about 3 fingerbreadths distal to the radial head. After identification of the nerve (possibly by splitting the muscle fibers), the supinator muscle with the nerve can be carefully detached close to the radius.

Henry approach: Enhance the view by rotating forearm.

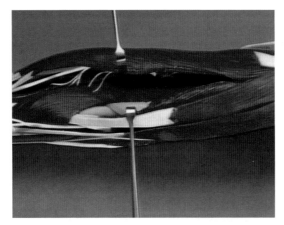

 Video AO22022

Palmar approach (Henry) [3]

The arm is placed on an arm rest with the elbow fully extended and in full supination.

Landmarks: Groove between brachioradialis muscle and distal biceps tendon. Styloid process of radius (**Fig. 4.3.2-4a**).

A straight skin incision is made on the palmar aspect of the arm, with a curve over the elbow joint. Incision of the subcutaneous fascia between the brachioradialis and flexor carpi radialis muscles. The anterior cutaneous nerve of the forearm and the superficial radial nerve run along the brachioradialis muscle. For deep dissection, the arterial branches of the radial artery supplying the brachioradialis muscle are carefully ligated (**Fig. 4.3.2-4b**). This muscle is retracted to the radial side and the radial artery and its accompanying veins to the ulnar side. The pronator teres muscle is preserved. After identification of the posterior interosseous nerve at its entrance into the supinator muscle (arcade of Frohse), this muscle together with the nerve on the radial side is detached in full supination and as close to the radius as possible. **At any point during this approach, the view may be enhanced by varying the rotation of the forearm** (**Fig. 4.3.2-4c**).

Fig. 4.3.2-4: Palmar approach to the radius (Henry).

a) Landmarks: Styloid process of radius (1), groove between m. brachioradialis and insertion of biceps tendon (2). Incision: Essentially straight, with an S-shaped curve over the elbow joint.

b) Deep dissection: Splitting of interval between m. brachioradialis and m. flexor carpi radialis—watch for the superficial (sensory) branch (3) of the radial nerve, as well as for the lateral cutaneous nerve of the forearm. Proximally, the arterial arch of the radial artery (4) must be ligated. The insertion of the supinator muscle (6) (watch for the deep branch of the radial nerve (5) can be separated to expose the bone at this level, as can the insertion of the pronator more distally.

c) To get better exposure of the radius, it is helpful to pronate the forearm. 7) Detached brachioradialis tendon, 8) radius fully exposed.

3.2 Reduction (tools and techniques) [5]

In general, open reduction is advised to guarantee an anatomically correct rotation. **Periosteal stripping should be limited to a minimum** (around 1 mm on each main fragment) and circumferential stripping is strictly to be avoided. Larger loose fragments stripped of their periosteum should be fixed to one main fragment by a lag screw, inserted either through the plate or separately (**Fig. 4.3.2-5**). After reduction and fixation of the main fragments, smaller devitalized fragments may be replaced by a cancellous bone graft.

A simple transverse fracture may be realigned by pulling on each main fragment with the aid of two small reduction forceps. The two fragments must interdigitate correctly to restore full rotation.

Minimize periosteal stripping during exposure and reduction.

a)

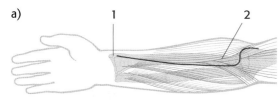

b)

c)

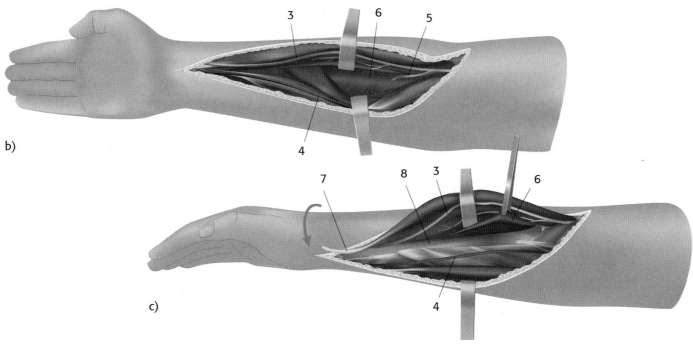

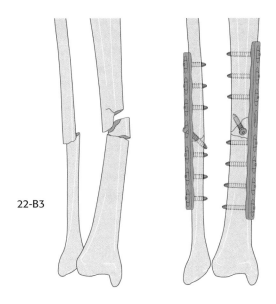

22-B3

Fig. 4.3.2-5: Simple both-bone fractures (22-B3). Stabilization with two LC-DCP 3.5 with interfragmentary compression. (Lag screw through the plate for the radius and separate 2.7 mm lag screw for the ulna.)

Implant of choice for the forearm bone: DCP or LC-DCP 3.5.

To neutralize torsional forces use 7-hole or 8-hole plates.

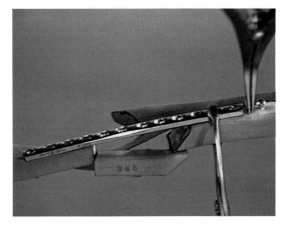

Video AO20099

Reduction can also be performed by fixing the plate on one main fragment and placing a screw in the other near the end of the plate. A spreader is then introduced between the plate and the screw and squeezed to distract the fracture site (**Video AO20099**)—push-pull technique (see **chapter 3.1, Fig. 3.1-13**).

In comminuted fractures (type C), preliminary distraction of the fracture by means of a unilateral external fixator may be useful. Fragments can then be approximately realigned with a dental pick.

3.3 Choice of implant

Up to this point in time, the defined goals of treatment (see **section 1.1**) have been achieved solely by open reduction and plate fixation.

Many years of clinical experience have proved **the plate 3.5 to be the ideal size for the forearm bones.** Available devices include the DCP (dynamic compression plate) or the more biologically shaped LC-DCP (limited contact-dynamic compression plate). Pursuing the concept of limited contact between plate and bone further has led to the development of the PC-Fix (point contact fixator) (see **chapter 3.4**).

One of the **purposes of the plate is neutralization of torsional forces** and, since the radius describes an important excursion around the ulna during rotation, **the plate must be long enough to achieve this**. Thus, there should be at least six cortices "holding", corresponding to three screws, in each main fragment. In simple fractures this usually means a 7-hole or 8-hole plate depending on the use of an additional plate-dependent lag screw.

Whenever possible an interfragmentary lag screw—whether independently or through a plate hole—should be introduced [6]. In the latter situation it may be expedient to use a screw of smaller diameter than 3.5 mm, for example, 2.7 mm.

The role of intramedullary locked nails is still to be defined while questions persist about their ability to control rotation.

<table><tr><td>4</td><td></td></tr></table>

4 Surgical treatment

If both bones have been fractured (**Fig. 4.3.2-6a**), **reduction is first performed on the bone with the simpler fracture pattern**. The plate is provisionally fixed with one or two screws or a reduction forceps. The other bone is exposed in turn and its fracture reduced. If reduction

proves to be impossible, the plate on the first bone is removed or loosened and the second bone is then reduced. After fixing it, the surgeon goes back to the first plate to complete the osteosynthesis. **Forearm rotation should be regularly checked throughout the procedure** (**Fig. 4.3.2-6b**).

If a simple transverse or short oblique fracture cannot be held reduced with a reduction forceps—and this is the case more often than not—the plate must be fixed on one main fragment (usually the proximal). Reduction is then carried out by bringing the other main fragment to the plate. In this case it is mandatory to fix the plate in such a way as to avoid torsion or uneven compression at the fracture site.

Prior to definitive fixation check forearm rotation regularly during surgery.

In both-bone fractures reduce the simpler fracture first.

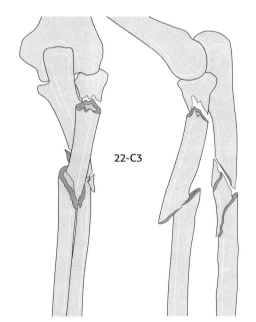
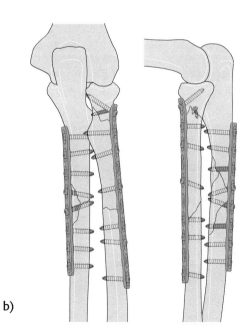

22-C3

a)   b)

Fig. 4.3.2-6: Complex both-bone fractures (22-C3). Stabilization with two long LC-DCPs 3.5, with separate 2.0 mm lag screw for the radial head. (Drawing from an actual case that healed uneventfully with a good functional outcome.)

Plan the plate position to allow correct placement of a lag screw through a plate hole.

In simple fractures, interfragmentary compression by a lag screw is a great advantage for stability of the fixation. If the intention is **to insert the lag screw through a central plate hole, the plate has to be positioned accordingly**.

It may be appropriate to prebend the plate (**Video AO00090a**) on simple forearm fractures; otherwise a fracture gap may develop on the

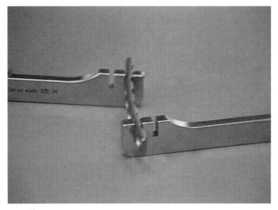

 Video AO00090a

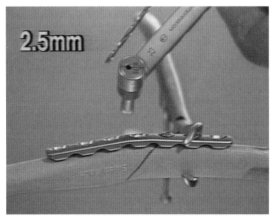

Video AO00090b

contralateral side and cause an uneven distribution of compression (see **chapter 3.2.2**). The required axial compression is achieved by eccentric drilling in the plate hole on one or both of the main fragments (**Video AO00090b**). Usually a certain amount of axial compression is applied before inserting the plate-dependent lag screw. In this way the surgeon can "play" with the interaction of interfragmentary and axial compression while tightening the plate screws.

Having completed the internal fixation, forearm rotation is once again assessed. Reduction and implant placement are verified under image intensification.

Wound closure: The fascia is usually not sutured. Wounds are closed over a suction drain. **It is rarely necessary to leave the skin open** but this may be done if there is considerable swelling.

Bone graft

In the past, the need for bone grafting on the forearm may have been overestimated. With very limited exposure of the fracture site and the care taken to avoid devitalizing third fragments, bone grafting has become less essential in many instances. During the postoperative course small fragments are often integrated into the healing fracture by callus formation.

If a bone graft is necessary, for example, in type C fractures, it should be placed away from the interosseous border.

Leaving skin open is rarely necessary.

5 Postoperative treatment

Following stable fixation, postoperative treatment is functional. A palmar splint or sugar tong splint may be used in unreliable patients. Immobilization in a circular cast may compromise the range of motion later. The operated arm is elevated. After 24–48 hours the suction drains can be removed. Active mobilization of fingers, wrist, and elbow including supervised forearm rotation are started on the first postoperative day. X-rays are taken at 6 and 12 weeks postoperatively and after 1 year. "Weight bearing" is usually allowed (in accordance with radiographic assessment after 6 weeks), for example, approximately 8 weeks after surgery.

Removal of the implants is not mandatory and is rarely indicated in an asymptomatic patient because of the risk of complications, including neurovascular injury and refracture [7]. If indicated it should not be performed for at least 2 years after internal fixation and then only after careful consideration by an experienced surgeon. Sometimes only one plate may need removal, (usually the ulnar one, because of the less abundant soft-tissue coverage). If both the radial and ulnar plates are to be removed, two-stage removal may be considered.

6 Pitfalls and complications

6.1 Open fractures

Grade 1 open fractures are treated according to the principles of closed fractures (see **chapter 5.1**).

Even higher grade open fractures of the forearm can be treated by immediate internal fixa-tion with results comparable to closed fractures [8–10] if meticulous débridement is carried out and soft-tissue coverage can be guaranteed. Open treatment of the wound, possibly with dressings soaked in antiseptic lotion, and accompanied by primary closure only of the iatrogenic extension of the wound may be safe. In these cases delayed wound closure is performed after a few days.

Techniques other than plating should be considered when covering of the plate cannot be achieved, because of soft-tissue loss [11]. Temporary external fixation is then recommended, possibly in combination with immediate internal fixation of the other bone in combined fractures.

Technique: Since both radius and ulna are of smaller diameter than other long bones, special Schanz screws for the tubular external fixator were designed with a thread diameter of 3.0 mm and a shaft diameter of 4.0 mm to fit into the normal adjustable clamp. To avoid nerve and vessel damage open pin insertion is recommended. The pin hole on the far cortex is drilled with a 2.5 mm drill bit and the near cortex is over-drilled with a 3.5 mm drill bit. The pins are then connected by either a single tube/carbon rod or by three tubes using tube-to-tube clamps to form a modular unilateral frame (see **chapter 3.3.3**).

As fracture consolidation with the external fixator alone often cannot be achieved [12] and pseudarthrosis and malrotation are considerable when using external fixation [13], sequential procedures with early secondary plate fixation are indicated, usually combined with cancellous bone grafting. If the conversion procedure can be performed within 3 weeks after initial treatment, an implant-free interval is not necessary. In large soft-tissue defects microvascular flaps might prove useful.

Routine implant removal is not recommended.

In Galeazzi fractures use an intraoperative x-ray to check that the ulna is back in place.

In recent Monteggia fractures the radial head usually reduces spontaneously.

6.2 Fracture dislocations of the forearm

The problem with these fractures is that they are often not recognized if the wrist and elbow are not included and inspected on the x-ray.

6.2.1 Monteggia fracture

A Monteggia fracture is a shaft fracture of the ulna, usually proximal, with an anterior or lateral dislocation of the radial head (Fig. 4.3.2-7). Delayed fixation compromises the functional outcome and immediate fixation is strongly recommended.

If the ulna is correctly reduced and fixed, the **radial head reduces spontaneously** in most cases. Pronation and supination are assessed clinically. If a tendency towards dislocation persists and if dorsal dislocation of the radial head is diagnosed, surgical inspection is indicated. This can be performed either by a separate lateral incision for the radial head or by extension of the original surgical approach and detachment of the anconeus and supinator muscles at their ulnar insertions. Interposed cartilage should be removed and the annular ligament sutured.

Postoperative treatment with a removable splint in supination for 3 weeks is then recommended to allow controlled mobilization of the elbow.

6.2.2 Galeazzi fracture

A Galeazzi fracture is a fracture of the radial shaft with dislocation of the distal radioulnar joint.

Correct reduction and fixation of the radial fracture is usually accompanied by **sponta-**

neous reduction of the ulna (Fig. 4.3.2-8). This **must be carefully checked on an intraoperative x-ray.** Thereafter, the wrist, forearm, and elbow may be splinted for 3 weeks to prevent rotation from the neutral position [14]. Other authors have disputed this procedure [15].

Exploration of the wrist by a dorsal approach is only recommended if stability after osteosynthesis is not guaranteed or if the reduction is unsatisfactory [15] and when these deficiencies cannot be put right at the time. Temporary

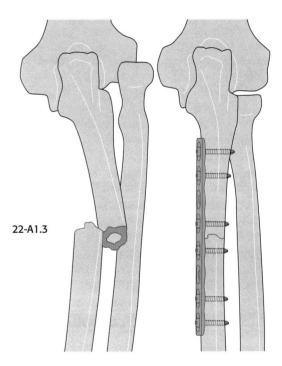

22-A1.3

Fig. 4.3.2-7: Isolated proximal ulnar fracture with dislocation of radial head (22-A1.3); Monteggia fracture. When the ulna is stabilized in correct rotation and length, the radial head displacement is usually reduced automatically.
Fixation of ulna by 8-hole LC-DCP 3.5 with axial compression. Repair of the annular ligament is optional.

transfixation of the ulna to the radius in supination by means of a K-wire for 3 weeks is another possible method [14]. In these cases, additional splinting of the forearm including elbow and wrist is mandatory. Otherwise, the K-wire will break during the 3 weeks before it is removed.

6.3 Synostosis and callus

Osteosynthesis of a forearm fracture is a demanding procedure. Several problems may result.

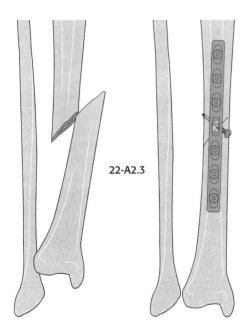

22-A2.3

Fig. 4.3.2-8: Isolated simple fracture of the distal third of the radius with dislocation of the distal radioulnar joint (22-A2.3), Galeazzi fracture. Anatomical stabilization of the radius using a LC-DCP 3.5 or DCP 3.5 will normally reduce the dislocation of the distal radioulnar joint which, usually, does not need any further treatment.

Posttraumatic radioulnar synostosis (cross-union) is an uncommon but very troublesome condition. Its incidence as reported in the literature ranges from 2.6% [4] to 6.6% [2].

Possible risk factors are:

1) Fractures of the radius and ulna at the same level [1], injury of the interosseous membrane [16], marked soft-tissue damage and comminution [17].
2) Delayed fixation of the fracture [2], a combined single approach for fixation of both bones [4], cancellous bone grafting [2], postoperative cast immobilization [2].
3) Concomitant head injury leading to increased propensity towards heterotopic bone formation [16, 17].

Several methods of treatment of synostosis have been proposed. These include resection of the distal part of the ulna—the Darrach procedure—excision and interposition of either foreign (Silastic®) or autogenous material [18], and excision combined with low dose irradiation [19].

Callus formation is usually not an issue after early fixation, but its postoperative incidence has been reported at up to 39% [20]. Callus formation usually peaks between the third and fourth postoperative months and often after 1 year has become partially resorbed. Technical imperfections and mechanical stress during functional treatment are frequently responsible. In this respect the importance of adequate compression of the fracture and of plates long enough to overcome torsional forces cannot be emphasized enough. External splints do not seem to influence callus formation [20].

Posttraumatic radioulnar synostosis is troublesome, but uncommon if fractures are stabilized within a few days after trauma.

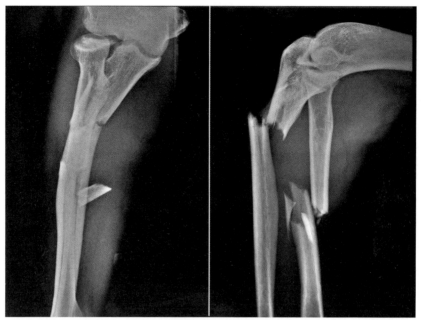

Fig. 4.3.2-9:
34-year-old male.
a) Complex both-bone forearm fracture with soft-tissue crushing (22-B3).

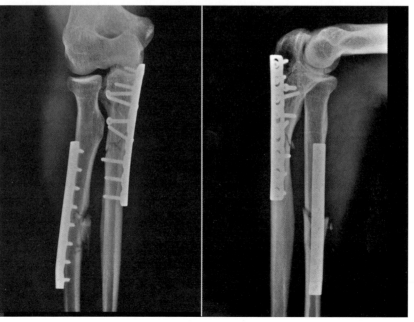

b) Postoperative x-rays: Internal fixation of ulna with LC-DCP 3.5, of radius with 8-hole PC-Fix (unicortical screw).

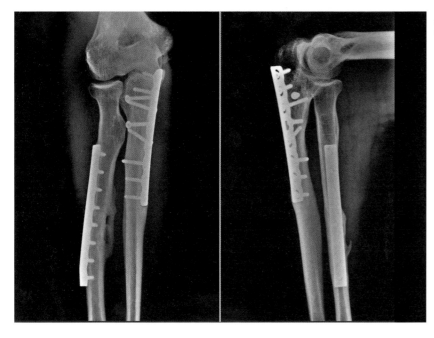

c) One-year result with functional restitution.

6.4   Non-union/ pseudarthrosis

The rates of non-union reported in the literature range from 3.7% [2] to 10.3%. Again, technical errors are most often responsible [20]. The benefits of more aggressive cancellous bone grafting have been discussed [20]. Once again, adequate plate length has to be emphasized. Bone grafting with or without repeat fixation usually leads to healing of the fracture [21].

6.5   Refracture after implant removal

Implant removal on the forearm is a recurrent topic because of the risk of refracture. The incidence rate reported is between 3.5% [22] and 25% and there is evidence that the use of the plate 3.5 has considerably decreased the rate of refracture [8].

Comminuted fractures, open fractures, bone defects, and technical failure (excessive stripping, inadequate compression) are considered to predispose to refracture. A further factor is the degree of initial displacement. It also seems evident that early plate removal, for example, within 12 months of internal fixation, increases the risk of refracture [22].

Implant removal on the forearm remains controversial. Before removal is carried out, close inspection of the x-rays for evidence of residual radiolucency at the fracture site is advocated, especially at the radius. Any signs of radiolucency are a clear contraindication to plate removal.

The general guidelines might be that implant removal on the forearm is to be performed only in symptomatic patients, after an interval of 2 years from internal fixation. The decision should be made by an experienced surgeon, who also performs the procedure.

7 Bibliography

1. **Vince KG, Miller JE** (1987) Cross-union complicating fracture of the forearm. Part I: Adults. *J Bone Joint Surg [Am]*; 69 (5):640–652.

2. **Oestern HJ, Tscherne H** (1983) [Results of a collective AO follow-up of forearm shaft fractures]. *Unfallheilkunde;* 86 (3):136–142.

3. **Henry AK** (1927) *Exposures of long bones and other surgical methods.* Bristol: John Wright.

4. **Bauer G, Arand M, Mutschler W** (1991) Post-traumatic radioulnar synostosis after forearm fracture osteosynthesis. *Arch Orthop Trauma Surg;* 110 (3):142–145.

5. **Mast J, Jakob R, Ganz R** (1989) *Planning and Reduction Technique in Fracture Surgery.* Berlin Heidelberg New York: Springer-Verlag.

6. **Claudi BF** (1979) *Untersuchungen zur Frage der Stabilitätsverbesserung von Druckplattenosteosynthesen durch schräge Zugschraube und Plattenüberbiegung.* München. (Thesis).

7. **Bednar DA, Grandwilewski W** (1992) Complications of forearm-plate removal. *Can J Surg;* 35 (4):428–431.

8. **Chapman MW, Gordon JE, Zissimos AG** (1989) Compression-plate fixation of acute fractures of the diaphyses of the radius and ulna. *J Bone Joint Surg [Am]*; 71 (2):159–169.

9. **Duncan R, Geissler W, Freeland AE, et al.** (1992) Immediate internal fixation of open fractures of the diaphysis of the forearm. *J Orthop Trauma;* 6 (1):25–31.

10. **Moed BR, Kellam JF, Forster RI** (1986) Immediate internal fixation of open fractures of the diaphysis of the forearm. *J Bone Joint Surg [Am]*; 68 (7):1008–1017.

11. **Müller ME, Allgöwer M, Schneider R, et al.** (1991) *Manual of Internal Fixation.* 3rd ed. Berlin Heidelberg New York: Springer-Verlag.

12. **Wild JJ, Jr., Hanson GW, Bennett JB, et al.** (1982) External fixation use in the management of massive upper extremity trauma. *Clin Orthop;* (164):172–176.

13. **Josten CH, Lies A, Knopp W** (1989) Verfahrenswechsel bei offener distaler Unterarmfraktur. *Hefte Unfallheilkd;* 201:116–119.

14. **Macule Beneyto F, Arandes Renu JM, Ferreres Claramunt A, et al.** (1994) Treatment of Galeazzi fracture-dislocations. *J Trauma;* 36 (3):352–355.

15. **Lechner J, Steiger R, Ochsner P** (1993) [Surgical treatment of Galeazzi fracture]. *Unfallchirurg;* 96 (1):18–23.

16. **Garland DE, Dowling V** (1983) Forearm fractures in the head-injured adult. *Clin Orthop;* (176):190–196.

17. **Stern PJ, Drury WJ** (1983) Complications of plate fixation of forearm fractures. *Clin Orthop;* (175):25–29.

18. **Failla JM, Amadio PC, Morrey BF**
(1989) Post-traumatic proximal radioulnar synostosis. Results of surgical
treatment. *J Bone Joint Surg [Am]*;
71 (8):1208–1213.

19. **Cullen JP, Pellegrini VD, Jr., Miller RJ,
et al**. (1994) Treatment of traumatic
radioulnar synostosis by excision and
postoperative low-dose irradiation.
J Hand Surg [Am]; 19 (3):394–401.

20. **Heim U, Zehnder R** (1989) Analyse von
Misserfolgen nach Osteosynthesen von
Unterarmschaftfrakturen. *Hefte
Unfallheilkd*; 201:243–258.

21. **Hertel R, Pisan M, Lambert S, et al.**
(1996) Plate osteosynthesis of diaphyseal
fractures of the radius and ulna. *Injury;*
27 (8):545–548.

22. **Rosson JW, Shearer JR** (1991)
Refracture after the removal of plates
from the forearm. An avoidable
complication. *J Bone Joint Surg [Br]*;
73 (3):415–417.

8   Updates

Updates and additional references for this chapter
are available online at:
http://www.aopublishing.org/PFxM/432.htm

4.3.3 Distal radius/wrist

Diego L. Fernandez

1 Fractures of the distal radius

1.1 Assessment of fractures and soft tissues

Fractures of the distal radius form a spectrum ranging from simple fractures requiring little management to complex multifragmented fracture dislocations of daunting complexity.

Minimally displaced intra-articular and extra-articular fractures as well as impacted stable fractures with minimal shortening can be managed adequately by closed reduction and cast or splint immobilization. However, more often than not, distal radius fractures will involve the radiocarpal joint and/or the distal radioulnar joint. They can be either partial articular (type B) or complete articular (type C). These require an anatomical reduction of the joint surface in order to reduce the incidence of posttraumatic arthrosis and to guarantee a successful functional outcome [1, 2].

Thus, intra-articular **fractures that cannot be reduced with closed methods will more often require operative treatment**.

A patient with an acute distal radius fracture should be evaluated for age, hand dominance, occupation, level of activity, and general medical condition. Fracture evaluation should determine whether it is open or closed and whether neurovascular compromise is present, as well as the degree of displacement of the fragments, and whether the fracture is intra-articular or extra-articular. Assessment of the mechanism of injury, which should include a grading from low-energy to high-energy trauma, and of the quality of bone (presence or absence of osteoporosis) is imperative. The associated ligamentous lesions, subluxations, or fractures of the neighboring carpal bones, and the concomitant soft-tissue damage, are all directly related to the quality and degree of violence sustained [3]. Furthermore, the mechanism of injury will dictate the reduction maneuvers which should be designed to reverse the force which caused the injury.

AP and lateral x-rays of the wrist usually suffice for the evaluation of extra-articular fractures and the assessment of shortening, direction of displacement and amount of metaphyseal comminution. Oblique films (45° pronated and supinated), in addition to the AP and lateral x-rays, permit a better view of the scaphoid and lunate facets respectively and allow better evaluation of intra-articular fractures. Finally,

Minimally displaced intra-articular and extra-articular fractures and impacted stable fractures with minimal shortening can be managed by closed reduction.

Fractures that cannot be reduced with closed methods will more often require operative treatment.

traction views or fluoroscopy following initial reduction with finger trap traction provide a better appreciation of intra-articular comminution. Trispiral tomograms can be helpful to show intra-articular displacement and are very useful for complex intra-articular fractures (type C). Computed tomography, especially coronal cuts, is useful to show lunate facet injuries including the involvement of the distal radioulnar joint (sigmoid notch), as well as associated distal radioulnar joint subluxation. Magnetic resonance imaging is reserved for late investigation of associated interacarpal ligament injuries and triangular fibrocartilage tears; it is seldom used in the acute stage.

Initial satisfactory closed reduction cannot always be maintained by splint.

The following radiological signs should alert the surgeon that an initial satisfactory closed reduction would not be maintained by a splint or cast [4, 5] (so-called unstable fractures):

- dorsal comminution exceeding more that 50% of the dorsal to palmar distance,
- palmar metaphyseal comminution,
- initial dorsal tilt more than 20°,
- initial displacement (fragment translation) more than 1 cm,
- initial shortening greater than 5 mm,
- intra-articular disruption,
- associated ulnar fracture,
- massive osteoporosis.

A treatment algorithm (**Table 4.3.3-1**) is based on types and groups of the comprehensive classification of fractures of long bones (**Fig. 4.3.3-1**). In distal radius fractures, assessment of associated soft-tissue lesions is just as important as assessing the fracture itself because these lesions affect initial management of the injury. **Table 4.3.3-2** shows a prognostic classification (which correlates with the "qualifications" proposed in the Müller AO Classification) of the associated

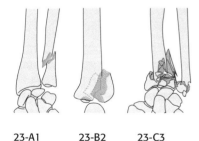

23-A1   23-B2   23-C3

Fig. 4.3.3-1: Müller AO Classification

distal radioulnar joint injuries, together with the recommendation for management. The classification parameters are based primarily on distal radioulnar joint stability and/or incongruity [6, 7]. Intercarpal ligament tears associated with distal radius fractures should also be carefully assessed since these co-exist with both intra-articular and extra-articular fracture types. Disruption of the extrinsic palmar ligaments inevitably accompanies radiocarpal fracture dislocations. Scapholunate ligament disruption is associated with displaced radius styloid fractures entering the ridge between the scaphoid and the lunate. Scapholunate tears occur in 30% of distal radial fractures and lunatotriquetral tears in 15% [8].

Patients with severely displaced distal radius fractures may present initially with some symptoms of median nerve compression. If initial closed reduction is satisfactory they should be observed for 48 hours. If symptoms persist, carpal tunnel decompression should be performed and stabilization obtained with the least invasive method appropriate to the fracture.

2 Surgical anatomy

The distal radius is superficial and readily surgically accessible from a dorsal, palmar, or combined approach. Palpable superficial landmarks are: the radial styloid process, Lister's tubercle, and the distal ulna. Superficial nerves include the superficial branch of the radial nerve and the dorsal cutaneous branch of the ulnar nerve. On the palmar aspect, the palmar cutaneous branch of the median nerve can be at risk when extending radial-side incisions into the palm.

The articular end of the radius slopes in an ulnar and palmar direction and has three concave articular surfaces: the sigmoid notch, the scaphoid fossa, and the lunate fossa. These articulate respectively with the ulnar head, the scaphoid, and the lunate. The palmar surface of the distal end of the radius is flat, with a gentle anterior curve. The dorsal aspect is, however, convex, and Lister's tubercle serves as a fulcrum for the extensor pollicis longus tendon (**Fig. 4.3.3-2**). The anatomical relationships of the extensor retinaculum, six extensor compartments, and the dorsal radial cortex are of extreme importance for the surgical approaches (**Fig. 4.3.3-3a**), as well as for the placement of plates on the dorsum of the radius.

Table 4.3.3-1: Treatment algorithm

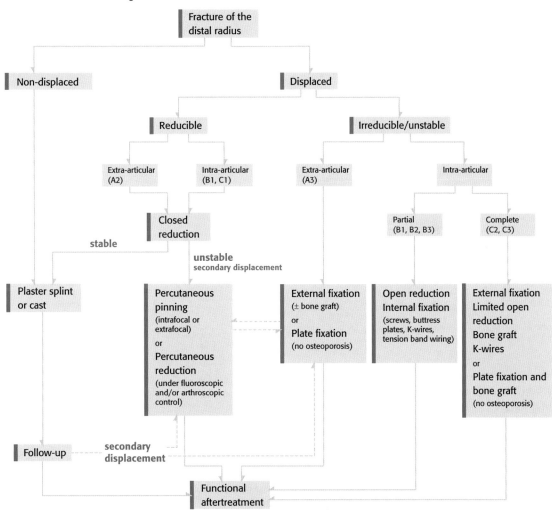

Table 4.3.3-2:

	Pathoanatomy of the lesion		Joint surface involvement	Prognosis	Recommended treatment
Type I stable (following reduction of the radius the distal radioulnar joint is congruous and stable)	**A** Fracture Tip ulnar styloid	**B** Stable fracture Ulnar neck	none	good	**A+B** Functional aftertreatment Encourage early pronation-supination exercises Note Extra-articular **unstable** fractures of the ulna at the metaphyseal level or distal shaft require stable fixation
Type II unstable (subluxation or dislocation of the ulnar head present)	**A** Tear of triangular fibrocartilage complex and/or palmar and dorsal capsular ligaments	**B** Avulsion fracture Base of the ulnar styloid	none	– Chronic instability – Painful limitation of supination if left unreduced – Possible late arthritic changes	**A** **Closed treatment** Reduce subluxation, sugar tong splint in 45° supination 4–6 weeks **A+B** **Operative treatment** Repair triangular fibrocartilage complex or fix ulnar styloid with tension band wiring. Immobilize wrist and elbow in supination (cast) or trans-fix ulna/radius with K-wire and forearm cast.
Type III potentially unstable (subluxation possible)	**A** Intra-articular fracture of the sigmoid notch	**B** Intra-articular fracture of the ulnar head	present	– Dorsal subluxation possible together with dorsally displaced die punch or dorsoulnar fragment – Risk of early degenerative changes and severe limitation of forearm rotation if left unreduced	**A** Anatomical reduction of palmar and dorsal sigmoid notch fragments. If residual subluxation tendency present, immobilize as in type II injury. **B** Functional aftertreatment to enhance remodeling of ulnar head. If distal radioulnar joint remains painful: Partial ulnar resection, Darrach or Sauvé-Kapandji procedure at a later date.

In the frontal plane, the ulnar inclination averages 23°, with a physiological range of 13–30°. In the sagittal plane, the palmar tilt or inclination averages 10–12° (range 4–22°). The ulnar variance or radioulnar index measures the length relationship between the ulna and radius. In approximately 61% of cases, the head of the ulna and the medial corner of the radius are at the same level bilaterally (neutral variance). Ulnar plus variance (longer ulna) and ulnar minus variance (shorter ulna) may be physiological, so that comparative x-rays of the uninjured wrist are usually necessary to determine normal length in each case.

The palmar aspects of the radius and distal ulna are the sites of origin of the extrinsic restraining ligaments supporting the carpus. Stout oblique radiocarpal and ulnocarpal ligaments maintain the normal kinematics of the radiocarpal joint. Weak and less important ligaments

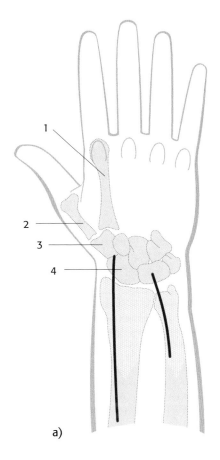

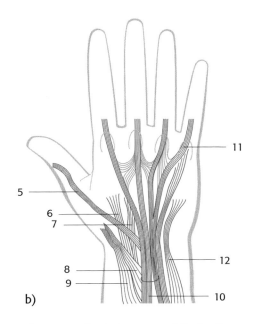

Fig. 4.3.3-2: Surgical anatomy of distal radius.
a) Dorsal approach: Skin incision. Os metacarpale II (1), os metacarpale I (2), os trapezium (3), os scaphoideum (4).
b) Surgical anatomy of dorsum of the wrist: 5) Extensor pollicis longus (EPL), 6) extensor carpi radialis longus (ECRL), 7) extensor carpi radialis brevis (ECRB), 8) extensor pollicis brevis (EPB), 9) abductor pollicis longus (APL), 10) extensor digitorum communis (EDC), 11) extensor digitorum minimi (EDQ), 12) extensor carpi ulnaris (ECU).

3 Preoperative planning

make up the dorsal supporting structures arising from the dorsal lip of the radius.

At the ulnar aspect of the lunate facet the triangular fibrocartilage arises which extends onto the base of the ulnar styloid process to serve as an important stabilizer of the distal radioulnar joint. Its other secondary stabilizers are the interosseous membrane, the pronator quadratus, and the tendon and sheath of the extensor carpi ulnaris muscle.

The preoperative plan must be done in advance and is essentially an "exercise in geometry" designed to correct the deformity (fracture displacement), achieve exposure, and obtain fixation. It consists of a free-hand tracing of the fracture pattern, followed by what it should look like when reduced (x-rays of the opposite side are helpful) with the appropriate implants in place. It should then list the instruments likely to be needed, special items and anything else that might be helpful, such as intraoperative x-rays, image intensifier, mini C-arm, or arthroscopic equipment. Next, the three stages of surgical intervention, position, incision, and dissection or exposure are set out as appropriate for the fracture.

4 Positioning and approaches

4.1 General observations

Approximately 35–40% of all distal radius fractures/injuries require operative treatment. The exposure, as a rule, should be extensile, atraumatic, and executed with great care and respect for the soft tissues. The goal is to achieve an anatomical reduction and obtain stable fixation with minimal disruption of supporting ligaments and with maintenance of the vascularity of the fragments. Surgery can usually be performed under regional axillary block. If iliac bone graft is needed, further local anesthesia or brief general anesthesia can be performed while the graft is harvested and the wound closed. General anesthesia is reserved for high-energy injuries or combined injuries for which a longer operative time is anticipated.

4.2 Surgical approaches to the distal radius

4.2.1 Dorsal approaches

(Fig. 4.3.3-3)

These are generally indicated for extra-articular and intra-articular fractures with dorsal displacement and dorsal metaphyseal comminution as well as fractures of the radial styloid and fractures involving the dorsoulnar aspect of the lunate facet. Dorsal surgical approaches are usually performed through straight longitudinal incisions centered between various extensor compartments [5, 9].

For radial/styloid fractures (B1.1 and B1.2) the approach is centered between the first and second extensor compartment (Fig. 4.3.3-3a). Great care should be taken to identify and protect the multiple branches of the superficial radial nerve and to avoid undue tension during the procedure. The radial artery is also at risk as it courses around the styloid into the anatomical snuffbox, especially if the incision is extended distally. Articular reduction can be best assessed through a partial arthrotomy of the wrist between the second and third compartment and one can also see if the scapholunate ligament has been disrupted when the radial styloid fracture is severely displaced proximally.

Internal fixation material (K-wires or cannulated screws) is inserted through the tip of the radial styloid dorsal to the tendons of abductor pollicis longus and extensor pollicis brevis.

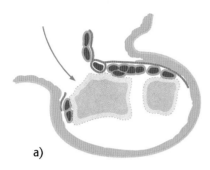

a)

Fig. 4.3.3-3: Dorsal approach to the wrist:
a) Between first and second extensor
compartment for fracture of radial styloid.

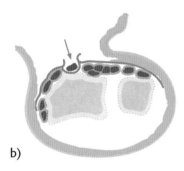

b)

b) Through the third dorsal compartment (EPL).

Exposure of the dorsal metaphysis and central articular fractures requires a longitudinal dorsoradial incision centered over the Lister's tubercle. The approach traverses the third dorsal compartment (**Fig. 4.3.3-3b**) with radial transposition of the extensor pollicis longus tendon. The second and fourth compartments are then subperiosteally elevated from the dorsal rim fragments. If plate fixation is planned, an ulnarly based flap of retinaculum is dissected just radial to the second compartment and elevated exposing the extensor pollicis longus and the radial half of the fourth compartment. Following application of the plate, part of the im-

plant comes to lie underneath the fourth compartment and the rest under the third and second compartments. During closure the retinaculum flap is used to cover the plate radially leaving the extensor pollicis longus in a subcutaneous position.

Finally, for internal fixation of the ulnar styloid process, repair of the triangular fibrocartilage, or reconstruction of fractures of the ulnar head, a dorsal ulnar incision between the fifth and sixth extensor compartments is used. The dorsal cutaneous branch of the ulnar nerve is at risk once the incision goes distal to the level of the ulnocarpal joint on the dorsum of the hand.

4.2.2   Palmar approaches

(**Fig. 4.3.3-4**)

These are indicated for all palmar displaced fractures (A2.3) and for palmar marginal fractures of the B3 group. Palmar approaches are also indicated for radiocarpal fracture dislocation, for primary repair of the torn wrist capsule, and whenever primary median nerve decompression or flexor compartment fasciotomy are needed. On the rare occasions where palmar and dorsal articular fragment displacement is present, a combined dorsal and palmar exposure may become necessary.

Two classical palmar approaches to the distal radius exist for exposure, reduction, and palmar plate application.

The first and most frequently used is the distal part of a classical Henry approach for palmar exposure of the whole radius. A longitudinal incision is made, slightly radial to the flexor carpi radialis tendon (FCR) (**Fig. 4.3.3-4a**). The space between the flexor carpi radialis

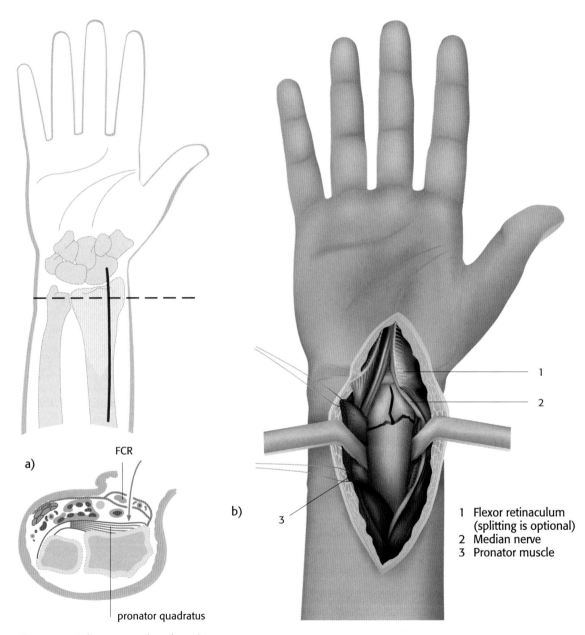

FCR

a)

pronator quadratus

b)

3

1 Flexor retinaculum
  (splitting is optional)
2 Median nerve
3 Pronator muscle

Fig. 4.3.3-4: Palmar approach to the wrist:
a) Palmar approach to distal radius (Henry). Note that the carpal tunnel cannot be easily reached!

b) Wide exposure of distal radius after detaching the pronator laterally.

tendon and the radial artery is dissected exposing the pronator quadratus, which is detached from the lateral border of the radius and elevated from the radial metaphysis towards the ulna (**Fig. 4.3.3-4b**). The tendon of the flexor pollicis longus (FPL) is visible more proximally in the wound and partial detachment of its radial attachment is necessary when applying longer plates to this part of the bone. This exposure is usually sufficient for the B3 group of fractures. If carpal tunnel decompression is necessary, it is preferable to make a separate palmar incision rather than to extend the Henry approach distally to the palm, as this would place the palmar cutaneous branch of the median nerve in jeopardy.

The second palmar exposure is one that is more extensile and is essentially a proximally extended carpal tunnel incision (**Fig. 4.3.3-5**). It is preferred when exposure of the ulnar palmar corner and distal radioulnar joint is required, such as for limited open reduction of four-part

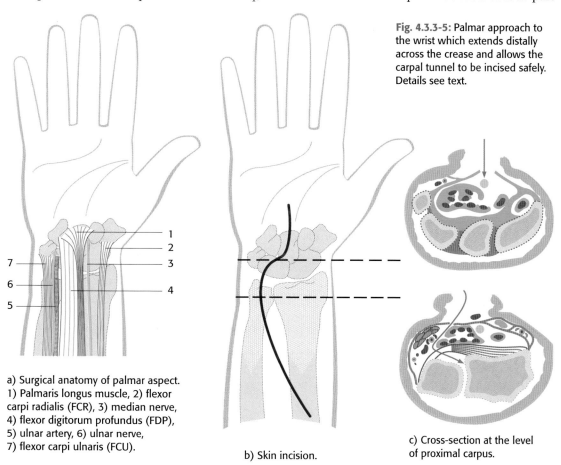

Fig. 4.3.3-5: Palmar approach to the wrist which extends distally across the crease and allows the carpal tunnel to be incised safely. Details see text.

a) Surgical anatomy of palmar aspect.
1) Palmaris longus muscle, 2) flexor carpi radialis (FCR), 3) median nerve,
4) flexor digitorum profundus (FDP),
5) ulnar artery, 6) ulnar nerve,
7) flexor carpi ulnaris (FCU).

b) Skin incision.

c) Cross-section at the level of proximal carpus.

fractures with a severely displaced palmar ulnar fragment. It can also be extended obliquely from ulnar to radial in the distal forearm for the treatment of more complex injuries such as radiocarpal fracture dislocations, the combination of distal radial fracture and perilunate injury, complex fractures with palmar displacement, and extensive metaphyseal and even diaphyseal comminution. For massive crush injury this incision can be extended to the elbow crease for primary fasciotomy of the palmar compartments.

The skin incision starts at the mid-palmar crease and zigzags across the wrist flexor crease on the ulnar aspect of the wrist. Proximally it can follow the radial border of the flexor carpi ulnaris and then cross in a more radial direction if proximal exposure of the radius is required. The median nerve can be decompressed at the carpal tunnel and the ulnar nerve at Guyon's canal. The exposure is carried through the interval between the ulnar neurovascular bundle and the deep flexor tendons, which are retracted ulnarly and radially respectively. The pronator quadratus can then be detached from either its ulnar or its radial insertion depending on the particular fracture pattern. This exposure does, however, restrict access to the most radial aspect of the distal radius, including the radial styloid process.

Finally, there is a third palmar approach intended for exposure of the distal ulna. An incision is made centered on the interval between the flexor carpi and extensor carpi ulnaris tendons. The dorsal cutaneous branch of the ulnar nerve should be identified as it crosses dorsally at the level of the ulnar styloid. This incision provides adequate exposure for internal fixation of the distal ulnar shaft, ulnar head, and ulnar styloid.

Skeletal fixation must be adapted to the particular fracture pattern, soft tissue, and quality of bone.

5 Management and surgical treatment—tricks and hints

5.1 General comments

Recommendations for management and fixation techniques will follow the Comprehensive Classification of Fractures. However, in selecting **skeletal fixation methods, the choice must remain wide and flexible and should be adapted to the particular fracture pattern characteristics, the local soft-tissue conditions and the quality of bone.**

5.2 Type A—extra-articular fractures

Group A1 (isolated extra-articular fractures of the distal ulna) fractures of the styloid process will require internal fixation when the lesion is associated with distal radioulnar joint instability (see **Table 4.3.3-2**). Isolated metaphyseal stable fractures may be treated either conservatively or with plate fixation; a DCP 3.5 or 2.7 is the implant of choice. The condylar plate 2.7 is an alternative implant when the fracture comminution starts just above the ulnar head.

The A2 extra-articular impacted or stable types of Colles' or Smith's fractures usually respond very well to conservative treatment. Dorsal metaphyseal comminution will make the fracture unstable (A3). In this situation, conventional extrafocal percutaneous pinning, or intrafocal as suggested by Kapandji [10, 11], may be used when bone quality is good (**Fig. 4.3.3-6a**). With extensive metaphyseal comminution there is a high risk of shortening and instability, so that for this fracture scenario closed reduction and external fixation will be the treatment of choice [12]. **Extra-articular unstable or irreducible fractures with good bone quality are treated with either dorsal or palmar plating depending on the direction of the deformity (Fig. 4.3.3-6c).** In these cases additional bone grafting must be considered. The advantage of plate fixation over external fixation is that early rehabilitation of the wrist is possible shortly after suture removal.

Unstable fracture patterns require surgical fixation.

5.3 Type B—partial articular fractures

The basic feature common to all fractures in this group is that a portion of the metaphyseal and epiphyseal area of the distal radius remains intact and in continuity with the uninvolved part of the joint surface. The displaced articular fragment can therefore be exactly reduced and solidly fixed to the intact column of the distal radius and for this reason the ultimate prognosis in these fractures is good. Furthermore, fractures with a distinct shearing component tend to occur in young individuals, whose dense cancellous bone offers ideal holding power for internal fixation material.

The B1 group, which includes fractures of the radial styloid and the medial cuneiform facet, will usually respond to closed reduction and percutaneous pinning or arthroscopically assisted percutaneous cannulated screw fixation (Fig. 4.3.3-6b). It is important to rule out scapholunate dissociation if the fragment is severely proximally displaced. If the fracture is irreducible, open reduction and internal fixation through the dorsal radial approach between the second and third compartment is recommended. Medial cuneiform or isolated "die punch" non-reducible fractures are exposed through a

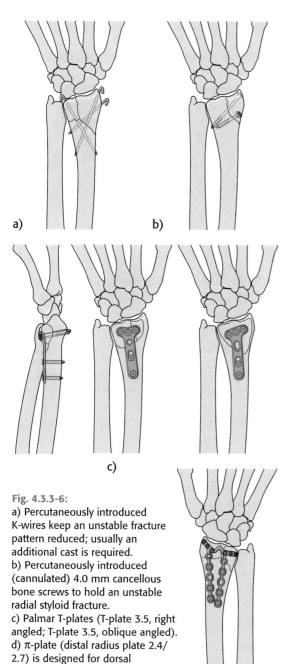

a)

b)

c)

d)

Fig. 4.3.3-6:
a) Percutaneously introduced K-wires keep an unstable fracture pattern reduced; usually an additional cast is required.
b) Percutaneously introduced (cannulated) 4.0 mm cancellous bone screws to hold an unstable radial styloid fracture.
c) Palmar T-plates (T-plate 3.5, right angled; T-plate 3.5, oblique angled).
d) π-plate (distal radius plate 2.4/2.7) is designed for dorsal application.

small incision between the fourth and fifth extensor compartments.

The B2 dorsal rim Barton type fracture does not commonly occur by itself but is often combined with a radial styloid fragment. Fixation techniques may involve K-wire or screw fixation depending on the fragment size. For unstable dorsal rim fractures a small buttress plate 2.7 may be used. This group includes the radio-carpal fracture dislocations (B2.3). These are high-energy injuries with small marginal avulsions, as well as ulnar and radial styloid fractures in association with a complete dislocation of the entire carpus. The recommended treatment includes initial closed reduction, palmar capsular repair, and decompression of the median nerve through an extended carpal tunnel approach. Stable fixation of the radial and ulnar avulsions using tension band wiring techniques and K-wires is advisable. Depending on the soft-tissue conditions, temporary neutralization with an external fixation frame for 4 weeks will permit cast-free aftercare.

Palmar marginal fractures (group B3) represent the classical indication for palmar buttress plating (**Fig. 4.3.3-7a**). The fracture is reduced with hyperextension of the wrist over a rolled towel and fixed with an oblique T-plate 3.5 which is pre-bent, so that a small space of 1–2 mm is maintained between it and metaphysis. Once it is confirmed that the plate abuts with the distal rim of the fracture, the most proximal screw is inserted first, and by driving the second screw in the central oval hole a very good buttressing effect is obtained (**Fig. 4.3.3-7b**) [3]. The palmar capsule should not be opened to control articular reduction, since the integrity of the radioscaphocapitate and radiolunotriquetral ligaments should be preserved. Interposed intra-articular fragments should be identified through the fracture site before preliminary

In the palmar approach it is recommended to release the carpal tunnel.

B3 fractures are the classical indication for palmar buttress plating.

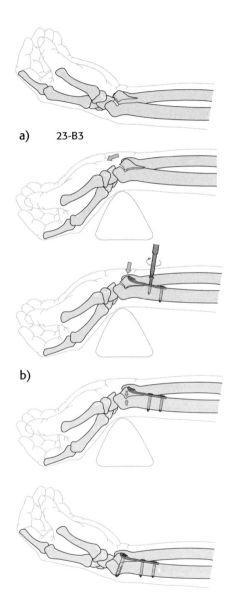

a)   23-B3

b)

Fig. 4.3.3-7: Technique of palmar plating of a B3 fracture:
a) Reduction by hyperextension of the wrist over a pad.
b) A small fragment T-plate 3.5 is placed in a buttress position. The first screw is placed in the most proximal hole. By tightening the second screw a good buttressing effect is obtained. The most distal screw(s) is/are optional.

reduction and temporary fixation with K-wires. Palmar intra-articular fractures with a separate radial fragment may require additional fixation with K-wires driven percutaneously through the radial styloid. The plate can usually be covered by suturing the pronator quadratus to the radial aspect of the shaft.

5.4 Type C—complete articular fractures

If the skeletal lesion has simple intra-articular components, with no metaphyseal comminution and no more than two fragments (group C1), these fractures usually respond well to closed or percutaneous reduction and rarely need formal open fixation. In percutaneous reduction the cartilage-bearing fragments are manipulated under fluoroscopic guidance with an awl or a periosteal elevator through a small skin incision with a minimum of soft-tissue dissection. They can be stabilized with percutaneous pinning (**Fig. 4.3.3-8**).

If the fracture presents with a **simple intra-articular component and extensive metaphyseal comminution (group C2), external fixation is the method of choice** to control radial shortening and metaphyseal angulation (**Fig. 4.3.3-9** and **Fig. 4.3.3-10**) (**Video AO22024**). If articular congruity is not adequately restored with ligamentotaxis following application of the

External fixation is the method of choice for fractures with simple intra-articular components and extensive metaphyseal comminution.

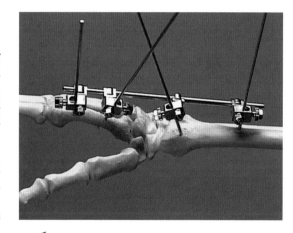

Video AO22024

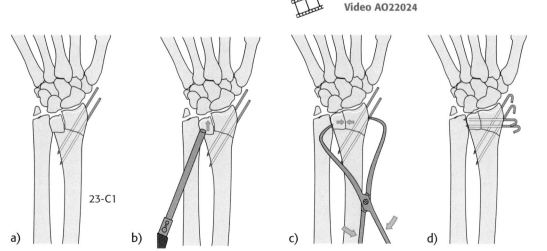

23-C1

a) b) c) d)

Fig. 4.3.3-8: Technique of percutaneous reduction and K-wire fixation of a C1 fracture.

Fig. 4.3.3-9: External fixator.

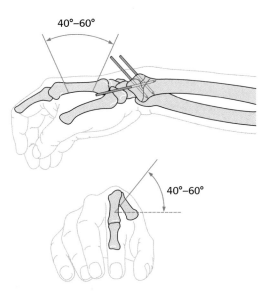

40°–60°

40°–60°

a) Reduction of the fracture with percutaneous K-wires. Definition of angle of 40–60° for the placement of the external fixator pins (in two planes).

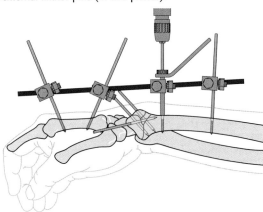

b) Placement of external fixator in a joint bridging fashion with two pins each in the distal redius and second metacarpal.

external fixator, then a percutaneous and/or limited open reduction in combination with bone grafting is advocated [13–15]. In this situation, a small dorsal approach between the third and fourth dorsal compartments is usually employed; the articular fragments are elevated against the carpus and stabilized with percutaneous pins. Autogenous bone grafting is strongly recommended, since it provides additional mechanical support to the small cartilage-bearing fragments—it increases the stability of the construct and accelerates bone healing. All this will permit removal of the fixator at 5 weeks [6].

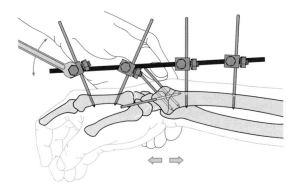

c) Definitive reduction of the fracture and securing of the construct.

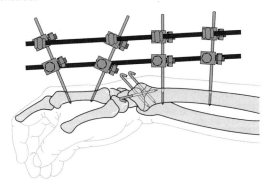

d) The addition of a second longitudinal bar increases the stability.

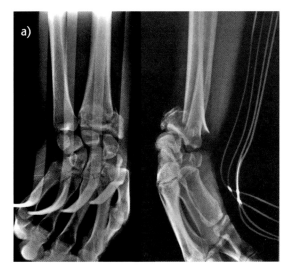

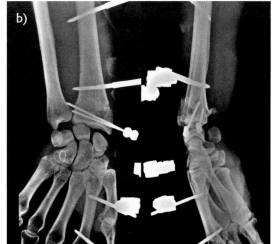

With increasing articular disruption (more than two fragments, group C3) and when the fracture does not respond to ligamentotaxis (since this does not always allow for disimpaction of the central articular fragments and does not always accomplish reduction of severely rotated palmar ulnar lip fragments), extensile open reduction and bone grafting become progressively necessary. This group includes those fractures that represent a difficult therapeutic challenge due to:

- the severity of the articular disruption,
- the increasing amount of metaphyseal comminution,
- inherent instability and irreducibility,
- the presence of important bone loss of the distal forearm (gunshot wounds, open wounds, crush injuries),
- association with carpal disruption and/ or fractures of the distal ulna or ipsilateral fractures of the upper extremity.

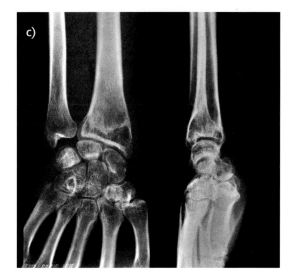

Fig. 4.3.3-10: External fixator:
a) Displaced, intra-articular distal radial fracture (23-C2).
b) Postoperative views after percutaneous K-wire fixation.
c) 3-year follow-up with almost symmetrical function.

Severely displaced four-part fractures may require both a palmar and a dorsal approach. In our experience it is best to stabilize the palmar ulnar fragments first and to restore the mechanical continuity of the palmar cortex with a palmar buttressing plate [5, 16]. This provides a solid base onto which the dorsoulnar and radial styloid fragments can be reduced, combining ligamentotaxis with a simple external fixator frame and limited dorsal open reduction with iliac bone graft.

In certain cases, plate fixation [16–18] may be used instead of external fixation provided that the following prerequisites are met:
- exact reduction of bony cortex opposite the plate,
- solid purchase of the screws in the distal fragments,
- associated primary bone grafting of defects or comminuted areas,
- ability to achieve primary soft-tissue coverage of the implants.

For dorsal plate fixation the π-shaped low-profile plate is preferred, because the transverse limb of the plate allows use of both smaller screws or pins. These can be threaded to the plate holes providing a condylar plate effect [18]. This feature facilitates independent fixation of articular fragments while the two longitudinal limbs of the plate (Fig. 4.3.3-11) (Video AO22043) bridge the metaphyseal fracture. Indirect reduction techniques are strongly encouraged for the application of the plate. This can be achieved with longitudinal intraoperative sterile finger trap traction, by using a fracture distractor, or with a temporary wrist external fixation device. Following temporary K-wire fixation of the fragments and controlled reduction with intraoperative fluoroscopy, the fracture is grafted and the plate applied. To prevent irritation of tendons in the third and second compartments,

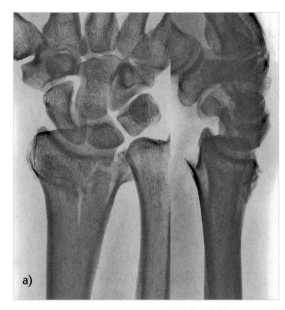

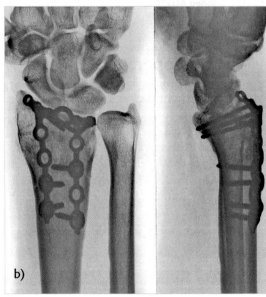

Fig. 4.3.3-11: a) Distal radius fracture type C2.1.
b) 6 months after fixation with the π-plate (distal radius plate 2.4/2.7).

the plate should be covered with an extensor retinaculum flap as described in the surgical approaches section.

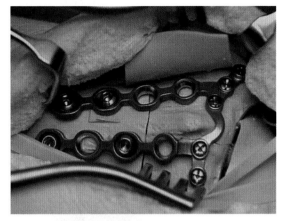

Video AO22043

6 Postoperative treatment

Depending on whether or not the fracture is associated with concomitant soft tissue, ligamentous, or other skeletal injuries (e.g., carpal fractures or ipsilateral fractures of the upper extremity), aftercare will vary somewhat from case to case. For simple extra-articular and articular fractures treated with percutaneous pinning or simple internal fixation with K-wires or small plates, a sugar tong splint is applied for a period of 2 weeks. This is followed for a further 3 weeks by a short forearm cast with a window to allow for pin care.

Group B fractures treated with palmar buttress plating and cannulated screw fixation, with good holding power, have functional aftercare after suture removal. For intra-articular fractures treated with open reduction, bone grafting, and external fixation, the frame is maintained for a period of 5 weeks. If the wrist was initially fixed in flexion and ulnar deviation, it is brought to a neutral position at 3 weeks to facilitate finger rehabilitation. Following removal of the frame, a protective wrist orthosis may be used intermittently for another 3 weeks.

The fracture of the distal radius may be associated with primary repair of the triangular fibrocartilage or ulnar styloid fixation. In this situation, the forearm is immobilized in a sugar tong splint for a period of 3 weeks in 45° of supination. This is to allow initial fibrous healing of the distal radioulnar joint ligaments, and is done in all cases whether or not external fixation is employed.

If the fracture is associated with primary scapholunate repair, when the frame has been removed at 5 weeks, cast fixation is continued for a total of 8 weeks postoperatively. For fractures of the distal radius with associated carpal bone injuries that have been treated with screw fixation, functional wrist aftercare is begun after removal of the wrist fixator at 5 weeks.

The only indications for maintaining a wrist fixator for longer than 5 weeks are:
- fractures which have not been grafted,
- complex injuries with massive soft-tissue defect requiring secondary plastic coverage, or
- fractures complicated by acute infection.

7 Pitfalls and complications

Most of the pitfalls that arise during treatment of fractures of the distal radius can be avoided if the surgeon has made a correct diagnosis of fracture type, has clearly analyzed the indications and contra-indications, and has profound knowledge of the anatomy of the wrist joint. Furthermore, before attempting to treat these fractures, surgeons should be very familiar with both internal and external fixation techniques. To avoid diagnostic pitfalls, special imaging of the wrist (CT scans, tomograms) should be undertaken if the fracture diagnosis is not clear in plain x-rays.

Preoperative evaluation should also include the investigation of associated soft-tissue lesions, carpal disruption, and carpal fractures, since concomitant injuries are commonly associated with severely displaced distal radius fractures as a result of high-velocity injuries in multiple trauma.

Neurovascular compromise or the presence of massive soft-tissue swelling and forearm compartment syndrome should be carefully ruled out. Adequate evaluation of the soft-tissue conditions is required to determine the ideal timing of surgery. Although surgical restoration of the articular surface is best carried out immediately after the accident, important soft-tissue swelling may jeopardize primary skin closure. For this scenario, surgery might be delayed for 5–6 days, provided that the initial displacement of the wrist is reduced and held in a plaster splint. Immediate surgery, on the other hand, is absolutely indicated if fractures are open or primary compression of the median nerve is present. In open fractures no attempt at primary soft-tissue coverage is made after fracture reduction. Usually the wound is left open and a mesh graft is applied, once the swelling has subsided and there are no signs of infection.

The most common pitfall encountered when dealing with the fracture itself is to find considerably more articular comminution on opening the joint than was expected from the study of the initial x-rays. In these situations the surgeon must be prepared to obtain the best possible joint congruity with minimal soft-tissue disruption and to graft subchondral bone defects. This must be followed by application of an external fixator that will at least restore radial length and maintain an adequate anatomical reduction of the distal radioulnar joint.

During insertion of percutaneous or external fixator pins, iatrogenic damage to tendons, nerves, and vascular structures should be avoided. The superficial branch of the radial nerve is at high risk during insertion of pins for a dorsoradial frame in the distal forearm. Generous incisions for pin insertion, careful separation of the cutaneous nerves and underlying tendons with blunt dissection by using the drill guide will diminish these complications. Prophylaxis of pin-track infection is achieved by preventing primary skin necrosis, making sure that the skin surrounding the pins is not under excessive tension, and instructing the patient on daily pin care.

Implant-related problems occur more often with dorsal implants because of the proximity and relationships of the extensor tendons and the bone. Adequate implant coverage is required and an extensor retinaculum flap is strongly recommended. Over-long screws inserted from palmar to dorsal in the metaphyseal area have been reported to cause extensive tendon attrition and rupture.

Complications associated with fracture treatment have usually been associated with pro-

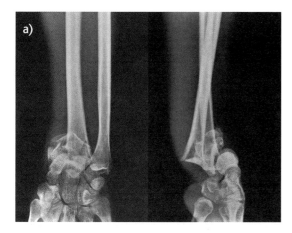
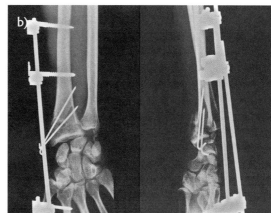
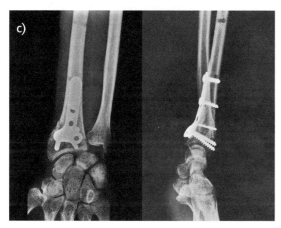
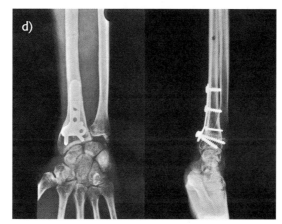

Fig. 4.3.3-12:
a) Complex, grossly displaced distal radial fracture 23-C2 in the dominant hand of a young man.
b) Initial closed reduction with small external fixator and percutaneous K-wires did not satisfy on lateral view.

c) After 2 weeks the fracture was revised through a palmar approach, a small fragment T-plate replacing the external fixator.
d) At 23 weeks the patient is pain-free with satisfactory function. The radial fracture is united.

longed use of external fixators, unphysiological wrist positioning, or extensive distraction. This produces median nerve neuropathy and metacarpophalangeal joint stiffness. It is claimed that excessive wrist flexion may trigger reflex sympathetic dystrophy. There is also risk of iatrogenic non-union of the distal radius if fractures are over distracted to obtain adequate radial length. Static external fixation should therefore be reduced to a minimum provided that the fracture has been bone grafted to accelerate bone healing and/or supplementary internal fixation techniques have been employed.

8 Results

Review of the relevant literature on operative treatment of distal radial fractures reveals that the more complex articular disruptions carry a more guarded prognosis than the simpler fractures. It has been inferred that the final outcome reflects how effectively the anatomy has been restored.

An acceptable final result requires:

- less than 2 mm of articular incongruity (the ideal being perfect anatomical reduction of the joint surface),
- radial shortening less than 5 mm, and
- residual dorsal tilt of less than 10°.

Long-term follow-up studies have demonstrated a strict correlation between wrist disability and posttraumatic deformity. Recent studies have shown the effectiveness of combined internal fixation, bone grafting, and external fixation techniques [9, 14, 15, 19]. In our own review of 40 intra-articular distal radius fractures managed by limited open reduction, we reported articular reduction to 1 mm or less in 92% of the patients, and radiocarpal arthritis at an average of 4 years follow-up to be present in only 5% of the cases. A recent report on operative treatment of 49 palmar marginal intra-articular fractures [20] showed 31 excellent, 10 good, and 8 fair results according to the system described by Gartland and Werley.

Management of complex articular distal radius fractures remains a difficult problem. However, in the last decade substantial improvement in results has been achieved, due to a combination of external and internal fixation techniques, bone grafting, and improved plate design (Fig. 4.3.3-12).

9 Bibliography

1. **Knirk JL, Jupiter JB** (1986) Intra-articular fractures of the distal end of the radius in young adults. *J Bone Joint Surg [Am]*; 68 (5):647–659.
2. **Melone CP, Jr.** (1986) Open treatment for displaced articular fractures of the distal radius. *Clin Orthop*; (202):103–111.
3. **Fernandez DL** (1993) Fractures of the distal radius: operative treatment. In: Heckmann JD, editor. *Instructional Course Lectures: Amer Acad Orthop Surg*; 42:73–88.
4. **Altissimi M, Mancini GB, Azzara A, et al.** (1994) Early and late displacement of fractures of the distal radius. The prediction of instability. *Int Orthop*; 18 (2):61–65.
5. **Fernandez DL, Jupiter JB** (1995) *Fractures of the Distal Radius*. Berlin Heidelberg New York: Springer-Verlag.
6. **Fernandez DL** (1995) Treatment of articular fractures of the distal radius with external fixation and pinning. In: Saffar P, Cooney WP, editors. *Fractures of the Distal Radius*. London: Martin Dunitz Ltd: 104–117.

7. **Geissler WB, Fernandez DL, Lamey DM**
(1996) Distal radioulnar joint injuries
associated with fractures of the distal
radius. *Clin Orthop;* (327):135–146.

8. **Fernandez DL, Geissler WB, Lamey DM**
(1996) Wrist instability with or following
fractures of the distal radius. In: Büchler U,
editor. *Wrist Instability.* London: Martin
Dunitz Ltd: 181–192.

9. **Hastings H, II, Leibovic SJ** (1993)
Indications and techniques of open
reduction. Internal fixation of distal
radius fractures. *Orthop Clin North Am;*
24 (2):309–326.

10. **Benoist LA, Freeland AE** (1995)
Buttress pinning in the unstable distal
radial fracture. A modification of the
Kapandji technique. *J Hand Surg [Br];*
20 (1):82–96.

11. **Kapandji AI** (1995) Treatment of
articular distal radial fractures by
intrafocal pinning with arum pins. In:
Saffar P, Cooney WP, editors. *Fractures of
the Distal Radius.* London: Martin Dunitz
Ltd: 160–166.

12. **Fernandez DL, Jakob RP** (1982) The
treatment of wrist fractures with the
small AO external fixation device. In:
Uhthoff HK, editor. *Current Concepts of
External Fixation.* Berlin Heidelberg New
York: Springer-Verlag: 307–314.

13. **Fernandez DL, Geissler WB** (1991)
Treatment of displaced articular fractures
of the radius. *J Hand Surg [Am];*
16 (3):375–384.

14. **Seitz WH, Jr., Froimson AI, Leb R,
et al.** (1991) Augmented external
fixation of unstable distal radius fractures.
J Hand Surg [Am] ;16 (6):1010–1016.

15. **Jakim I, Pieterse HS, Sweet MB**
(1991) External fixation for intra-
articular fractures of the distal radius.
J Bone Joint Surg [Br]; 73 (2):302–306.

16. **Axelrod TS, McMurtry RY** (1990)
Open reduction and internal fixation of
comminuted, intra-articular fractures of
the distal radius. *J Hand Surg [Am];*
15 (1):1–11.

17. **Rikli DA, Regazzoni P** (1996) Fractures
of the distal end of the radius treated by
internal fixation and early function. A
preliminary report of 20 cases.
J Bone Joint Surg [Br]; 78 (4):588–592.

18. **Ring D, Jupiter JB, Brennwald J,
et al.** (1996) Multicenter prospective trial
of a new distal radius plate. *Book of
Abstracts.* Boston: Orthopedic Trauma
Assoc: 263–264.

19. **Steffen T, Eugster T, Jakob RP** (1994)
Twelve years follow-up of fractures of the
distal radius treated with the AO external
fixator. *Injury;* 25 (Suppl 4):44–54.

20. **Jupiter JB, Fernandez DL, Toh CL,
et al.** (1996) Operative treatment of volar
intra-articular fractures of the distal end
of the radius. *J Bone Joint Surg [Am];*
78 (12):1817–1828.

10 Updates

Updates and additional references for this chapter
are available online at:
http://www.aopublishing.org/PFxM/433.htm

4.3.4 Hand fractures: assessment and concepts of surgical management

Jesse B. Jupiter

1 Treatment goals and fracture patterns

Nowhere in the body does function follow form as closely as in the hand. The stability of its small articulations, the balance between its extrinsic and intrinsic motors and the complexity of the tendon systems require a stable and well-aligned supporting skeleton. The outcome of skeletal injuries in the hand may be judged more on the return of function of these soft-tissue structures rather than on skeletal union.

Every effort must be made to obtain the cooperation of the patient in assessing preoperative tendon, motor, sensory, and vascular status all of which should be carefully documented. **The goals in treatment of metacarpal and phalangeal fractures remain the same regardless of the method employed.** These include [1–5]:

- Restoration of articular anatomy.
- Elimination of angular or rotational deformity.
- Stabilization of fractures.
- Surgically acceptable wounds.
- Rapid mobilization.

While many fractures of the tubular skeleton in the hand can be effectively treated by non-operative means, there are numerous fractures which, because of their nature, situation, or associations, require stable skeletal fixation. These include the following groups [6–10]:

- Fractures which are:
  multifragmented,
  severely displaced,
  multiple metacarpal,
  short oblique or spiral metacarpal,
  accompanied by soft-tissue injury.
- Fractures at particular sites:
  subcondylar, proximal phalanx,
  palmar base middle phalanx.
- Displaced articular fractures:
  Bennett's,
  Rolando,
  unicondylar and bicondylar.
- Certain injury types:
  complete or incomplete amputations,
  some fracture dislocations.

In any given fracture, stability is based upon its specific pattern, location, and response to motion, together with any associated injuries (**Fig. 4.3.4-1**).

Nowhere in the body does function follow form as closely as in the hand.

The goals in treatment of metacarpal and phalangeal fractures remain the same regardless of the method employed.

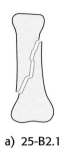 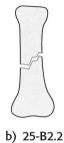 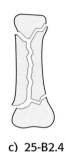 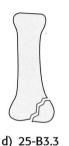 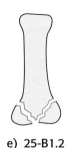

a) 25-B2.1   b) 25-B2.2   c) 25-B2.4   d) 25-B3.3   e) 25-B1.2

Fig. 4.3.4-1: Common fracture patterns in the hand.
a) Spiral metacarpal fracture.
b) Oblique metacarpal fracture.
c) Multifragmented metacarpal fracture.
d) Simple articular fracture.
e) Bicondylar fracture.

2 Surgical anatomy

The four metacarpals form the breadth of the hand, with the rigid central pillar extending through the index and middle metacarpals. The distal transverse arch of the hand is located along the deep metacarpal ligaments which interconnect the metacarpal heads. The thumb and the ring and little finger metacarpals are the mobile units (**Fig. 4.3.4-2**).

The metacarpal shaft extends distally with a gentle dorsal convexity. The concave palmar cortex is denser than the dorsal cortex. This indicates a compression side on the palmar aspect, with tensile stresses normally present dorsally.

Fig. 4.3.4-2: Longitudinal and transverse arches of the hand with the metacarpals.

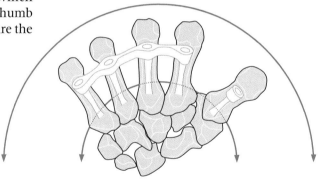

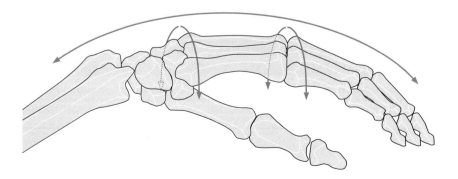

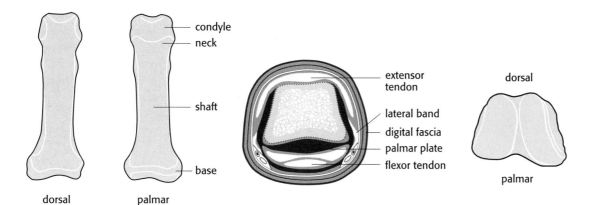

Fig. 4.3.4-3: The surgical anatomy of the proximal phalanx.

Fig. 4.3.4-4: The relationship of the gliding tendons with the phalangeal skeleton.

Fig. 4.3.4-5: The anatomy of the distal articular surfaces of the proximal phalanx.

The proximal and middle phalanges are structurally divided into the base, shaft, neck, and head (condyles). In contrast to the metacarpals, the phalanges are enveloped by the gliding surfaces of the overlying intrinsic and extrinsic tendons (**Fig. 4.3.4-3** and **Fig. 4.3.4-4**).

The distal articular anatomy of the proximal interphalangeal joint is condylar in configuration and when viewed tends to resemble a grooved trochlea. The palmar aspect is nearly twice as wide as the dorsal margin. Dynamic stability results from compressive forces within a joint which increase with pinch and grip, while passive stability derives from collateral ligament tension which increases with joint flexion (**Fig. 4.3.4-5**).

When viewed in the sagittal plane, the metacarpal head displays a curve of increasing diameter. When viewed in the coronal plane, it is pear-shaped. **Because of the eccentric origin of the collateral ligaments on this oddly shaped metacarpal head, the joint is stable in flexion and lax in extension** (**Fig. 4.3.4-6**).

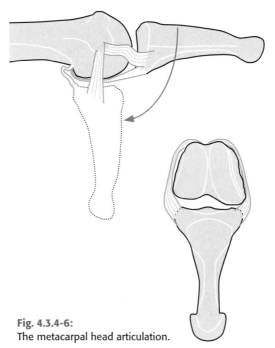

Fig. 4.3.4-6:
The metacarpal head articulation.

Because of the eccentric origin of the collateral ligaments on this oddly shaped metacarpal head, the joint is stable in flection and lax in extension.

The carpometacarpal joint of the thumb is a reciprocally biconcave saddle joint. The thumb is allowed to have its extensive degree of free movement because of the relationship of the reciprocal concave and convex arcs of the bases of its metacarpal and trapezium, oriented almost at 90° to each other (**Fig. 4.3.4-7**).

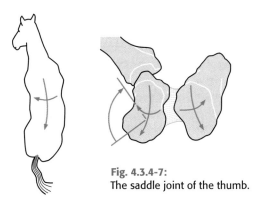

Fig. 4.3.4-7:
The saddle joint of the thumb.

3 Preoperative planning

The normal considerations of preoperative planning apply to the management of hand fractures. Because of the limited bone stock and the problems of access, implant selection is of critical importance.

3.1 Implants

(**Fig. 4.3.4-8**)

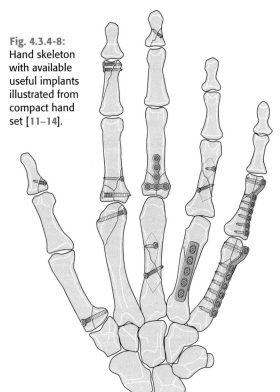

Fig. 4.3.4-8:
Hand skeleton with available useful implants illustrated from compact hand set [11–14].

Implant: Screws

Indications	Size
Distal or mid phalanx	1.1 mm
Distal or mid phalanx	1.3 mm
Unicondylar fracture	
phalangeal diaphysis	1.5 mm
Metacarpal diaphysis	2.0 mm
Metacarpus or carpus	2.4 mm
Metacarpus or carpus	2.7 mm

Implant: Plates

Indications	Size
Mid or proximal phalanx	Cage 1.5
Mid or proximal phalanx replantation	H-plate 1.5
Mid or proximal phalanx diaphysis	Straight 1.5
Base proximal phalanx	T-plate 1.5
Base or neck proximal phalanx	Mini condylar 1.5
Metacarpal diaphysis	Straight 2.0
Metacarpal diaphysis	LC-DCP 2.0
Metacarpal neck or base	Mini condylar 2.0
Metacarpal base	T-plate 2.0
Metacarpal replantation	H-plate 2.0
Thumb metacarpal	Different adaptation plates 2.4

4 Surgical treatment

4.1 Approaches

Incisions are straight, with limited end curvatures if needed. Dorsal venous drainage must be respected.

4.1.1 Metacarpals

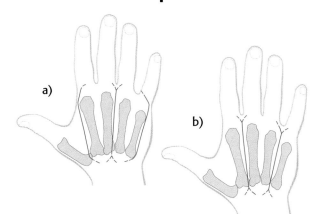

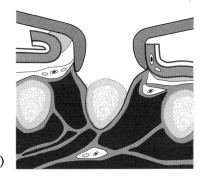

Fig. 4.3.4-9: Metacarpals:
a) Incisions for individual metacarpal exposure.
b) Incisions for exposure of all four metacarpals.
c) Exposure to the metacarpal with minimal elevation of the interosseus muscles.

4.1.2 Proximal phalanx

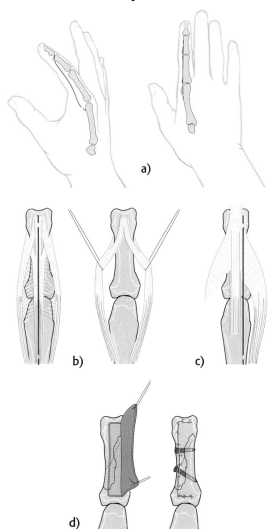

Fig. 4.3.4-10: Proximal phalanx:
a) Mid-axial or dorsal longitudinal incision.
b) Exposure of the phalanx by splitting the extensor apparatus.
c) Exposure of the phalanx between the lateral band and extensor apparatus.
d) Elevation of the periosteum in a wide flap, which is sutured back after fixation.

4.1.3 Dorsal approach to proximal interphalangeal joint

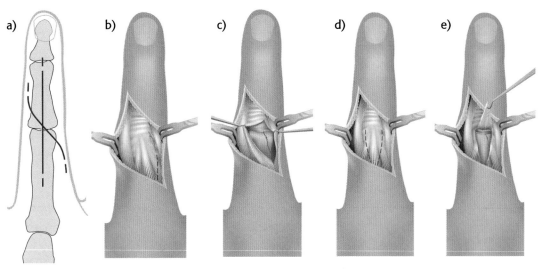

a)   b)   c)   d)   e)

Fig. 4.3.4-11: Proximal interphalangeal joint:
a) The longitudinal skin incision is preferable.
b/c) Exposure of the joint between the lateral band and central extensor slip.

d/e) Exposure of the joint through a distally-based flap of the central slip.

4.1.4 Palmar approach to base of thumb

Technique:
- Elevate origins of abductor pollicis brevis and opponens pollicis off base of metacarpal.
- Open carpometacarpal joint and reduce fracture under direct vision.
- Temporary K-wire fixation.
- Interfragmentary screw fixation with 2.7 or 2.0 mm screw (**Fig. 4.3.4-8**).

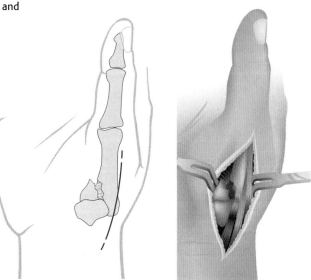

Fig. 4.3.4-12: Modified extensile approach of base of thumb.

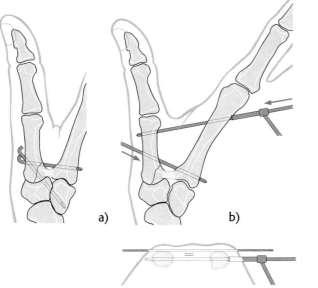

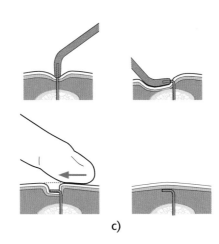

Fig. 4.3.4-13: Bennett's fractures [15]:
a) Direct, percutaneous K-wire transfixation.
b) Indirect reduction and percutaneous fixation.
c) How to bend, cut, and sink a K-wire.

4.2 Rigid internal fixation in phalangeal fractures

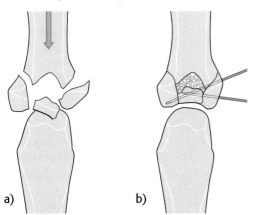

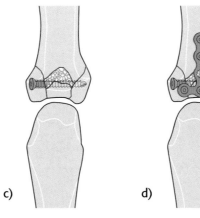

Fig. 4.3.4-14: Compression fracture at the base of the proximal phalanx—extensile exposure through the extensor apparatus.
a) The central impacted fragment with displacement of the medial and lateral joint surfaces.

b) Reduction of the articular fragments is held with small K-wires.
c) Cancellous bone graft is used to support the articular reduction along with a 1.5 mm lag screw.
d) A T-adaption plate 1.5 is used to buttress the articular reconstruction.

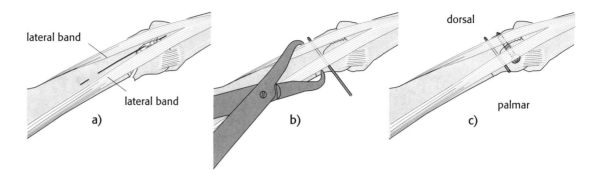

Fig. 4.3.4-15: Unicondylar fracture—head of proximal phalanx.
a) Access between the lateral band and the extensor tendon (omitted for clarity).
b) The fragment is reduced and secured with a small K-wire.

c) For screw fixation, the fragment must be at least three times the diameter of the screw thread. The placement of the screw should be slightly dorsal and proximal to the origin of the collateral ligament.

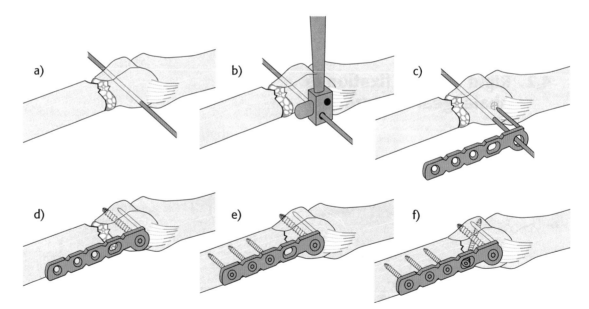

Fig. 4.3.4-16: Bicondylar fracture—head of proximal phalanx.
a) The condylar fragments are reduced and held with a small K-wire placed parallel to the joint line.
b) Using a guide, a 1.5 mm drill bit is used to make a seating hole for the blade.
c) The mini condylar plate 1.5 (pin left) is seated over the K-wire and a seating hole marked.

d) The plate is contoured to fit the shaft, and the blade introduced. A 1.5 mm lag screw is placed across the condylar fragments.
e) Three proximal screws (1.5 mm) are placed through the plate.
f) A final interfragmentary screw may be introduced obliquely through the remaining plate hole.

5   Postoperative treatment

For most injuries if stable internal fixation is achieved, a splint is initially used for comfort with **active digital mobility started within 2–3 days following surgery.**

6   Techniques, pitfalls, and complications

6.1   Lag screw

- Fractures to be fixed by lag screws alone should have a fracture line at least equal in length to twice the diameter of the bone.
- The fracture should be opened and inspected to seek out hidden fracture lines or combinations; optimal screw placement is determined before fracture reduction.
- Anatomical reduction of the fracture to interdigitate the fracture lines will help to prevent shearing displacement when the lag screws are tightened.
- Repeated drilling or tapping of screw holes is to be avoided.
- Screws should optimally be placed perpendicular to the fracture line rather than at an angle dictated by the surgical exposure.
- Screw fixation of a single fragment should be considered only if its width is at least three times the thread diameter of the screw.

6.2   Pitfalls in plate fixation

- The plate is too large for location on bone.
- The plate is not accurately contoured before securing it to the bone.
- The bulk of the plate may interfere with the gliding tendons around the phalanges, requiring a second operation.

7   Results

The development of better techniques to achieve stable internal fixation has led to substantially improved results, especially in skeletal injuries combined with soft-tissue and/or gliding tendon or joint involvement. The bibliography identifies a number of studies demonstrating enhanced outcome due in large part to stable skeletal management which has permitted earlier and more thorough functional aftercare [4, 6, 11, 16–19]. One must caution, however, that plate and screw fixation of the tubular skeleton in the hand is technically demanding, with some studies reporting problems should a second procedure be required to remove the plate and perform tenolyses and/or joint releases [1, 8].

Active movement of fingers and hand should start within 2–3 days following surgery.

8 Bibliography

1. **Chen SH, Wei FC, Chen HC, et al.** (1994) Miniature plates and screws in acute complex hand injury. *J Trauma;* 37 (2):237–242.

2. **Jupiter JB, Silver MA** (1988) Fractures of the metacarpals and phalanges. In: Chapman M, editor. *Operative Orthopedics.* Philadelphia: J.B. Lippincott Co.

3. **Jupiter J, Axelrod T, Belsky M** (1997) Fractures and dislocations of the hand. In: Browner B, Jupiter J, Levine A, editors. *Skeletal Trauma.* 2nd ed. Philadelphia: W.B. Saunders Co.

4. **Rüedi TP, Burri C, Pfeiffer KM** (1971) Stable internal fixation of fractures of the hand. *J Trauma;* 11 (5):381–389.

5. **Segmüller G** (1988) Principles of stable internal fixation in the hand. In: Chapman M, editor. *Operative Orthopedics.* Philadelphia: J.B. Lippincott Co.

6. **Breen TF, Gelberman RH, Jupiter JB** (1988) Intra-articular fractures of the basilar joint of the thumb. *Hand Clin;* 4 (3):491–501.

7. **Crawford GP** (1988) Screw fixation for certain fractures of the phalanges and metacarpals. *J Bone Joint Surg [Am];* 58 (4):439–451.

8. **Dabezies EJ, Schutte JP** (1986) Fixation of metacarpal and phalangeal fractures with miniature plates and screws. *J Hand Surg [Am];* 11 (2):283–288.

9. **Segmüller G** (1977) *Surgical Stabilization of the Skeleton of the Hand.* Baltimore: Williams & Wilkins.

10. **Segmüller G, Schönenberger F** (1980) Fractures of the hand. In: Weber BG, Brunner C, Freuler F, editors. *Treatment of Fractures in Children and Adolescents.* New York: Springer-Verlag.

11. **Büchler U, Fischer T** (1987) Use of a minicondylar plate for metacarpal and phalangeal perariticular injuries. *Clin Orthop;* (214):53–58.

12. **Freeland AE, Jabaley ME, Hughes JL** (1987) *Stable Fixation of the Hand and Wrist.* New York: Springer-Verlag.

13. **Hastings H II** (1987) Unstable metacarpal and phalangeal fracture treatment with screws and plates. *Clin Orthop;* (214):37–52.

14. **Nunley JA, Goldner RD, Urbaniak JR** (1987) Skeletal fixation in digital replantation. Use of the "H" plate. *Clin Orthop;* (214):66–71.

15. **Heim U, Pfeiffer KM** (1988) *Internal fixation of small fractures.* Berlin, Heidelberg, New York: Springer-Verlag.

16. **Black DM, Mann RJ, Constine RM, et al.** (1986) The stability of internal fixation in the proximal phalanx. *J Hand Surg [Am];* 11 (5):672–677.

17. **Foster RJ, Hastings H II** (1987) Treatment of Bennett, Rolando, and vertical intraarticular trapezial fractures. *Clin Orthop;* (214):121–129.

18. **Hastings H II, Carroll C** (1988) Treatment of closed articular fractures of the metacarpophalangeal and proximal interphalangeal joints. *Hand Clin;* 4 (3):503–527.

19. **Vanik RK, Weber RC, Matloub HS, et al.** (1984) The comparative strengths of internal fixation techniques. *J Hand Surg [Am];* 9 (2):216–221.

9 Updates

Updates and additional references for this chapter
are available online at:
http://www.aopublishing.org/PFxM/434.htm

4.4 **Pelvic ring injuries: assessment and concepts of surgical management**

Tim Pohlemann

1 Assessment of fractures and soft tissues

Pelvic injuries are rare when compared to fractures in other body regions. Their overall incidence is estimated at about 3% of all fractures or 19–37 injuries per 100,000 inhabitants per year. Among "polytrauma" patients, the incidence has risen to about 25% and in the group of traffic-related fatalities a pelvic fracture was detected in as many as 42% of individuals. A pelvic injury must, therefore, be looked upon as an indicator of a major trauma until associated injuries can definitely be excluded. The close proximity of osteoligamentous structures to pelvic organs, neurovascular, hollow-viscera, and urogenital structures may lead to a wide range of severe complications and late sequelae if not diagnosed and treated early. The evaluation of a pelvic injury has to be based on repeated checks of the patient's vital parameters (hemodynamics), a detailed clinical examination (pelvic stability, concomitant peripelvic injuries, neurology) and a structured radiographic evaluation. Emergency decisions can be based on a pelvis AP x-ray, whereas the detailed classification is assigned after additional oblique projections ("inlet" and "outlet" views, **Fig. 4.4-1a/b**) and a CT examination. In all situations which are unclear,

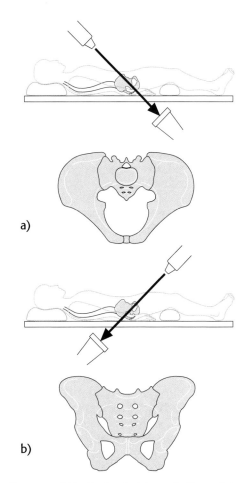

Fig. 4.4-1: a) Positioning for inlet projection and drawing of the x-ray appearance obtained from the inlet projection. b) Positioning for outlet projection and drawing of the x-ray appearance obtained from the outlet projection.

or where a lesion within the posterior pelvic ring is suspected or diagnosed, CT examination is the present diagnostic "gold standard".

Additional diagnostic techniques such as ultrasound, cysto-urethrograms, EMG, etc. must be included in the early or late phase if a specific lesion is suspected.

Decision making can be divided into two phases:

I: Detection and treatment of life-threatening situations ("emergency algorithm").
II: Diagnosis and detailed classification of the osteoligamentous injury and operative planning and surgery, if required.

As pelvic surgery has many potential risks, a detailed period of training in decision making, anatomy, and operative techniques is very strongly recommended, preferably organized as a fellowship in a suitable clinic. In this chapter a short overview is presented of the currently accepted concepts and techniques. Further information can be obtained from standard textbooks [1–3].

Patients admitted with a blood loss of more than 2,000 ml require attention as a specific group.

2 Surgical anatomy

2.1 Osteoligamentous structure

The pelvis has a stiff osteoligamentous ring structure with the pelvic joints (SI-joints and pubic symphyses) allowing only very limited movement under load. By far the greatest proportion of load goes through the posterior ring structures, giving them the key role when pelvic stability is assessed. The pelvic bones themselves have no inherent stability and therefore the integrity of the ligamentous structures is crucial to the preservation or the loss of stability (**Fig. 4.4-2**).

2.2 Soft tissues and neurovascular structures

Besides the essential contribution of the ligaments to pelvic integrity, the large number and the high density of peripelvic organs and soft tissues play an important role in relation to the acute (e.g., hemorrhage) and late (e.g., neurological, urologic injuries) prognosis. A clear understanding of structures at risk is necessary for the treatment of pelvic fractures.

The combination of osteoligamentous and concomitant peripelvic soft-tissue injuries (hollow-visceral, urogenital, and neurovascular) results in a significantly increased mortality and is therefore defined as "complex pelvic injury". Mortality is further increased in cases where a life-threatening hemorrhage results in unstable hemodynamics. **Therefore, patients admitted with a blood loss of more than 2,000 ml require attention as a specific group.**

Fig. 4.4-2: Osteoligamentous anatomy of the pelvic ring.
a) Important ligamentous structures for pelvic stability.

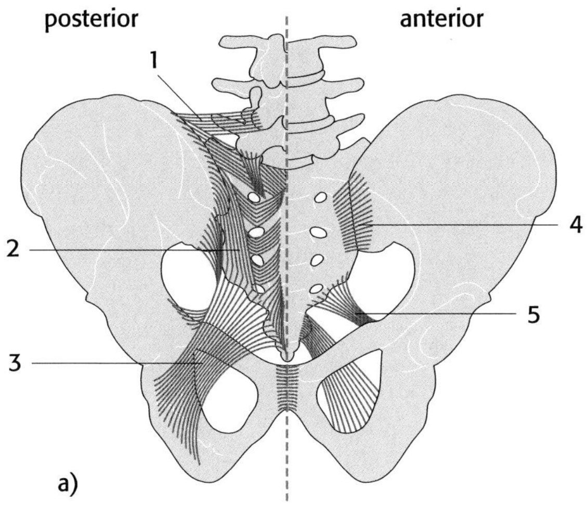

b) The posterior sacro-iliac ligaments play a key role in the evaluation of posterior stability.

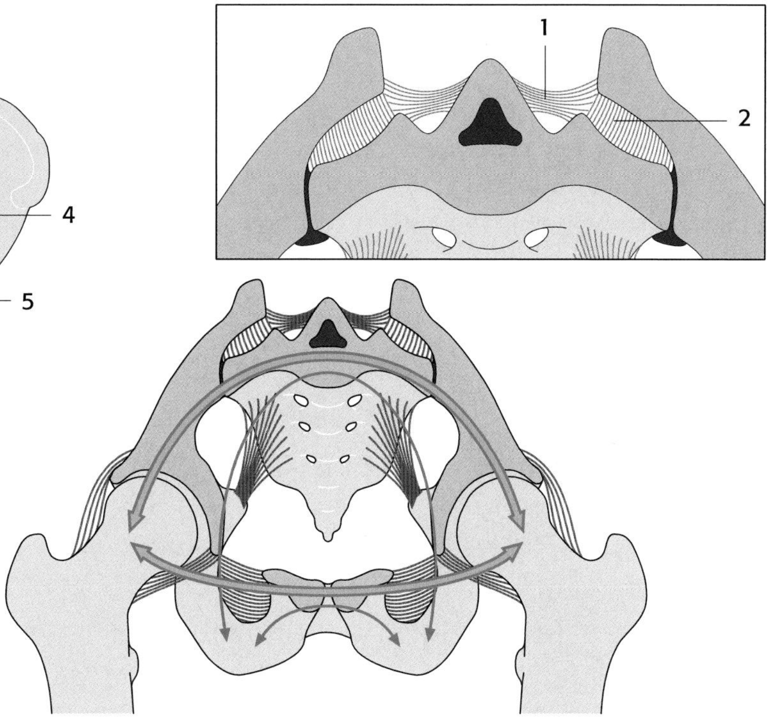

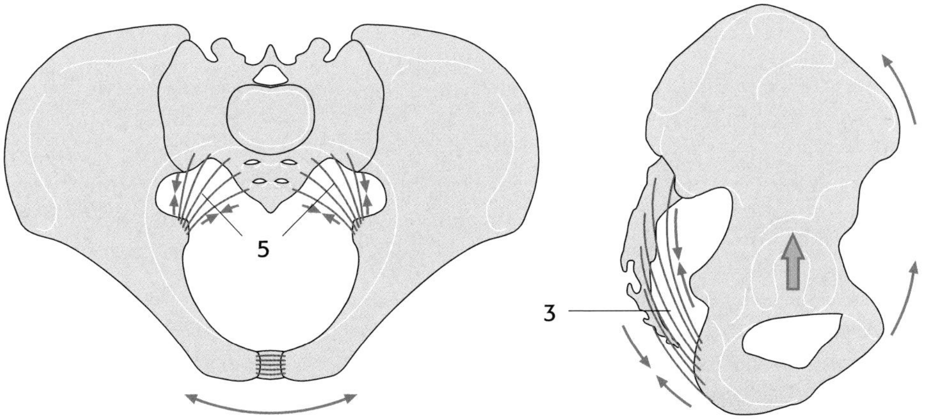

posterior   anterior

a)

1 Iliolumbar ligament
2 Dorsal sacroiliac ligament
3 Sacrotuberous ligament
4 Ventral sacroiliac ligament
5 Sacrospinous ligament

c) Forces acting on pelvic structures and direction of displacement under load.

3　Terminology and classification

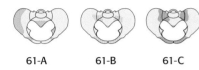

61-A　　61-B　　61-C

Fig. 4.4-3: Müller AO Classification.

Clinical and radiological evaluation of the pelvis based on the identification of the **grade of stability or instability is the platform for further decision making.** Transition between stability and instability is a continuum. For practical reasons and as a basis for indications, three different degrees of stability/instability are differentiated [4]:

- Mechanical structure of the pelvic ring intact: type A injury, incidence 50–70% of patients.
- Partial posterior stability, rotational instability: type B injuries, incidence 20–30% of patients.
- Combined anterior and posterior instability, translational instability: type C, incidence 10–20% of patients.

The decision on whether or not to operate can be based on the fracture types:

- Type A injuries: surgical stabilization is only exceptionally indicated.
- Type B injuries: stabilization of the anterior pelvic ring alone is sufficient.
- Type C injuries: adequate stabilization of the ring is required, to minimize the risk of secondary displacement.

Differentiation between partial or complete posterior instability (type B or C) can be difficult. The primary evaluation must be rechecked and followed, if necessary, by review of diagnosis and classification and the consequent therapeutic decisions.

More than 40 classification systems or major modifications have been published over the last 30 years. In contrast to other body regions, the possible variations of pelvic injury can include multiple lesions of the anterior and/or posterior ring, of the right and/or left side, and a great variety of involved fracture patterns and anatomical segments.

The present classification of pelvic injuries based on the Müller AO system (**Fig. 4.4-3**) comes from the evaluation of the mechanism of injury and the resulting "stability/instability" of the pelvic ring [4, 5]. By extending the three basic fracture types A, B, C by groups, subgroups, and specific modifiers, every injury and combination of injuries can easily be classified in an alphanumeric notation (see **chapter 1.4**).

4　Primary evaluation and decision making

The primary goals in the assessment of pelvic injuries are:

- In case of severe "internal" hemorrhage: is this caused by a pelvic fracture?
- The clinical and radiological assessment of the degree of mechanical stability of the pelvic ring.
- The diagnosis of peripelvic soft-tissue and organ injuries.

The diagnosis of hemodynamic instability of pelvic origin must result in immediate surgical resuscitation procedures, preferably by following a "protocol" or "algorithm" as described in (**Fig. 4.4-4**).

In the vast majority of the cases of pelvic injury, hemodynamics are affected only minimally or not at all. However, a detailed clinical and radiological work-up for detection and grading of a pelvic injury is still necessary.

Clinical examination

Manual examination of pelvic stability is by AP and lateral compression, sometimes supplemented by occasional push-pull examination of the leg. Repeated examinations should be avoided in unstable situations, to prevent further induction of blood loss.

Radiological examination

The diagnosis is based on the radiological examination. **The AP pelvic view is mandatory and can provide a reliable working diagnosis in about 90% of the cases.**
For three-dimensional analysis, oblique views (inlet and outlet films) are included to evaluate anterior, posterior, craniocaudal, and rotational displacement.
A CT examination is performed in all cases to further define the posterior pelvic injury and any possible associated acetabular fracture. CT is not a method of emergency evaluation and can in most cases be delayed until the general condition of the patient is stabilized.

5 Instability of the pelvic ring combined with hemodynamic instability

In this situation primary therapy has to concentrate on immediate control of pelvic hemorrhage. Several treatment protocols for emergency hemostasis have been published favoring a wide variety of methods (**Table 4.4-1**). No single method is effective by itself in controlling the bleeding. Only a combination of interventions (early pelvic stabilization followed by surgical hemostasis if necessary) following a priority orientated "algorithm" can have a beneficial impact on the patient's survival. Continued evaluation of resuscitation algorithms is necessary to evaluate their efficiency in saving lives.

5.1 Treatment protocol

A standardized protocol for primary clinical treatment is used for all patients being admitted in polytrauma situations. If the pelvic fracture causes hemodynamic instability, this protocol is expanded by a "complex pelvic fracture module". This is based on three simple decisions to be made within 30 minutes after admission (**Fig. 4.4-4**). Whereas the rare case of severe pelvic hemorrhage has to result in immediate surgical intervention, most patients will undergo a primary diagnostic evaluation (clinical examination, pelvis AP x-rays, ultrasound abdomen). **If the unstable hemodynamics come from a pelvic instability, emergency stabilization is performed immediately.** The pelvic C-clamp or the simple external fixator can allow effective stabilization as early as

AP pelvic view provides diagnosis in about 90% of cases.

CT examination is performed in all cases but not as an emergency evaluation.

Unstable hemodynamics resulting from pelvic instability require emergency fixation of the pelvic ring.

Fig. 4.4-4:
Emergency algorithm for
pelvic injuries.

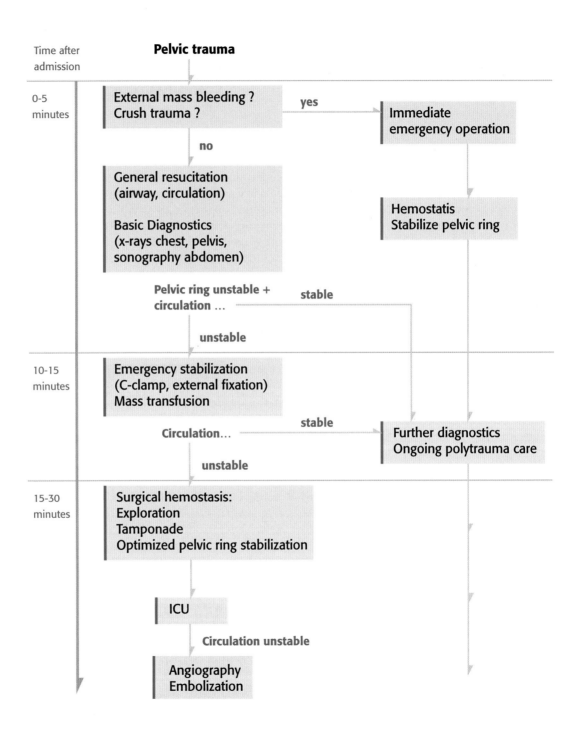

Time after
admission

Pelvic trauma

0-5
minutes

External mass bleeding ?
Crush trauma ?

yes

Immediate
emergency operation

no

General resucitation
(airway, circulation)

Basic Diagnostics
(x-rays chest, pelvis,
sonography abdomen)

Hemostatis
Stabilize pelvic ring

Pelvic ring unstable +
circulation …

stable

unstable

10-15
minutes

Emergency stabilization
(C-clamp, external fixation)
Mass transfusion

Circulation…

stable

unstable

Further diagnostics
Ongoing polytrauma care

15-30
minutes

Surgical hemostasis:
Exploration
Tamponade
Optimized pelvic ring stabilization

ICU

Circulation unstable

Angiography
Embolization

10–15 minutes after admission in the shock-room (**Fig. 4.4-4** and **Fig. 4.4-5**). If these devices are not readily available, other non-invasive techniques (traction and ring closure with a sheet or pelvic sling, pneumatic anti-shock garment and vacuum splints) are used for emergency stabilization. Frequently, mechanical stabilization will reduce the amount of pelvic blood loss, but will not provide complete hemostasis. If the patient's hemodynamics remain unstable 10–15 minutes after application, immediate surgical hemostasis with revision and repair of the pelvic retroperitoneum has to follow.

5.2 Technique of pelvic packing in a hemodynamically unstable patient

The patient is positioned supine with the entire abdomen and pelvis draped. If little or no intra-peritoneal free fluid was detected either on initial or on control ultrasound examination and the origin of bleeding can therefore clearly be centered to the pelvic region, a lower midline incision is used. With additional intraperitoneal hemorrhage, a formal laparotomy is performed and the incision is extended to the pubic symphysis region.

Method	Value
"Self-tamponade"	Effective in uncomplicated pelvic fractures, but not effective in major disruptions with instability, as in these cases all "compartment borders" are disrupted ("chimney effect") [6].
Anti-shock trousers	No impact on survival rate, severe complications reported (compartment syndrome, extremity loss), timely application [7].
Embolization	Arterial lesions only present in 10–20% of cases [8], specialist required, time delay in unstable hemodynamics (blood loss > 2,000 ml!), method of secondary choice.
Pelvic stabilization	Beneficial effect both in the acute situation and for the late outcome [9, 10]. Devices for emergency stabilization are the pelvic C-clamp [11] and/or external fixation and in rare occasions (contraindication for the pelvic C-clamp in comminuted iliac fractures) a definitive internal stabilization.

Table 4.4-1: Pros and cons of different methods for hemorrhage control after pelvic fractures.
The number of patients with hemodynamic instability directly related to an unstable pelvic fracture is small. While the individual variations are high and generally accepted standards for classification of associated injuries are missing, the literature is frequently misleading. The table can therefore only provide an overview of the value of the individual procedure. The aim of every protocol must be to provide timely early pelvic stabilization with effective control of hemorrhage, usually by surgical means.

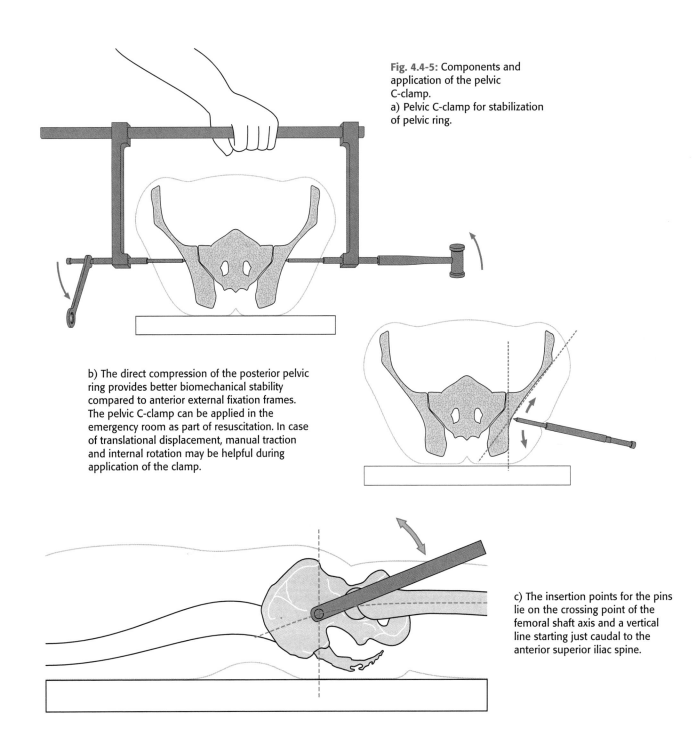

Fig. 4.4-5: Components and application of the pelvic C-clamp.
a) Pelvic C-clamp for stabilization of pelvic ring.

b) The direct compression of the posterior pelvic ring provides better biomechanical stability compared to anterior external fixation frames. The pelvic C-clamp can be applied in the emergency room as part of resuscitation. In case of translational displacement, manual traction and internal rotation may be helpful during application of the clamp.

c) The insertion points for the pins lie on the crossing point of the femoral shaft axis and a vertical line starting just caudal to the anterior superior iliac spine.

In the majority of cases all parapelvic fascial planes have already been disrupted and direct manual access through the right or left paravesical space down to the presacral region is obtained without further dissection. Primary orientation includes looking for a rare arterial bleeding, which is managed either by clamping, ligature, or a vascular repair. In mass bleeding a temporary clamping of the infrarenal aorta may be helpful (laparotomy required!). In most cases, however, diffuse bleeding stems from venous plexus and from the fracture surfaces, where a specific source cannot be identified. In external rotation-type injuries the sources of bleeding are generally located close to the anterior pelvic ring; in type C injuries the origin of bleeding is most frequently located in the presacral region. Hemorrhage is controlled by application of tight presacral and paravesical packing. Tamponade can only be effective if the posterior pelvic ring is sufficiently stable (C-clamp) (**Video AO53030**). If major posterior displacement is still present (check by palpation), the reduction is optimized by clamp loosening and

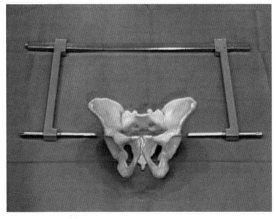

 Video AO53030

further reduction by hand before the tamponade is reapplied.

- At the end of the procedure the anterior pelvic ring is stabilized by a symphysis plate or, in transpubic instabilities, an external fixator.
- Additional intra-abdominal organ injuries are repaired according to general surgical rules. Care has to be taken that further surgery is matched to the patient's general condition. In many cases only emergency "damage control" procedures are advisable in the early stage (e.g., suprapubic urine drainage, insertion of a transurethral catheter, and suture of the bladder after urological injuries or, in rectal injuries, a diverting colostomy with prograde wash-out and drainage).
- The tamponade packs are left for 24–48 hours and are removed or replaced in planned "second look" operations.
- Angiography and embolization are recommended if, after effective tamponade, a subsequent, significant pelvic blood loss still persists.

6   The unstable pelvic ring in a hemodynamically stable patient

This is the situation most frequently encountered. In the hemodynamically stable patient, detailed evaluation of the nature of the pelvic ring injury is required before deciding about indications for and selection of appropriate stabilization techniques. A complete diagnostic work-up must be completed before definitive decisions can be made (see **chapter 2.1** and **5.3**).

6.1 Indications and decision making

The indications for surgical stabilization or non-operative treatment are based on the fracture type:

Type A ("stable" ring)

Surgical stabilization is not normally required. Functional treatment will not produce further displacement. Treatment consists of a few days of bed-rest and early ambulation.

Indications for open reduction and internal stabilization are exceptional (open or grossly displaced iliac crest fractures, displaced pubic rami fractures, avulsion fractures in young professional athletes, etc.).

Type B (rotational instability, partial dorsal stability)

Stabilization of the anterior pelvic ring is usually sufficient for early ambulation with partial weight bearing. The differentiation between the "type B injury" and the "type C injury" can be misleading in the primary evaluation, especially in minimally displaced "lateral compression type fractures" with a transforaminal sacral fracture line. Therefore, radiological controls must be made 8 and 14 days after injury or after ambulation to ensure that no posterior displacement has occurred.

Type C (anterior and posterior instability)

The pelvic ring requires combined posterior and anterior stabilization for anatomical reduction, early ambulation, and to avoid complications.

Every part of the pelvic ring where an actual "instability" (not only a fracture line!) can be diagnosed should be addressed by surgical sta-bilization to provide stability and sufficient safety for early ambulation. As an example, in type C injuries an additional stabilization of the anterior ring is recommended after posterior osteosynthesis. The method of fixation, however, is chosen according to the specific fracture pattern.

6.2 Preparation and choice of fixation

6.2.1 Instruments, implants, and timing

Pelvic surgery embraces complex operations where, because of the anatomy, there is a high risk of causing additional damage (vascular injuries, neurological injuries, neighboring organs, soft tissues, etc.). Detailed analysis of every case, with individual decision making and planning, is therefore strongly recommended. Comprehensive knowledge is required of anatomical relations, reduction and stabilization techniques, to avoid complications. The basic rules for management of pelvic trauma must, however, be common to all trauma surgeons. Pelvic surgery is "specialist surgery" and a transfer of a "stable" patient has to be considered if only limited personal experience is available.

The following precautions and preparations are mandatory for more extensive surgery:
- availability of postoperative ICU therapy,
- availability of sufficient blood replacement,
- strategies to minimize blood loss (operative technique, cell saver),
- experienced operative team with adequate assistance,

- standard and pelvic instruments (e.g., a pelvis set with reduction instruments and implants).

The timing of surgery depends on the patient's general condition. The indications for emergency stabilization have already been discussed; in general, an unstable pelvic injury should be stabilized as early as possible. As a high percentage of these patients are polytraumatized, early definitive stabilization will not only facilitate management, but will also have a beneficial effect on the general prognosis. In patients with stable hemodynamics definitive surgery should be completed within 14 days, and preferably within 7 days, after injury. After 14 days the difficulty of anatomical reduction increases significantly, leading to a high number of inadequate reductions. To prevent disability from malunion or non-union, which represent complex problems for late surgical correction, early decisions for anatomical reduction and stabilization should be made. The alternative is to consider early transfer to an appropriate unit.

Therefore, the use of external and internal fixation devices should always be looked upon as "integrated methods" rather than as "concurrent methods". Some techniques of pin placement and frame construction are illustrated in **Fig. 4.4-6 (Video AO52004)**.

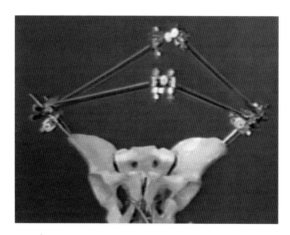

 Video AO52004

6.2.2 External vs. internal stabilization

Discussion about the indications for external or internal stabilization in the different types of pelvic injuries remains inconclusive. The external fixator certainly has a place in the emergency treatment of pelvic instability and can be used as an additional fixation device in certain fracture patterns, for example, rotational instability, open book. Its role as a definitive fixation device remains, however, to be established [2].

6.3 Preferred methods of fixation

The techniques for internal stabilization of pelvic fractures are many and varied. The methods described have delivered reliable results in all cases where indications and techniques were correct.

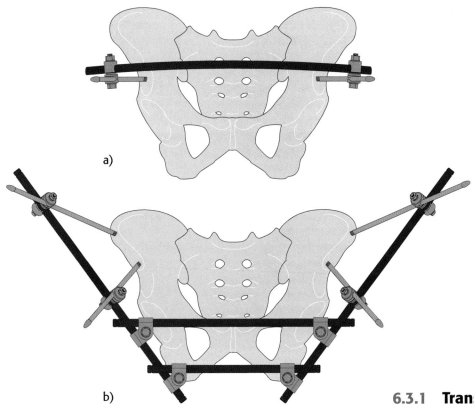

a)

b)

Fig. 4.4-6: External fixation of the pelvis.
a) Demonstration of a simple external fixator with one bar in the supra-acetabular region ("low route") providing optimal holding power for the Schanz screws in the anterior inferior iliac spine—caveat hip joint penetration!
b) Example of a pelvic frame with iliac crest fixation ("high route"). Despite the advantage of simple identification of the iliac crest, misplacements of the Schanz screws are frequent.

6.3.1 Transsymphyseal instability (disruption of the pubic symphysis) with stable posterior ring

The standard method of stabilization here is open reduction and internal fixation (ORIF) with a 2-hole or 4-hole dynamic compression plate (DCP 4.5) (see **Fig. 4.4-7** for approach). For smaller individuals, DCP 3.5 or reconstruction plates are acceptable. To achieve optimal stability, care has to be taken to position the plate screws in a craniocaudal direction, affording them the longest possible bone contact in the pubic bone (**Fig. 4.4-8a–d**, **Video 53027**).

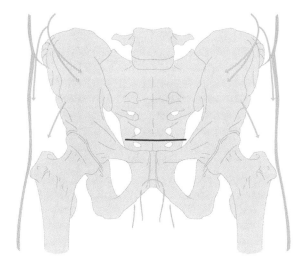

a)

Fig. 4.4-7: Approach to the symphysis pubis.
a) Horizontal Pfannenstiel type incision (7–12 cm
long) about 2 fingerbreadths above the symphysis
exposes the abdominal wall with the strong fascia of
rectus muscles.
b) Splitting the fascia usually exposes the injury with
only a little more dissection to be done. Quite often
the insertion of the rectus muscle is avulsed on one
side only. There is no need to detach the other side
to place a plate.

b)

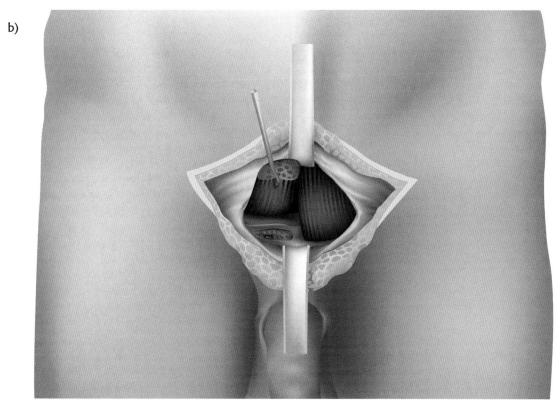

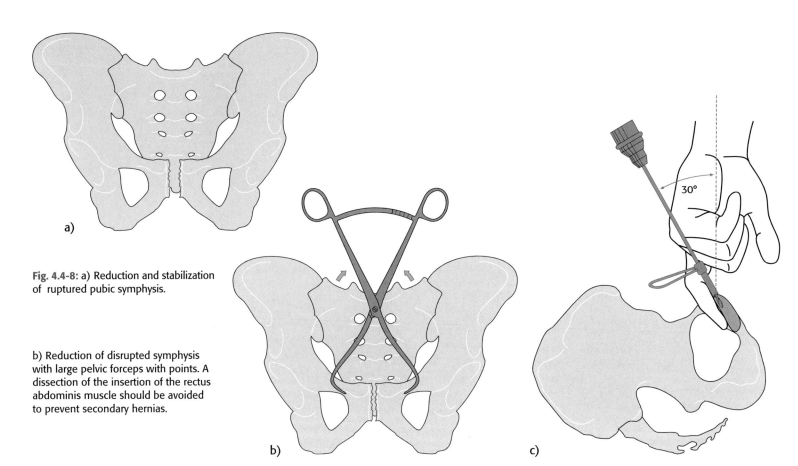

Fig. 4.4-8: a) Reduction and stabilization of ruptured pubic symphysis.

b) Reduction of disrupted symphysis with large pelvic forceps with points. A dissection of the insertion of the rectus abdominis muscle should be avoided to prevent secondary hernias.

c) Insertion of screws under the guidance of the index finger along the internal aspect of the pubic rami.

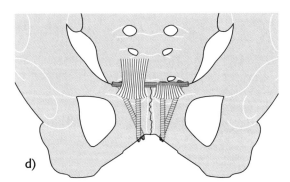

d) Position of the DCP 4.5 or 3.5, or LC-DCP 4.5 or 3.5 "on top" of the symphysis.

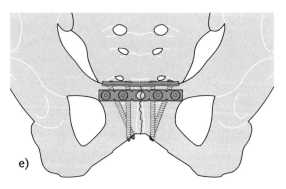

e) If two plates are used to increase stability, a 4-hole plate 3.5 is placed "on top" and a reconstruction plate 3.5 anteriorly.

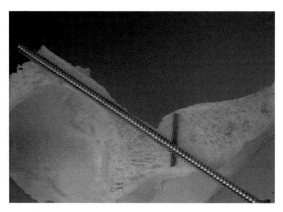

 Video AO53027

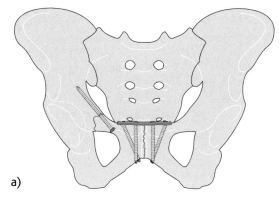

a)

6.3.2   Fixation of the pubic rami

Pubic rami fractures are benign fractures; extensive muscle coverage promotes rapid healing with sufficient stability approximately 3 weeks after injury. Strong periosteum, ligaments, and the muscle envelope will provide adequate stability in most cases. Surgical stabilization is therefore only necessary with wide diastasis of the fracture or severe displacement of the pubic rami or if, after osteosynthesis of posterior lesions (type C injuries), the anterior ring has to be stabilized as well. The standard device—especially in emergencies—is a simple two-pin external fixator (see **Fig. 4.4-6a**).

A "transpubic instability" that is combined with a ruptured symphysis can be stabilized by the use of an extra long screw (3.5 or 4.5 mm cortex screw) placed into the pubic ramus (**Fig. 4.4-9**). Care has to be taken to prevent the screws from penetrating the hip joint. Intraoperative use of an image intensifier is therefore recommended (see also **Video AO53027**).

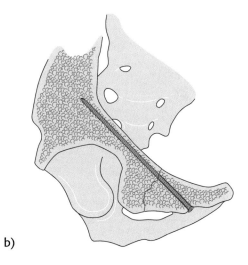

b)

Fig. 4.4-9: Screw fixation of a transpubic instability/ fracture. In case of transpubic instability, combined with a ruptured symphysis, a stabilization of the pubic ramus can be done using the same approach without further dissection with a long 3.5 mm cortex screw placed within the pubic ramus. For correct aiming, fluoroscopy is required.
a) View of the whole pelvis with the screw in place.
b) Cross-section showing the correct screw position in the anterior column.

6.3.3 Instability of the iliac wing

Transiliac fractures have a wide variety of configurations, so individual planning of the internal fixation is required for each case. In the region of the iliac crest, lag screws (3.5 mm) have been suggested. At the region of the pelvic brim DCP 3.5 or reconstruction plates are used (**Fig. 4.4-10**).

6.3.4 Sacroiliac instability

Sacroiliac instability can occur with either disruption of the sacroiliac joint (SI-dislocation) or fracture dislocation involving the ilium (transiliac) or the sacrum (transsacral).

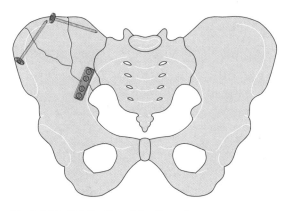

Fig. 4.4-10: Stabilization of the iliac wing.
As there is wide variation in fracture patterns of iliac wing injuries, the type of fixation has to be planned individually. The iliac crest is usually stabilized by 3.5 mm cortex lag screws (exceptionally 6.5 mm screws).

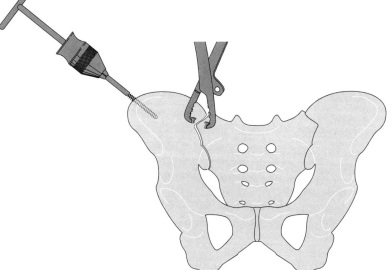

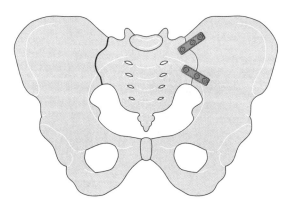

Fig. 4.4-11: Anterior plate fixation of the SI-joint. The SI-joint is exposed by an anterolateral approach to the iliac fossa (see ilioinguinal approach, **chapter 4.5**). Care has to be taken to avoid an injury to the lumbosacral nerve root L5, which runs very closely (10–15 mm) across the ala of the sacrum (see **Video Still AO53028**). Usually the reduction can be performed by manual lateral compression or the insertion of a Schanz screw into the iliac wing. In delayed cases with difficult reduction, a pelvic reduction forceps (small or medium) can be applied.
Narrow 3-hole DCPs 4.5 or 3.5 are the preferred implants. An angle of 60–90° between the two plates enables fixation in areas of dense bone and prevents shearing. The holes for the sacral screws are drilled under direct vision and parallel to the joint.

Depending on the surgeon's preference, an anterior or posterior approach is chosen. **One method is an anterior plate fixation, as the anterolateral approach to the iliac fossa affords excellent exposure of the sacroiliac joint** (Fig. 4.4-11). In the majority of cases, the reduction is facilitated because the anterior lesion (e.g., symphysis disruption) can be exposed simultaneously. The supine position has additional advantages in polytrauma situations because patient monitoring is facilitated and simultaneous operations are possible.

This position provides an excellent orientation for inspection of the SI-joint, while the screw holes can be drilled into the sacrum under direct vision. Two standard DCP 3.5 or 4.5 (3-holes or 4-holes) are preferred as implants. An angle of 60–90° between the plates facilitates iliac fixation in the dense bone at the pelvic rim and the dorsal iliac crest (**Video AO53028**). **Careful dissection is needed to avoid injury to the lumbosacral trunk (particularly L5),**

which is usually only 1.5 cm from the region of the ventral SI-joint.

If a sacroiliac fracture dislocation exists, internal stabilization depends upon the fracture configuration. Combinations of screw and plate fixation using the anterolateral approach are preferred.

An alternative and very valid technique is transiliosacral lag screw fixation (6.5 mm cancellous bone or 7.3 mm cannulated screw) in supine or prone position. The use of an image intensifier as proposed by Matta [12] is highly recommended to minimize the risk of iatrogenic injuries of the sacral plexus (see Fig. 4.4-13). This technique can even be performed percutaneously.

6.3.5 **Transsacral instability**

The surgical treatment of sacral fractures is still under discussion. A specific problem is the combination of pelvic instability with a fracture pattern directly involving the cauda equina. The neurological complication rate is therefore high and treatment should be focused on the early recognition of potential risk factors for neurological damage (displaced fractures, neurological deficits on clinical examinations, fragment interference with nerve roots in CT scans) while achieving an adequate stabilization of the injury.

For this reason, in our own protocol, unstable sacral fractures are exposed by a posterior approach (Fig. 4.4-12) allowing direct vision of the fracture line, as well as decompression of the sacral plexus. For stabilization, "safe zones" on the sacrum are used for a direct plate fixation within the sacral bone ("local stabilization").

Preferred method is an anterior plate fixation.

Avoid injury to the lumbosacral trunk (particularly L5).

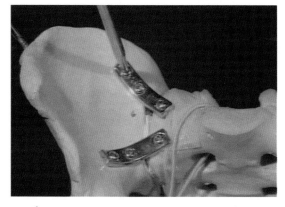

Video AO53028

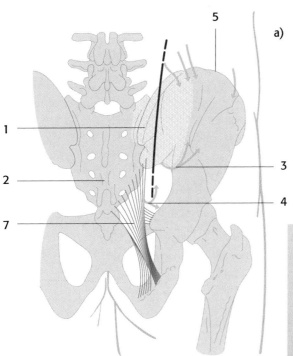

a)

Fig. 4.4-12: Posterior approach to the SI-joint.
a) The skin incision starts 1–2 fingerbreadths distal and lateral to the posterior superior iliac spine (1) and runs in a straight line proximally (about 10–15 cm).
b) The origin of the gluteus maximus muscle (6) is detached from the posterior iliac crest (5). This exposes the iliac wing and the gluteus medius muscle. The latter can be retracted. Care has to be taken not to injure the gluteal vessels (8) and nerves that come out of the greater sciatic notch.

1 Posterior superior iliac spine
2 Medial sacral crest
3 Superior gluteal nerve
4 Inferior gluteal nerve
5 Iliac crest
6 Gluteus maximus muscle
7 Sacrotuberous ligament
8 Gluteal vessels

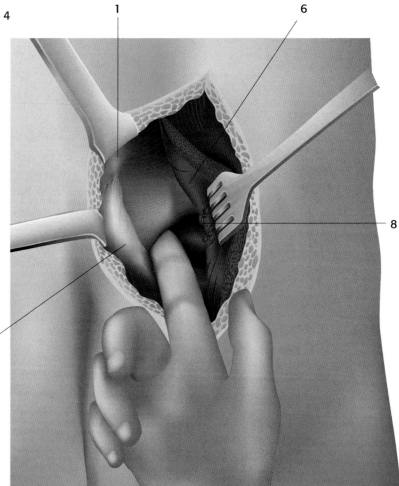

b)

Fig. 4.4-13: Technique of iliosacral screw fixation from behind.

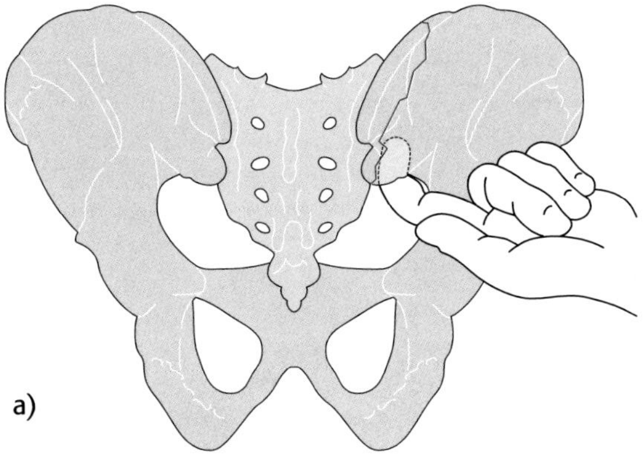

c) The technique of Matta uses the fluoroscope (inlet and outlet views), which allows better control of screw insertion into the body of S1. This technique also allows stabilization of sacral fractures.

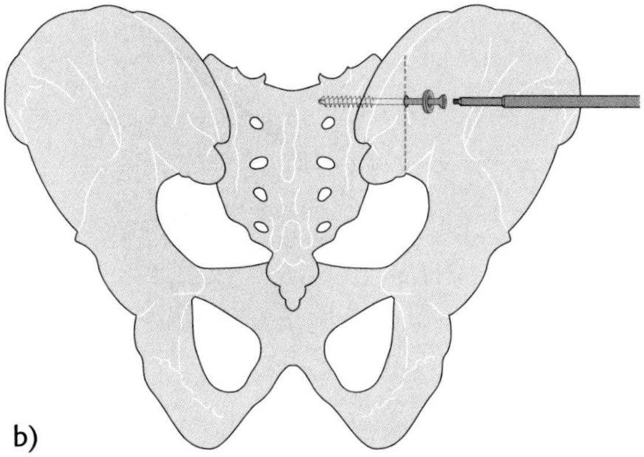

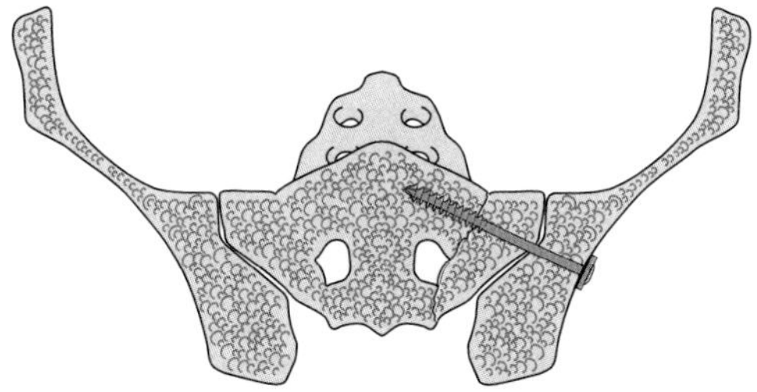

d) Correct position of a 6.5 mm cancellous bone screw in the body of S1, which is the recommended location in the treatment of SI-disruptions. The S2 body should only be used if it is ascertained that pedicle diameter is adequate.
e) The technique has a relatively high risk of neurological and vascular injuries with severe sequelae. More recently computer guidance has been proposed especially for percutaneous screw placement.

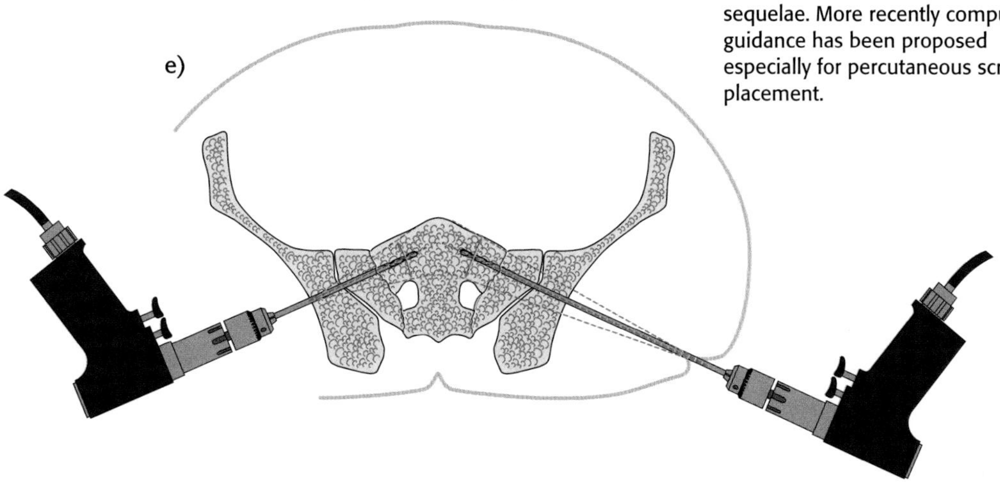

a) Orientation and starting points for transiliosacral screw insertion (middle third on a line 15 mm anterior to the gluteal crest).
b) For pure SI-dislocations, screws can be inserted under manual control by palpation of the ala through the greater sciatic notch [1].

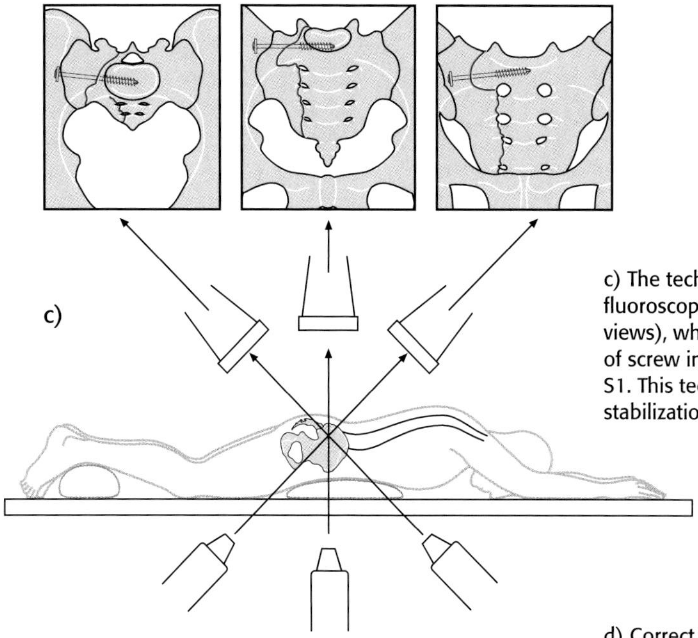

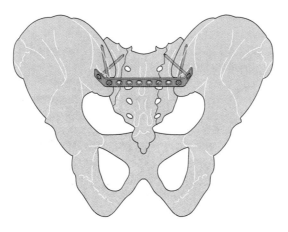

Fig. 4.4-14: Posterior transsacral plate or screw fixation.
a) In cases of bilateral sacral fractures or severe comminution, where a single screw does not provide sufficient
stability, an ilioiliac transsacral plate can be applied as a
salvage procedure. The screws are anchored in the solid
posterior ilical crest.

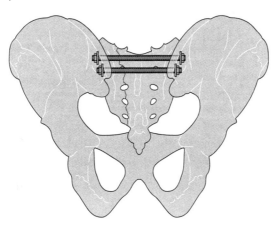

b) Alternatively, sacral bars have been proposed. These,
however, do not provide the same stability as a plate.

Alternative techniques for stabilization are
the use of transiliosacral lag screws (**Fig. 4.4-13,**)
ilioiliac plate fixations (**Fig. 4.4-14**), internal
fixators, and the application of ilioiliac sacral
bars. The latter require one stable SI-joint, as
otherwise they tend to shear and move. Whatever method of fixation is chosen, complete
decompression and absolute anatomical reduction of the sacrum with stable fixation must
be ensured.

7 Postoperative treatment

The goal of pelvic stabilization is the early mobilization of the patient. The methods of fixation
described will provide sufficient stability for
mobilization under partial weight bearing, pre-
suming the operative technique was correct.

Radiographic controls should be made after
mobilization to check for late displacement due
to errors in classification (type B or C injury?)
or technique. The duration of partial weight
bearing is limited to 6 weeks in type B injuries
and 8–10 weeks after type C injuries.

Implant removal is often recommended
6–12 months after operation when pelvic joints
have been surgically transgressed (pubic symphyses and sacroiliac joint); this is, however, not
mandatory.

8   Pitfalls and complications

Surgical complications after pelvic injuries can include the entire range of possibilities:

- As **pelvic injuries are accompanied by a high rate of thromboembolic complications**, a "high risk" prophylaxis should be applied continuously together with extended preoperative screening (color-coded Doppler ultrasound, MRI, venography).
- Precise surgical technique and the administration of perioperative antibiotics are recommended to minimize the risk of infections. Postoperative hematomas should be evacuated immediately after detection.
- Iatrogenic neurological and vascular injuries must be prevented by exact planning and knowledge of anatomy and approaches (cadaver studies, fellowships), as well as the correct use of image intensification.

In the majority of cases, pitfalls are caused by inadequate primary diagnostics, mistaken classification, and difficult fracture patterns. These can lead to inappropriate indications and choice of stabilization methods. Exact preoperative analysis and complete understanding of the "nature" of the injury are the keys to successful surgical treatment. Given the complexity of pelvic stability, only a few guidelines can be given:

- External fixation alone is not sufficient for posterior stabilization in type C injuries.
- Additional implants in the anterior pelvic ring will not compensate the lack of fixation of a complete posterior lesion.
- Even in "lateral compression type injuries" a complete posterior instability can be present (type C injury).
- The differentiation between type B (no posterior stabilization necessary) and type C injuries (posterior stabilization required) can be difficult. Early radiographic controls can show secondary displacement and will enable early (and therefore easy) surgical correction (< 14 days).
- Early surgical reduction and stabilization prevent risky and technically demanding late corrections.

9   Results and long-term assessment

Pelvic fractures, especially the unstable types, lead to a high rate of late sequelae. Recent studies, including a multicenter study, have shown that by using standard indications and the techniques described here, a rate of over 80% of anatomical reconstructions can be achieved even in type C injuries [13]. Despite this, however, in clinical terms, good and excellent results are still found in less than 60% of cases. Frequently, long-term neurological and urological deficits are responsible for patients' complaints, but a non-specific pain in the posterior pelvic ring is also commonly reported.

Therefore, patients after pelvic trauma should be seen in a specific follow-up program, which is preferably organized within an interdisciplinary structure.

Pelvic injuries are often accompanied by thromboembolic complications.

10 Bibliography

1. **Letournel E, Judet R** (1981) *Fractures of the Acetabulum.* Berlin Heidelberg New York: Springer-Verlag.
2. **Tile M** (1995) *Fractures of the Pelvis and Acetabulum.* Baltimore: Williams & Wilkins.
3. **Tscherne H, Pohlemann T** (1998) *Becken und Acetabulum.* Berlin Heidelberg New York: Springer-Verlag.
4. **Tile M, Pennal GF** (1980) Pelvic disruption: principles of management. *Clin Orthop*; (151):56–64.
5. **Pennal GF, Tile M, Waddell JP, et al.** (1980) Pelvic disruption: assessment and classification. *Clin Orthop*; (151):12–21.
6. **Trentz O, Bühren V, Friedl HP** (1989) [Pelvic injuries]. *Chirurg*; 60 (10):639–648.
7. **Flint LM, Jr., Brown A, Richardson JD, et al.** (1979) Definitive control of bleeding from severe pelvic fractures. *Ann Surg*; 189 (6):709–716.
8. **Huittinen VM, Slatis P** (1973) Postmortem angiography and dissection of the hypogastric artery in pelvic fractures. *Surgery*; 73 (3):454–462.
9. **Goldstein A, Phillips T, Sclafani SJ, et al.** (1986) Early open reduction and internal fixation of the disrupted pelvic ring. *J Trauma*; 26 (4):325–333.
10. **Ward EF, Tomasin J, Vander Griend RA** (1987) Open reduction and internal fixation of vertical shear pelvic fractures. *J Trauma*; 27 (3):291–295.
11. **Ganz R, Krushell RJ, Jakob RP, et al.** (1991) The antishock pelvic clamp. *Clin Orthop*; (267):71–78.
12. **Matta JM** (1996) Fractures of the acetabulum: accuracy of reduction and clinical results in patients managed operatively within three weeks after the injury. *J Bone Joint Surg [Am]*; 78 (11):1632–1645.
13. **Pohlemann T, Gänsslen A, Hartung S** (1998) *Beckenverletzungen/Pelvic injuries: Results of the German Multicenter Study Group.* Berlin Heidelberg New York: Springer-Verlag.

11 Updates

Updates and additional references for this chapter are available online at:
http://www.aopublishing.org/PFxM/44.htm

4.5 Acetabular fractures
Evaluation/classification/treatment concepts and approaches

David L. Helfet & Craig S. Bartlett, III

1 Introduction

The treatment of acetabular fractures has rapidly evolved over the past three decades, leading to decreased morbidity and improved outcomes [1–6]. To a great extent, this can be attributed to the revolutionary techniques introduced by Judet [7, 8] and Letournel [1, 5]. However, accurate diagnosis, appropriately chosen approaches, and proper surgical techniques are still necessary to offer the patient the best chance of a good surgical outcome.

2 Evaluation and diagnosis

2.1 The patient

As for all trauma cases, the essentials of airway, breathing, and circulation are the initial priorities for a patient with an acetabular fracture, followed by a secondary survey. The latter is mandatory, as these high-energy fractures are associated with pelvic ring and long bone fractures, spinal and head trauma, and abdominopelvic visceral injuries—often fatal in themselves [1]. Acetabular fractures most frequently result from indirect trauma, transmitted via the femur, after a blow to the greater trochanter, to the flexed knee, or to the foot with the knee extended. There is, therefore, a **frequent association with fractures of the lower extremity.** Contusions and abrasions in the area of the greater trochanter or iliac crest may herald the presence of the "Morel-Lavalle" lesion. This area is usually fluctuant, a large hematoma, with fat necrosis, having developed under degloved skin in subcutaneous tissues. Although technically they are closed injuries, these lesions have high rates of secondary bacterial contamination and require surgical decompression, débridement, and drainage prior to definitive fracture care.

Rectal and vaginal examinations are required to rule out the presence of an open fracture. Hematuria, although frequent in the trauma patient even without pelvic fracture, must be carefully assessed. Injuries to the superior gluteal artery often occur in association with fractures that enter the sciatic notch but may also result from an insult during surgery [1, 3, 9]. Patients with unexplained hemodynamic instability or

Acetabular and lower limb fractures are often associated.

Accurate neurological
examination is also critical.

Associated hip dislocations
must be promptly reduced.

a drop in hematocrit should undergo pelvic angiography to exclude pelvic vascular injuries. An **accurate neurological examination is also critical.** Following a fracture of the acetabulum, the incidence of sciatic nerve compromise detected preoperatively (most frequently in the peroneal division) has ranged from 12–38% [1, 2, 10–12].

An associated hip dislocation is an orthopedic emergency and requires prompt reduction. If there is any tendency toward renewed dislocation, then either proximal tibial or distal femoral skeletal traction is indicated—the latter is preferred if the ligamentous status of the knee has not been determined. The traction weight should be no more than one-sixth of the patient's body-weight. The hip must be kept extended and externally rotated to assist in maintaining reduction.

2.2 The fracture

An AP view of the pelvis is required for all patients sustaining significant trauma (**Fig. 4.5-1**). In those diagnosed with, or suspected of having, a fracture of the acetabulum, three additional views are necessary:
1) An AP view of the involved hip.
2) An iliac oblique view (**Fig. 4.5-2**), obtained by rolling the patient 45° towards the injured side. This provides an "en face" view of the iliac wing and a profile of the obturator ring. (This is used to assess the posterior column and anterior wall.)
3) An obturator oblique view (**Fig 4.5-3**), obtained by rotating the pelvis 45° towards the uninjured side, provides an "en face" view of the obturator ring, and a profile of the iliac wing. (This is

Patient's position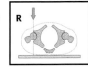

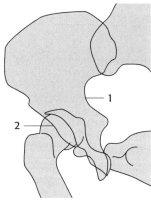

Fig. 4.5-1: The six fundamental radiographic landmarks of Letournel:
1) Posterior wall (border or lip) of acetabulum
2) Anterior wall (border or lip) of acetabulum
3) Roof (dome or sourcil)
4) Teardrop
5) Ilioischial line (posterior column)
6) Brim of pelvis (anterior column)

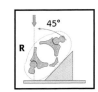

Fig. 4.5-2:
Right iliac oblique view (Judet).
1) Posterior column
2) Anterior lip

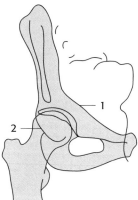

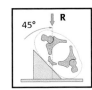

Fig. 4.5-3:
Right obturator oblique view (Judet).
1) Anterior column
2) Posterior lip

used to assess the obturator ring, anterior column, and posterior wall.)

Axial and 3-D **computed tomography (CT) improves understanding of the extent of injury** (**Fig. 4.5-4**), especially in identifying the size and number of posterior wall fragments, marginal impaction injuries, rotation of the columns, and the presence of intra-articular fragments or femoral head fractures. This modality can also identify injuries to the posterior aspect of the pelvis, such as sacroiliac joint disruption or a sacral fracture. A better appreciation of fracture line orientation will also facilitate the proper placement of implants.

3 Classification

Judet and Letournel [8] proposed a classification system for acetabular fractures (**Fig. 4.5-5**, **Fig. 4.5-6**) that is still widely accepted and based on the anatomical concept that the acetabulum is composed of two pillars or columns (**Fig. 4.5-7**). This has been incorporated into the more detailed Müller AO Classification [13] (**Fig. 4.5-8**):

Type A: Partial articular, involving only one of the two columns
    A1 Posterior wall fracture
    A2 Posterior column
    A3 Anterior column or wall

Type B: Partial articular, involving a transverse component
    B1 Pure transverse
    B2 T-shaped
    B3 Anterior column and posterior hemitransverse

Type C: Fractures (complete articular: both columns)
    C1 High variety, extending to the iliac crest
    C2 Low variety, extending to the anterior border of the ilium
    C3 Extension into the sacroiliac joint

Computed tomography (CT) improves understanding of the extent of injury.

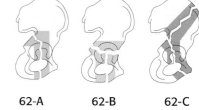

62-A   62-B   62-C

Fig. 4.5-8: Müller AO Classification

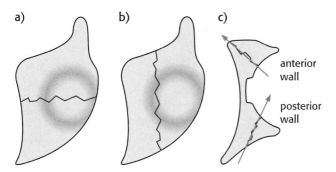

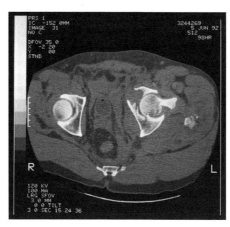

anterior wall

posterior wall

Fig. 4.5-4: Axial CT can be used for fuller clarification of the fracture pattern. a) Vertical (coronal) fracture line through dome, b) transverse fracture line, c) fracture lines traversing anterior and posterior walls.

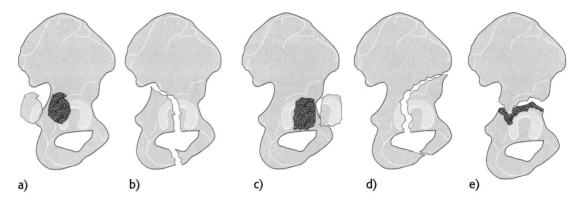

Fig. 4.5-5: The five elemental fracture types (Letournel). a) Posterior wall, b) posterior column, c) anterior wall, d) anterior column, e) transverse.

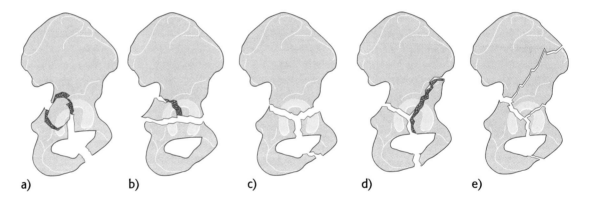

Fig. 4.5-6: The five associated fracture types (Letournel). a) Posterior column and wall, b) transverse and posterior wall, c) anterior column and posterior hemitransverse, d) T-type, e) both columns.

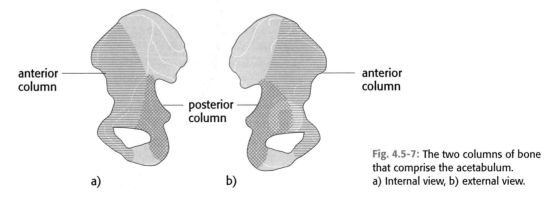

Fig. 4.5-7: The two columns of bone that comprise the acetabulum. a) Internal view, b) external view.

4   Treatment

4.1   Surgical indications and timing

The decision to proceed with surgical stabilization, depends upon several factors, including the fracture pattern, availability of an experienced surgeon, stabilization of associated visceral, skeletal, and soft-tissue injuries, and completion of all imaging studies necessary for preoperative planning. However, a femoral head dislocation or fracture as well as an incarcerated intra-articular fragment following a closed reduction must be addressed promptly to minimize the incidence of avascular necrosis of the femoral head and posttraumatic arthritis.

Other indications for operative intervention include displacement of the articular surface, joint incongruity, and unacceptable roof arc measurements. These are based on the **principle that performing an accurate reduction of the articular surface, thereby obtaining a congruent hip joint, will restore normal joint mechanics.** This is supported by the observation that long-term clinical outcomes closely correlate with the quality of the surgical reduction [1, 2, 14, 15]. **Malreduction or subluxation of the hip joint will lead to abnormal loading of the articular cartilage and subsequent joint arthrosis.** While the amount of incongruity that is acceptable is still open to debate, it seems to be agreed that displacement or incongruity greater than 1–2 mm is unsatisfactory [1, 2, 14].

Because most non-displaced fractures will have a stable and concentric hip joint, surgery can often be avoided. Conservative management may also be prudent for some displaced fractures. These include fractures not extending into the weight-bearing dome, low anterior column fractures, small posterior wall fractures (not associated with a dislocation or involving the posterosuperior portion of the acetabulum), and certain low transverse fractures with roof-arc angles greater than 45° on all three radiographic views. For individuals with low demand, both-column fractures that demonstrate excellent secondary congruence will often have a good functional outcome from non-operative treatment.

Severe osteoporosis limits the ability to achieve rigid and permanent fixation, and is probably the single greatest contraindication to internal fixation. If either significant osteoarthritis or femoral head damage is present, then primary total hip arthroplasty should be considered. Certain pre-existing medical conditions can increase the risks of prolonged anesthesia or blood loss and thus indicate conservative management. However, **non-operative treatment presents its own risks,** and subsequent late reconstruction of an acetabular malunion or non-union is quite difficult.

4.2   Preoperative preparation

Using the preoperative x-rays and axial CT images, the fracture should be reconstructed on a 3-D model. Medical conditions must be aggressively managed to permit surgical intervention, if indicated. **Prophylaxis for deep vein thrombosis [16] is effective but to date there is no evidence-based proof that it is also effective in reducing the risk of fatal pulmonary embolism.** It is appropriate to consider screening the pelvic veins with duplex ultrasound, magnetic resonance veno-

The greatest contraindication to surgery is severe osteoporosis.

Non-operative treatment presents its own risks, and late reconstructions are most difficult.

Normal joint mechanics will only result from accurate reduction leading to a congruent hip joint.

Malreduction or persistent subluxation will lead to posttraumatic osteoarthritis.

Be aware of deep vein thrombosis as a potential source for pulmonary embolism.

graphy or contrast enhanced CT scans on high-risk patients, and to delay surgery when findings are positive. Appropriate treatment, including Greenfield filter placement, can then be undertaken.

4.2.1 Selection of proper approach

Operative experience and the likelihood of anatomical reduction and stabilization will govern the choice of approach.

The approach utilized is often dictated by the experience of the operating surgeon, but should provide the greatest chance of anatomical reduction and stabilization of the joint surface. Mayo [3] has stressed five factors which affect this selection: the fracture pattern, local soft-tissue conditions, presence of associated major systemic injuries, age and projected functional status of the patient, and delay to surgery.

The three most frequently used approaches are:

The four most frequently used approaches are:
1) Kocher-Langenbeck
2) Ilioinguinal
3) Extended iliofemoral
4) Combination of 1) and 2).

1) The **Kocher-Langenbeck approach** (**Fig. 4.5-9**), which gives access to the retro-acetabular surface of the innominate bone from the ischium to the greater sciatic notch. Access to the quadrilateral surface is possible by palpation through the greater and lesser sciatic notches, allowing assessment after the reduction of fractures involving the quadrilateral plate and anterior column. The greater sciatic notch also provides a window for the placement of clamps to manipulate and reduce these fractures. The superior gluteal neurovascular bundle limits access to the superior iliac wing in this approach.

2) The **ilioinguinal approach** (**Fig. 4.5-10**) introduced by Letournel, [1, 4, 5], which offers a direct view of the iliac wing, anterior sacroiliac joint, the entire anterior column, and the pubic symphysis.

3) The **extended iliofemoral approach** (**Fig. 4.5-11**), also introduced by Letournel [1, 5], which is an anatomical approach and follows an internervous plane, reflecting anteriorly the femoral nerve-innervated muscles and posteriorly the muscles innervated by the superior and inferior gluteal nerves. The posterior flap is mobilized as a unit without damaging its neurovascular bundles [1]. This approach provides direct exposure of the whole outer aspect of the ilium, the posterior column down to the ischium, and the hip joint. With further retraction of the iliopsoas and abdominal muscles medially (and some risk of devascularization), exposure of the internal aspect of the ilium is also possible.

4) A combination of 1) and 2).

The Müller AO Classification can be used to provide general guidelines as to the selection of the proper approach:

A1 (posterior wall) Kocher-Langenbeck approach—lateral decubitus.

A2 (posterior column) Kocher-Langenbeck approach.

A3 (anterior wall and/or column) Ilio-inguinal approach.

B1 (pure transverse) The proper approach depends on the obliquity of the transverse component, the direction of rotation, and the column with the major displacement. For most fractures, a Kocher-Langenbeck approach (prone) will be successful. For transtectal pure transverse (B1.2) and difficult associated transverse and posterior wall fractures (B1.3), an extensile approach may provide greater utility.

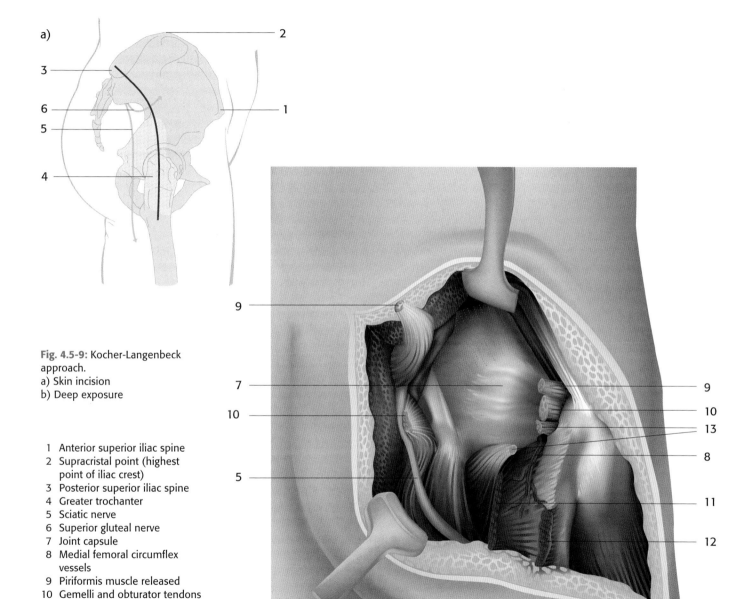

Fig. 4.5-9: Kocher-Langenbeck
approach.
a) Skin incision
b) Deep exposure

1   Anterior superior iliac spine
2   Supracristal point (highest
    point of iliac crest)
3   Posterior superior iliac spine
4   Greater trochanter
5   Sciatic nerve
6   Superior gluteal nerve
7   Joint capsule
8   Medial femoral circumflex
    vessels
9   Piriformis muscle released
10 Gemelli and obturator tendons
    (here illustrated as conjoined)
    released
11 Quadratus femoris
12 Gluteus maximus tendon
    released
13 obturator externus

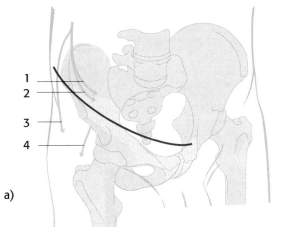

a)

Fig. 4.5-10: Ilioinguinal approach.
a) Skin incision
b) Deep exposure

1 Iliohypogastric nerve
2 Ilioinguinal nerve
3 Lateral cutaneous branch of iliohypogastric nerve
4 Lateral cutaneous nerve of thigh
5 Penrose drain around femoral iliopsoas muscle and lateral femoral cutaneous nerve
6 Penrose drain around femoral vessels
7 Penrose drain around the contents of the inguinal canal

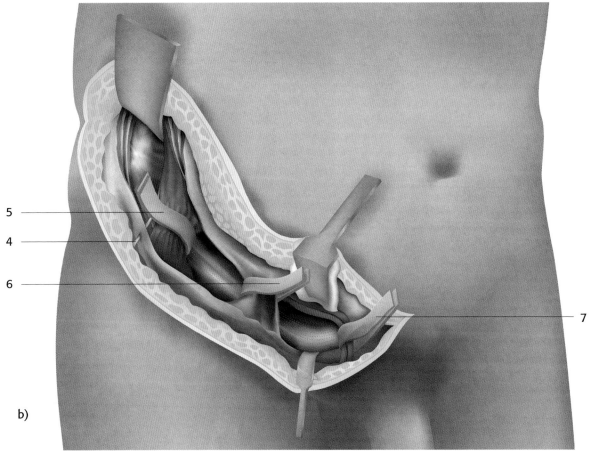

b)

a)

2

3

6

5

4

Fig. 4.5-11: Extended iliofemoral approach.
a) Skin incision
b) Deep exposure

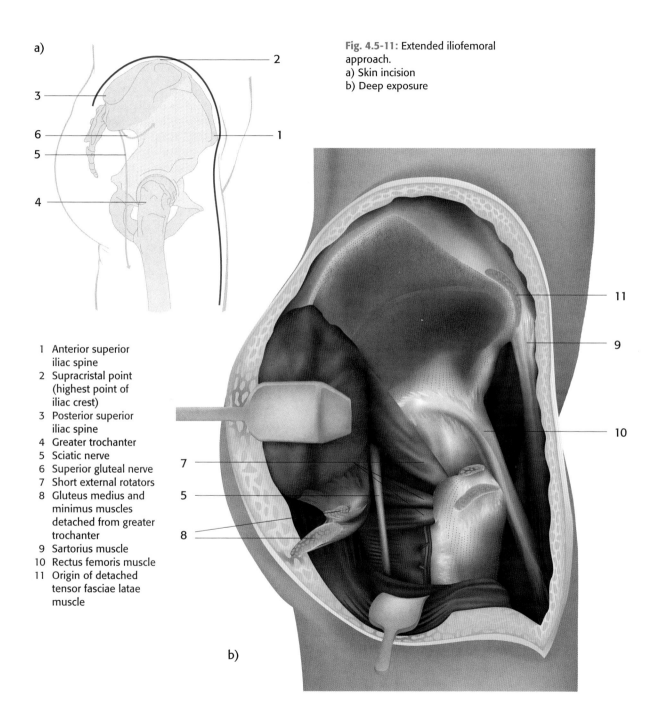

11

9

1

7

5

10

8

1 Anterior superior iliac spine
2 Supracristal point (highest point of iliac crest)
3 Posterior superior iliac spine
4 Greater trochanter
5 Sciatic nerve
6 Superior gluteal nerve
7 Short external rotators
8 Gluteus medius and minimus muscles detached from greater trochanter
9 Sartorius muscle
10 Rectus femoris muscle
11 Origin of detached tensor fasciae latae muscle

b)

B2 (T-shaped) If the major displacement is posterior, particularly in the infratectal or juxtatectal type, and there is an associated posterior wall fracture, then the Kocher-Langenbeck approach should be utilized. However, when the major displacement or rotation is primarily anterior, then the ilioinguinal approach should be employed. The patient should be prepped for both exposures, in case a supplemental approach is required.

B3 (anterior column posterior hemi-transverse) Ilioinguinal approach if the anterior column shows major displacement and the posterior column is high. If the posterior column is low and displaced, we may need simultaneous double incisions or extended iliofemoral approach.

C1/C2 (associated both column = complete articular fracture) Ilioinguinal approach, unless there is complex involvement of the posterior column/and or wall, which will necessitate an extensile approach.

C3 (associated both column extending into SI joint) Extended iliofemoral approach.

The majority of acetabular fractures can be managed through a single surgical approach, but combined approaches are also feasible.

When open treatment is indicated, **the majority of acetabular fractures can be managed through a single surgical approach,** after a thorough preoperative evaluation of the fracture [14, 17]. For more complex fracture patterns, involving both acetabular columns, an extensile or combined anterior and posterior approach may be necessary for exposure and reduction [1, 5, 11, 18, 19]. Compared to single anterior or posterior approaches, extensile exposures involve greater patient morbidity, including increased operative time and blood loss, with

risk of infection, nerve injury, abductor weakness, joint stiffness, and heterotopic ossification [1–3, 11, 19–21]. However, concerns about abductor muscle flap necrosis may be more theoretical than clinical [1, 15]. The extensile approach may be preferred in the presence of nearby suprapubic catheters and colostomies, where infection rates with the ilioinguinal approach rise rapidly, and when surgical treatment of the acetabular fracture is delayed beyond 2–3 weeks [1, 22]. The major technical limitation of the extended iliofemoral exposure is access to the low anterior column [3], where the procedure becomes more difficult and dangerous as the surgeon dissects medial to the iliopectineal eminence.

4.2.2 Operating room preparation

The patient is placed on a radiolucent operating table, which allows intraoperative traction and fluoroscopy. All cases should be performed under general anesthesia, with the option of hypotensive anesthesia to decrease blood loss. Epidural catheterization is optional as a method of decreasing the inhalational agents required, blood loss, and postoperative pain. A Foley catheter should be placed in the patient's bladder, and vascular access established with two large-bore intravenous catheters. Patients of advanced age or with significant medical conditions may require placement of an additional arterial or central line. An intraoperative cell saver permits recycling of about 20–30% of the effective blood loss and minimizes patient exposure to banked blood.

Both somatosensory-evoked potentials and electromyography [10] may provide a degree of protective surveillance. The use of nerve monitoring has not been proven to be of any more benefit than appropriately performed surgery.

4.3   Approaches

4.3.1   Posterior: Kocher-Langenbeck

(Fig 4.5-9)

The patient is positioned in either the lateral decubitus or prone position. The former simplifies intraoperative management, particularly for the anesthesia team, and is used primarily for type A1 and simple type A2 fractures. In this position, the weight of the leg often hinders the reduction of type B1 fractures, so prone positioning is to be favored. The maintenance of knee flexion (at 90°) and hip extension throughout the procedure reduces tension on the sciatic nerve.

The incision is centered over the posterior half of the greater trochanter, extends distally along the shaft of the femur for approximately 8 cm, and curves proximally toward the posterior superior iliac spine for another 8 cm. The fascia lata and fascia over the gluteus maximus are incised and the muscle gently split by blunt dissection. The sciatic nerve can be consistently identified along the medial aspect of the quadratus femoris fascia. A portion of the gluteus maximus insertion may require release, to decrease tension (**Video 4.5-1**).

The short external rotators are placed on stretch by internal rotation of the hip, tagged, and reflected from their femoral insertions. Retraction of the obturator internus tendon provides access to the lesser sciatic notch and protects the sciatic nerve, which passes superficial to the tendon. Retraction of the piriformis tendon provides access to the greater sciatic notch, but fails to protect the sciatic nerve, which exits deep to the tendon. Blunt retractors

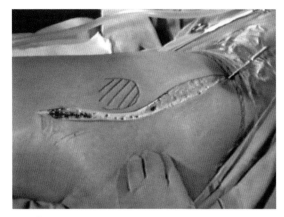

 Video 4.5-1

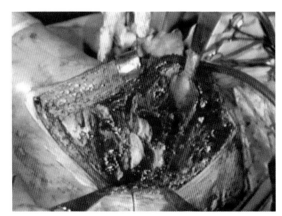

 Video 4.5-2

are carefully placed into these two locations to provide a view of the entire retroacetabular surface. Care should be taken to identify and protect the superior gluteal neurovascular bundle as it exits the greater sciatic notch. For fractures such as high transtectal transverse or T-type fractures, an osteotomy of the greater trochanter is occasionally required, to gain access to the superior weight-bearing surface of the acetabulum (**Video 4.5-2**). However, this carries the disadvantage of potential non-union and an increased risk of heterotopic ossification.

At closure, the external rotators are sutured to the cuff of tissue on the posterior aspect of the greater trochanter, or are reattached through drill holes. If a release of the gluteus maximus insertion has been required, this too is repaired. Deep and superficial drains are placed if felt necessary by the surgeon. The fascia lata and fascia over the gluteus maximus are repaired followed by the superficial closure.

4.3.2 Anterior: ilioinguinal

(Fig. 4.5-10)

With the patient in a supine position, the incision starts at the midpoint of the iliac crest, curves towards the anterior superior iliac spine, continues parallel to the inguinal ligament, and ends 2 cm above the pubic symphysis. The avascular fascial periosteal layer at the iliac crest is identified and divided sharply, the abdominal and iliacus musculature is elevated in continuity subperiosteally, and the internal iliac fossa packed with a sponge. Anteriorly, the incision is carried down to the level of the external oblique aponeurosis, and the contents of the inguinal canal identified and mobilized. The external oblique aponeurosis is incised 5 mm from its insertion on the inguinal ligament, from the anterior superior iliac spine to the external inguinal ring. Laterally, the conjoint tendon is incised from the inguinal ligament with a 2 mm cuff, while carefully preserving the underlying lateral femoral cutaneous nerve. As the incision proceeds medially, the reflection of the iliopectineal fascia will be encountered. Extreme care must be exercised, as the femoral vascular bundle lies just medial to this structure. By leaving the conjoint tendon intact, where it covers the femoral artery, vein, and lymphatics, unnecessary dissection is avoided and these structures protected. Medial to the vessels, the conjoint tendon can be incised, if required, and the ipsilateral rectus abdominis muscle released from the pubic tubercle to the pubic symphysis, allowing access to the space of Retzius. **Keeping the bladder decompressed with a Foley catheter decreases the risk of injuring it.** Associated anterior pelvic ring injuries may require fixation across the pubic symphysis, necessitating a partial release of the contralateral rectus abdominis muscle.

Laterally, the iliopsoas muscle and the femoral nerve, and medially the femoral vasculature and lymphatics, are delicately separated from the iliopectineal fascia. Once this structure has been isolated, it is excised along the pelvic brim from the pectineal eminence to just anterior to the sacroiliac joint. Carefully, the femoral vessels are mobilized from the underlying ramus, but not before inspecting this area to avoid injuring an inconstant, but dangerous retro-pubic communication between the external iliac and the obturator or deep epigastric arteries ("corona mortis").

During closure, drains are inserted into the space of Retzius, over the quadrilateral surface and along the internal iliac fossa, if necessary due to the excessive wound bleeding. The recti abdomini are reattached to the cuff of tissue remaining on the anterior aspect of the pubis. The floor of the inguinal canal is repaired by suturing the conjoint tendon to the inguinal ligament with non-absorbable sutures. The roof of the inguinal canal is restored by repairing the external oblique aponeurosis and external inguinal ring. The skin is closed over a superficial suction drain.

Keeping the bladder decompressed with a Foley catheter decreases the risk of injuring it.

4.3.3 Extensile: extended iliofemoral

(**Fig. 4.5-11**)

The patient is supported in the lateral decubitus position. The incision is in the form of an inverted "J", beginning at the posterior superior iliac spine and extending along the iliac crest toward the anterior superior iliac spine, where it continues distally along the anterolateral aspect of the thigh for 15–20 cm [1, 3]. The avascular fascial periosteal layer at the iliac crest is identified and divided, and the musculature along the external surface of the iliac wing released up to the superior border of the greater sciatic notch and anterosuperior aspect of the hip-joint capsule. Care must be taken to identify and protect the superior gluteal neurovascular bundle as it exits the greater sciatic notch.

In order to protect the lateral femoral cutaneous nerve and the majority of its branches, the distal limb of the incision is carried through the fascial sheath of the tensor fascia lata muscle. Reflecting the muscle off its posterior fascia and retracting it laterally, the rectus sheath and fascia are exposed. Small vessels from the superficial circumflex artery are divided and coagulated between the superior and inferior spines, [1] the rectus fascia is divided, and the reflected and direct heads of the muscle are retracted medially to expose the aponeurosis over the vastus lateralis muscle, where a small vascular pedicle often requires coagulation [1]. The aponeurosis over the vastus lateralis can be divided longitudinally to expose the ascending branches of the lateral circumflex vessels, which must be isolated and ligated. Next, the thin sheath of the iliopsoas muscle is exposed and longitudinally incised. An elevator is used to strip the muscle from the anterior and inferior aspects of the hip capsule. The gluteus minimus and medius tendons are tagged and transected, leaving small cuffs, and the abductor muscle flap is retracted to expose the external rotators of the hip. From this point, the dissection is similar to the Kocher-Langenbeck. Further access to the internal iliac fossa and acetabulum can be obtained by subperiosteal dissection of the sartorius and direct head of the rectus, or by osteotomy of the iliac spines. In the absence of capsular disruption, the acetabular articular surface is exposed with a marginal capsulotomy, leaving a cuff of tissue for repair. Distraction is achieved with either a Schanz screw placed into the femoral neck or with a femoral distractor (**Fig. 4.5-12**). This approach creates significant soft-tissue flaps which it is important to keep moist throughout the procedure.

Prior to closure, suction drains are placed along the external surface of the iliac wing, in the vicinity of the posterior column and vastus lateralis muscle. If the internal iliac fossa has been exposed, a third drain is placed here. All drains should exit anteriorly. The hip capsule is repaired first, followed by reattachment of the tendinous insertions of the short external rotators and gluteal muscles to the greater trochanter. Finally, the tensor fascia lata and gluteal muscles are reattached to their origins on the iliac crest. If a medial exposure has been performed, then the origins of the sartorius and direct head of the rectus femoris muscles are reattached through drill holes (or by lag screws if osteotomies have been performed). The fascia overlying the proximal thigh is repaired, a subcutaneous drain placed, and a superficial closure performed.

The extended iliofemoral approach is most demanding and has inherent hazards that have to be taken into account.

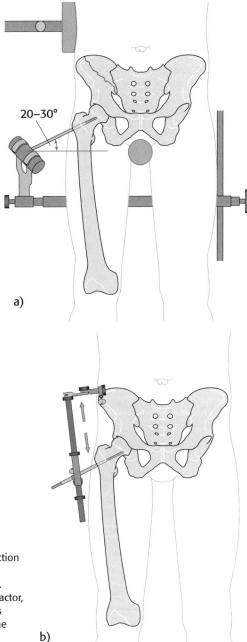

20–30°

Traction may reduce fragments with retained soft-tissue attachments.

a)

Fig. 4.5-12: Essential reduction tools are:
a) The classical Judet table.
b) The universal large distractor, where one Schanz screw is placed in the trochanter, the other into the pelvis.

b)

4.3.4 Others

Various other exposures have been proposed [23, 24]. Of these, the most useful are the extensile triradiate of Mears and Rubash [23], and the modified Stoppa (anterior) approach of Cole and Bolhofner.

4.4 Reduction techniques and internal fixation

Intraoperative traction brings about an indirect reduction of those fragments which have retained their capsular or soft-tissue attachments. It also moves the femoral head, to permit inspection of the joint. This can be achieved either with a Judet fracture table [1], or by positioning the patient on a radiolucent table, with the leg draped free, followed by direct manual traction through the thigh, by a Schanz screw placed laterally into the femoral head, or with the large distractor (**Fig. 4.5-12**).

A wide variety of reduction tools is available for use along the bony pelvis. Several of these may be needed to correct each of the displacement vectors. "King Tong" and "Queen Tong" clamps are designed for application from the outer and inner pelvic surfaces, or from the greater sciatic notch, to the anterior inferior iliac spine. The Lambotte-Farabeuf and the large pelvic reduction forceps are designed to anchor to screw heads on each side of a major fracture line, providing substantial leverage and rotational control of fragments.

Several columns of bone exist for placement of screws, including the iliac crest, gluteal ridge, sciatic buttress, anterior column, and posterior column. **A dislocated sacroiliac joint or displaced sacral fracture is usually reduced**

first and fixed, prior to the reduction of the acetabular fracture.

4.4.1 ORIF through the posterior approach

In this approach, distraction of the hip joint is best achieved with a universal large distractor, with a 5 mm Schanz screw in the sciatic buttress proximally, and a second pin into the femur at the level of the lesser trochanter. This allows exposure of the joint, removal of loose fragments, and the reduction of any marginal impaction fractures. After traction has been released, the femoral head provides a template for the articular reduction. Autogenous cancellous bone, obtained through a small window in the greater trochanter, is then used to buttress the reduced marginal fragments (**Fig. 4.5-13**).

For type A1 fractures, the medial aspect of each cortical wall fragment should be cleared of enough soft tissue to permit the reduction to be seen, while retaining as much capsular attachment as possible to preserve the blood supply. These fragments are then reduced and held in place by the straight ball spike pusher, followed by provisional fixation with K-wires. A reconstruction plate 3.5 is applied in buttress mode over the reduced posterior wall and anchored to the ilium proximally and ischium distally. Under-contouring (under-bending) of this plate,

A dislocated sacroiliac joint or displaced sacral fracture is usually reduced first and fixed, prior to the reduction of the acetabular fracture.

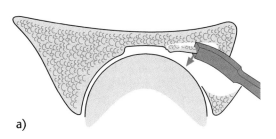
a)

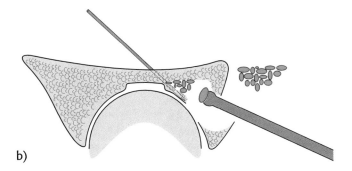
b)

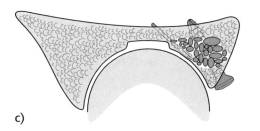
c)

Fig. 4.5-13: Posterior wall fracture.
a) In case of a circumscribed impaction of the articular surface, this area must be carefully elevated and molded against the femoral head.
b) The resulting defect must be filled with cancellous autograft or a bone substitute.
c) To hold the reduction, resorbable pins, K-wires, or a screw may be used.

in relation to the posterior wall, will aid in reduction of the construct and compress the fracture (**Fig. 4.5-14**) (**Video AO20134**). To prevent fracture displacement, one or more lag screws should be placed through the plate and posterior wall into the posterior column. Should significant fragmentation prevent capture of

each of the articular fragments with a lag screw, then spring hook plates are used (**Fig. 4.5-15**). When under-contoured, these further act to reduce small fragments to the femoral head. Be careful to ensure that the hooks of the spring plate do not impale the labrum and are far enough away from the edge of the joint not to

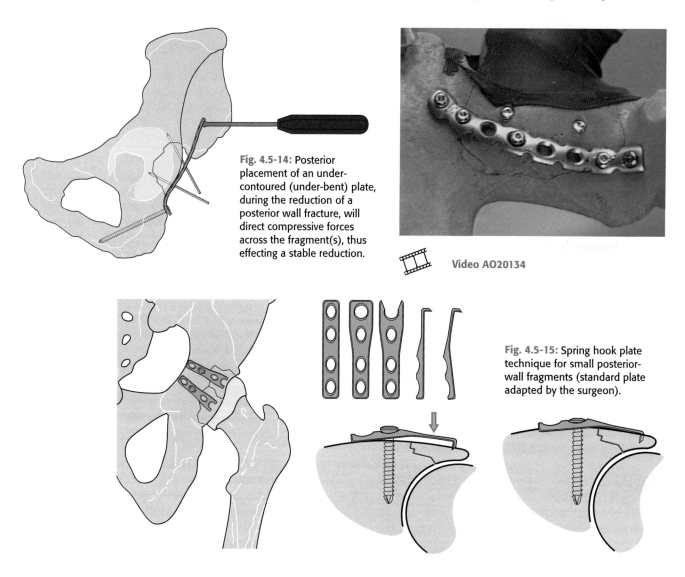

Fig. 4.5-14: Posterior placement of an under-contoured (under-bent) plate, during the reduction of a posterior wall fracture, will direct compressive forces across the fragment(s), thus effecting a stable reduction.

Video AO20134

Fig. 4.5-15: Spring hook plate technique for small posterior-wall fragments (standard plate adapted by the surgeon).

scratch the femoral head. It might be best not to place the hooks on the end of the plates and just use them in buttress mode.

In type A2 fractures, the posterior column is typically displaced postero-medially and internally rotated. Reduction is usually accomplished by screw-holding forceps applied to 4.5 mm bicortical screws inserted into each of the main column fragments. Additional derotation of the inferior portion of the posterior column fragment can be achieved with a 5 mm Schanz screw inserted into the ischium or by pelvic reduction forceps with pointed ball tips placed into the sciatic notch (**Video AO20135**). The gluteal neurovascular bundle can be damaged during this maneuver, and must be monitored. After reduction and provisional fixation with a K-wire, a reconstruction plate 3.5 is applied from the ischium to the ilium. A lag screw across the fracture, into the anterior column, will prevent renewed displacement.

Type A2 fractures seldom occur in isolation and are frequently associated with a posterior wall fracture. In these cases, the wall fragment should be treated next with a separate buttress plate.

Type B1 fractures require techniques similar to those used for type A2 fractures, except that the reduction is more difficult due to the additional anterior column involvement. An elegant maneuver is first to secure a plate into one of the fracture fragments, then to use the plate as a reduction tool. After provisional fixation and inspection, stabilization is obtained with a reconstruction plate 3.5 applied to the retroacetabular surface and lag screw(s). This plate should be over-contoured, to compress the anterior column segments as it is tightened down to the posterior column (**Fig. 4.5-16**).

In acetabular fractures correct contouring of the plates is most essential.

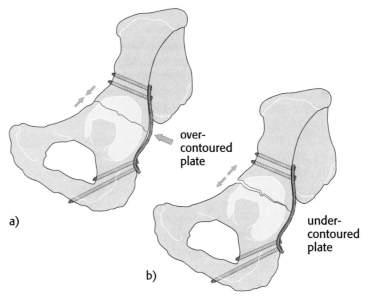

over-contoured plate

a)

b)

under-contoured plate

Fig. 4.5-16: a) Posterior placement of an over-contoured (over-bent) plate during the fixation of a transverse fracture will result in compressive forces over the anterior portion of the fracture and an optimal reduction.
b) In contrast, placement of an under-contoured (under-bent) plate during the reduction of a transverse fracture will lead to distraction of the fracture anteriorly.

Video AO20135

Under-contouring, as performed for type A1 fractures, will actually lead to distraction of the anterior column in type B1 fractures. A posterior to anterior column lag screw will prevent displacement of the anterior column. This screw can usually be placed through the posterior buttress plate and must be oriented parallel to the quadrilateral surface to avoid joint penetration (**Fig. 4.5-17**). In case of a circumscribed impaction of the articular surface, this area must be reduced anatomically and the resulting bone defect must be filled with cancellous autograft (or bone substitute). Temporary reduction can be obtained by a resorbable pin, a K-wire, or a screw (see **Fig. 4.5-13**).

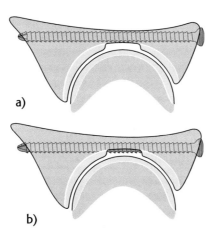

a)

b)

Fig. 4.5-17: Demonstration of acceptable positioning of lag screw parallel to the quadrilateral plate. A screw which crosses deep within the cotyloid fossa may be retained until healing of the fracture.

Type B2 (transverse and T-shaped) fractures are among the most difficult of all fracture types to manage, as the inferior segment has been separated into anterior and posterior fragments by a vertical stem component. Successful fixation of this fracture, through a posterior approach, is dependent upon the surgeon's ability to palpate the anterior column and stem component through the greater sciatic notch. It is impossible to control the separate anterior column fragment by manipulation of the posterior column fragments. Thus, the surgeon must be familiar with the placement of instruments into the sciatic notch and with their use to manipulate the anterior column fragment after the provisional stabilization of the posterior column. Posterior column implants that cross into the anterior column will make such a reduction difficult, if not impossible. Definitive fixation is accomplished with a posterior buttress plate and lag screws, as in type B1 fractures.

4.4.2 ORIF through an anterior approach

Reduction is facilitated by hip flexion, in order to relax structures crossing anterior to the hip joint. Manual traction with a Schanz screw, inserted through the lateral aspect of the femur into the femoral head, will effect fracture reduction through ligamentotaxis. Every step is critical to the outcome of the procedure, including an accurate reduction of all fracture fragments, since the articular surface is not directly seen through this approach. Each fracture line should be carefully irrigated and debrided to remove hematoma and small fragments. The hip joint is also irrigated and loose fragments removed through the displaced portion of the articular fracture.

Reconstruction of type A3, B3, and C fractures begins with reduction of the individual peripheral fracture fragments to portions of the intact pelvis. Working from the periphery towards the articular surface, fragments are sequentially reduced and provisionally stabilized. This process requires patience and a three-dimensional understanding of the pelvic anatomy. The crest is stabilized by any combination of lag screws or reconstruction plates 3.5.

In type A3 and B3 fractures, the anterior column is next reduced to the intact iliac wing and temporarily stabilized with a K-wire or 3.5 mm lag screw into the sciatic buttress. Finally, any anterior wall or superior pubic ramus fractures are reduced and provisionally fixed.

For type C fractures, the reconstruction must be performed perfectly, from the iliac crest to the symphysis pubis, in order to provide an anatomical template for subsequent reduction of the posterior column to the reduced anterior column. An incomplete anterior column fracture may require completion to permit an adequate reduction. The anterior column segment is typically shortened and externally rotated. In order to reduce this segment to the intact iliac wing ("spur" sign), a significant amount of longitudinal traction is often required.

Definitive fixation of most fracture types involves a reconstruction plate 3.5 molded along the iliac fossa, across the iliopectineal eminence to the pubic tubercle and pubic column (**Fig. 4.5-18**). This should not cross the symphysis pubis, unless there are associated ramus fractures or involvement of the symphysis pubis with an associated pelvic ring injury. This plate must be perfectly contoured, otherwise its fixation to the pelvis can lead to

Reconstruction of type A3, B3, and C fractures begins with reduction of the individual peripheral fracture fragments.

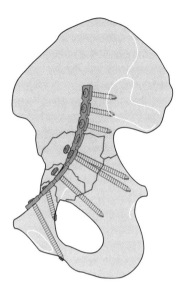

Fig. 4.5-18: In general, anterior fixation includes at least two screws into the pubis, two into the intact iliac wing, and any number of bicortical or lag screws through a reconstruction plate contoured along the pelvic rim. In this example, three screws, one through the plate and two outside the plate, have been used to lag the posterior column.

poor reduction of the acetabular fracture. The plate is fixed to the internal iliac fossa, superior to the acetabulum, with 3.5 mm cortex screws, and medially to the pubic tubercle and ramus. Screw placement within the thin central area of the iliac fossa should be avoided. In contrast, the sciatic buttress and quadrilateral plate, proximal to the acetabulum, provide optimal purchase for stabilization of the anterior column to the iliac wing and posterior column. Aiming the screws parallel to the quadrilateral plate best prevents joint penetration.

In type C and B3 fractures, following anatomical reduction and stabilization of the anterior column, the rotated and medially displaced posterior column is reduced to the restored

Definitive fixation of most fractures requires a reconstruction plate 3.5 contoured along the iliac fossa.

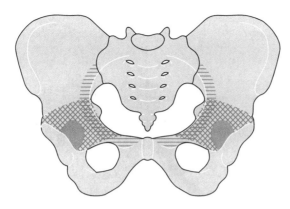

Fig. 4.5-19: The danger zone of screw placement, through the ilioinguinal approach, extends from the anterior border of the iliopectineal eminence to the anterior border of the anterior inferior iliac spine. Screws placed in this region can easily violate the joint. Therefore, if they are required, screws must be placed perfectly (parallel to the quadrilateral plate) or be unicortical.

4.4.3 ORIF through an extensile approach

For type B2 and the more comminuted variants, the anterior column may be reduced first with respect to the residual acetabular "roof" portion of the ilium [23]. The screw-holding forceps and 4.5 mm cortex screws proximal and distal to the posterior column fracture will improve distraction, débridement of the fracture surfaces, and reduction. A laminar spreader in the fracture site is also useful. For additional control, a Schanz screw is placed in the ischium, or a pelvic clamp in the greater sciatic notch. Prior to definitive reduction, a gliding hole inserted into the proximal aspect of the posterior column, from superior to inferior, will assure optimal positioning of a 4.5 or 3.5 mm cortex lag screw in the middle of the posterior column. Additional stabilization is accomplished with a reconstruction plate 3.5 molded to the posterior column. A lag screw can also be inserted from the lateral aspect of the iliac wing, and angled from posterosuperior to anteroinferior directly down the superior pubic ramus to secure the anterior column of the acetabulum. Care must be taken to assure that this screw remains extra-articular and does not penetrate the anterior aspect of the superior ramus in the area of the iliopectineal eminence, where the femoral vasculature is closely adherent.

Type C fractures require sequential reconstruction from the periphery toward the acetabulum. Once the iliac wing is stabilized with lag screws and/or reconstruction plates 3.5, the posterior column is reduced to the iliac wing by looking directly at the acetabular articular surface. Next, the anterior column is reduced to the intact posterior column, with 4.5 mm lag

Type C fractures require sequential reconstruction from the periphery toward the acetabulum.

anterior column. This often requires lateral and anterior traction of the hip, via the Schanz screw in the femoral head, and specially designed pelvic reduction clamps. One tine of the clamp is placed on the outer surface of the ilium, through a small limited exposure, and the other tine is placed on the quadrilateral plate and/or posterior column. With a small supplemental bone hook, slipped down the quadrilateral plate to the ischial spine, the posterior column can be pulled up to the anterior column. Upon reduction of the posterior column, 3.5 mm lag screws are inserted through the pelvic brim superior to the acetabulum into the posterior column. These should parallel the quadrilateral surface, aiming for the ischial spine (**Fig. 4.5-18**, **Fig. 4.5-19**). For other valuable maneuvers and tricks see **chapter 3.1**.

screws inserted from the anterior superior spine into the sciatic buttress, and/or anterior column lag screws from the lateral aspect of the iliac wing.

4.5 Assessment of reduction and fixation

Prior to closure, the reconstructed acetabulum must be assessed using fluoroscopic imaging and intraoperative radiographs (anteroposterior pelvic, obturator, and iliac oblique views) to confirm that a satisfactory reduction has been achieved, and to ensure there has been no inadvertent intra-articular hardware placement. Depending on the exposure used, the adequacy of the reduction of the posterior column to the anterior column is determined by digital palpation along the quadrilateral surface, or through the greater and lesser sciatic notches. Moving the hip while a finger touches the quadrilateral surface can detect the presence of any crepitation in the joint, indicative of residual bony fragments or intra-articular hardware.

4.6 Postoperative management/ rehabilitation

Postoperatively, patients are maintained on intravenous cefazolin for 48–72 hours. Thromboembolic prophylaxis should be discussed with the patient. At the present time there is no evidence-based data to prove that prophylaxis will prevent fatal pulmonary embolism. There are serious complications that will occur if prophylaxis is used uncritically. After Kocher-Langenbeck approaches, extended iliofemoral

approaches, and ilioinguinal approaches where the external surface of the iliac wing has required stripping, Indomethacin (75 mg sustained release) orally once daily for 6 weeks, provides prophylaxis against heterotopic bone formation.

Early mobilization should be stressed and patients encouraged to sit up within the first 24–48 hours following surgery. After the removal of drains, usually by the third day, patients are allowed toe-touch weight bearing using crutches. Strengthening exercises and gait training are initiated by the physical therapist. However, weight bearing is not advanced for 6–8 weeks. In the case of an extended iliofemoral approach or a trochanteric osteotomy, active abduction is avoided for 6–8 weeks. During the third month, depending on radiographic evidence of healing, the patient is allowed to progress to full weight bearing as tolerated.

Intraoperative x-rays may be inadequate to demonstrate residual joint incongruity, penetrating hardware, or loose fragments. Therefore, postoperative x-rays (anteroposterior pelvis, obturator, and iliac oblique views) are recommended but CT scan is only needed if the plain x-rays do not confirm an adequate reduction or show that the screws are all out of the joint.

4.7 Complications

4.7.1 Early

Intraoperative complications include neurovascular injury, inadequate reduction, articular penetration by hardware, and pulmonary embolism (PE). Early postoperative complications include deep vein thrombosis (DVT), skin necrosis, infection, loss of reduction,

The reconstructed acetabulum should be radiologically assessed prior to closure.

Joint incongruity, misplaced hardware, and loose fragments may not show on intraoperative x-rays, therefore postoperative x-ray assessment is mandatory.

Neurovascular injury, inadequate reduction, articular penetration by hardware, and pulmonary embolism may complicate surgery.

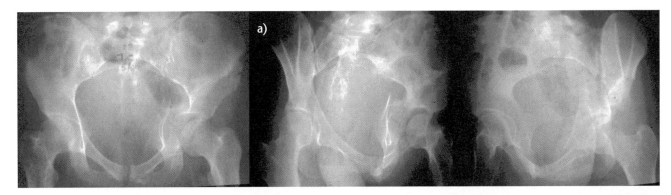

Fig. 4.5-20:
22-year-old female, unrestrained driver involved in a motor vehicle accident.
a) Radiographic views (AP/ obturator-oblique/iliac-oblique; respectively) revealing a displaced (left) associated both-column acetabular fracture. The iliac oblique view demonstrates the pathognomonic spur sign.

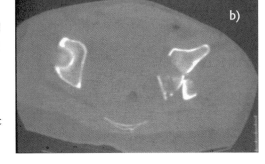

b) CT scan showing displacement/rotation of the two columns.

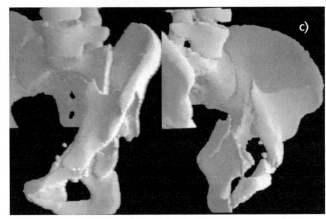

c) 3-D CT reconstruction images demonstrating the malrotation and displacement of the two columns.

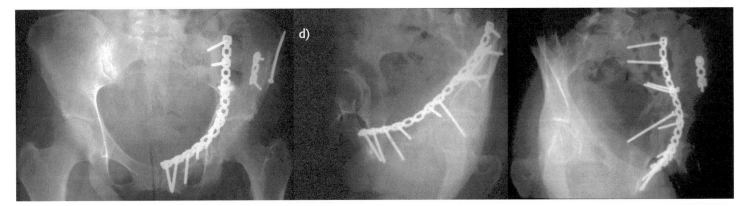

d) Follow-up x-rays (AP/obturator-oblique/iliac-oblique; respectively) showing an anatomic reduction via an anterior approach with restoration of the joint surface and fracture healing.

arthritis, and death. The incidence of infection is between 4–5% [1, 2, 14, 15]. An iatrogenic sciatic nerve injury or worsening of a pre-existing deficit can cause significant problems. While correlated with the experience of the surgical team [1, 2], even the most experienced surgeons still report rates of 2–3% [2]. The incidence of DVT detected by proximal screening has been reported to be ±30% and plays a major role in postoperative morbidity and mortality. However, improved treatment protocols and preoperative detection of venous thromboembolism by magnetic resonance venography [25] has lead to a lower incidence of PE.

4.7.2 Late

Late complications include heterotopic ossification, chondrolysis, avascular necrosis, and posttraumatic arthrosis. Heterotopic ossification is the most common complication following the operative fixation of acetabular fractures, with an incidence ranging from 18–90% [1, 2, 21], most commonly in association with the extensile approaches [1, 2, 15, 21]. Both Indomethacin [1] and low dose radiation therapy (single or multiple fractions) [1, 21] have displayed prophylactic efficacy when given early. The incidence of avascular necrosis of the femoral head following operative treatment of acetabular fractures has generally ranged from 3–9% [1, 2]. **Posttraumatic arthrosis is directly related to the quality of reduction—the better the latter, the greater the chance of a good or excellent result.**

5 Bibliography

1. **Letournel E, Judet R** (1993) *Fractures of the Acetabulum.* 2nd ed. Berlin Heidelberg New York: Springer-Verlag.
2. **Matta JM** (1996) Fractures of the acetabulum: accuracy of reduction and clinical results in patients managed operatively within three weeks after the injury. *J Bone Joint Surg [Am];* 78 (11):1632–1645.
3. **Mayo KA** (1990) Surgical approaches to the acetabulum. *Tech Orthop;* 4:24–35.
4. **Letournel E** (1987) Surgical treatment of acetabular fractures. *Hip;* 157–180.
5. **Letournel E** (1980) Acetabulum fractures: classification and management. *Clin Orthop;* (151):81–106.
6. **Tscherne H, Pohlemann T** (1998) *Tscherne Unfallchirurgie. Becken und Acetabulum.* Berlin Heidelberg: Springer-Verlag.
7. **Judet R, Lagrange J** (1958) La voie postero externe de Gibson. Presse Med; 66:263–264.
8. **Judet R, Judet J, Letournel E** (1964) Fractures of the acetabulum: classification and surgical approaches for open reduction. *J Bone Joint Surg;* 46:1615–1646.
9. **Johnson EE, Eckardt JJ, Letournel E** (1987) Extrinsic femoral artery occlusion following internal fixation of an acetabular fracture. A case report. *Clin Orthop;* (217):209–213.
10. **Helfet DL, Anand N, Malkani AL, et al.** (1997) Intraoperative monitoring of motor pathways during operative fixation of acute acetabular fractures. *J Orthop Trauma;* 11(1):2–6.

Late complications include heterotopic ossification, chondrolysis, avascular necrosis, and posttraumatic arthrosis.

Posttraumatic arthrosis is directly related to the quality of reduction—the better the reduction, the greater the chance of a good or excellent result.

11. **Pennal GF, Davidson J, Garside H, et al.** (1980) Results of treatment of acetabular fractures. *Clin Orthop;* (151):115–123.

12. **Matta JM, Mehne DK, Roffi R** (1986) Fractures of the acetabulum. Early results of a prospective study. *Clin Orthop;* (205):241–250.

13. **Tile M, Helfet DL, Kellam JF, et al.** (1995) *Comprehensive Classification of Fractures in the Pelvis and Acetabulum.* Berne: Maurice E. Müller Foundation.

14. **Helfet DL, Schmeling GJ** (1994) Management of complex acetabular fractures through single nonextensile exposures. *Clin Orthop;* (305):58–68.

15. **Alonso JE, Davila R, Bradley E** (1994) Extended iliofemoral versus triradiate approaches in management of associated acetabular fractures. *Clin Orthop;* (305):81–87.

16. **Geerts WH, Code KI, Jay RM, et al.** (1995) A prospective study of venous thromboembolism after major trauma. *N Engl J Med;* 332:1448–1449.

17. **Helfet DL, Bartlett CS, Lorich D** (1997) The use of a single limited posterior approach and reduction techniques for specific patterns of acetabular fractures. *Op Tech Orthop;* 7:196–205.

18. **Routt ML, Jr., Swiontkowski MF** (1990) Operative treatment of complex acetabular fractures. Combined anterior and posterior exposures during the same procedure. *J Bone Joint Surg [Am];* 72 (6):897–904.

19. **Tile M, Burgess A, Helfet DL, et al.** (1995) *Fractures of the Pelvis and Acetabulum.* Baltimore: Williams & Wilkins.

20. **Leenen LP, van der Werken C, Schoots F, et al.** (1993) Internal fixation of open unstable pelvic fractures. *J Trauma;* 35 (2):220–225.

21. **Bosse MJ, Poka A, Reinert CM, et al.** (1988) Heterotopic ossification as a complication of acetabular fracture. Prophylaxis with low-dose irradiation. *J Bone Joint Surg [Am];* 70 (8):1231–1237.

22. **Johnson EE, Matta JM, Mast JW, et al.** (1994) Delayed reconstruction of acetabular fractures 21–120 days following injury. *Clin Orthop;* (305):20–30.

23. **Mears DC, Rubash HE** (1983) Extensile exposure of the pelvis. *Contemp Orthop;* 6:21–31.

24. **Reinert CM, Bosse MJ, Poka A, et al.** (1988) A modified extensile exposure for the treatment of complex or malunited acetabular fractures. *J Bone Joint Surg [Am];* 70 (3):329–337.

25. **Montgomery KD, Potter HG, Helfet DL** (1995) Magnetic resonance venography to evaluate the deep venous system of the pelvis in patients who have an acetabular fracture. *J Bone Joint Surg [Am];* 77 (11):1639–1649.

6 Updates

Updates and additional references for this chapter are available online at:
http://www.aopublishing.org/PFxM/45.htm

4.6.1 Femur: proximal

Reinhard Hoffmann & Norbert P. Haas

1 Introduction

According to the Müller AO Classification (**Fig. 4.6.1-1**), fractures of the proximal femur are devided into three groups:

- Type 31-A: Extracapsular trochanteric fractures
- Type 31-B: Intracapsular, femoral neck fractures
- Type 31-C: Intracapsular, femoral head fractures

2 Trochanteric fractures (31-A)

2.1 General considerations

Trochanteric fractures are the most frequent fractures of the proximal femur and occur predominantly in geriatric patients. The early perioperative mortality is, therefore, rather high. Trochanteric fractures are always extracapsular and the vascularity of the femoral head is rarely compromised. Operative treatment is generally indicated and leads to a good clinical result in the majority of cases.

Considering different classification systems, the commonly used terms stable and unstable basically address the fact that some fractures are simple and easy to fix, while others are more complex and demanding. The Müller AO Classification subdivides trochanteric fractures into three groups. A1 fractures are simple two fragment fractures with a good support at the medial cortex. A2 fractures are multifragmentary with the medial and dorsal cortices broken at several levels, but with an intact lateral cortex. In A3 fractures the lateral cortex is also broken (reversed fracture type). If the center of the fracture line is below the transverse line at the level of the distal end of the lesser trochanter which marks the defined inferior limit of the trochanteric region, it is a subtrochanteric fracture, to be discussed in **chapter 4.6.2.**

2.2 Surgical treatment

Standard AP and axial x-rays of the proximal femur are required for evaluation of the fracture. If a proximal femur nail (PFN) is planned for an unstable fracture, the femoral shaft must be included for measurement of the width of

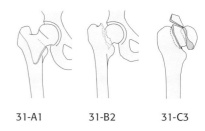

31-A1   31-B2   31-C3

Fig. 4.6.1-1: Müller AO Classification

Trochanteric fractures are the most frequent fractures of the proximal femur.

the medullary cavity and assessment of dia-physeal morphology. With excessive anterior bowing of the femur it may be impossible to use a PFN because its tip may perforate the anterior cortex of the shaft and cause a fracture.

As soon as the general condition of the patient is under control, internal fixation should be carried out. The fractures are usually reduced and fixed either on a radiolucent or a fracture table (**Fig. 4.6.1-2**). Both techniques have their advantages and disadvantages. However, intraoperative x-ray control with an image intensifier in two planes is mandatory.

Successful treatment of trochanteric frac-tures requires a mechanically stable osteo-synthesis based on proper use of implants and instrumentation. Internal fixation of these frac-tures has advanced greatly in recent decades and the different concepts of fixation overall provide good results, if applied correctly [1–5]. **The DHS (dynamic hip screw) is the im-plant of choice for stable fractures (A1, A2.1).** It allows secondary impaction of the fracture along the axis of the gliding femoral neck screw (**Fig. 4.6.1-3**), which must be placed in the center of the femoral head [6]. A position in the superior quadrant may lead to failure by pull-out, particularly in osteoporotic bone. To avoid malposition of the DHS, correct placement of the guide wire is essential and has to be checked carefully in two planes (**Video AO20156**).

For stable fracture patterns the DHS is the implant of choice.

Internal fixation should be done as early as possible.

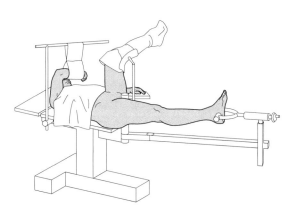

Fig. 4.6.1-2:
Positioning on a fracture table. Alternatively, a radiolucent table with simple supine positioning may be used.

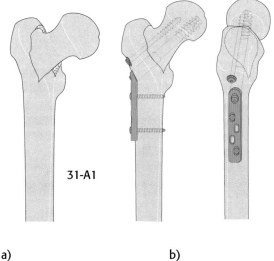

31-A1

a)   b)

Fig. 4.6.1-3:
a) Trochanteric two-fragment fracture (A1).
b) The fracture can be fixed with a DHS. The additional insertion of a cancellous bone screw provides increased rotational stability.

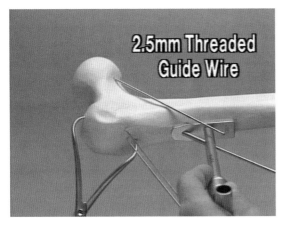

 Video AO20156

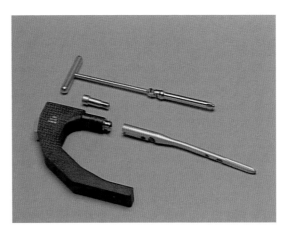

 Video AO20173B

Due to its biomechanical characteristics, the new PFN is especially suitable for highly unstable multifragmentary fractures (A2.3 and A3) (**Fig. 4.6.1-4, Fig. 4.6.1-5**). Distal locking should be static (**Video AO20173B**).

The DCS and condylar plate as well as the DHS with the trochanter-stabilizing plate (**Fig. 4.6.1-4c**) [7, 8] may be valid alternative options in selected cases. Of the three, the DCS may be easier to insert (**chapter 4.6.2**).

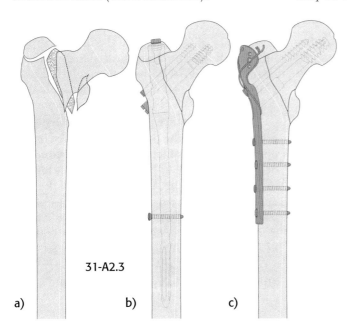

31-A2.3

a)   b)   c)

Fig. 4.6.1-4:
a) Multifragmentary trochanteric fracture (A2.3).
b) Typical unstable fracture morphology to be treated with the PFN. The shaft of the nail safely prevents lateral displacement of the fragments.
c) The fracture can also be fixed with the DHS. If the DHS is used, it should be combined with the trochanter stabilizing plate to prevent shaft medialization by lateral displacement of the fragments. The greater trochanter can additionally be fixed with small fragment screws through the plate and/or a tension band wire.

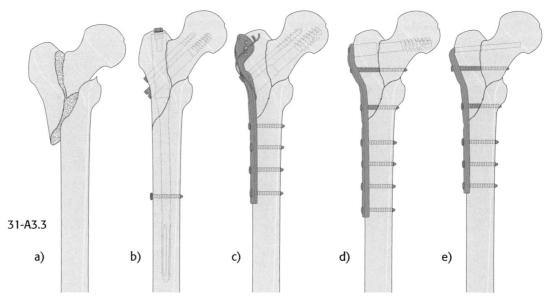

31-A3.3

a)   b)   c)   d)   e)

Fig. 4.6.1-5:
a) Reversed intertrochanteric fracture (A3.3).
b) This fracture is preferably fixed with the PFN.
c) Alternatively the DHS with an additional trochanter-stabilizing plate and a tension band wire can be used.

d/e) The fracture can also be fixed with the DCS or a condylar plate. The DCS compression screw or the blade of the plate is placed high in the proximal fragment. The plates have to be put under tension.

It is possible that a patient with pre-existing symptomatic osteoarthritis can be managed with a total hip replacement. However, primary arthroplasty in trochanteric fractures is difficult and associated with a high rate of complications. In most of these patients, initial internal fracture fixation is more appropriate. If the patient's arthritis is symptomatic after the fracture has healed, an arthroplasty can be performed more easily than in a fresh fracture.

2.3 Postoperative management

After internal fixation, mobilization of the patient starts on the first postoperative day with walking in a walker or on crutches.

After a good internal fixation the patient should be mobilized within 1–2 days postoperatively.

The rigidity of fixation should allow for almost full weight bearing since most elderly patients have difficulties with partial weight bearing. Fracture healing should be completed within 3–5 months.

If the implants are used correctly, they work properly even in the presence of marked osteoporosis. If failure of fixation or loss of reduction occurs, the choice of how to proceed is related to the type of failure, the bone quality, the age, and the requirements and expectations of the patient. In younger patients revision of the internal fixation is considered if the femoral head still has good bone stock, intact cartilage, and good blood supply. In geriatric patients an arthroplasty is usually more appropriate.

3 Femoral neck fractures (31-B)

3.1 General considerations

Old age, vertigo, dementia, tumor malignancy, and cardiopulmonary disease, as well as high-energy injuries in the younger patient are all associated with an increased risk of femoral neck fracture. **These fractures are intracapsular, which adversely affects the blood supply to the femoral head (Fig. 4.6.1-6).** The severity of the damage to the crucial lateral epiphyseal artery depends mainly on the extent of displacement of the fragments. Early anatomical reduction, as well as stable internal fixation of the fractures are associated with a lower rate of avascular necrosis of the femoral head [9, 10]. The increased intracapsular pressure from the fracture hematoma may occlude venous drainage of the capsular vessels and also decrease the arteriolar flow in the femoral neck.

The intracapsular hematoma may be evacuated via capsulotomy [10–13]. Open reduction and capsulotomy also facilitate anatomical reduction under direct vision. The capsule should be left open. The vitality of the head may be assessed intraoperatively by drilling holes with a 2 mm drill bit before reduction. **If preservation of the femoral head of displaced fractures is considered, internal fixation should be carried out as soon as the patient is medically stable.** To enable follow-up MRI studies for femoral-head vitality, the use of titanium implants is advisable.

In cases where immediate intervention is not possible, needle aspiration of the intra-articular hematoma may be performed. The hip should be kept in a semi-flexed and externally rotated position. Lateral or basicervical femoral neck fractures (B2.1) in children or elderly adults are partially extracapsular and the femoral head vitality may be jeopardized by the intracapsular hematoma rather than by the disruption of the blood supply to the head.

Open reduction and internal fixation of neck fractures must be performed within hours after the injury.

Femoral neck fractures are at risk due to vulnerable blood supply.

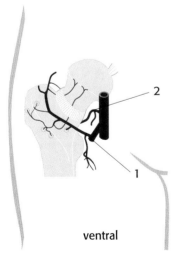 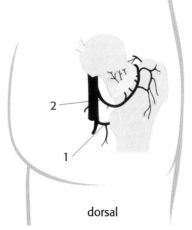

Fig. 4.6.1-6: The blood supply of the femoral head.
Most of the blood supply of the femoral head comes from the medial circumflex artery (1), which in the trochanteric fossa gives rise to three or four branches, the retinacular vessels. These run posteriorly and superiorly along the neck in a synovial reflection until they reach the cartilaginous border of the head. The obturator artery gives rise to the vessels within the ligamentum teres. An ascending branch of the lateral circumflex femoral artery (2) supplies the greater trochanter and forms branches with the medial femoral circumflex artery.

ventral

dorsal

3.2 Surgical treatment

X-rays in two planes should be obtained in all cases. Retroversion of the head and posterior comminution can easily be evaluated by a cross-table lateral view. Undisplaced or valgus impaction subcapital fractures (B1), the so-called **abduction fractures, may be stable enough for non-operative treatment**. The stability of the fracture should be checked under image intensifier and regularly monitored thereafter. However, secondary displacement does occur and increases the risk of head necrosis. Therefore, internal fixation is strongly recommended for these fractures, particularly in younger individuals and active elderly patients.

In unstable and displaced femoral neck fractures the choice of treatment depends mainly on the general and biological conditions of the patient. A reasonable treatment algorithm should address the age and the activity level, the bone density, additional diseases, the estimated life expectancy, and the compliance of the patient [10]. Patients who are less than 65 years old and do not have a chronic illness should have urgent open reduction and internal fixation if medically stable. Patients who are 75–80 years old should have prosthetic replacement. **Internal fixation is the treatment of choice for patients with high functional demands and a good bone stock.** In those who have low functional demands, chronic illness, severe osteoporosis, or who are non-compliant, a bipolar or total hip arthroplasty is recommended. Patients of any age with severe chronic illness or a limited life expectancy should be managed with a cemented prosthesis. With a life expectancy of less than one year a unipolar prosthesis can be used. In general, the biological rather than the chronological age should determine the management.

The same principles apply for polytrauma patients, where the fixation of a displaced femoral neck fracture must have a high priority in the management protocol. When a prosthetic replacement is indicated, this can be done within the first 24 hours after stabilizing the patient's general condition to reduce postoperative morbidity.

Closed reduction can usually be obtained with traction and internal rotation under image intensifier. In cases that do not reduce easily, repeated and vigorous attempts must be avoided and open reduction is indicated. With the patient in a supine position, a lateral approach to the hip is chosen and an anterior capsulotomy is performed. The femoral head, which is usually displaced posteriorly and inferiorly, is carefully disimpacted by additional abduction of the leg or by lateral traction with a bone hook. After reduction this is secured with one or two 2.0 mm K-wires. In young patients we aim for anatomical alignment of the fragments; in elderly patients with osteoporosis, however, the fractures may also be impacted in a slightly valgus position. Correct reduction is verified with the image intensifier in two planes.

The crucial element for fracture fixation and the choice of implant is the quality of bone. Any fixation method used in these critical fractures should be safe and easy to apply. With regard to complications and outcome, the DHS has proved to be superior to fixation by screws only or by angled blade plates [14] (**Fig. 4.6.1-7**). To achieve rotational stability and good buttressing at the fracture site, an additional screw cranial to the DHS should be inserted, especially in case of marked dorsal fragmentation. An angled blade plate 130° may also be used, but the technique is more demanding because good fragment contact has to be obtained and fracture distraction must be avoided especially

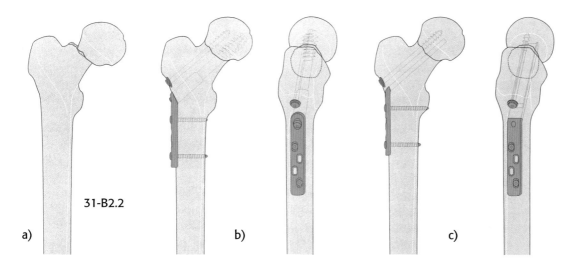

31-B2.2

a)

b)

c)

Fig. 4.6.1-7: a) Displaced femoral neck fracture (31-B2.2).
b) The fragments have been reduced and impacted with slight over-correction into valgus and without retro-version. Fixation with the DHS plate 135° and 4-hole side plate. Alternatively a 2-hole plate could have been used. An additional, cancellous bone screw was inserted in parallel to prevent rotation of the head fragment. The thread of this screw should engage fully in the head fragment. As some sintering of the fracture may occur during weight bearing, some backing out of the screws is possible.
c) The same fracture can also be treated with an angled blade plate 130° with one or two screws. An additional cancellous bone screw may be inserted to increase the initial stability of the fixation, to close the fracture gap, and put it under compression intraoperatively. The blade of the plate should be inserted into the lower half of the head.

in the young patient with dense cancellous bone. An additional compression screw may be implanted to ensure good fragment contact from the outset. With good bone quality three 7.0 or 7.3 mm cannulated cancellous bone screws can be used for fragment fixation (**Fig. 4.6.1-8**). These should be inserted parallel to each other with the help of the aiming device to allow for gliding and secondary impaction of the fracture.

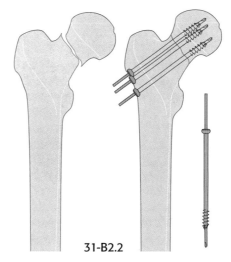

31-B2.2

Fig. 4.6.1-8: A similar fracture treated with three large 7.0 or 7.3 mm cancellous bone screws. The screws should run parallel and the threads of all screws must engage completely in the head fragment. Cannulated screws facilitate correct placement and may even be inserted percutaneously if closed reduction can be obtained.

Care must be taken that the threads of all three screws are placed well within the head fragment and do not cross the fracture line, as only then compression can be exerted. The screws must be tightened carefully and repeatedly during the procedure (**Video AO00087**). (If a fracture table is used, traction must be released.) This procedure can also be performed percutaneously through stab incisions.

In the rare instance of a vertical shear fracture that may be difficult to reduce, a valgus osteotomy and fixation with an angled blade plate 120° may be considered (**Fig. 4.6.1-9**). Although still controversial, if a femoral head arthroplasty is considered, a cemented bipolar prosthesis is preferable to a unipolar prosthesis because acetabular abrasion and the dislocation rate seems lower [**10, 15**]. In case of limited life expectancy, in debilitated patients or those with minimum activity, the use of a unipolar prosthesis is recommended. For very active patients with pre-existing osteoarthritis a total hip replacement is more appropriate (**Fig. 4.6.1-10**). In joint replacement after femoral neck fractures the posterior capsule should be preserved in order to avoid secondary dislocation of the hip.

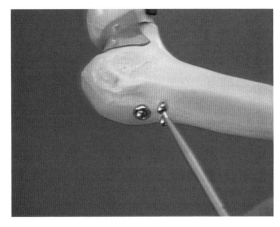

Video AO00087

3.3 Postoperative management

Depending on the strength of fixation achieved, the patient can be mobilized within 24 hours with partial or full weight bearing. However, it should be kept in mind that in elderly patients partial weight bearing may be difficult. They need either reliable internal fixation or a prosthetic replacement that allows for immediate full weight bearing.

If failure of fixation or loss of reduction should occur, the choice of how to proceed is

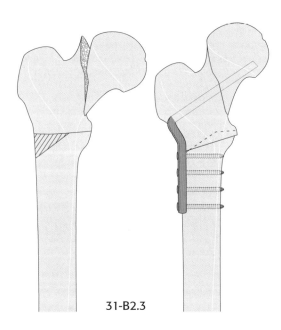

31-B2.3

Fig. 4.6.1-9: In the presence of a vertical fracture plane, the shearing forces can be transformed into compressive forces by performing an intertrochanteric valgus osteotomy of some 30–40° and fixation with the 120° double angled blade plate.

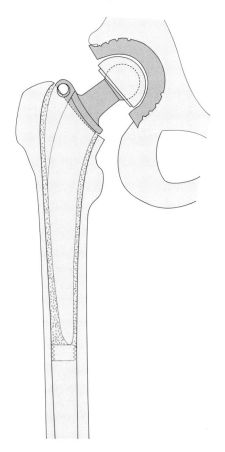

Fig. 4.6.1-10: In geriatric patients with dislocated femoral neck fractures and limited life expectancy, a femoral head prosthesis, a bipolar prosthesis, or a total hip prosthesis are preferred treatment options.

bipolar or total hip arthroplasty is the procedure of choice. If a femoral head necrosis develops in younger patients and the area of head collapse involves less than 50% of the head, an intertrochanteric flexion osteotomy may provide relief of pain and relatively good function. Hip fusion is an alternative, but is technically more difficult in the presence of avascular bone; total hip replacement may be a preferable solution.

4 Femoral head fractures (31-C)

4.1 General considerations

A substantial force is required to produce a fracture of the femoral head. Traumatic hip joint dislocations or fracture dislocations are often associated. Therefore, femoral head or Pipkin fractures commonly represent just one aspect of a combined and most serious lesion of the hip joint. Additional fractures of the femoral neck and acetabulum are quite frequent. The injury mostly occurs in motor vehicle collisions and is often accompanied by multiple trauma or other injuries, in particular to the lower extremity. One plain AP x-ray of the pelvis is mandatory to rule out a dislocation or a fracture of the hip. If the hip is dislocated, reduction of the dislocated femoral head must be performed as urgently as the patient's condition permits. This is best achieved under general anesthesia with muscle relaxation. If there is a femoral head fracture, primary open reduction with internal fixation is usually appropriate. After reduction, the joint stability has to be examined and a standard AP view of the pelvis is taken

related to the type of failure, the bone quality, the age, and the requirements of the patient. In younger patients, revision of the internal fixation is considered if the head appears viable. With a non-union or varus deformity a valgus osteotomy may be indicated. In patients with poor bone quality and limited functional demands a

under some axial load and with the legs slightly abducted. The width and congruency of the joint space are compared with the opposite side. On the injured side, interposed fragments, a torn and inverted labrum, or a folded ligamentum teres may cause the joint space to appear wider. Additional CT scans of the hip will permit assessment of impaction or flake fractures of the femoral head. Simultaneously, the reduction can be checked, loose bodies localized, and the acetabulum may be evaluated for a precise classification (see **Fig. 4.6.1-1**). Biplanar CT scan reconstructions can be especially helpful in demonstrating the femoral head alignment in the weight-bearing area and may reveal prognostically important bone bruises that cannot be diagnosed otherwise.

Small fragments may be removed while larger ones must be reduced and fixed.

4.2 Surgical treatment

Small fragments (< 1 cm^2) below the round ligament do not need anatomical reduction unless they interfere with joint motion. If they do, **small fragments may be removed while larger ones must be reduced and fixed** with small fragment screws (**Fig. 4.6.1-11**). Since these fragments are usually still attached to the inferior joint capsule, care has to be taken to preserve this potential vascular supply during internal fixation. Surgery is clearly indicated in cases where loose fragments or soft tissues are interposed in the joint, otherwise rapid joint destruction will follow. Special attention has to be paid on CT scans to a (usually) small bone fragment within the fossa of the acetabulum.

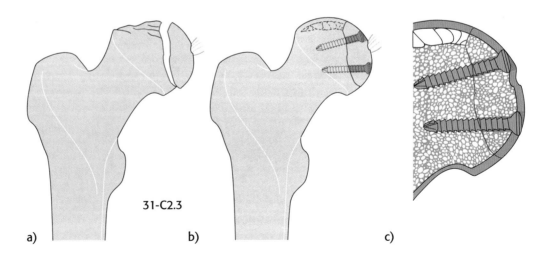

31-C2.3

a)   b)   c)

Fig. 4.6.1-11: Split depression fracture (C2.3) of the femoral head. Elevation of impacted area, cancellous bone graft, and transchondral screw fixation of the split fragment.

This fragment is often firmly attached to the ligamentum teres, as it had been avulsed from the femoral head and therefore does not dislocate into the true joint space. If no other indication for surgery exists, it can be left untouched. The position of this fragment in the fossa can easily be monitored by a CT scan after one week.

Osteochondral fragments cranial to the ligamentum teres are usually part of the weight-bearing surface of the femoral head (C1.3, C3.1), which makes anatomical reduction mandatory. Even if apparently reduced after closed reduction, fragment instability usually persists, thus open reduction and internal fixation is indicated. Taking care to preserve the vascular supply, the fragment is fixed with 3.5 or 2.7 mm small fragment screws or with the 3.0 mm cannulated screw with a threaded washer system. The screw heads should be buried beneath the level of the cartilage. Any additional impaction fracture of the head can be elevated and the defect filled with autogenous cancellous bone. The same procedure may be considered for fractures with significant depression (C2.1–C2.3).

Split fractures combined with a femoral neck fracture (C3.2, C3.3) have the worst prognosis because in most of the cases the main fragment of the femoral head loses its vascular supply [16]. This combination is therefore best treated with a primary total joint replacement or, in selected cases, by an arthrodesis. Some information about the vascularity of the main head fragment may be obtained by making drill holes, which may produce bleeding. This test is, however, unreliable. If there is hope that the vascular supply is still intact, the femoral neck fracture can be fixed with 6.5 or 7.0 mm cancellous bone screws before the head fracture is fixed. In young patients especially, the bias should be

towards preserving the joint. Titanium implants may be used to facilitate MRI follow-up studies for femoral head vitality [17].

The presence of an acetabular fracture determines the further management according to the established principles of treatment for such injuries (see **chapter 4.5**).

If needed, **open reduction and internal fixation must be carried out as soon as the general condition of the patient permits.** If the joint remains unstable after emergency reduction or if loose fragments are trapped within the joint space but immediate surgery is not yet possible, the leg must be put in femoral skeletal traction until surgery can be performed.

Isolated split fractures of the head can be managed through an anterior or posterior approach to the hip joint. If a femoral neck or acetabular fracture needs to be fixed at the same time, the injury determines the choice of the surgical approach. The advantages of the anterior Smith-Petersen approach are a significant decrease in operative time and blood loss, as well as an improved exposure for the fixation of the small fragments. Through the anterior approach split fractures can be fixed directly with screws. The attachment of the fragments to the joint capsule or ligamentum teres can be preserved. With the posterior Kocher-Langenbeck approach visual control of exact reduction is difficult and the fixation of the fragment usually has to be done indirectly if the vascularity is to be preserved. Any attempt at an anatomical fragment fixation through the posterior approach demands redislocation of the femoral head and detachment of the fragment from its capsular or ligamentous attachments. This, of course, destroys the remaining blood supply. However, according to some reports, the long-term results with the anterior approach may be poorer because it provokes more heterotopic ossification

Type C femoral head fractures are serious injuries requiring urgent treatment.

Osteochondral fragments cranial to the ligamentum teres are usually part of the weight-bearing surface, making anatomical reduction mandatory.

Fig. 4.6.1-12:
a) Unstable intertrochanteric A3 fracture with diaphyseal extension in a 55-year-old woman after skiing accident.
b) Postoperative views after emergency stabilization with long proximal femoral nail (PFN). Full weight bearing within 6 weeks and complete restitution of function.
c) One-year follow-up.

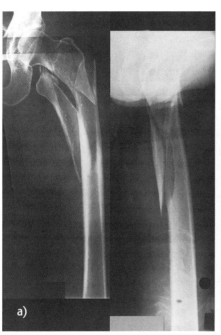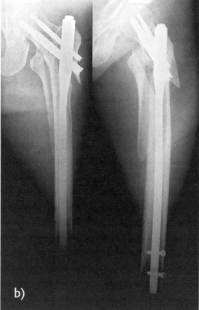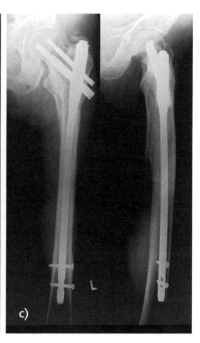

The outcome of these injuries remains unpredictable even after anatomical joint restoration.

compared to the posterior approach [18]. Another option may be to fix minimally displaced split fractures with cannulated screws through a lateral approach or even percutaneously. In these instances, CT-guided imaging techniques may prove indispensable.

4.3 Postoperative management

This includes early mobilization, CPM, partial weight bearing for 6–12 weeks, according to the type of injury, and administration of indomethacin as prophylaxis of heterotopic ossification [18]. In patients with a high risk of heterotopic ossification (e.g., a polytrauma patient with head injury plus anterior approach) an additional single dose of radiation to the hip may be considered.

The outcome of these injuries remains unpredictable for the individual patient even after anatomical joint restoration. The incidence of posttraumatic arthrosis or avascular femoral head necrosis is determined by the initial damage caused to the cartilage and the subchondral bone by the impact of trauma. In severe impaction fractures of the femoral head or, if symptomatic partial head necrosis develops, intertrochanteric osteotomy may be indicated. In complete avascular head necrosis, or painful arthrosis, a total joint replacement or a hip arthrodesis are secondary treatment options.

5 Bibliography

1. **Bridle SH, Patel AD, Bircher M, et al.** (1991) Fixation of intertrochanteric fractures of the femur. A randomised prospective comparison of the gamma nail and the dynamic hip screw. *J Bone Joint Surg [Br];* 73 (2):330–334.

2. **Davis TR, Sher JL, Horsman A, et al.** (1990) Intertrochanteric femoral fractures. Mechanical failure after internal fixation. *J Bone Joint Surg [Br];* 72 (1):26–31.

3. **Larsson S, Friberg S, Hansson LI** (1990) Trochanteric fractures. Influence of reduction and implant position on impaction and complications. *Clin Orthop;* (259):130–139.

4. **Leung KS, So WS, Shen WY, et al.** (1992) Gamma nails and dynamic hip screws for peritrochanteric fractures. A randomised prospective study in elderly patients. *J Bone Joint Surg [Br];* 74 (3):345–351.

5. **O'Brien PJ, Meek RN, Blachut PA, et al.** (1995) Fixation of intertrochanteric hip fractures: gamma nail versus dynamic hip screw. A randomized, prospective study. *Can J Surg;* 38 (6):516–520.

6. **Baumgaertner MR, Curtin SL, Lindskog DM, et al.** (1995) The value of the tip-apex distance in predicting failure of fixation of peritrochanteric fractures of the hip. *J Bone Joint Surg [Am];* 77 (7):1058–1064.

7. **Babst R, Martinet O, Renner N, et al.** (1993) [The DHS (dynamic hip screw) buttress plate in the management of unstable proximal femoral fractures]. *Schweiz Med Wochenschr;* 123 (13):566–568.

8. **David A, Hüfner T, Lewandrowski KU, et al.** (1996) [The dynamic hip screw with support plate—a reliable osteosynthesis for highly unstable "reverse" trochanteric fractures?]. *Chirurg;* 67 (11):1166–1173.

9. **Pauwels F** (1935) Der Schenkelhalsbruch, ein mechanisches Problem. Grundlagen des Heilungsvorganges, Prognose und kausale Therapie. *Z Orthop Chir;* 6 (Suppl 3).

10. **Swiontkowski MF** (1994) Intracapsular fractures of the hip. *J Bone Joint Surg [Am];* 76 (1):129–138.

11. **Bonnaire F, Gotschin U, Kuner EH** (1992) [Early and late results of 200 DHS osteosyntheses in the reconstruction of pertrochanteric femoral fractures]. *Unfallchirurg;* 95 (5):246–253.

12. **Gerber C, Strehle J, Ganz R** (1993) The treatment of fractures of the femoral neck. *Clin Orthop;* (292):77–86.

13. **Manninger J, Kazar G, Fekete G, et al.** (1989) Significance of urgent (within 6h) internal fixation in the management of fractures of the neck of the femur. *Injury;* 20 (2):101–105.

14. **Bonnaire F, Kuner EH, Lorz W** (1995) [Femoral neck fractures in adults: joint sparing operations. II. The significance of surgical timing and implant for development of aseptic femur head necrosis]. *Unfallchirurg;* 98 (5):259-264.

15. **Bray TJ, Smith-Hoefer E, Hooper A, et al.** (1988) The displaced femoral neck fracture. Internal fixation versus bipolar endoprosthesis. Results of a prospective, randomized comparison. *Clin Orthop;* (230):127–140.

16. **Pipkin G** (1957) Treatment of grade IV fracture dislocation of the hip. A review. *J Bone Joint Surg [Am]*; 39:1027–1042.

17. **Stockenhuber N, Schweighofer F, Seibert FJ** (1994) [Diagnosis, therapy and prognosis of Pipkin fractures (femur head dislocation fractures)]. *Chirurg*; 65 (11):976–981; discussion 981–982.

18. **Dreinhofer KE, Schwarzkopf SR, Haas NP, et al.** (1996) [Femur head dislocation fractures. Long-term outcome of conservative and surgical therapy]. *Unfallchirurg*; 99 (6):400–409.

6 Updates

Updates and additional references for this chapter are available online at:
http://www.aopublishing.org/PFxM/461.htm

4.6.2 Femur: shaft (incl. subtrochanteric)

Dankward Höntzsch

1 Diagnosis

The diagnosis of femoral shaft fractures, including subtrochanteric fractures, is made straightforward by the presence of such clinical signs as axial deviation, shortening, abnormal function, and pain.

An assessment of soft-tissue damage is an integrated part of every clinical examination. Open fractures are less common because of the dense soft-tissue cover. Lacerations of the muscle layers can be present and subcutaneous degloving injuries should not be overlooked despite an intact integument. Assessment of neurovascular functions is mandatory (see **chapter 2.1**).

Standard x-ray examinations consist of views in two planes. Adjacent joints must be included so that ipsilateral fractures of the femoral neck or tibial head are not missed. A femur fracture in a young individual is always the consequence of a considerable trauma and may involve other injuries. More extensive examinations are required in the polytrauma patient or if concomitant injuries to the pelvis, spine, or knee joint are suspected, since such additional injuries will affect the treatment concept [1] (see **chapter 5.3**).

2 Classification

(Fig. 4.6.2-1)

Classification must take the fracture and the soft-tissue damage into account (see **chapter 1.4**). In the Müller AO Classification the femoral shaft is identified by the number 32 [2]. This includes the subtrochanteric region (distal to lesser trochanter) and extends to the supracondylar area.

3 Anatomy

The greater trochanter, the lateral femoral condyle, the patella, and the knee-joint space are the main landmarks of the femur. **The most important soft-tissue structures on the lateral aspect are the fascia lata, the iliotibial tract, and the vastus lateralis muscle; these act as tension band.** Depending on the choice of operative approach, the vastus lateralis muscle is retracted ventrally away from the linea aspera or is just gently elevated and "tunneled" for minimally invasive fixation techniques.

In most indirect procedures additional landmarks on the pelvis and tibia are important in order to evaluate the axis, rotation, and length of the limb. In complex fractures the contralateral limb should be draped for intraoperative comparison.

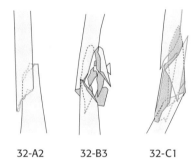

32-A2   32-B3   32-C1

Fig. 4.6.2-1: Müller AO Classification

Iliotibial tract and fascia lata act as tension band.

Main goals: correct length and rotation as well as axial alignment.

Rotation is easier to evaluate if the hip and knee joints are so draped that they can be bent to at least 60° during the operation.

4 Preoperative planning

Preoperative planning is not efficient for simple fractures, but complex patterns require careful analysis. Good x-rays in two planes are needed. Fractures in the proximal shaft or in the sub-trochanteric region are often highly unstable and painful. It is recommended to take lateral x-rays from the opposite side by flexing the intact hip joint to 90° and directing the x-ray beam horizontally. For femoral shaft and proximal femoral fractures, which are to be fixed by intramedullary nailing, good imaging of the pelvis and proximal end of the bone are essential to exclude hidden fractures in the trochanteric/femoral neck region. Once good x-rays are available preoperative planning can start (see **chapter 2.4**). In complex fractures it may be helpful to have an AP x-ray of the contra-lateral side for comparison.

Correct length and axial alignment (ante-recurvatum deformity, varus and valgus, as well as rotation) are the principal objectives. In simple fractures, more or less anatomical reduction will guarantee correct length. Varus, valgus, and ante-recurvation have to be assessed radiographically and clinically (see **chapter 3.3.1**).

Rotation is easier to evaluate if the hip and knee joints are so draped that they can be bent to at least 60° during the operation.

Fig. 4.6.2-2: Positioning options for fixation of femoral shaft and subtrochanteric fractures. Viewing the normal limb permits comparison when overcoming difficulties with length, rotation, and axial displacements.
a) Normal supine position.
b) Lateral decubitus on the normal table for intramedullary nailing (rare today).
c) Fracture table for intramedullary nailing of shaft and proximal femoral fracture in the supine position.
d) Position on the fracture table for nailing in lateral decubitus (more complicated).

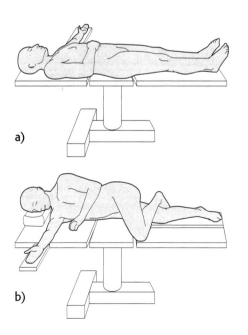
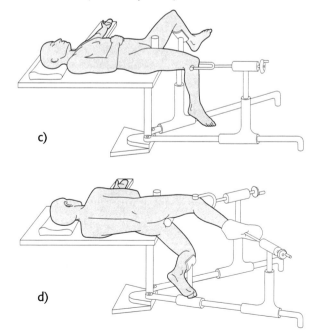

a)

b)

c)

d)

4.1 Positioning and reduction

Depending on the preference and experience of the surgeon, the patient is operated on an ordinary radiolucent table or on a fracture table in supine or lateral position. For intramedullary nailing the proximal end of the femur must be reached by the image intensifier in two planes (**Fig. 4.6.2-2**).

Closed reduction of femoral shaft fractures can be achieved by manual traction or distraction using the fracture table or distractor (**Fig. 4.6.2-3**). With the distactor, and depending on the level of the fracture, abduction or adduction may be applied relatively simply. In intramedullary nailing a short nail may be used as a "joystick" to manipulate the proximal fragment (see **chapter 3.3.1**). Complex fractures can be reduced by ligamentotaxis.

4.2 Approaches

For antegrade femoral nailing, a relatively small (3–5 cm) longitudinal incision placed approximately 12–15 cm proximal to the tip of the greater trochanter is usually sufficient (see **Fig. 3.3.1-3** and **Video 3.3.1-3**). The exact entry point—which varies according to the nail designs—can be exposed by blunt dissection down to the tip of

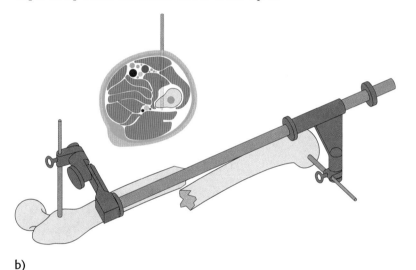

a)
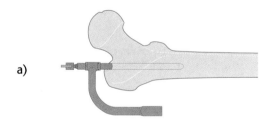

b)

Fig. 4.6.2-3: Application of the distractor in femoral shaft fractures with well-placed Schanz screws, especially on the distal and proximal sides.
a) "Dummy nail" with handle for joystick reduction maneuvers or to mount aiming device for Schanz screw insertion.
b) The proximal Schanz screw is inserted with the help of a special aiming device for later nailing, so as not to interfere with the nail. The cross-section demonstrates that with this technique the femoral neurovascular structures are not violated.
c) The two Schanz screws for the distractor may also be placed in the same frontal plane.

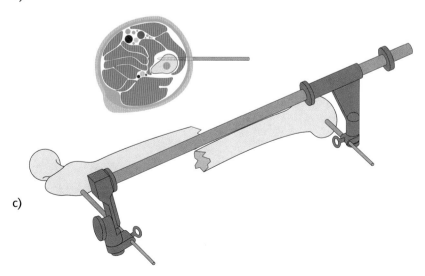

c)

the greater trochanter (**Fig. 4.6.2-4**). For conventional antegrade locked nailing of mid-third and distal diaphyseal fractures, it is important to use flouroscopy to align the proximal starting point in two planes with the medullary canal of the femur.

For open plating the skin incision lies on the lateral side of the thigh between the greater trochanter and the lateral femoral condyle. The fascia lata is split, the vastus lateralis muscle is retracted along the intermuscular septum down to the linea aspera and the perforating vessels are preserved if possible (**Fig. 4.6.2-5**).

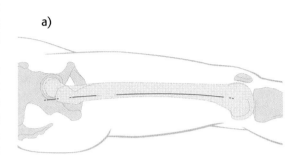

a)

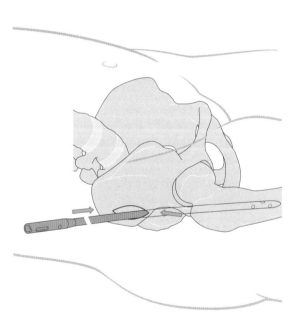

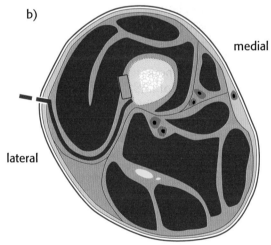

b)

medial

lateral

Fig. 4.6.2-5:
a) The standard approach to the femoral shaft is by a straight incision on the lateral side of the thigh.
b) Deep dissection follows the intermuscular septum down to the linea aspera. We expose as little bone as is required for plate placement in order to preserve the vacularitity of the fragments.

Fig. 4.6.2-4: Proximal approach to the greater trochanter in the line of the medullary canal. Usually a short (3–5 cm) incision 8–10 cm proximal to the tip of the greater trochanter is sufficient.

For plating with less invasive exposures the plate entry point is usually at the lateral femoral condyle, where a 3–5 cm long incision is placed anterolaterally. Once the fracture has been indirectly reduced (femoral distractor), the submuscular route for plate insertion along the shaft of the femur is prepared with an elevator. Fixation screws are introduced via small separate incisions.

4.3   Choice of implant

The choice of implant depends on a number of factors:

- Fracture location and configuration.
- Size of the medullary canal, presence of other implants (prosthesis).
- Soft-tissue conditions (see **chapter 1.5**).
- Condition of the patient (polytrauma, ISS, see **chapters 2.1** and **5.3**).
- Personal experience and preference.
- Availability of implants, instruments, and intraoperative imaging.

For subtrochanteric fractures, the choice is between condylar plates, dynamic condylar screws (DCS), proximal femoral nails (PFN) [**3**], and solid femoral nails (UFN) using the spiral blade device [**4**]. Diaphyseal fractures are the domain of intramedullary nailing [**5**, **6**]. Simple fractures (type A and B) of the mid-third are preferably fixed with the universal or the new cannulated nail after reaming of the canal and with interlocking technique [**5**], while complex type C fractures and fractures of the proximal and distal third may be stabilized with the solid or cannulated intramedullary nail. In the rare event of plating of the femur we use the broad LC-DCP 4.5, the long condylar plates, or the dynamic condylar screw (**Fig 4.6.2-6**).

In case of severe soft-tissue injury, whether open or closed [**2**, **7**, **8**], external fixation or unreamed or minimally reamed intramedullary nailing are recommended. As the external fixator causes the least local and systemic interference, it is recommended for fracture fixation in the severely polytraumatized patient with an ISS greater than 40 (see **chapter 5.3**). Due to the risk of pin-track infection, conversion to a more stable internal fixation device should be performed within 1–2 weeks.

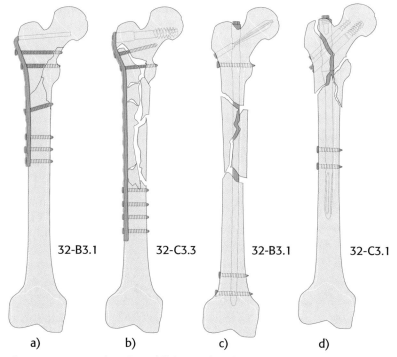

32-B3.1   32-C3.3   32-B3.1   32-C3.1

a)   b)   c)   d)

Fig. 4.6.2-6: Four options for stabilizing a subtrochanteric fracture:
a) 95° angled blade plate, with anatomical reconstruction and rigid fixation.
b) Dynamic condylar screw (DCS) bridging the complex fracture area. The side plate can be introduced with a tunneling technique.
c) Femoral nail with spiral blade (UFN).
d) Proximal femoral nail (PFN) introduced from the tip of the trochanter gives a very stable construct. For more complex 32-B3.1 configurations, especially with a more distal segmentation, the long PFN offers an alternative to the UFN with spiral blade.

5 Surgical treatment— tricks and hints

5.1 Osteosynthesis for subtrochanteric fractures

Plate

Today, indirect reduction procedures and less invasive operative techniques are preferred because these methods cause less damage to the blood supply to the fragments and thus contribute positively to the healing process. Bone grafting, even in complex multifragmented fractures, will rarely be needed [9].

The advantages, disadvantages, and technical feasibility must be carefully evaluated. In either case, **simple fractures can be anatomically reduced and stably fixed by the principles of absolute stability with interfragmentary compression. The multifragmentary fracture is best handled by indirect reduction and bridge plating.** If in doubt, leave the lag screw out. The position of the blade for the condylar plate is prepared with the seating chisel. The position of the DCS compression screw is prepared with a special guide wire (see **chapter 4.6.1**).

In either case, the position is checked on the image intensifier in anteroposterior and lateral views. Axial monitoring is achieved either with the laterally placed image intensifier or the Lauenstein technique. Once the seating chisel and/or guide wire has been correctly positioned, the next steps can start, for example, length measurement of the condylar plate, insertion of the condylar blade, and preparation of the path for the dynamic compression screw using the special reamer.

Although bridge plating with minimal access can be done with the plates mentioned, a new device, the LISS (less invasive stabilization system), has been developed, featuring screws that are locked in a plate at a fixed angle (see **chapter 3.4**).

Proximal femoral nail (PFN)

Alternatively, subtrochanteric fractures can be treated with the proximal femoral nail (PFN) (**Video AO20173B**), but also with the solid femoral nail (UFN) with a spiral blade [10] (**Video AO20154**) (see **chapter 3.3.1**). The PFN is most suitable in unstable fracture patterns or in case of poor bone stock (see **chapter 4.6.1, Fig. 4.6.1-5b**).

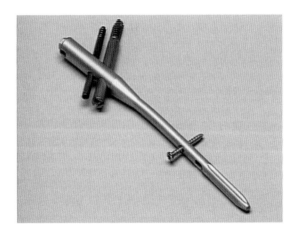

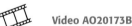 Video AO20173B

Reduce simple fractures anatomically and fix rigidly; complex fractures are aligned and bridged.

5.2 Diaphyseal fractures

The femoral shaft is the domain of the intra-medullary nail with or without reaming of the medullary cavity (**Fig. 4.6.2-7a**) (see **chapter 3.3.1**).

The solid femoral nail can be applied in conventional or in locking technique. The un-reamed femoral nail must always be locked proximally and distally (**Video AO20153a/b**).

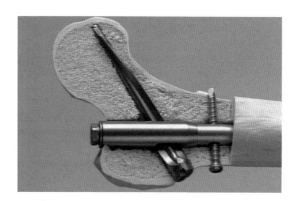

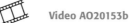 Video AO20154

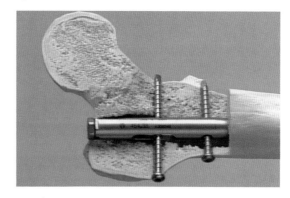

Video AO20153a

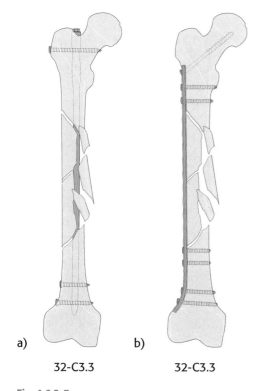

a)   b)

32-C3.3   32-C3.3

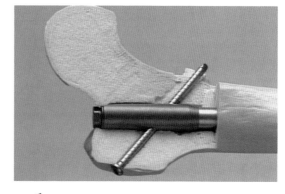

Video AO20153b

Fig. 4.6.2-7:
a) For complex, multifragmented diaphyseal fractures of the femur, the locked intramedullary nail reamed, unreamed, or cannulated is the implant of choice.
b) If for any reason nailing cannot be performed, a bridge plate (broad DCP 4.5 or broad LC-DCP 4.5) can be used—preferably after indirect reduction and using the tunneling technique.

In addition to nailing of femoral shaft fractures, plate osteosynthesis is also utilized for special indications, for example, ipsilateral femoral shaft and femoral neck fractures, polytrauma, and correction osteotomy. Plate osteosynthesis can be performed as an open or semi-closed technique (**Fig. 4.6.2-7b**) (see **chapter 3.3.2**).

6 Aftercare

After internal fixation of the proximal femur, the hip joint should be kept extended to prevent flexion contractures while, following fixation of a diaphyseal fracture, a 90°–90° position may be helpful to prevent contracture and facilitate knee motion. After osteosynthesis of the distal femur, flexion of the knee joint between 30–60° on a CPM-machine is advantageous and will ease later mobilization (see also **chapter 5.7**).

Physiotherapy should start immediately, no later than on the second postoperative day.

Ambulation is generally started after a few days, depending on the overall condition of the patient, concomitant injuries, and patient compliance. Partial weight bearing (10–15 kg) should be possible in practically all situations, provided the patient can follow instructions. Increasing the load depends on the fracture pattern and the type of fixation and must be prescribed by the surgeon on an individual basis.

Physiotherapy must start immediately.

7 Pitfalls and complications

7.1 Intraoperative intramedullary nailing

The pitfalls and complications of intramedullary nailing are described in detail in **chapter 3.3.1**. The nail entry point at the greater trochanter is crucial, especially for proximal or subtrochanteric fractures. The instructions for the different nail types and designs must be carefully studied and followed. Special attention in nailing must also be given to the correct rotational alignment of the fragments, as wrong alignment is probably the most frequent cause of malposition or malunion.

7.2 Plate fixation

In open plating the biggest danger lies in the devitalization of fracture fragments by attempts at anatomical reduction. Only simple fractures should be reduced precisely and fixed rigidly by interfragmentary compression (see **chapter 3.2.2**). In all other, and especially in complex situations, the fracture focus should be left untouched and bridged by a long plate [11]. The biggest challenge in subtrochanteric fractures is fatiguing of the plate, especially if there is no medial buttress within the bone. Bone grafting may become necessary to win the race between fracture healing and implant failure.

7.3 External fixator

As exact alignment of the Schanz screws is rather difficult in the femur, the modular technique with three tubes and the tube-to-tube connecting clamps should be used in order to facilitate reduction of the fracture. This also allows easy adjustments at a later time, for example, in a polytraumatized patient. For temporary fixation, such as in polytrauma, pin placement must respect a likely secondary procedure. Even in a more definitive application of an external fixator it is important not to violate the vastus lateralis muscle. In the latter situation the pin should be inserted laterally from posterior to anterior in the plane of the intermuscular septum (**Fig 4.6.2-8**) (see **chapter 3.3.3**).

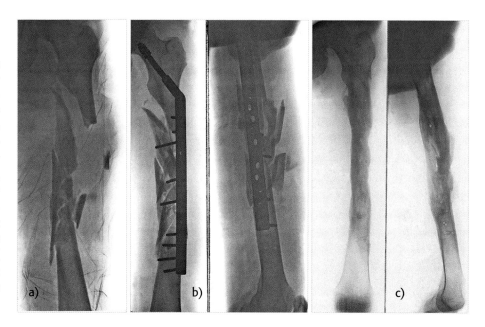

Fig. 4.6.2-9: a) Shattered proximal two thirds of left femur in a 22-year-old male after car accident. Acute compartment syndrom of thigh requiring extensive lateral release.
b) Postoperative view after minimally invasive bridge plating with longest available DHS. No attempt was made to reduce the fragments. Axial alignment by clinical judgement. Two weeks later closure of iliotibial tract and skin incision. Uneventful recovery with full weight bearing after 3 months.
c) X-ray follow-up 2 years after the injury and shortly after plate removal.

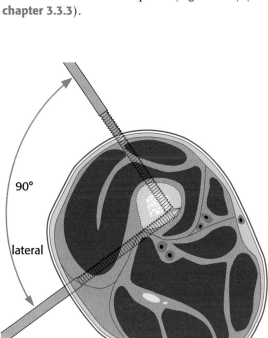

Fig. 4.6.2-8: Placement of Schanz screws in femoral fractures fixed with external fixator:
• For temporary fixation there will be little interference with later plating.
• For definitive treatment with an external fixator, for example, in children, the Schanz screws must be introduced from posterolateral along the intermuscular septum so as not to interfere with muscle movement.

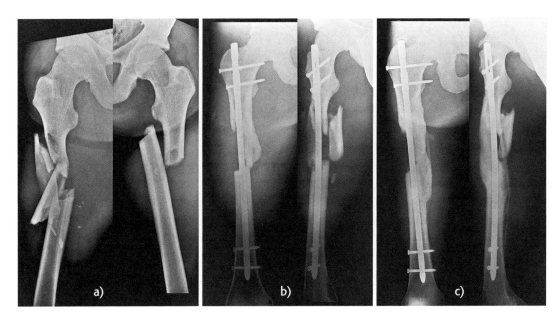

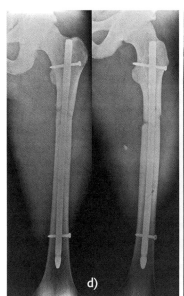

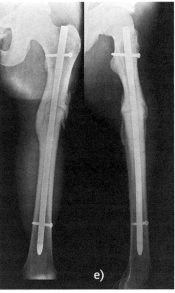

Fig. 4.6.2-10: a) Bilateral femur fractures in an 18-year-old male after motorbike accident. The right side shows a C3 subtrochanteric fracture, on the left we see an A2 shaft fracture. Both femura were stabilized shortly after the injury by locked unreamed nails (UFNs).
b) Postoperative views of the right subtrochanteric fracture after closed nailing with static locking.
c) Right side at 5 months. The patient was back to work as an apprentice laborer—no pain or limitations.
d) Postoperative views of the left femur.
e) 5-months follow-up of left side—well healed.

8 Bibliography

1. **Friedl HP, Stocker R, Czermak B, et al.** (1996) Primary fixation and delayed nailing of long bone fractures in severe trauma. *Techniques Orthop;* 11 (1):59.

2. **Müller ME, Nazarian S, Koch P, et al.** (1990) *The comprehensive classification of fractures of long bones.* Berlin Heidelberg New York: Springer-Verlag.

3. **Simmermacher RK, Bosch AM, Van der Werken C** (1999) The AO/ASIF-proximal femoral nail (PFN): a new device for the treatment of unstable proximal femoral fractures. *Injury;* 30 (5):327–332.

4. **Krettek C, Schandelmaier P, Miclau T, et al.** (1998) Techniques for control of axes, rotation and length in minimal invasive osteosynthesis. *Injury;* 29 (Suppl 2).

5. **Krettek C, Rudolf J, Schandelmaier P, et al.** (1996) Unreamed intramedullary nailing of femoral shaft fractures: operative technique and early clinical experience with standard locking option. *Injury;* 27 (4):233–254.

6. **Küntscher G** (1958) *Praxis der Marknagelung.* Wien: W. Maudrich.

7. **Gustilo RB, Mendoza RM, Williams DN** (1984) Problems in the management of type III (severe) open fractures: a new classification of type III open fractures. *J Trauma;* 24 (8):742–746.

8. **Oestern HJ, Tscherne H** (1983) [Physiopathology and classification of soft-tissue lesion]. *Hefte Unfallheilkd;* 162:1–10.

9. **Kinast C, Bolhofner BR, Mast JW, et al.** (1989) Subtrochanteric fractures of the femur. Results of treatment with the 95° condylar blade plate. *Clin Orthop;* (238):122–130.

10. **Hoffmann R, Südkamp NP, Müller CA, et al.** (1994) [Osteosynthesis of proximal femoral fractures with the modular interlocking system of unreamed AO femoral intramedullary nail. Initial clinical results]. *Unfallchirurg;* 97 (11):568–574.

11. **Heitemeyer U, Hierholzer G, Terhorst J** (1986) [Value of bridging plate osteosynthesis in multiple fragment fracture damage of the femur in a clinical comparison]. *Unfallchirurg;* 89 (12):533–538.

9 Updates

Updates and additional references for this chapter are available online at:
http://www.aopublishing.org/PFxM/462.htm

4.6.3 Femur: distal

Lothar Kinzl

1 Introduction

Fractures of the distal femur represent only 6% of all femoral fractures. They typically occur after high-energy trauma in younger patients, as well as in the elderly with osteoporotic bone. One third of the younger patients are polytraumatized and in only one fifth of the cases do distal fractures occur as an isolated injury.

There is usually considerable soft-tissue damage and almost one half of the intraarticular fractures are open injuries.

lateral condyle. The joint capsule and the strong collateral ligaments originate on the femoral condyles.

Due to the close proximity of neurovascular structures, vascular lesions are found in about 3% and nerve injuries in about 1% of distal femoral fractures.

Lesions of the menisci and osteochondral fractures can be observed in 8–12%, while there are associated fractures of the patella in approximately 15%.

Fractures of distal femur are rare, however, they often have considerable associated injuries.

2 Anatomical characteristics

In addition to the articular capsule, the insertions of tendons and ligaments at the femoral condyles contribute to the function and stability of the knee joint as a complex system of force transmission.

The gastrocnemius muscle originates at the back of the femoral condyles; the cruciate ligaments are located in the central notch, and the tendon of the popliteus muscle inserts at the

3 Clinical findings and diagnostic tools

Usually, the diagnosis of a distal femoral fracture can be made clinically. Careful examination of the neurovascular status is essential. It may be necessary to verify the patency of the popliteal artery with a Doppler ultrasound or, more accurately, by angiography. If a compartment syndrome is suspected, early measurement of the compartment pressure is advisable.

Examination of the stability of ligamentous structures prior to osteosynthesis is usually quite painful and not reliable. It should be done under anesthesia prior to surgery, and again after the fracture has been stabilized.

If multiple injuries of the lower extremity are suspected, AP and lateral x-rays of both femur and tibia must be taken as well as focused views of the knee joint. CT scans or MRI, as well as 3-D reconstructions, offer additional information but are rarely essential.

3.1 Classification of fractures

The fractures are classified as (**Fig. 4.6.3-1**):
- Extra-articular fractures (type A)
- Partial articular fractures (type B)
- Complete articular fractures (type C)
(see **chapter 1.4**)

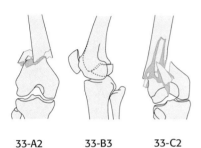

33-A2   33-B3   33-C2

Fig. 4.6.3-1: Müller AO Classification
A2 Extra-articular fracture, metaphyseal wedge
B3 Partial articular fracture, frontal ("Hoffa" fracture)
C2 Complete articular fracture, bicondylar fracture with supracondylar comminution

| 4 | **Principles of operative treatment** |

Standard treatment consists of operative reduction and fixation of the fracture.

Standard treatment consists of operative reduction and fixation of the fracture. Conservative treatment is only justified in impacted undisplaced extra-articular distal femoral fractures or in patients who are deemed inoperable. The aims of operative treatment are:
- Anatomical reconstruction of the articular surfaces,
- Restoration of rotational and axial alignment,
- Stable fixation of the condyles to the shaft of the femur,
- Early functional aftercare.

When the knee joint is fully extended, the pull of the gastrocnemius muscle on the one hand, and of the adductor magnus muscle on the other, leads to recurvation and shortening.

The traditional concept of internal fixation, which requires an extended approach to the fracture zone, is presently being challenged by a more biological, atraumatic approach with careful handling of the soft-tissue envelope. However, it is still mandatory to make a precise reconstruction of the anatomy of the condyles; this requires a direct view into the knee joint through an appropriate exposure.

4.1 Timing of the operation

In isolated injuries definitive treatment is indicated as soon as clinically feasible. In polytrauma patients the early stabilization of all long-bone fractures is decisive to provide the conditions for successful intensive-care management (see **chapter 5.3**).

In open fractures with severe soft-tissue damage, or under conditions that prevent an early definitive operation (e.g., polytrauma), transarticular bridging external fixation is a quick and effective method of stabilization.

4.2 Operative technique

4.2.1 Positioning and reduction

Anatomical reduction of the articular fracture with adequate restoration of length and alignment must be achieved before internal fixation. **When the knee joint is fully extended, the pull of the gastrocnemius muscle on the one hand, and of the adductor magnus muscle on the other, leads to recurvation and shortening.** With the knee flexed at approximately 60° over a knee support this malalignment of

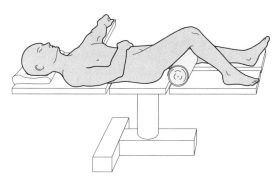

Fig. 4.6.3-2: Positioning of the leg during reduction and operation of the distal femoral fracture.

the distal femur can be corrected (**Fig. 4.6.3-2**). The shortening is best approached by manual traction or with a distractor. In case of extensive fragmentation, restoration of anatomy may be extremely difficult. Careful planning, using the contralateral side, is helpful. In some instances it may be useful to accept some shortening, particularly in osteopenic bone and complex fractures where impacted metaphyseal fragments are preferable to exact length. To facilitate reduction, Schanz screws can be anchored in larger fragments (joystick technique).

a)

Fig. 4.6.3-3: Lateral approaches to the distal femur.
a) Incision of skin and fascia.
b) Minimal detachment of the vastus lateralis muscle. Avoid denuding the bone!

b)

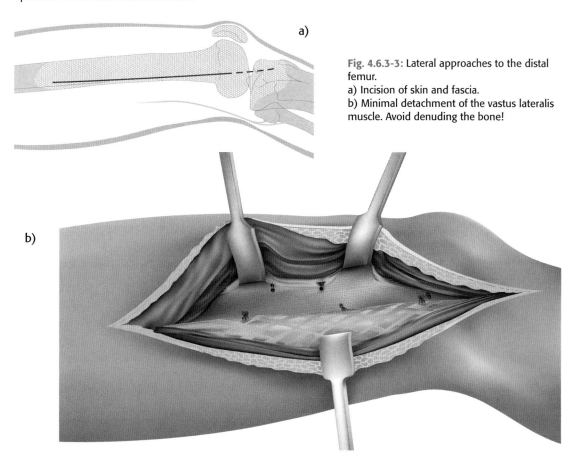

4.2.2 Approaches

The standard lateral approach (**Fig. 4.6.3-3**) simplifies anatomical reduction of the shaft and metaphyseal area, with the disadvantage of extensive soft-tissue exposure and stripping of fragments.

In case of intra-articular fragmentation, where exact reconstruction of the joint congruity is mandatory, additional small medial or lateral parapatellar incisions may be helpful. As an alternative, a more anterior parapatellar approach (**Fig. 4.6.3-4a/b**) has been described [1]. By pulling the patella medially, the reconstruction of the condylar components is facilitated. This incision may also be used for the submuscular introduction of a long bridging side plate—DCS (dynamic condylar screw) or LISS (less invasive stabilization system). The approach with detachment of the patellar ligament at the tibial tuberosity or patellar tendon Z-plasty should only be used in exceptional circumstances. Open fractures often have insufficient soft-tissue cover. If a tension-free closure of the defect is not feasible, secondary contamination of the wound must be avoided by using a skin substitute and early local or free flaps (see **chapters 5.1** and **5.2**).

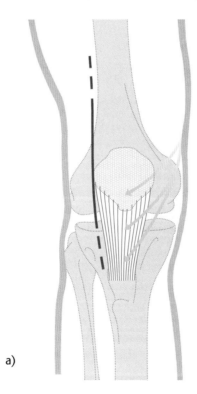

a)

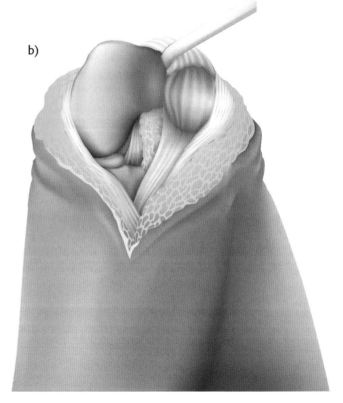

b)

Fig. 4.6.3-4:
Lateral parapatellar approach.
a) Skin incision.
b) Exposure of the femoral condyles by pulling the patella medially.

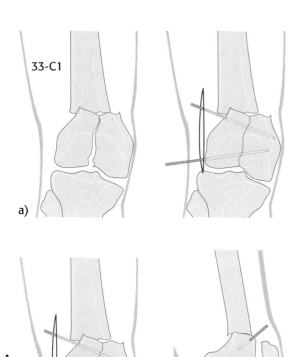

a)

33-C1

a')

A

A

A

4.3 Special fixation techniques and implants

The principle in treating intra-articular distal femur fractures lies in the reduction of the joint fragments under direct vision [1, 2] (see **chapter 2.3**). After temporary stabilization with K-wires (**Fig. 4.6.3-5**), fixation is achieved either by compressing the fragments with lag screws (usually 6.5 mm cancellous bone screws), or by bridging the defect with cortex screws (without lagging). The subsequent fixation of the articular block to the distal femur is done with additional implants, depending on the type of fracture.

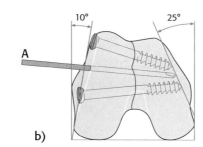

b)

A

10°   25°

Fig. 4.6.3-5: Intra-articular distal femur fractures.
a) AP view of the intra-articular 33-C1 fracture of the femoral condyles, reduction, and temporary fixation with K-wires.
a') The guide wire A for the DCS runs parallel to the joint line.
b) Frontal view of the definitive lag screw fixation of the articular fragments. The distal femur in cross section is a trapezoid. The anterior and posterior surfaces are not parallel and the medial and lateral walls are inclined. The guide wire for the DCS or blade plate enters the condyles anteriorly and runs in a posterior direction and must be at a right angle to the lateral condylar wall.
c) The position of the lag screws (one or two) and their washers must not interfere with the windows for the blade plate or DCS. These windows are in the middle third of the anterior half of the distal femur. The window of the condylar plate is 1.5 cm and the window for the DCS 2 cm proximal to the joint line.

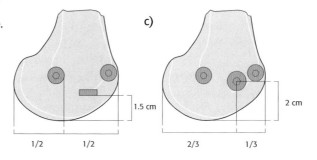

c)

1.5 cm

1/2   1/2

2 cm

2/3   1/3

4.3.1 Screw fixation

Large and small screws, which can be solid or cannulated, are used for the reconstruction of the articular block at the condyles. Except for type B fractures, the stability of the fixation must be increased by a plate with buttress function (**Fig. 4.6.3-6**).

In type B fractures it may be possible to insert the screws through small stab incisions or under arthroscopic control; for reconstruction of complex intra-articular fractures a formal arthrotomy is usually required.

4.3.2 Condylar plate/dynamic condylar screw (DCS)

In the treatment of complex extra-articular fractures (33-A3 fractures, and simple intra-articular fractures (type C1.2) the classical implants, the **condylar plate 95° (Video AO00051), and the DCS have proven to be reliable and effective.** Thanks to the step-by-step assembly, the

DCS (**Video AO20155**) is somewhat less demanding than the condylar plate and can be implanted with minimal soft-tissue exposure [3].

After reduction of the articular fragments, the condylar screw is inserted over a correctly placed guide pin under fluoroscopic control (**Fig. 4.6.3-7**). The side plate can then be slid underneath the vastus lateralis muscle along the linea aspera of the femur. With the impactor the side plate is seated against the shaft of the bone and then locked to the condylar screw. To fix the plate to the femur, a short incision has to be made at its proximal end.

It is possible, but more demanding, to insert the condylar plate in a similar fashion using longer incisions and reflecting the vastus lateralis (**Video AO20194**). After the implant is inserted with the blade parallel to the joint line, it is fixed to the distal femur, maintaining correct frontal and sagittal alignment. Additional stability of the blade can be achieved if cancellous bone screws are inserted through the plate into the condyles (**Fig. 4.6.3-8**).

The condylar plate 95° and the DCS have proven to be reliable and effective.

Fig. 4.6.3-6: Screw fixation of 33-B fractures.
a) B1 fracture with small condylar fragments: two 6.5 mm cancellous bone screws.
b) B1 fracture with larger fragment and buttress (anti-glide) plate fixation (here T-plate 4.5).
c) B3 "Hoffa" fracture (frontal plane) fixed with two 6.5 or 4.0 mm cancellous bone screws.

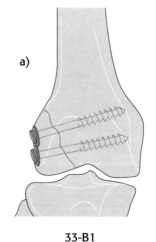
a)

33-B1

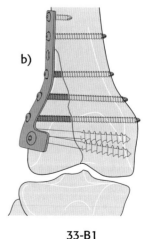
b)

33-B1

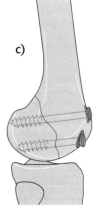
c)

33-B3

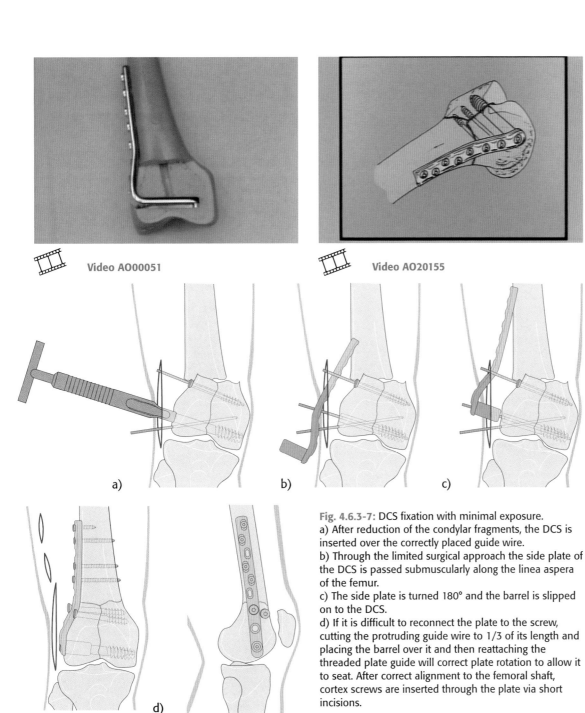

Video AO00051

Video AO20155

a)

b)

c)

d)

Fig. 4.6.3-7: DCS fixation with minimal exposure.
a) After reduction of the condylar fragments, the DCS is inserted over the correctly placed guide wire.
b) Through the limited surgical approach the side plate of the DCS is passed submuscularly along the linea aspera of the femur.
c) The side plate is turned 180° and the barrel is slipped on to the DCS.
d) If it is difficult to reconnect the plate to the screw, cutting the protruding guide wire to 1/3 of its length and placing the barrel over it and then reattaching the threaded plate guide will correct plate rotation to allow it to seat. After correct alignment to the femoral shaft, cortex screws are inserted through the plate via short incisions.

The condylar buttress plate is
the preferred implant for
complex fractures (33-C3)
with additional fracture lines in
the frontal plane.

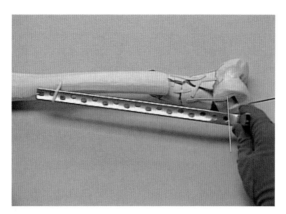

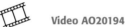
Video AO20194

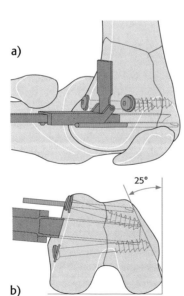

a)

b)

25°

4.3.3 Condylar buttress plate

The condylar buttress plate is the preferred implant for complex fractures (33-C3) with additional fracture lines in the frontal plane [4–6]. Compared to the condylar plate and the DCS, this plate offers the advantages of individual placement of screws over a wide area and of buttressing of the lateral femoral condyle. If the correct level is chosen for fixation of the plate to the distal femur, the large, tongue-shaped and prebent head of the plate usually does not need additional contouring (**Fig. 4.6.3-9**). Since there is no angular stability between the screws and the plate, it may be difficult to control varus malalignment if the medial bony buttress is absent. To overcome this problem the use of a medial plate may be necessary. This is usually done as a staged process and bone grafting may be required because of the soft-tissue dissection medially. The angular

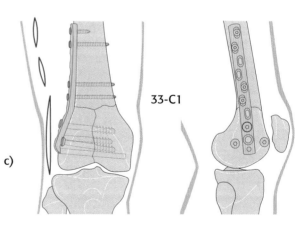

33-C1

Fig. 4.6.3-8: Condylar plate fixation.
a) Insertion of the seating chisel parallel to the joint line and to the correctly orientated K-wire. The intra-articular fracture has to be fixed prior to this by one or two lag screws.
b) Position of the lag screws and the seating chisel in the femoral condyles, as viewed in horizontal plane.

c) The supracondylar fracture has been reduced to the plate. Plate fixation to the femur with cortex screws. In transverse supracondylar fractures, axial compression should be applied using the tension device.

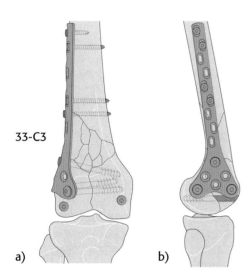

33-C3

a)   b)

Fig. 4.6.3-9: Complex distal femur fracture (33-C3).
a) Condylar buttress plate with 6.5 mm cancellous bone
screws. If there is no bony support opposite to the plate,
varus deformity may arise.
b) Condylar fractures in the frontal plane have to be fixed
by separate screws (6.5 or 4.0 mm).

stability produced by the newly designed LISS
internal fixator (**chapter 3.4**) may help to overcome this problem.

4.3.4   Retrograde nailing

Retrograde nailing is suitable for extra-articular
(33-A) and sometimes also for simple articular
fractures (33-C1, 33-C2) [1, 7–9]. Under fluoroscopic guidance, with the knee flexed, a medial
parapatellar arthrotomy is used to gain transarticular access [10]. The medullary canal is
opened just anterior to the notch, respecting the
cruciate ligament origin, and the slightly bent
solid distal femoral nail (DFN) is inserted into the
medullary cavity with the mounted aiming
device (**Fig. 4.6.3-10**).

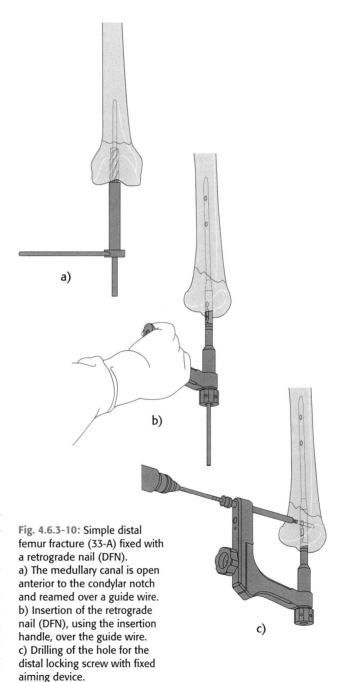

a)

b)

c)

Fig. 4.6.3-10: Simple distal
femur fracture (33-A) fixed with
a retrograde nail (DFN).
a) The medullary canal is open
anterior to the condylar notch
and reamed over a guide wire.
b) Insertion of the retrograde
nail (DFN), using the insertion
handle, over the guide wire.
c) Drilling of the hole for the
distal locking screw with fixed
aiming device.

To prevent misplacement of the interlocking bolts, locking is done from distal to proximal. If necessary, it is possible to adapt the distal to the proximal fragment by careful axial compression. Due to its axial and bending stability, the locked intramedullary nail, unlike the blade plate or DCS, provides adequate long-term stability without additional bone grafting, even in multifragmentary supracondylar fractures [11, 12].

On the other hand, the correct alignment of intra-articular fragments may be hazardous.

4.3.5 External fixation

The indications for temporary joint bridging external fixation are polytrauma patients, open fractures, or closed fractures with severe soft-tissue damage. If possible, the articular block is reconstructed with minimal internal fixation using conventional or cannulated lag screws. Then the joint bridging external fixator is mounted with Schanz screws, which are inserted laterally in the femur and anteromedially in the tibia. Both elements are then connected in a tube-to-tube fashion (**Fig. 4.6.3-11**), thus providing sufficient stability until definitive treatment is feasible.

5 Additional treatment

Cancellous bone grafting is seldom necessary as long as the metaphyseal fracture has not been exposed and devitalized during surgery (indirect reduction technique and biological fracture bridging). However, bone grafting is indicated to stimulate new bone formation in larger defects or to provide stability within a comminuted condyle. Exceptionally, bone cement may be applied to provide implant purchase in very osteopenic bone.

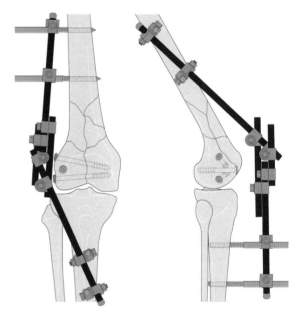

Fig. 4.6.3-11: Temporary external fixation bridging the knee joint with tube-to-tube fixator. Insertion of the Schanz screws at the femur laterally and at the tibia anteromedially. Flexion of the knee joint approx. 20°. The articular block is fixed by lag screws only.

Concomitant lesions of the medial, lateral, and cruciate ligaments are rarely encountered. If present, they should be treated primarily, because secondary interventions to the ligamentous structures seldom yield a good result in this situation.

6 Complications

Axial and rotational malalignment are typical problems observed while treating distal femoral fractures.

Due to the pull of the gastrocnemius and the adductor magnus muscles there is a risk of genu recurvatum with subsequent hyperextension and laxity of the knee joint. Flexion of the knee during surgery can help to prevent this.

Varus malalignment and malrotation are encountered more frequently after fixation with the condylar plate, or DCS, than with buttress plates. **If the insertion point of the blade (or DCS) is too far posterior, the condylar block is shifted medially,** which invariably produces a varus deformity.

The use of the retrograde nail seems to cause such problems less often, because insertion of the implant requires the knee to be flexed with the lower leg hanging down. This positioning can lead to a partial "self-reduction" of the fracture. However, very few intra-articular fractures are suitable for nailing!

The indication for a corrective osteotomy depends on the degree of malalignment and the severity of symptoms. Valgus/varus-malalignment greater than 10° and/or rotational deformity greater than 15° should be corrected.

If the insertion point of the blade (or DCS) is too far posterior, the condylar block is shifted medially.

Fig. 4.6.3-12: 36-year-old male with a 33-C3 fracture after motorbike accident.
a) Preoperative condition.
b) Postoperative control after reconstruction with condylar plate and 6.5 mm cancellous bone screws.
c) 4-months follow-up with satisfactory functional result.

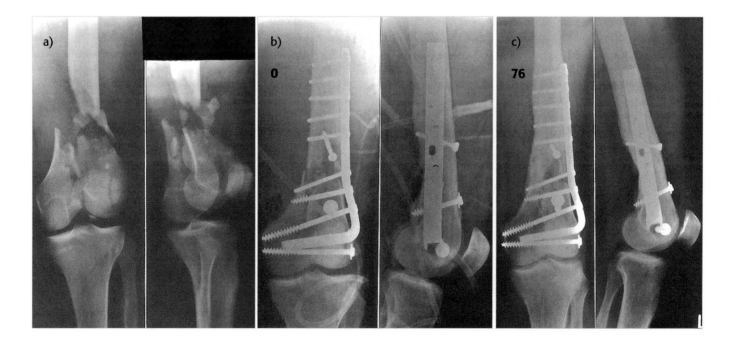

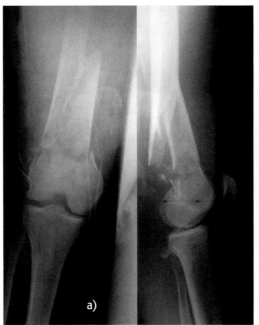

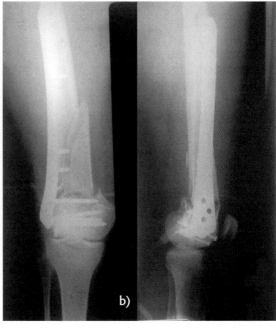

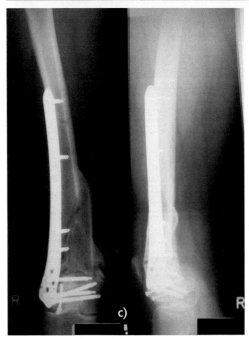

Fig. 4.6.3-13: 28-year-old polytraumatized female with distal femur fracture type 33-C2 and contralateral femur shaft fracture, bilateral humeral fractures, and complex foot injury on left side.
a) Accident view of right femur.
b) Postoperative aspect after minimally invasive fixation with LISS-DF plate.
c) 5-months follow-up with consolidated fractures and satisfactory axial alingment.

7   Bibliography

1. **Krettek C, Schandelmaier P, Tscherne H** (1996) [Distal femoral fractures. Transarticular reconstruction, percutaneous plate osteosynthesis and retrograde nailing]. *Unfallchirurg;* 99 (1):2–10.

2. **Stocker R, Heinz T, Vecsei V** (1995) [Results of surgical management of distal femur fractures with joint involvement]. *Unfallchirurg;* 98 (7):392–397.

3. **Sanders R, Regazzoni P, Rüedi TP** (1989) Treatment of supracondylar-intracondylar fractures of the femur using the dynamic condylar screw. *J Orthop Trauma;* 3 (3):214–222.

4. **Baumgaertel F, Gotzen L (1994)** [The "biological" plate osteosynthesis in multi-fragment fractures of the para-articular femur. A prospective study]. *Unfallchirurg;* 97 (2):78–84.

5. **Bolhofner BR, Carmen B, Clifford P** (1996) The results of open reduction and internal fixation of distal femur fractures using a biologic (indirect) reduction technique. *J Orthop Trauma;* 10 (6):372–377.

6. **Ostrum RF, Geel C** (1995) Indirect reduction and internal fixation of supracondylar femur fractures without bone graft. *J Orthop Trauma;* 9 (4):278–284.

7. **Danziger MB, Caucci D, Zecher SB, et al.** (1995) Treatment of intercondylar and supracondylar distal femur fractures using the GSH supracondylar nail. *Am J Orthop;* 24 (9):684–690.

8. **Iannacone WM, Bennett FS, DeLong WG, Jr., et al.** (1994) Initial experience with the treatment of supracondylar femoral fractures using the supracondylar intramedullary nail: a preliminary report. *J Orthop Trauma;* 8 (4):322–327.

9. **Moed BR, Watson JT** (1995) Retrograde intramedullary nailing, without reaming, of fractures of the femoral shaft in multiply injured patients. *J Bone Joint Surg [Am];* 77 (10):1520–1527.

10. **Herscovici D, Jr., Whiteman KW** (1996) Retrograde nailing of the femur using an intercondylar approach. *Clin Orthop;* (332):98–104.

11. **David SM, Harrow ME, Peindl RD, et al.** (1997) Comparative biomechanical analysis of supracondylar femur fracture fixation: locked intramedullary nail versus 95-degree angled plate. *J Orthop Trauma;* 11 (5):344–350.

12. **Firoozbakhsh K, Behzadi K, DeCoster TA, et al.** (1995) Mechanics of retrograde nail versus plate fixation for supracondylar femur fractures. *J Orthop Trauma;* 9 (2):152–157.

8   Updates

Updates and additional references for this chapter are available online at:
http://www.aopublishing.org/PFxM/463.htm

4.7 Patella

Michael Nerlich & Bernhard Weigel

1 Assessment of fractures and soft tissues

1.1 Anatomy

The patella is the largest sesamoid bone in the human body. It is located in the extensor apparatus of the knee. Anatomical features include the cranial base and the extra-articular caudal apex as well as the anterior extra-articular and the posterior articular surfaces. The rectus femoris and intermedius muscles insert at the base and the vastus medialis and lateralis muscles on either side. The patellar tendon originates from the apex patellae and inserts at the tibial tuberosity.

1.2 History and examination

Patellar fractures make up about 1% of all fractures [1] and are mostly caused by direct trauma to the front of the knee, for example, a fall from a height, a direct fall, or a blow, usually onto the flexed knee. Bony avulsions of the adjacent tendons are caused by indirect forces.

Typical signs are swelling, tenderness, and limited or lost function, especially of the extensor mechanism. **Preservation of active knee extension does not rule out a patellar fracture if "the auxiliary extensors of the knee" [2] are intact.** If displacement is significant, the physician can palpate a defect between the fragments. Usually a hemarthrosis is present. The examination must include evaluation of the soft tissues, so as not to overlook an injury to the patellar bursa or to omit grading the injury if the fracture is open.

1.3 X-ray evaluation

In addition to the standard x-rays of the knee in two planes, a tangential view of the patella may be useful. In the AP view the patella normally projects into the midline of the femoral sulcus. Its apex is located just above a line drawn across the distal profile of femoral condyles. In the lateral view the proximal tibia must be visible to exclude a bony avulsion of the patellar ligament from the tibial tuberosity. A rupture of the patellar ligament or an abnormal position of the patella (patella alta, e.g., high-riding or patella baja, e.g., shortening of the tendon) can

Preservation of active knee extension does not rule out a patellar fracture.

be recognized with the help of the Insall method [3] of relating the greatest diagonal lengths of the patella and the patellar tendon. This ratio is normally $r = 1$. A ratio $r < 1$ suggests high-riding patella (patella alta) or ligamentous rupture. The third important plane is the 30° tangential view, which is obtainable in 45° knee flexion. If a longitudinal or osteochondral fracture is suspected, the 30° tangential view will be a helpful diagnostic adjunct.

Tomography is helpful in special cases, such as stress fractures, in elderly patients with osteopenia and hemarthrosis [4], and also in cases of a patellar non-union or malunion [5]. Computed tomography is recommended only for the evaluation of articular incongruity in cases of non-union, malunion, and femoropatellar alignment disorders. Scintigraphic examination can be helpful in the diagnosis of stress fractures; leukocyte scan can reveal signs of osteomyelitis [6].

Tendon ruptures, patellar dislocation, and growth abnormalities (bipartite patella) must be ruled out. Isolated rupture of the quadriceps or patellar tendon must be excluded by clinical evaluation (palpation). The lateral x-ray may indicate an abnormal position of the patella.

Dislocation, most commonly occurring to the lateral side, may result in osteochondral shear fractures with lesions of the medial margin of the patella.

Bipartite or tripartite patella result from lack of assimilation of the bone during growth. Located on the proximal lateral quadrant of the patella, the condition is usually bilateral and has a characteristic x-ray feature with rounded, sclerotic lines rather than the sharp edges and lines of a fracture.

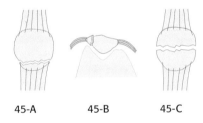

45-A   45-B   45-C

Fig. 4.7-1: Classification OTA

Most types of fracture need open reduction and osteosynthesis. Patellectomy is reserved for fractures that cannot be reconstructed.

1.4 Fracture classification

The major fracture types are illustrated in **Fig. 4.7-1**. Each fracture type has its own code consisting of three elements—e.g., 45-C1.3:

The first element, 45, identifies the bone. The OTA classification describes the different fracture types:

A   Extra-articular, extensor mechanism disrupted: therapy operative.

B   Partial articular, extensor mechanism intact, for example, often vertical fractures: therapy non-operative or operative in case of intra-articular incongruency or danger of secondary dislocation.

C   Complete articular, disrupted extensor mechanism: therapy operative.

1.5 Decision making

The choice of treatment depends on the type of fracture (**Fig. 4.7-1**). There are four possible treatment options.

Non-operative treatment is generally possible in the case of closed, non-displaced fractures with an intact extensor mechanism (45-B).

Simple fractures with gaps and steps in the articular surface may be stabilized by percutaneous screw fixation under arthroscopic control.

Most types of fracture need open reduction and osteosynthesis.

Patellectomy is reserved for fractures that cannot be reconstructed (45-C3). The recommended therapy for each fracture-pattern is included in the following **Table 4.7-1**.

Table 4.7-1: Summary of indications

45-A Extra-articular "pole" fractures

- Lag screw plus tension band wire or cerclage to tuberosity
- Transosseous suture of avulsed tendon plus cerclage between patella and tibial tuberosity to secure suture

45-B Partial articular, vertical fracture

- Non-displaced → Non-operative
- Displaced, simple → Transverse lag screw, plus cerclage
- Multifragmentary (stellate) → Circumferential cerclage plus tension band

45-C Complete articular, transverse

- K-wire plus tension band wire
- Plus third fragment → Lag screw or K-wire plus tension band
- Four or more fragments → K-wires, screws plus tension band
- Partial or total patellectomy

2 Surgical anatomy

The anterior surface is surrounded by an extraosseous arterial ring, which receives inflow from branches of the genicular arteries. This anastomotic ring supplies the patella through midpatellar vessels, which penetrate the middle third of the anterior surface, and the polar vessels, which enter the apex [7, 8]. Avascular necrosis is rare but can occur when excessive bilateral incisions are made and the patella is injured.

The infrapatellar branch of the saphenous nerve crosses from medial to the ventrolateral aspect of the tibial head close to the apex of the patella. It runs in the subcutaneous tissue layer and may be at risk in transverse incisions.

2.1 Biomechanics

(see chapter 3.2.3)

The patella serves as the fulcrum of the extensor mechanism within the two lever arms, the quadriceps tendon as extension of the largest muscle in the body, and the patellar tendon inserting in the tibial tuberosity. Enormous forces are transmitted across the femoropatellar joint. Maximal forces measured within the quadriceps tendon ranged up to 3,200 N, within the patellar tendon 2,800 N, and in young, physically fit men up to 6,000 N [9]. This corresponds to three to seven times the body weight and indicates the load-bearing capacity required of an osteosynthesis. At 4–5 mm in depth the patellar cartilage is the thickest in the human body [10]. This is due to the high pressures created by knee flexion and especially by arising from a squatting position. The shape of the femoropatellar joint, and hence the posterior surface of the patella, varies widely. Patellar tracking also depends on the configuration of the extensor mechanism and on the balance of the quadriceps muscles. The congruency of the articulation of the patella with the femur changes considerably from extension to flexion. From full extension to 45° of flexion the articular surface of the patella is in contact with the anterior femur. In a knee flexed more than 45° the posterior surface of the quadriceps

Be aware of infrapatellar branch of saphenous nerve when using a transverse incision.

Forces transmitted across the femoropatellar joint correspond to three to seven times the body weight.

tendon articulates with the patellar facets of the femur [10]. This increases the lever arm, for example, the distance from quadriceps tendon-patellar tendon linkage to the axis of knee rotation. **The increased lever arm of the extensor mechanism, due to the height of the patella, adds an additional 60% of the force needed to gain full (e.g., the final 15°) extension** [11]. This fact must be taken into account if patellectomy is performed, since full extension power will be markedly reduced postoperatively.

Due to the increased lever arm of the extensor mechanism an additional force is needed to gain full extension.

3 Preoperative planning

3.1 Positioning and approaches

The patient is placed supine on a radiolucent table. A cushion under the patient's ipsilateral buttock is helpful to rotate the leg internally. A tourniquet around the thigh, inflated to about 250 mmHg, gives better visibility. The surgeon has to take into account that **the inflated tourniquet can complicate the reduction of the fracture by fixing the quadriceps in a shortened position**. To avoid this, the knee should be carefully flexed beyond 90° and the patella manually pushed distally to gain as much length as necessary before the tourniquet is inflated [6]. In some cases it may be helpful to deflate the tourniquet while reducing the fracture.

The inflated tourniquet can inhibit the reduction of the fracture.

Clinical examination under anesthesia

Clinical examination of the knee under anesthesia is of the utmost importance. Associated lesions, such as ligamentous damage or dislocation and instability, must be ruled out.

Approach

Either a longitudinal or a transverse incision can be used (**Fig. 4.7-2**). We prefer the midline longitudinal incision over the patella, because it can be extended proximally or distally and it does not interfere in case of later revision. The transverse approach gives the best cosmetic result since it lies within Langer's lines, but may injure the infrapatellar branch of the saphenous nerve. Parapatellar incisions are also possible, especially in the case of an open fracture when one may be able to incorporate skin lesions into the approach. After incision of the superficial fascia, the extensor apparatus is exposed and tears in the auxiliary extensors can be identified. If necessary to inspect the knee joint, a medial parapatellar arthrotomy is made. Intra-articular surgery can be performed as needed. In the case of an open fracture or a pre-existing chronic bursitis, the prepatellar bursa may be excised; this is normally not required in closed fractures.

3.2 Reduction techniques and tools

The knee joint and fracture lines must be irrigated and cleared of small debris to allow exact reconstruction. The larger fragments are reduced using a large pointed bone reduction forceps. In type A or C fractures, reduction is easier in a full or hyperextended position of the knee. Longitudinal type B fractures are sometimes better reduced with the knee flexed. Anatomical reduction of the articular surface is monitored by palpating the joint from inside, as neither inspection nor the x-ray will reveal a minor step off. If an inside-out technique is planned, K-wires are inserted in an open manner before the reduction is done. The wires can also

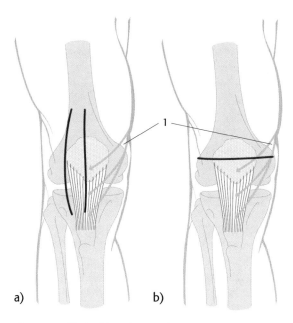

Fig. 4.7-2: Skin incisions/approaches.
a) Midline/vertical: allows for extensions and respects infrapatellar nerve (1). A parapatellar incision is also possible.
b) Transverse: respects Langer's line and allows easy access laterally and medially. Usually severs infrapatellar nerve (1). Choice of approach should respect the skin contusion/abrasion which is often present.

be used as joysticks to help in reducing the fragments. Reduction is held by one or two reduction forceps.

3.3 Choice of implant

The forces being transmitted through the patella require implants that withstand high tensile stress. Tension band wiring, being highly effective in transforming distraction forces into compressing forces, is most widely used. Single lag screws, if applied properly, will add to stability but should not be used without a

tension band except in longitudinal type B fractures. Articular osteochondral flake fractures can be kept in place with biodegradable pins until healed.

Tension band wiring

1.0 mm or, exceptionally, 1.25 mm stainless steel wire in combination with 1.6, 1.8, or 2.0 mm K-wires are the implants of choice.

Lag screws

The small fragment 3.5 mm cortex screw, used as a lag screw, is preferred. The 4.0 mm cancellous bone screw can also be used, but it has some disadvantages. Because of the high density of the patellar bone, reduction may be lost during screw insertion (high torque). Removal of a shaft screw may be difficult.

Biodegradable implants

Osteochondral fragments can be fixed with biodegradable pins of 1.6–2.0 mm diameter instead of K-wires. These implants consist of polyglycolic acid (PGA), polydioxanone (PDS), or polylactic acid (PLA). PGA starts to lose stability after 1–2 weeks; while PLA holds for 6 months. These implants are useful only for adaptation of unloaded fragments and are not recommended in areas of high mechanical stress. The same applies to resorbable suture material, which cannot match the tensile strength of metallic wires. Different factors contribute to the biocompatibility of these implants, and local foreign-body reactions remain a matter of concern [12]. Their advantage is that implant removal can be avoided.

The patella requires implants that withstand high tensile stress.

4   Surgical treatment— tricks and hints

4.1   Open fractures

Open fractures are generally emergency cases and require surgery as soon as possible. **Débridement of contused or contaminated soft tissue should be combined with irrigation or in severe cases with jet lavage.** Soft-tissue stripping from the bony fragments must be avoided for the sake of maintaining blood supply (see **chapter 5.1**).

> Débridement of contused or contaminated soft tissue is essential in open fractures.

Procedure

First, the complete extent of the injury must be identified, since the preoperative x-ray may not always reveal all fracture lines. Any extra-articular fracture lines will be detected by clearing a very small amount of overlapping tissue (1 or 2 mm) at the fracture edges. Steps, gaps, and the amount of destroyed or impacted cartilage are noted and any loose fragments are removed from the knee. The joint is irrigated and the articular surface of the corresponding femoral condyle is examined.

4.2   Tension band wiring

> Tension band principle: Tensile forces are converted to compression.

The principle is to convert the tension force into compression as the knee is flexed (**Fig. 4.7-3**) (**Video AO51049**).

Reduction and fixation can be achieved in two ways, either by first reducing the fracture and then drilling the K-wires through the reduced fragments (outside-in technique) or by first drilling the wires into the unreduced fragments

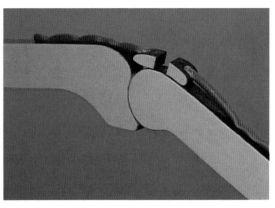

 Video AO51049

followed by reduction and completion of the fixation (inside-out technique).

Using the outside-in technique, the first wire is drilled in an axial direction, the second one parallel to the first, through the reduced fragments. It may be difficult to find the right direction and position for the wires. Alternatively, drilling the two wires from the fracture side inside out should be considered. Before reduction, the blunt ends of the wires must be cut obliquely, to make them pointed. After this, the main fragments will be manually reduced and held with a pointed reduction forceps. Then the K-wires are drilled forward through the opposite main fragment. (If the bone is very dense, the holes for the K-wires can be predrilled.) The ideal level for the pins lies in the center of the patella, approximately 5 mm below its anterior surface. Often the K-wires are closer to the articular than to the anterior surface. Nevertheless, the principle of tension banding is not disturbed.

A sufficiently long (ca. 30 cm), 1.0 or 1.25 mm thick cerclage wire is pushed manually as closely as possible to the edge between the bone and the protruding pin tips. The cerclage is placed

Fig. 4.7-3:
a) 45-C transverse fracture.
b) Reduction with large reduction forceps with points and pre-liminary fixation with two parallel 1.6–2.0 mm K-wires.
c) To pass the "cerclage" wires through the ligamentous structures and around the K-wires close to the bone it may be helpful to use a curved large bore needle or cannula.
d) The cerclage wire should lie anteriorly to the patella so as to act as a tension band. A circular wire is preferable to a figure-of-eight.

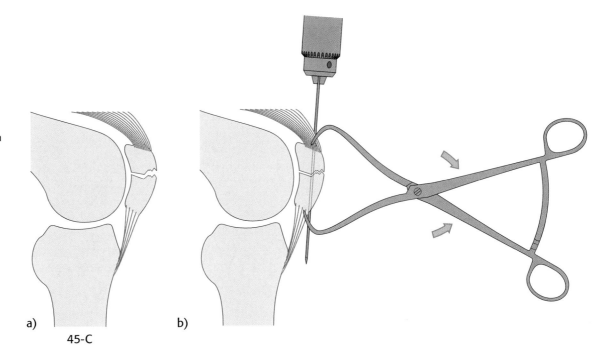

a)

45-C

b)

e) The lateral view demonstrates the tension band principle, where by flexing the knee, tensile forces are converted into compressive ones (arrows).

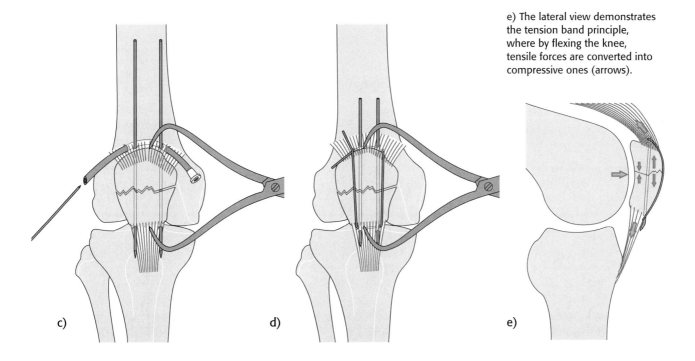

c)

d)

e)

in the form of a figure-of-zero or figure-of-eight. The wire should be as close as possible to the bone throughout its whole course. The use of a curved large bore injection needle may be helpful (**Fig. 4.7-3c**). The figure-of-zero of the cerclage has more stability against torsion forces, but if the pins are located near the bone limits, the cerclage can cut into the retinacula. As a result the principle of tension banding might be lost. A figure-of-eight is therefore preferred by some authors, although it does "squeeze" the underlying tissues. The ends of the cerclage are located medially or laterally.

While tightening the cerclage with the knee in extension, the reduction is checked by palpating the retropatellar surface. After tightening the cerclage, the proximal pin ends will be bent, shortened and turned towards the quadriceps tendon, and driven into the patella to prevent skin irritation and loosening. The distal pin ends are only trimmed, not bent, for easier removal.

Additional cerclage

Even comminuted fractures can be reduced and stabilized with the tension band technique if they are not too badly displaced (type B3 stellate fracture) (**Fig. 4.7-4**). In such cases, with many small fragments, the tension band technique must be combined with an additional circumferential cerclage around the fractured patella. The placement of this cerclage should be the initial step of stabilization to avoid further displacement as tension band wiring is carried out.

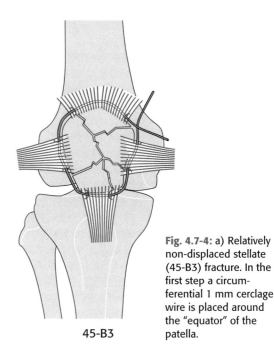

45-B3

Fig. 4.7-4: a) Relatively non-displaced stellate (45-B3) fracture. In the first step a circumferential 1 mm cerclage wire is placed around the "equator" of the patella.

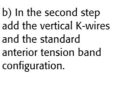

b) In the second step add the vertical K-wires and the standard anterior tension band configuration.

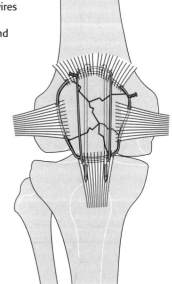

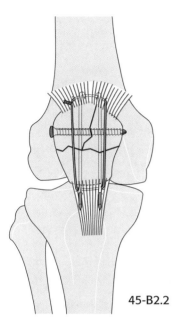

45-B2.2

Fig. 4.7-5: 45-C2.2 fracture. A combination of a transverse 4.0 mm lag screw with the standard tension band (see **Fig. 4.7-3**) is used to fix the transverse and vertical fracture pattern.

Combined tension banding plus lag screws or K-wires

In transverse fractures, the two main fragments are themselves often further fragmented (**Fig. 4.7-5**). Tension band wiring is possible only if the two main fragments have been reconstructed by lag screws. After reduction of fragments and temporary fixation by a pointed reduction forceps, the screws are implanted as demonstrated in **chapter 3.2.1**. Lag screws are inserted closer to the retropatellar surface leaving enough space for the K-wires. For fragments too small to hold a screw, 1.6 mm K-wires are used. Interfragmentary compression is done later by an additional cerclage.

Lag screws plus an anterior band wiring

Fractures of a pole of the patella are best stabilized by lag screws (**Fig. 4.7-6**). As implant pull-out or failure is inevitable, the bending forces must be neutralized by additional anterior tension band wiring. Upper pole fractures are stabilized in this manner, if necessary combined with additional transosseous sutures of the quadriceps tendon.

Transosseous sutures for tendon repair

Very small fragments should be excised and tendon repair is done by transosseous sutures alone (**Fig. 4.7-6a**). We prefer non-resorbable heavy suture material for the main adaptation and resorbable material for the additional fine sutures.

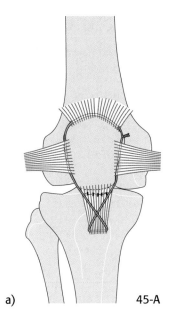
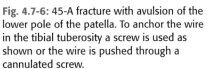
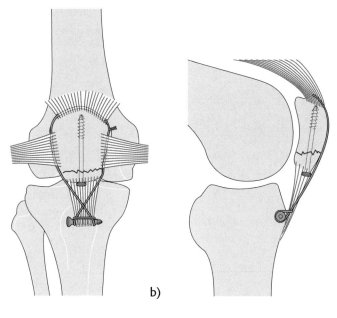

a)   45-A   b)

Fig. 4.7-6: 45-A fracture with avulsion of the lower pole of the patella. To anchor the wire in the tibial tuberosity a screw is used as shown or the wire is pushed through a cannulated screw.

a) The fragment is discarded and the transosseous sutures reattaching the patellar ligament are protected by a figure-of-eight wire between patella and tibial tuberosity.

b) The fragment is preserved and fixed with a 4.0 mm cancellous bone screw. Again, this must be protected by a figure-of-eight wire.

4.3   Patellotibial cerclage

Partial patellectomy is preferred to total patellectomy.

Management is the same as for lower pole fractures, but if fixation of patellar tendon origin is inadequate because of a small fragment or multiple parts, the necessary transosseous sutures must be protected by a patellotibial cerclage between patella and tibial tuberosity (**Fig. 4.7-6b**). The anchoring at the tuberosity can occur around a 3.5 mm cortex screw or through the hole of a cannulated screw. When tightening this, it is necessary to ensure that the knee can flex to 90°. This means that in full extension there will be some redundancy of the cerclage wire.

4.4   Partial patellectomy

Partial patellectomy is preferred to total patellectomy, whenever possible, as it keeps the lever arm intact (**Fig. 4.7-7**). A comminuted upper or lower pole and even a comminuted zone in the middle of the patella can be managed best by taking out all small particles. If the damaged zone is in the middle of the patella, an osteotomy proximally as well as distally and reduction of the main fragments, as in a transverse fracture, can be done. If the comminuted area is marginal, the bony particles should be removed in order to prevent osteophyte formation. Then the neighboring tendon

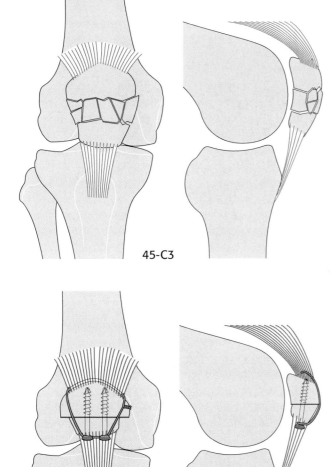

45-C3

Fig. 4.7-7: In the case of a severe central comminution of the patella, as a salvage procedure the injured segment may be removed by osteotomy. The two remaining portions are joined together by two lag screws and a tension band wire.

part is sutured keeping the extensor axis in mind, otherwise patellar balance could be disturbed. Distally, sutures have to be protected by a patellotibial cerclage as described above.

4.5 Patellectomy

In case of severe comminution and extended cartilage damage, patellectomy may be the only way to manage the injury (**Fig. 4.7-8**). All bony fragments and shredded tissue are removed by sharp dissection leaving as much extensor apparatus as possible. Tendinous reconstruction then follows. A defect zone of 3–4 cm can be bridged by direct adaptation. Shortening of the extensor apparatus is beneficial as it increases the muscle preload. If a direct suture proves impossible, then inverted V-plasty is recommended [6]. However, one should always take into consideration the fact that retention of even one larger fragment would maintain the lever arm.

Wound closure

A suction drain is placed into the joint. The arthrotomy is closed and tears in the retinacula are adapted by resorbable sutures and the skin is closed. In open fractures the small implants can usually be covered by adjacent soft tissue and the skin can be mobilized considerably, so even large skin defects do not pose any problem.

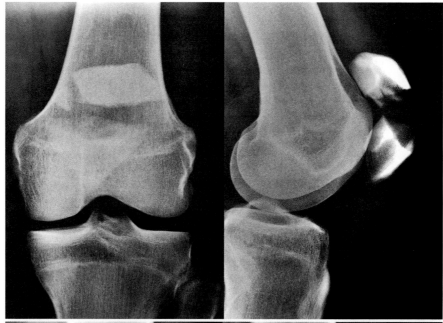

Fig. 4.7-8:
45-C closed fracture.
a) Closed fracture of
the patella.

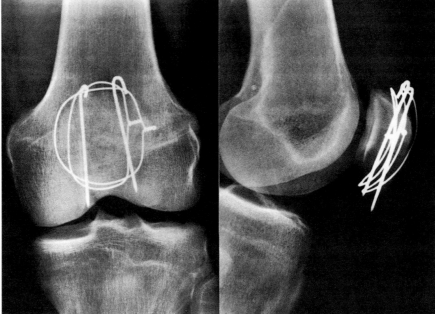

b) After ORIF with
tension band wiring.

5 Postoperative treatment

The osteosynthesis is stable and implants (not only K-wires but also lag screws) are protected by anterior banding against bending forces. Therefore, it may not be necessary to use casts or braces. When the patient is walking, a knee brace is helpful until quadriceps control is regained. Early motion, especially active assisted, is beneficial to articular cartilage health. This may be facilitated by continuous passive motion (CPM). Drains are removed on the first or second postoperative day, depending on the amount of wound drainage. Then the patient begins with isometric exercises and mobilization. Partial weight bearing to 15 kg or half body weight for 6 weeks and active assisted motion from full extension to 90° of knee flexion are allowed, assuming there are no wound problems. Knee flexion is most important for changing anterior traction forces into retropatellar compression forces, which supports bone healing.

Implant removal will take place after 1 year on average (6–24 months). A patellotibial cerclage should be removed within 12 weeks if 90° knee flexion is not obtained or after breakage if painful.

6 Pitfalls and complications

Disturbed wound healing

The optimal plane of tissue dissection lies between the subcutaneous fascia and the extensor apparatus. For an undisturbed blood supply of the skin, it is very important not to commit the common error of separating the tissue layers between skin and subcutaneous fascia. The inevitable result will be the necrosis of the wound margins. Improper use of wound hooks can also produce such problems.

Deep infection

Revision with débridement and irrigation is indicated every other day until wound healing is secured. With deep infection, long-term anti-biotic application (6 weeks) is recommended (see chapter 5.5).

Synovitis by biodegradable implants

Crystalline decomposition products can create mild to severe sterile synovitis, which may be hard to distinguish from an infection. An arthroscopic intervention may be necessary [12].

Skin irritation by wire tips

The irritating end of a pin or a cerclage should be shortened before the soft-tissue layer becomes perforated; otherwise the patient is threatened with infection.

Patella baja

This complication can cause a severe limitation of knee flexion. If there is the need for a cerclage wire to protect the patellar ligament, a patella baja could be produced by misjudging the exact length of the patellar tendon. The opposite knee will indicate the correct position of the patella as described under x-ray evaluation.

Shorten ends of pin and cerclage before soft tissue is perforated.

The optimal plane of tissue dissection lies between the subcutaneous fascia and the extensor apparatus.

Implant failure

Implant failure requires a revision only if the main fragments are displaced or the articular surface is showing incongruity. A common complication is proximal K-wire migration. To prevent this, the wire ends should be bent to a loop and the tension band wire is then pulled through the two proximal loops holding the K-wires in stable position [13]. A rare complication is the intra-articular migration of a broken wire [14].

Loss of motion

In the case of limited flexion, intensive physiotherapy is indicated. If the range of motion does not improve within months, an arthroscopic arthrolysis will be the next step, removing scar contractions from the upper recess. If patellectomy has been performed, tendon rupture is a later possibility.

Posttraumatic arthritis

This can follow if the patellar ligament is attached too anteriorly, rotating the distal pole backwards, or if the patella becomes elongated as a comminuted fracture heals. In the first situation the origin of the tendon should be corrected by transposing it, in the second case patellectomy is indicated.

7 Bibliography

1. **Bostrom A** (1972) Fracture of the patella. A study of 422 patellar fractures. *Acta Orthop Scand Suppl;* 143:1–80.
2. **Carson WG, Jr., James SL, Larson RL, et al.** (1984) Patellofemoral disorders: physical and radiographic evaluation. Part II: Radiographic examination. *Clin Orthop;* (185):178–186.
3. **Insall JN** (1984) *Anatomy of the knee. Surgery of the Knee.* New York: Churchill-Livingstone: 1–20.
4. **Weber BG, Cech O** (1976) *Pseudarthrosis.* New York: Grune & Stratton: 224–225.
5. **Sanders R** (1992) Patella fractures and extensor mechanism injuries. In: Browner BD, Jupiter JB, Levine AM, et al., editors. *Skeletal Trauma.* Philadelphia: W. B. Saunders Co.: 1685–1710.
6. **Arnoczky SP** (1985) Blood supply to the anterior cruciate ligament and supporting structures. *Orthop Clin North Am;* 16 (1):15–28.
7. **Scapinelli R** (1967) Blood supply of the human patella. Its relation to ischaemic necrosis after fracture. *J Bone Joint Surg [Br];* 49 (3):563–570.
8. **Huberti HH, Hayes WC, Stone JL, et al.** (1984) Force ratios in the quadriceps tendon and ligamentum patellae. *J Orthop Res;* 2 (1):49–54.
9. **Kapandji IA** (1985) *Funktionelle Anatomie der Gelenke.* Stuttgart: Enke Verlag.
10. **Goodfellow J, Hungerford DS, Zindel M** (1976) Patello-femoral joint mechanics and pathology 1. Functional anatomy of the patello-femoral joint. *J Bone Joint Surg [Br];* 58 (3):287–299.

11. **Hoffmann R, Weller A, Helling HJ, et al.** (1997) [Local foreign body reactions to biodegradable implants. A classification]. *Unfallchirurg*; 100 (8):658–666.

12. **Gotzen L, Ishaque B, Morgenthal F, et al.** (1997) [External patello-tibial transfixation. I: Indications and technique]. *Unfallchirurg*; 100 (1):24–28.

13. **Us AK, Kinik H** (1966) Self locking tension band technique in transverse patellar fractures. *Int Orthop*; 20:357–358.

14. **Chen YJ, Wu CC, Hsu RW, et al.** (1994) The intra-articular migration of the broken wire: a rare complication of circumferential wiring in patellar fractures. *Chang Keng I Hsueh Tsa Chih*; 17 (3):276–279.

8   Updates

Updates and additional references for this chapter are available online at:
http://www.aopublishing.org/PFxM/47.htm

4.8.1 Tibia: proximal

J. Tracy Watson

1 Introduction

A surgeon considering operative management of a proximal tibial end-segment fracture should decide the course of treatment on the basis of the patient's age, level of activity, previous medical conditions, and expectations. The need to avoid the undesirable outcomes of instability, malalignment, and articular incongruity of the knee will often dictate surgical management. Indications for surgery include:

- Open plateau fractures,
- Fractures with an associated compartment syndrome or acute vascular lesion,
- Articular fractures with displacement greater than 10 mm although in young or active patients 2 mm [1–6] may be unacceptable,
- Axial malalignment.

2 Assessment of fractures and soft tissues

It is important to determine the force of the injury, as **high-energy fractures** are associated with considerable **soft-tissue injuries** [7, 8]. Physical examination should focus on the integrity of the soft-tissue envelope, especially the presence of blisters or superficial abrasions, which indicate areas to be avoided in a surgical approach until the soft tissues have resolved. If lacerations and compromised skin cannot be avoided, any intervention must be delayed. The fracture is temporarily stabilized by bridging external fixation, and the fixation is carried out in stages. Some attempt, however limited, to reassemble the articular surface is mandatory. Especially in open fractures with soft-tissue loss or severe closed soft-tissue injury, this articular reconstruction can be protected by a spanning external fixator. After soft-tissue recovery, a secondary procedure can be safely accomplished to achieve metaphyseal stabilization.

Neurovascular status should be assessed and, in the presence of a high-energy fracture pattern, compartment syndrome and arterial injury must be ruled out, usually by compartment-pressure monitoring and/or arteriography [9, 10].

High-energy fractures are associated with considerable soft-tissue injuries.

2.1 Imaging studies

X-rays should include AP, lateral, and internal and external oblique views. Traction x-rays are an additional method to determine the efficacy of distraction techniques and will determine if a ligamentotaxis—indirect reduction—is possible. They are useful to plan the extent and location of surgical incisions. In many parts of the world CT scanning is the imaging study of choice, although linear tomography still has its place if CT is not available (**Fig. 4.8.1-1**)[11]. CT scans with axial, coronal, and sagittal reconstruction assist in delineating the severity and orientation of condylar fracture lines (**Fig.4.8.1-2**). This is useful when using minimally invasive techniques associated with indirect reduction where direct exposure of the fracture lines is to be avoided.

MR imaging has been shown to be superior to CT scans when assessing associated soft-tissue injuries, such as meniscal and ligamentous disruptions; however, MR imaging may not be widely available and is seldom indicated [12, 13].

Arteriography should be considered whenever there is a serious possibility of an arterial lesion. Fracture patterns most commonly associated with **arterial injuries** are the higher energy 41-B1.3 and 41-B3.3 fractures. These fractures frequently present with a very unstable knee or even an actual **fracture dislocation.** High-energy-type fracture patterns, including 41-C1, 41-C2, and 41-C3 fractures, especially if there is a posterior medial corner fragment, should lower the surgeon's threshold for obtaining an arteriogram.

Arterial injuries are associated with high-energy fractures or fracture dislocation.

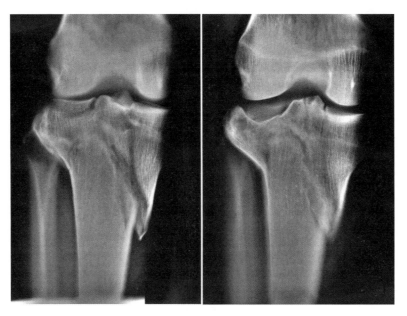

Fig. 4.8.1-1: 41-C3.1 Bicondylar fracture.
a) Standard AP view.
b) Same fracture in linear tomography with considerable impaction of the articular surface.

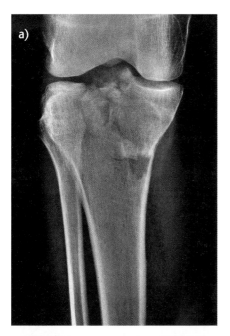

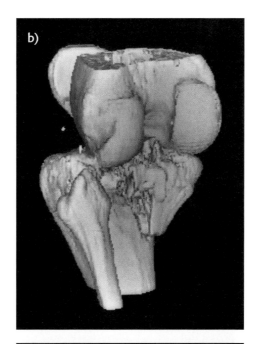

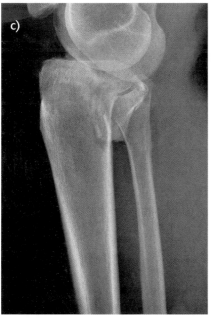

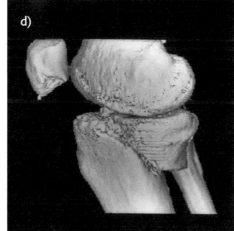

Fig. 4.8.1-2: The rare case of a 41-B3.2 fracture.
a) Standard AP view.
b) 3-D reconstruction as seen from behind.
c) Lateral view.
d) Lateral 3-D reconstruction.

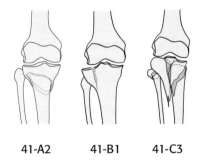

41-A2   41-B1   41-C3

Fig. 4.8.1-3: Müller AO Classification

2.2   Classification

The Müller AO Classification distinguishes between extra-articular (type A), unicondylar (type B), and bicondylar (type C) fractures (**Fig. 4.8.1-3**).

3   Surgical anatomy

The medial plateau is the larger of the two articular surfaces. It is also concave from front to back, as well as from side to side. The lateral plateau is smaller and higher than the medial, it is convex from front to back and from side to side, which also helps to identify it on a lateral x-ray (**Fig. 4.8.1-4**). This is important to note, so that screws inserted from lateral to medial do not enter the concave medial joint surface. The intermediate, non-articular intercondylar eminence serves as a tibial attachment of the ante-rior cruciate ligament. Fractures of this area, when present as isolated injuries, represent an avulsion of the anterior cruciate ligament and are not usually discussed under fractures of the tibial plateau (41-A1). The tibial tubercle and Gerdy's tubercle are bony prominences located in the subcondylar region and serve as points of attachment for the patellar tendon and ilio-tibial band respectively. These landmarks are important when planning surgical incisions. The medial condyle, including its articular surface, is stronger than the lateral. As a result, fractures of the lateral plateau are more common and may present articular impaction and frag-mentation. Medial plateau fractures occur more often "en bloc" and are invariably associated with more violent injuries (**Fig. 4.8.1-5**). They have a higher degree of soft-tissue injury, such as disruption of the lateral/collateral ligament complex and neurovascular lesions.

The proximal tibiofibular joint is located posterolaterally on the lateral tibial condyle. The fibular head provides attachment for the fibular collateral ligament and biceps tendon, as well as acting as a buttress for the proximal lateral portion of the tibial plateau.

The outer portion of each plateau is covered by a cartilaginous meniscus. The lateral meniscus covers a much larger portion of the articular surface than does the medial. Meniscotibial ligaments attach the menisci to the periphery of the tibial plateaus. **These are important to identify at surgery, so that a submeniscal exposure or peripheral meniscal rim tear can be correctly sited and repaired.** In case of meniscal detachment through the injury, it is recommended that its periphery be tagged with stay sutures prior to reduction of the fracture, as the siting of sutures can be difficult afterwards.

Meniscal tears or avulsion must be identified and repaired.

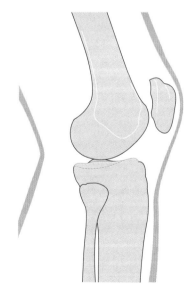

Fig. 4.8.1-4: Normal anatomy of medial and lateral tibial condyles as seen in the sagittal plane. NOTE: The lateral joint line is convex, the medial concave!

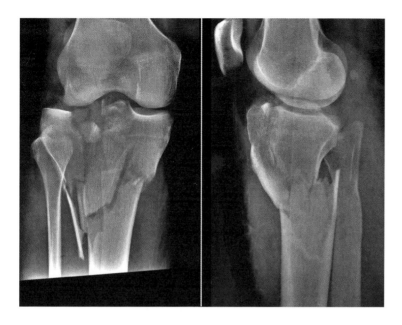

Fig. 4.8.1-5: 41-C3.1 fracture in a 44-year-old female after a skiing accident. In bicondylar fractures the medial plateau is mostly sheared off "en bloc" without major damage to the articular surface.

4 Preoperative planning

A complete understanding of the routine and traction x-rays, and CT or MR scans is essential to develop a preoperative plan. This confirms that the appropriate implants and reduction instruments are available. It also clarifies the need for supplemental bone grafts. Additionally, the surgical tactics should include the operative approach to ensure that the exposure is completed with the least soft-tissue dissection [14].

4.1 Surgical approach

The patient is positioned supine on a radiolucent operating table, preferably one which "breaks" so that the knee can be flexed to 90°. Alternatively, this can be achieved using a large sterile bolster or a beanbag patient positioner.

Knee flexion allows the iliotibial band to slip posteriorly off the lateral condyle of the femur, affording a better view of the posterolateral plateau. This is helped by allowing the dependent weight of the leg to apply a distraction force. A C-arm image intensifier should be available and brought in from the opposite side of the operating table.

Since the majority of plateau fractures primarily involve the lateral side, a straight lateral parapatellar incision is usually the first option (Fig. 4.8.1-6). This incision can be extended proximally and distally as more exposure is needed. The deep dissection should go straight down to the bone by detaching the lateral muscle origins and splitting the fibers of the iliotibial tract. The knee joint is then opened below the lateral meniscus in order to get a good view of the articular surface. An avulsed meniscus should be reattached rather than

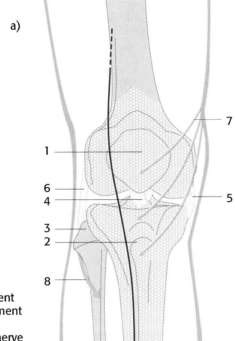

a)

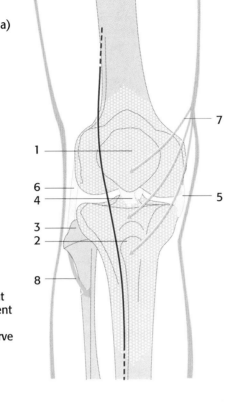

1	Patella
2	Tibial tuberosity
3	Fibular head
4	Cruciate ligament
5	Tibial collateral ligament
6	Fibular collateral ligament
7	Saphenous nerve
8	Superficial peroneal nerve
9	Iliotibial tract
10	Muscle origins
11	Meniscus

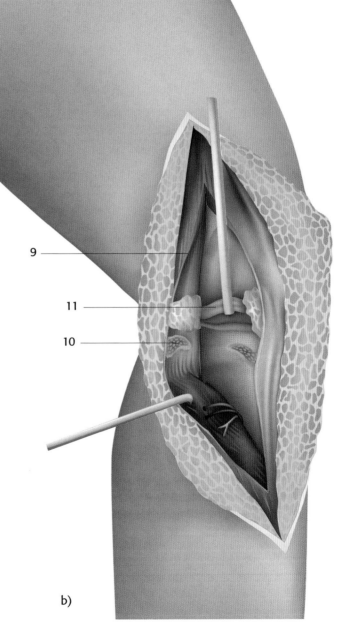

b)

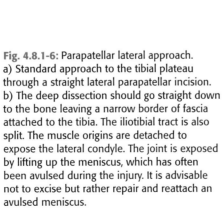

Fig. 4.8.1-6: Parapatellar lateral approach.
a) Standard approach to the tibial plateau through a straight lateral parapatellar incision.
b) The deep dissection should go straight down to the bone leaving a narrow border of fascia attached to the tibia. The iliotibial tract is also split. The muscle origins are detached to expose the lateral condyle. The joint is exposed by lifting up the meniscus, which has often been avulsed during the injury. It is advisable not to excise but rather repair and reattach an avulsed meniscus.

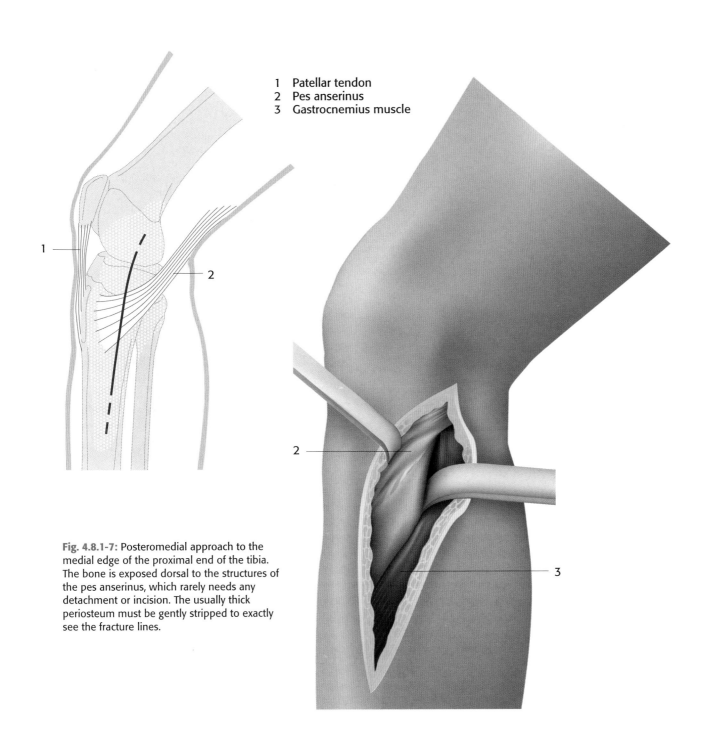

1   Patellar tendon
2   Pes anserinus
3   Gastrocnemius muscle

Fig. 4.8.1-7: Posteromedial approach to the medial edge of the proximal end of the tibia. The bone is exposed dorsal to the structures of the pes anserinus, which rarely needs any detachment or incision. The usually thick periosteum must be gently stripped to exactly see the fracture lines.

In bicondylar fractures an additional posteromedial incision may be recommended.

excised. It is, furthermore, advisable not to dissect across the tibial tuberosity—unless absolutely necessary—because of the very delicate skin cover on the medial side. Care must be taken not to place incisions over the proposed sites of plates or screws or where there is risk of devitalizing sensitive structures. This requires good planning. When treating fractures with a **bicondylar component** (41C), where perfect reduction and buttressing of the usually large posteromedial fragment is needed, an **additional posteromedial incision** [15] is preferred to an extensive exposure from anteriorly (**Fig. 4.8.1-7**). The posteromedial incision is planned in such a way as to expose the medial edge of the tibial plateau dorsal to the tendons of the pes anserinus. The usually simple fracture can be anatomically reduced and buttressed by a DCP 3.5, LC-DCP 3.5, or one-third tubular plate. The infrapatellar Z-plasty is no longer recommended, while posterior approaches are rarely indicated [16]. Any additional subperiosteal exposure, either laterally or medially, carries the risk of devitalizing the fracture fragments and should not be done.

4.2 Reduction techniques and tools

Fracture reduction techniques in the proximal tibia rely on the concept of indirect reduction to realign the fracture fragments attached to soft-tissue hinges such as ligaments. These techniques require use of one or two large distractors bridging the slightly flexed knee. Ligamentotaxis can reduce a considerable portion of the fracture, primarily large condylar fragments, as well as realign the diaphyseal-metaphyseal shaft extension.

Large pointed reduction forceps are applied percutaneously to achieve compression between the different fracture lines (**Fig. 4.8.1-8**).

To gain exposure and to reconstruct a depressed articular fragment, it is best to exploit the primary fracture line. The lateral condylar fracture fragment can be hinged back on its soft-tissue attachment, much like opening the cover of a book (**Video AO20144a**). One can then see the joint depression, which usually consists of a centrally impacted area. If the injury has caused a central depression with no split, the

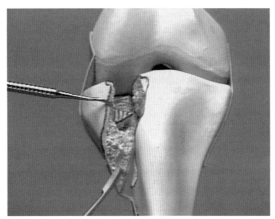

 Video AO20144a

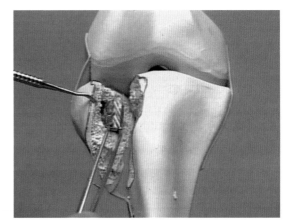

 Video AO20144b

Fig. 4.8.1-8: Indirect reduction of lateral 41-B3 fracture with the large distractor and compression using the long pelvic reduction forceps. Preliminary fixation with K-wires.

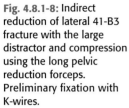
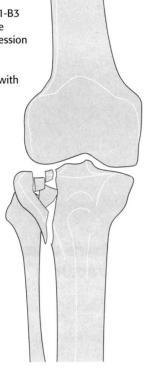
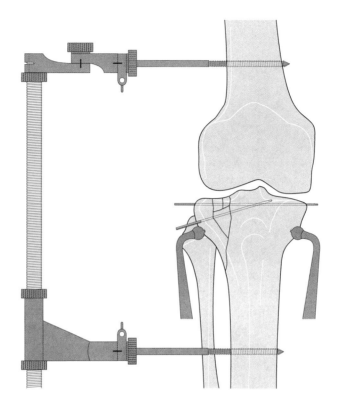

depressed area can be approached from below through a window made in the anterolateral cortex of the tibial condyle. The articular surface is then seen indirectly through a standard submeniscal articular exposure. Reduction of the articular surface must be accomplished by elevating the fragments "en masse" from below (Fig. 4.8.1-9). The resulting defect in the metaphyseal area must be filled with cancellous autograft or a corticocancellous bloc to support the elevated fragments (Video AO20144b). Alternatively, newer bone substitutes have been used successfully in this situation.

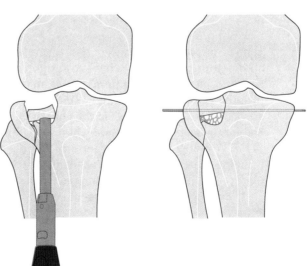

Fig. 4.8.1-9: The impacted articular surface must be elevated gently with a pusher that can be introduced through the fracture or by creating a small cortical window. Most importantly, the resulting bony defect must be filled with a cancellous or cortico-cancellous autograft to prevent secondary collapse. Alternatively, bone substitute can be used.

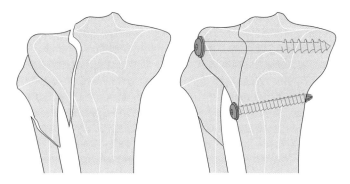

Fig. 4.8.1-10: A simple condylar split fracture 41-B1 may be stabilized by lag screws, given good bone quality and a compliant patient. The distal 4.5 mm cortex screw with a washer is actually preventing the tip of the fragment from displacing distally.

For split fractures (41-B1) with no fragmentation, multiple 6.5 mm cannulated screws can be used to stabilize the condylar fragment, associated with an antiglide screw or small plate at the apex of the fragment (**Fig. 4.8.1-10**). For more fragmented fracture types (41-B3 and C2) or osteoporotic bone, cancellous bone lag screws may not provide enough support and a buttress plate is necessary. The concept of a "raft-plate" allows multiple 3.5 mm screws to support the elevated, depressed fragment. These may be inserted separately or through a buttress plate applied as closely as possible to the joint margin. Significant metaphyseal-diaphyseal dissociation (41-C3) injuries require larger and stronger bridging plates like the lateral tibial buttress plates to span these zones of fragmentation.

In extensive comminution or soft-tissue injury large exposures must be avoided.

If extensive comminution or soft-tissue injury is present, additional dissections are contraindicated to avoid wound problems. To stabilize the posteromedial condyle a simple half-pin external fixator may be applied or alter-

natively a medial plate through a separate small incision. When severe soft-tissue contusions are combined with significant metaphyseal-diaphyseal extension and fragmentation, the joint must be reduced by minimally invasive techniques and stabilized by interfragmental compression while the metaphyseal-diaphyseal stabilization may be by hybrid external fixation (**Fig. 4.8.1-11**) (see **chapter 3.3.3**) [3, 17–22] or else delayed until the soft tissues are suitable for internal fixation.

5 Surgical treatment

5.1 Extra-articular type A fractures

41-A1 fractures are extra-articular avulsion-type injuries, which in general can be treated non-operatively or with simple lag screw fixation. Type A2 fractures are simple metaphyseal injuries, frequently allowing conservative management by skeletal traction [23] casts and orthotics. With higher-energy fractures (41-A2.3) and the multifragmentary metaphyseal injuries (41-A3), operative intervention is needed. If soft tissues permit, simple DCP plating or the use of the lateral tibial buttress plate is indicated. High-energy injuries with compromised soft tissues are suitable for hybrid external fixation. Secure proximal fracture fixation is accomplished with two or three transfixion wires and distal fixation can be achieved with two well-spread Schanz pins. A simple frame can be constructed that will allow immediate weight bearing, as tolerated, and rapid fracture consolidation.

5.2 Condylar split fractures (type B1)

A pure split, or a wedge fracture of the lateral plateau (41-B1) is often amenable to a percutaneous approach, using either arthroscopic control and or fluoroscopy to confirm the reduction. Fixation is accomplished with one or two 6.5 mm cancellous bone screws placed just below the joint margin and one antiglide screw or plate at the apex of the fracture fragment (see **Fig. 4.8.1-10**).

When the condylar fragment is **fragmented** (41-B1.3), a **lateral buttress or anti-glide plate** should be used instead of multiple lag screws.

5.3 Pure impaction fracture (type B2)

41-B2.1 and 41-B2.2 are circumscribed impactions of the lateral plateau and may involve any portion of the articular surface, usually centrally or laterally. CT or MR scanning will indicate the location and depth of the depression. During

"Screws only" for split or wedge fractures. All other situations require buttressing, usually by a plate.

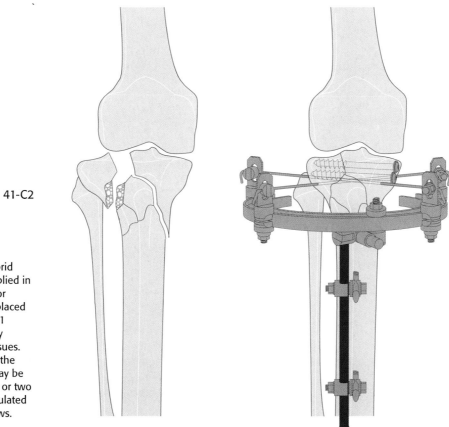

41-C2

Fig. 4.8.1-11: The hybrid ring fixator is best applied in extra-articular 41-A3 or simple minimally displaced intra-articular B1 or C1 fractures with severely compromised soft tissues. In this 41-C2 fracture the articular fragments may be approximated by one or two regular or large, cannulated cancellous bone screws.

surgery the quality of reduction can be observed through direct vision or the arthroscope [24–27]. A limited lateral exposure is used to develop a small metaphyseal cortical window through which a small guide wire may be passed to the area of joint impaction. A curved bone impactor allows elevation of the fragment from below. A graft is introduced and stabilized by percutaneous cannulated screws (see **Fig. 4.8.1-9**).

5.4　Split-compression fractures (type B3)

More extensive injuries involve a combination of a lateral condyle fracture with impaction of its articular surface (41-B3.1). Preoperative imaging studies are crucial to determine the extent and location of the impacted articular

surface. Associated injuries such as ligamentous injuries or meniscal tears may be present and must be considered separately. Provisional K-wire fixation is useful to stabilize the articular surface following reduction of the impacted fragment(s) (**Video AO20144c**). Fixation of the condyle is best achieved with interfragmental compression by cancellous bone lag screws and a buttress plate. The lag screws may be incorporated into the plate or inserted separately, allowing a straight plate to be contoured to act in buttress mode. Other specially designed plates for buttressing these fractures are the L-plate and T-plate allowing the incorporation of screws into the plate (**Fig. 4.8.1-12**) (**Video AO20144d**). With extensive articular impaction, "raft-plate" fixation using 3.5 mm cortex screws provides excellent subchondral support and prevents secondary displacement of the reconstructed articular surface [28]. **Any**

41-B3.1

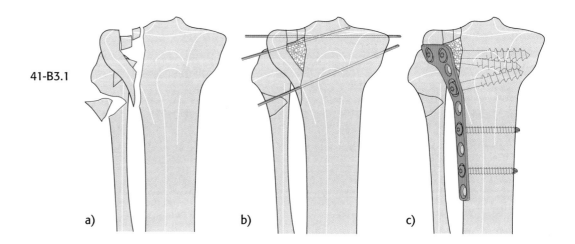

Fig. 4.8.1-12:
a) Typical 41-B3 fragment fracture with impaction of articular surface.
b) Reduction and temporary fixation with K-wires. The subchondral defect must be filled with a cancellous or corticocancellous autograft.
c) Final aspect after application of a lateral tibial head buttress plate.

bony defect should be filled with an auto-genous cancellous or corticocancellous bone graft or other bone substitute.

5.5 Medial plateau fractures (41-B2.2/B3.2)

Isolated medial plateau injuries are rare and often occur as a result of a high-energy force. They may be associated with meniscal tears, ligament rupture, neurovascular lesions, and compartment syndrome. For fractures with little or no condylar comminution or displacement, reduction with a large reduction forceps and fixation by percutaneous screws and a buttress plate is usually successful. Fractures with fragmentation extending into the intercondylar region preclude percutaneous treatment, especially if there is an associated posterior split-wedge fracture of the medial plateau. Intracondylar fragmentation should be repaired and the avulsed ligament fixed with lag screw or wire-suture loop placed through drill holes in the anterior tibial cortex.

5.6 Bicondylar fractures (type C)

These are characterized by involvement of both the medial and lateral plateaus (41-C1, 41-C2, and 41-C3) and often result from high-energy injuries. In addition to bicondylar fragmentation, there may be dissociation of the shaft from the metaphysis. A major concern in the surgical management of these severe injuries should be the limitation of additional damage to an already tenuous soft-tissue envelope. Distraction often improves alignment of the condyles by ligamentotaxis, and large percutaneously applied reduction forceps may improve the position of the intercondylar fragments or even achieve complete reduction. Based on this information the surgeon should carefully plan the approach or approaches, the reduction, and fixation techniques.

Analogous to fixing the fibula first in injuries about the ankle, a case may be made for fixing the (usually large) medial plateau fragment first, through a separate posteromedial incision

Any bone defect must be filled with a bone graft or bone substitute.

Type C fractures involve both tibial condyles.

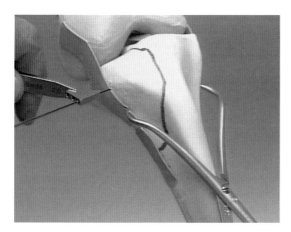

 Video AO20144c

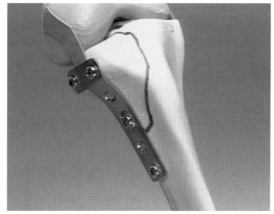

 Video AO20144d

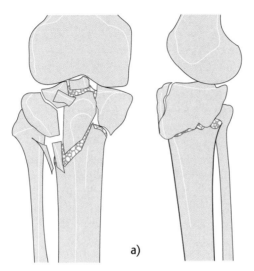

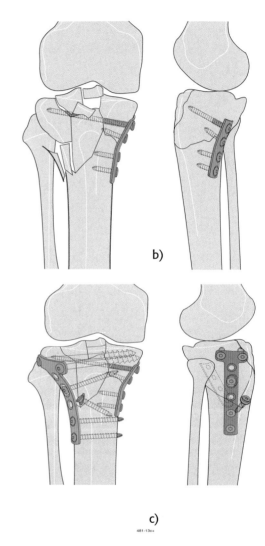

(see **Fig. 4.8.1-7**). This helps to establish the correct height of the joint line and offers a buttress against which to reduce the rest of the fracture. To secure the reduced medial plateau a LC-DCP 3.5 or one-third tubular plate 3.5 in an antiglide mode is applied (**Fig. 4.8.1-13**) (**Video AO20190a**). Next, the more fragmented lateral plateau is approached through a standard lateral para-patellar incision. Care must be taken to leave the most delicate soft-tissue cover over and medial to the tibial tuberosity untouched. The reconstruction of the lateral plateau follows the principles already mentioned above, using a heavier implant (L-plate, tibial buttress plate, or LC-DCP) to buttress this side (**Fig. 4.8.1-14**) (**Video AO20190b**). It is imperative to remember that the metaphyseal fixation of these fractures is the problem. It must be well planned and done when the soft tissues will allow for definitive fixation, either external or internal.

Fig. 4.8.1-13: a) High-energy bicondylar plateau fracture 41-C3.1 (see **Fig. 4.8.1-5**).
b) First step: Reduction and fixation of the medial block by a one-third tubular plate through a separate postero-medial approach (**Fig. 4.8.1-7**).
c) Reduction of lateral side through a standard lateral approach. Reduction and bony buttressing with bicortical graft, followed by fixation with a lateral T-plate 4.5 in buttress position.

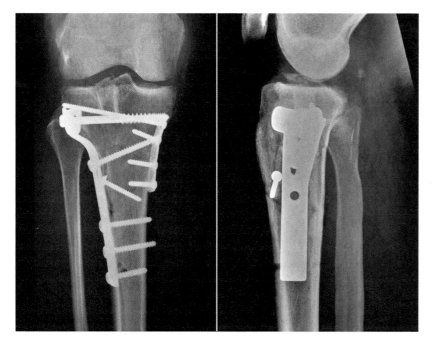

Fig. 4.8.1-14: AP and lateral x-ray view of the case shown in Fig. 4.8.1-5 7 weeks postoperatively. Note the well incorporated bicortical bone graft on the lateral side.

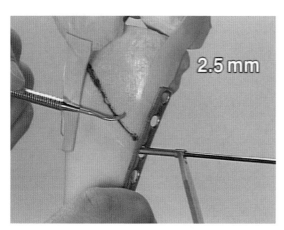

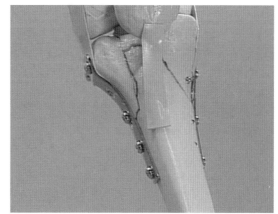

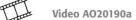 Video AO20190a

Video AO20190b

6 Postoperative management

Postoperatively, the limb is elevated on a frame for up to 5 days or on a CPM machine set at 20–60° of flexion [29]. Alternatively, the leg is placed in a knee immobilizer and active assisted range of motion is commenced about the third postoperative day. The knee immobilizer is discontinued when the patient regains quadriceps control. Usually by 7–10 days at least 90° of flexion is obtained. A cephalosporin antibiotic is administered for a maximum of 24–48 hours following surgery. Suction drainage, if indicated, is maintained for at least 24 hours. If there is significant swelling or tension on the suture line, physical therapy may be delayed until it has subsided. Depending on their compliance, patients with type B and C fractures are maintained with partial weight bearing (10–15 kg) or non-weight bearing for approximately 6–8 weeks [30]. The goal in pursuing active movement is to achieve 120° of knee flexion at the latest at 1 month postoperatively. Weight bearing is advanced to 50% body weight at 6–8 weeks depending on x-ray evidence of fracture consolidation. In higher-energy fracture patterns (B3 and C3 injuries), full weight bearing must often be delayed to 12–16 weeks. For low-energy injuries, full weight bearing is achieved by 8–12 weeks, and patients can expect to resume most simple activities at 4–6 months. Union at the metaphyseal-diaphyseal junction is often slow. If not progressing, the area should be bone grafted. Higher-grade injuries often take 12–18 months before the patients are able to resume routine daily activities.

7 Pitfalls and complications

The primary complications associated with the treatment of high-energy tibial plateau fractures are wound complications [31]. These can be minimized by careful evaluation of the soft-tissue envelope, the precise timing of surgery, development of full-thickness flaps, extraperiosteal dissection of fracture fragments, and minimizing soft-tissue stripping at the fracture site. Should superficial wound breakdown occur, immediate surgical intervention is indicated. Repeat irrigation and débridement with secondary closure, rotational flap, or, rarely, vascularized free flap may be indicated.

Malunion can occur with late joint collapse or deformation at the metaphyseal shaft junction. If the mechanical axis is affected, then an osteotomy to restore the normal mechanical axis is indicated. If the major articular fragment has displaced in the early postoperative period, this should be revised immediately; once the large articular fragment unites in the displaced position, it is impossible to free and reduce it anatomically.

Arthrofibrosis may occur in severe fractures or if early range of motion is not instituted immediately. Arthroscopic lysis of adhesions combined with gentle manipulation under anesthesia is indicated for those patients who fail to achieve 90° of flexion within the first 4 weeks after surgery.

8 Results

For low-energy tibial plateau fractures (41-B1.1, 41-B2, and 41-C1.1) treated surgically, multiple studies report excellent results. Patients with low-energy fractures treated with internal fixation techniques had from 75–90% satisfactory results [6, 32, 33]. In general, those patients who underwent internal fixation for low-energy-type fractures with minimal comminution and competent soft tissues have an excellent prognosis to return to full and restricted activities with only minimal limitations. Studies of patients with comminuted high-energy fractures requiring extensile approaches with single or double buttress plates have reported significant complications with wound slough, deep infection, and malunion/non-union.

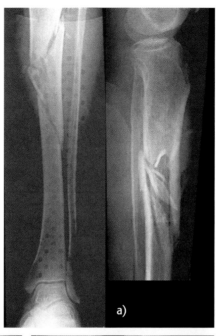
a)

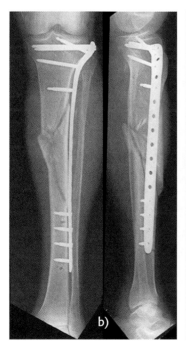
b)

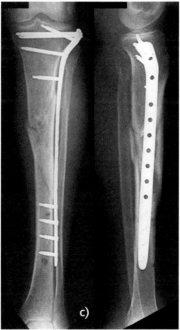
c)

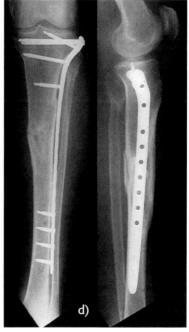
d)

Fig. 4.8.1-15:
60-year-old male with an isolated open type II lower leg fracture (42-B3) with extension and comminution of diaphysis.
a) Accident view.
b) After initial external fixation a 13-hole LISS-PLT plate was applied bridging the fracture zone.
c) Follow-up after 4 months, and
d) after 14 months. There were no complications and a good functional outcome.

Patients experiencing a high-energy-type plateau fracture treated with limited internal fixation with anti-glide plates and bridge plates, as well as limited posteromedial extraperiosteal plate application, have significantly reduced complications and have improved clinical outcomes.

Studies on patients with significant articular comminution or metadiaphyseal extension using limited articular fixation in combination with hybrid external fixation have also demonstrated minimal complications with an overall 70–80% rate of good to excellent outcomes for these severe fracture patterns.

9 Bibliography

1. **Benirschke S** (1991) Open reduction internal fixation of complex proximal tibial fractures. *J Orthop Trauma;* 5:236.

2. **Bolhofner BR** (1995) Indirect reduction and composite fixation of extraarticular proximal tibial fractures. *Clin Orthop;* (315):75–83.

3. **Duwelius PJ, Rangitsch MR, Colville MR, et al.** (1997) Treatment of tibial plateau fractures by limited internal fixation. *Clin Orthop;* (339):47–57.

4. **Hohl M, Luck V** (1956) Fractures of the tibial condyle. *J Bone Joint Surg [Am];* 38:1001–1018.

5. **Honkonen SE** (1994) Indications for surgical treatment of tibial condyle fractures. *Clin Orthop;* (302):199–205.

6. **Schatzker J, McBroom R, Bruce D** (1979) The tibal plateau fracture. The Toronto experience 1968–1975. *Clin Orthop;* (138):94–104.

7. **Bennett WF, Browner B** (1994) Tibial plateau fractures: a study of associated soft tissue injuries. *J Orthop Trauma;* 8 (3):183–188.

8. **Tscherne H, Gotzen L** (1984) *Fractures with Soft Tissue Injuries.* Berlin Heidelberg New York: Springer-Verlag.

9. **Andrews JR, Tedder JL, Godbout BP** (1992) Bicondylar tibial plateau fracture complicated by compartment syndrome. *Orthop Rev;* 21 (3):317–319.

10. **Watson JT** (1994) High-energy fractures of the tibial plateau. *Orthop Clin North Am;* 25 (4):723–752.

11. **Chan PS, Klimkiewicz JJ, Luchetti WT, et al.** (1997) Impact of CT scan on treatment plan and fracture classification of tibial plateau fractures. *J Orthop Trauma;* 11 (7):484–489.

12. **Barrow B, Fajman WA, Parker LM, et al.** (1994) Tibial plateau fractures: evaluation with MR imaging. *Radiographics;* 14 (3):553–559.

13. **Brophy D, O'Malley M, Lui D, et al.** (1996) MR imaging of tibial plateau fractures. *Clin Radiol;* 51 (12):873–878.

14. **Mast J, Ganz R, Jakob R** (1989) *Planning and Reduction Techniques in Fracture Surgery.* Berlin Heidelberg New York: Springer-Verlag.

15. **Georgiadis GM** (1994) Combined anterior and posterior approaches for complex tibial plateau fractures. *J Bone Joint Surg [Br];* 76 (2):285–289.

16. **De Boeck H, Opdecam P** (1995) Posteromedial tibial plateau fractures. Operative treatment by posterior approach. *Clin Orthop;* (320):125–128.

17. **Blake R** (1993) Treatment of complex tibial plateau fractures with the Ilizarov external fixator. *J Orthop Trauma;* 7:167–168.

18. **Gaudinez RF, Mallik AR, Szporn M** (1996) Hybrid external fixation of comminuted tibial plateau fractures. *Clin Orthop;* (328):203–210.

19. **Marsh JL, Smith ST, Do TT** (1995) External fixation and limited internal fixation for complex fractures of the tibial plateau. *J Bone Joint Surg [Am];* 77 (5):661–673.

20. **Murphy CP, D'Ambrosia R, Dabezies EJ** (1991) The small pin circular fixator for proximal tibial fractures with soft tissue compromise. *Orthopedics;* 14 (3):273–280.

21. **Stamer DT, Schenk R, Staggers B, et al.** (1994) Bicondylar tibial plateau fractures treated with a hybrid ring external fixator: a preliminary study. *J Orthop Trauma;* 8 (6):455–461.

22. **Weiner LS, Kelley M, Yang E, et al.** (1995) The use of combination internal fixation and hybrid external fixation in severe proximal tibia fractures. *J Orthop Trauma;* 9 (3):244–250.

23. **Apley A** (1956) Fractures of the lateral tibial condyle treated by skeletal traction and early mobilization. *J Bone Joint Surg [Br];* 38:699–702.

24. **Fowble CD, Zimmer JW, Schepsis AA** (1993) The role of arthroscopy in the assessment and treatment of tibial plateau fractures. *Arthroscopy;* 9 (5):584–590.

25. **Holzach P, Matter P, Minter J** (1994) Arthroscopically assisted treatment of lateral tibial plateau fractures in skiers: use of a cannulated reduction system. *J Orthop Trauma;* 8 (4):273–281.

26. **Perez Carro L** (1997) Arthroscopic management of tibial plateau fractures: special techniques. *Arthroscopy;* 13 (2):265–267.

27. **Vangsness CT, Jr., Ghaderi B, Hohl M, et al.** (1994) Arthroscopy of meniscal injuries with tibial plateau fractures. *J Bone Joint Surg [Br];* 76 (3):488–490.

28. **Koval KJ, Polatsch D, Kummer FJ, et al.** (1996) Split fractures of the lateral tibial plateau: evaluation of three fixation methods. *J Orthop Trauma;* 10 (5):304–308.

29. **Gausewitz S, Hohl M** (1986) The significance of early motion in the treatment of tibial plateau fractures. *Clin Orthop;* (202):135–138.

30. **Segal D, Mallik AR, Wetzler MJ, et al.** (1993) Early weight bearing of lateral tibial plateau fractures. *Clin Orthop;* (294):232–237.

31. **Young MJ, Barrack RL** (1994) Complications of internal fixation of tibial plateau fractures. *Orthop Rev;* 23 (2):149–154.

32. **Christensen K, Powell J, Bucholz R** (1990) Early results of a new technique for treatment of high grade tibial plateau fractures. *J Orthop Trauma;* 4:226.

33. **Waddell JP, Johnston DW, Neidre A** (1981) Fractures of the tibial plateau: a review of ninety-five patients and comparison of treatment methods. *J Trauma;* 21 (5):376–381.

10 Updates

Updates and additional references for this chapter are available online at:

http://www.aopublishing.org/PFxM/481.htm

4.8.2 Tibia: shaft

Raymond R. White & George M. Babikian

1 Assessment of fractures and soft tissues

The soft-tissue envelope is the most important component in the evaluation and subsequent care of tibial fractures. One third of the tibia has no muscle cover and lies directly beneath the skin. Therefore, every tibial fracture is associated with an injury to this most delicate skin cover.

The extent and location of swelling and bruises are assessed first. Fracture blisters are a sign of massive soft-tissue swelling and should be a warning to delay any intervention. The skin must next be assessed for intradermal swelling. When this occurs, the normal skin lines are lost and the skin appears shiny. This situation is not safe for routine surgery, which must be delayed until the skin starts to "wrinkle" again. It may be appropriate to consider some form of soft-tissue stabilization, traction, or a bridging external fixation while awaiting resolution of the swelling.

The pulses are assesed. A missing pulse in an otherwise healthy leg must raise suspicion of vascular damage, especially in a displaced fracture of the proximal tibia. The Doppler signal may be helpful but is not always reliable. If in doubt, an arteriogram should be performed. This is also advisable in the aged patient with established or potential vascular disease. In tibial fractures, nerve injuries are less common than arterial injuries, but the limb must still be closely checked.

Compartment syndromes occur more often with tibial fractures than with other long bone fractures. The cause can be swelling, bleeding, ischemia, or rebound edema following restoration of vascularity (ischemia reperfusion injury). The anterior compartment is most commonly involved. The usual signs of severe pain, pain with passive stretch, and localized loss of sensation must call for immediate action, either measurement of compartment pressure or operative fascial release, which must be combined with appropriate fracture fixation (see **chapter 1.5**).

X-ray imaging of the tibia is usually confined to standard AP and lateral x-rays, which should include the knee and ankle joints. Additional imaging is rarely required in fresh fractures.

The soft-tissue envelope is the most important component in the evaluation and subsequent care of tibial fractures.

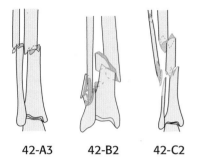

42-A3   42-B2   42-C2

Fig. 4.8.2-1: Müller AO Classification

Unstable and displaced fractures of the tibia seem to benefit from operative fracture fixation.

Displaced, unstable fractures of the proximal and distal thirds of the tibia provide the best indications for plating.

1.1 Classification

In the diaphysis, the A,B,C classification distinguishes between simple (A), wedge (B), and complex (C) fractures (**Fig. 4.8.2-1**). For further details see **chapters 1.4** and **2.2.**

1.2 Non-operative treatment

Fractures of the tibial shaft which are stable and only minimally displaced can be treated, with good functional results, by initial immobilization in a cast followed by early weight bearing in a PTB (patellar tendon bearing) cast. When the patient is able to bear weight, a PTB cast or brace is applied. This is worn until union occurs.

However, in most cases, **unstable and displaced fractures of the tibia seem to benefit from operative fracture fixation,** provided this is performed according to today's standards.

2 Plate fixation

Displaced, unstable fractures of the proximal and distal thirds of the tibia—with or without articular involvement—**provide the best indications for plating,** particularly when they are difficult to nail or require anatomically accurate reduction, for example, in high performance athletes and skiers (**Fig. 4.8.2-2** and **Fig. 4.8.2-3**).

Plating is contraindicated, however, in unreliable patients or when the soft tissues are damaged or deficient. If the possibility of early weight bearing is more important than perfect alignment, intramedullary nailing is preferred [1]. The following principles as described by Tscherne are relevant:

- Place plate under viable soft-tissue coverage.
- Create a stable bone-plate construct, allowing efficient healing.
- To apply the plate do not strip the periosteum and soft tissues any more than the injury did.

2.1 Surgical anatomy

The tibia is well suited to plate fixation, especially along its medial subcutaneous surface, where a plate does not interfere with the critical blood supply to the bone. Moreover, the flat medial surface makes contouring of the plate easy (see **chapter 3.2.2**).

The lateral surface is also accessible, but the exposure requires separation of the muscles and respect for the nerves and vessels. Plate contouring is more demanding on this side.

2.2 Preoperative planning and approaches

Tibial plating requires the basic instrument set, a range of narrow DCPs 4.5 or LC-DCPs 4.5, and reduction instruments. The patient is positioned supine on a regular, and preferably radiolucent, operating table. The use of a tourniquet is rarely necessary, but it may be an advisable precaution to have an uninflated cuff on the thigh.

The standard approach to the tibia lies 1–2 cm lateral (or in exceptional situations only, medial) to the tibial crest (**Fig. 4.8.2-4**). An incision placed directly over the crest will end up over the medial surface after skin closure and when the swelling has subsided, because of the extra bulk of the plate.

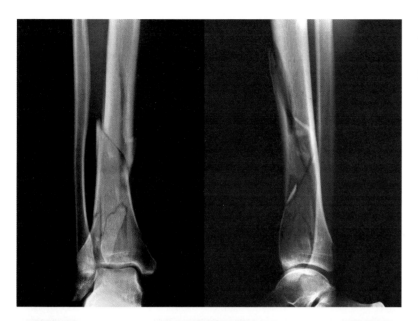

Fig. 4.8.2-2: Tibial shaft fracture of the distal third (42-C1), extending into the joint. Not considered suitable for nailing but a good indication for plating.

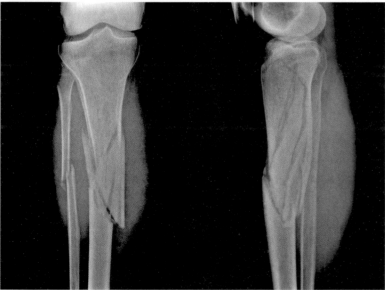

Fig. 4.8.2-3: Proximal tibial fracture (42-C1) as an indication for plating.

In the proximal and mid-shaft areas the incision is straight, while distally it is curved gently in the direction of the medial malleolus. The incision is carried down straight to the fascia without undermining the subcutaneous tissues. The paratenon of the tibialis anterior must be avoided. The periosteum should be pushed away at the level of the fracture gap no more than is needed to clear it and judge the reduction; elsewhere the plate will be placed on top of the undisturbed periosteum. Exceptionally, as when plating is delayed, a case can be made for subperiosteal placement.

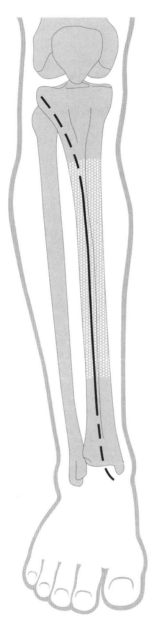

Fig. 4.8.2-4: a) Standard approach to the tibia 1–2 cm lateral to the crest, at the distal end, the incision crosses the crest in a gentle curve in the direction of the medial malleolus.

b) The cross-section of the lower leg shows the best way of approach to the medial as well as lateral side of the tibia.

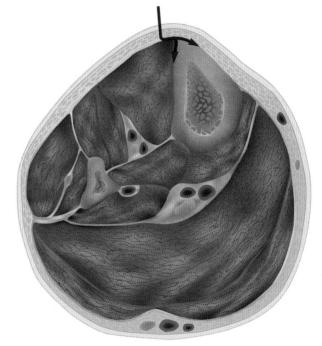

The newer plates, i.e., the narrow LC-DCP 4.5 and the PC-Fix (see **chapter 3.2.2**), lend themselves to extraperiosteal positioning because their minimal contact with the bone is designed to preserve the periosteal blood supply.

The skin incision for the lateral approach to the tibia is the same as for the medial side. The fascia overlying the muscle is incised a few millimeters away from the crest to leave a fringe for later reattachment. In order to position the plate, the muscles are gently separated from the tibia.

2.3 Reduction techniques

Selection of the correct reduction technique is probably the most important part of internal fixation. Whether by direct or indirect means (see **chapter 3.1**), the goal is to achieve alignment of the limb axis in all planes, including rotation. Manipulations to obtain reduction must be gentle and atraumatic in order not to compromise the essential blood supply to the fracture fragments.

With a simple fracture pattern, for example, spiral, oblique, and bending or spiral wedges, direct anatomical reduction should be followed by plating with interfragmentary lag screw fixation following classical AO principles (**Fig. 4.8.2-5**).

In case of complex fragmentation (type C) exact reduction is not required and the plate should only bridge the fracture area, [2, 3] following minimal exposure and indirect reduction technique (biological or bridge plating) (**Fig. 4.8.2-6c**) (see **chapter 3.3.2**). Appropriate length, rotation, and axial alignment must be restored.

> Selection of the correct reduction technique is critical.

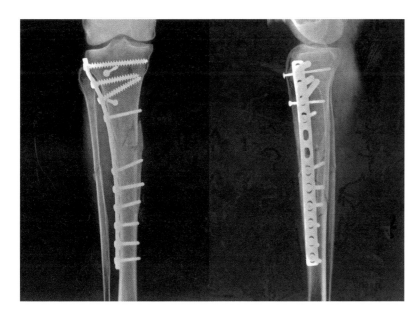

Fig. 4.8.2-5: Internal fixation of the fracture in Fig. 4.8.2-3 by the classical principles of interfragmentary compression with two 3.5 mm cortex lag screws and addition of a DCP 4.5 neutralization plate. Due to the soft-tissue conditions the plate was applied to the lateral aspect of the tibia.

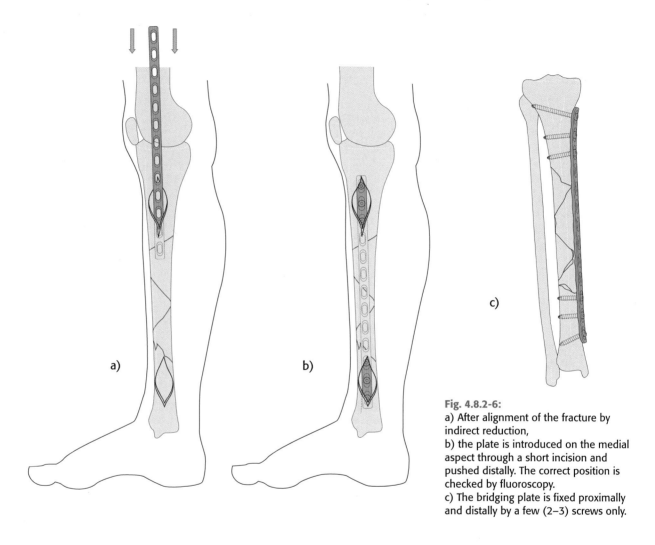

Fig. 4.8.2-6:
a) After alignment of the fracture by indirect reduction,
b) the plate is introduced on the medial aspect through a short incision and pushed distally. The correct position is checked by fluoroscopy.
c) The bridging plate is fixed proximally and distally by a few (2–3) screws only.

2.4   Choice of implant

A longer plate may be used. Not every hole need be filled.

In diaphyseal fractures of the tibia the narrow DCP 4.5 or LC-DCP 4.5 is most commonly used [4, 5]. Standard plating requires fixation in at least six cortices on either side of the fracture. Broad plates should not be used; they are too stiff and too bulky. Smaller plates (DCP 3.5) are occasionally indicated in the distal tibia but are not strong enough for use as single implants; the six cortex rule applies.

Currently **the trend is to use longer plates (8-hole to 10-hole) and not to fill every hole.** Two to three screws above and two to three below the fracture are considered sufficient provided they are spaced apart and anchored in good quality bone. To use more screws is not wrong but probably unnecessary (see **chapter 3.2.2**).

2.5 Tricks and hints

Percutaneous plate application is a technique which has recently been described as an alternative to classical ORIF [6]. It requires practice and experience in indirect reduction techniques, (with either a large distractor or external fixator) as correct axial alignment is mandatory before the plate is applied. In distal tibial fractures, indirect reduction and further stability may be achieved by plating the fibula. The reduction must be exact or the tibia will be reduced into malalignment. Once the fracture is reduced and the plate is contoured to fit the bone, the skin incision to introduce the plate is sited either proximally or distally to the fracture (**Fig. 4.8.2-6a/b**). With a sharp periosteal elevator a tunnel is prepared through which the plate is then introduced. Its correct position is checked under fluoroscopy and subsequently the screws are inserted through stab incisions (see **chapter 3.4**) (**Video AO20191**).

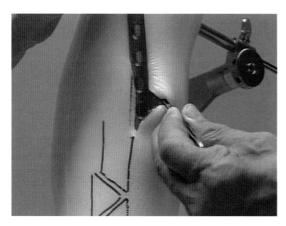

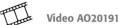
Video AO20191

2.6 Postoperative management

The leg is elevated with the ankle at 90° for about 5–7 days or until active dorsiflexion has been regained. Immediate active ankle and knee movement is encouraged with the help of a therapist. As soon as the swelling has subsided the patient, if appropriately compliant, is allowed to get up with immediate toe-touch weight bearing (10–15 kg). Otherwise the limb, after ankle motion is established, is protected by a short leg splint or cast. At 4–6 weeks weight bearing is increased. Depending on the original fracture pattern and on the radiological and clinical follow-up, full weight bearing should be reached by 10–12 weeks postoperatively. X-rays are obtained after 6 and 12 weeks. While callus—a sign of some motion at the fracture site—is welcome after bridge plating, it should not appear after a simple fracture has been treated by open reduction and fixation aimed at absolute stability.

2.7 Pitfalls and complications

The greatest concern after plating of fractures about the tibia is to obtain uneventful healing of the soft-tissue cover, particularly the skin, which is very sensitive to poor handling. **To avoid skin problems, correct timing of surgery, gentle soft-tissue technique and wound closure without tension,** as well as an atraumatic suture technique (modified Donati suture according to Allgöwer) are essential (**Fig. 4.8.2-7**).

To avoid skin problems wound closure without tension is required.

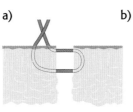

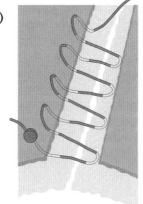

Fig. 4.8.2-7: Allgöwer stitch modified from Donati.
a) interrupted stitch
b) running suture.

3   Intramedullary nailing

3.1   Indications

In the central diaphysis the intramedullary nail is the implant of choice.

Intramedullary nailing is indicated for the majority of closed mid-shaft fractures of the tibia, as well as for open fractures with adequate soft-tissue cover [7–9]. In metaphyseal fractures it may be difficult to control and hold the correct alignment of the short fragment, so many surgeons prefer plates in such situations. Reamed intramedullary nails are preferred for closed fractures, allowing the use of stronger implants of larger diameter and offering a higher chance of undisturbed healing. The solid, so-called "unreamed" nail is presently preferred to the external fixator as the implant of choice for most open tibial fractures [10] (see **chapter 3.3.1**).

Fig. 4.8.2-8: Positioning for intramedullary nailing of tibia.
a) On a fracture table.
b) On a radiolucent table, knee fully flexed.
c) On a padded knee support, flexed as far as possible.

3.2   Preoperative planning

Based on the surgeon's preference and experience, the patient is placed on a fracture table or on a radiolucent table, with the leg draped so as to be freely mobile. A support can be placed under the thigh or the knee can be held fully flexed (**Fig. 4.8.2-8**). Surgical access to the ankle for distal locking must be assured.

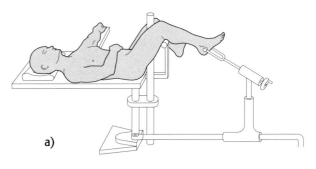

a)

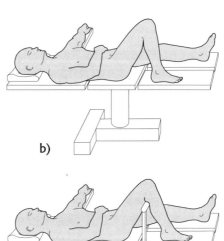

b)

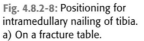

c)

For intramedullary nailing without reaming, the size of the medullary canal must be carefully measured in order to choose the correct nail diameter. Similarly careful measurement of the solid nail length is needed. This is more difficult as no guide wire for direct measurement is available; a ruler is used instead (see **chapter 3.3.1**).

3.3 Surgical anatomy and approach

As the proximal nail entry point is not in line with the medullary canal in the sagittal plane, its exact position varies depending on the nail design and nail stiffness. The recommendations for the different types of nails must therefore be carefully considered. Generally, in the frontal plane the entry point, which should remain extra-articular, must be centered over the canal, especially if there is a short proximal fragment. Eccentric nail insertion will result in a valgus or varus tilt of the proximal fragment.

The safest incision is therefore the one directly in line with the patellar ligament, which is split in the middle and gently held apart

(**Fig. 4.8.2-9a**). Some authors prefer to go medial to the patellar ligament (**Fig. 4.8.2-9b**) in order not to violate it. This may result in an eccentric starting point if not monitored by fluoroscopy. A lateral parapatellar incision is suggested as an alternative to assure proper insertion in proximal fractures, as the medullary canal tends to align to the lateral side of the tibia.

The locking bolts are usually inserted from the medial aspect or in an AP direction. During distal locking the saphenous vein and nerve can be injured if care is not taken to avoid them.

3.4 Reduction techniques

A diaphyseal fracture of the tibia can be reduced for nailing in a variety of ways: on a fracture table, manually, with percutaneous forceps, with the large distractor, or with an extra wide tourniquet. The fracture table gives excellent leg control and x-ray access, but is usually not really necessary as it adds considerable time and expense to the procedure. Once the leg is draped, a fresh fracture can often be reduced by manual traction, while the reaming rod or nail is passed

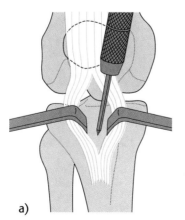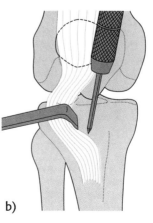

Fig. 4.8.2-9: Longitudinal approach for intramedullary nailing:
a) patellar tendon splitting,
b) medial to the tendon.

a)

b)

Getting rotation right is difficult.

across the fracture gap. If little or no traction is needed, percutaneously placed pointed reduction clamps or an extra wide tourniquet can reduce and hold the fracture for nail insertion. However, no reaming should be done with the tourniquet inflated. Good axial alignment prior to nail insertion is important when using the solid unreamed nail, as this relatively thin implant will not accomplish the fracture reduction "automatically" as can be the case with an universal tibial nail (**Fig. 4.8.2-10**). In delayed cases with some shortening, the distractor is most useful to gain length. The application of the distractor is shown in **Fig. 4.8.2-11**. Depending on which side it is applied, care must be taken to avoid varus or valgus deformation.

The most difficult part is determining the correct rotation. Keys to this are matching of cortical thickness on x-rays, placement of pointed fragments in correct position, and ensuring that the tension lines of the skin are not "twisted". In severely comminuted fractures it is advisable to prepare the opposite leg to allow intraoperative comparison of length and rotation.

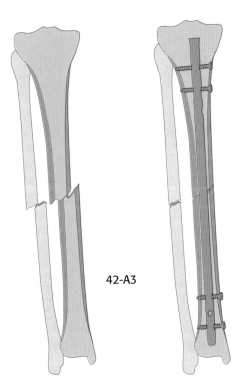

42-A3

Fig. 4.8.2-10: Reduction of a displaced transverse fracture with a reamed universal tibial nail that tightly fits into the medullary canal.

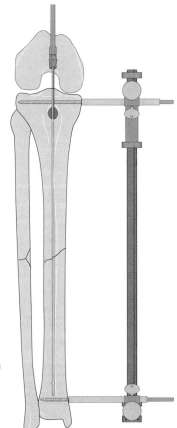

Fig. 4.8.2-11: Reduction by the large distractor with correction of length, axial and rotational alignment prior to nailing.

3.5 Choice of implant

The nails are either solid or cannulated. Reamed and unreamed nails are, in essence, similar implants which splint the bone from within; the difference lies in the technique of insertion. Reamed nails are tubular and tend to be used with a larger diameter. They have a long, proven record of success and are to be favored for closed fractures and non-unions. Unreamed nails are solid (UTN) or cannulated and are smaller (8–10 mm). They are becoming more popular for open fractures and are gaining some use in closed fractures with considerable soft-tissue involvement (**Fig. 4.8.2-12**) (**Video AO20149Bb/AO20139**).

Interlocking of the nail with bolts is **mandatory for small diameter nails** to enhance their stability in a wide medullary canal. Interlocking is recommended in all other situations unless the nail has achieved excellent endosteal contact above and below a stable mid-diaphyseal fracture. The amount of reaming should be adjusted to ensure that the nail will pass the narrow isthmus easily on one side and to permit the insertion of a large enough nail to provide stability on the other. In most cases, this means a nail of 11–12 mm in acute fractures. In delayed unions or non-unions, even larger nails are required for better stability.

Interlocking is mandatory for small diameter nails.

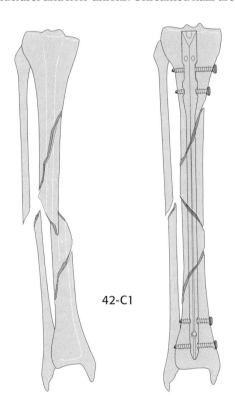

42-C1

Fig. 4.8.2-12: Segmental 42-C1 fracture stabilized with 9 mm unreamed solid tibial nail (UTN).

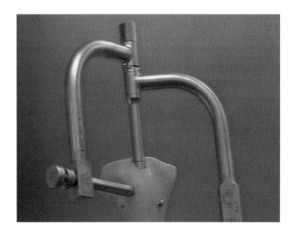

 Video AO20149Bb/AO20139

As interlocking can inhibit or prevent beneficial fracture loading, it is suggested that, depending on the fracture type, only dynamic locking is performed. In statically locked nails dynamization is rarely required unless there is delayed union of the hypertrophic type at 4–6 months. If there is an atrophic or poorly vascularized healing response, other methods of stimulating fracture union are necessary.

In distal fractures that also involve the fibula it is advisable [11] to fix it with a one-third tubular plate to add to stability and assure the reduction (**Fig. 4.8.2-13**).

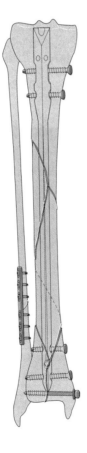

Fig. 4.8.2-13: In the case of a distal both-bone fracture, a one-third tubular plate in the fibula may help to control alignment of tibial fragment.

3.6   Tricks and hints for medullary nailing

(see **chapter 3.3.1**)

3.7   Postoperative management

The leg is elevated for the first few days until swelling has subsided and the patient is comfortable with active ankle and knee movement. The timing of weight bearing depends on the fracture pattern and patient compliance. In axially stable fractures fixed with a large nail, immediate weight bearing as tolerated is allowed. In axially unstable fracture patterns, partial weight bearing with 20–25 kg is begun immediately, while full weight bearing should be reached within 8–10 weeks. If by that time the fracture is not showing any callus and the patient complains of pain, the nail must either be dynamised and may even need to be exchanged.

3.8   Pitfalls and complications

About 30% of patients will have some knee pain which is usually due to an inappropriate nail entry point. A nail left proud can cause considerable irritation of the patellar ligament. Any incision about the anterior aspect of the knee usually leads to pain and discomfort, especially in kneeling.

Breakage of interlocking screws is not uncommon, especially with the use of smaller nails and in open fractures where the time to union takes longer. One of the features of closed nailing is the high rate of union and the low incidence of infection; therefore, these complications are not separately considered in this chapter.

4 External fixation

External fixation is advocated in severe open fractures (Gustilo types IIIB and IIIC), open fractures involving bone loss, and fractures where other implants, such as plates and nails, would remain exposed. **External fixation is, furthermore, indicated in life-threatening polytrauma situations where the fractures must be stabilized expediently with no additional insult to the patient.** External fixation can also be applied as an adjunct to internal fixation (lateral bridge plate—medial external fixator) or as a joint bridging device. In all these situations external fixation is intended to provide temporary fixation, to be followed by some means of internal fixation.

4.1 Surgical anatomy

In the tibia the pertinent anatomy for external fixation concerns the "safe zones" through which half pins, transfixing pins, or Schanz screws can be placed without involving muscles, tendons, nerves, or vessels [12]. The zones for half pins are an arc of about 220° proximally, 140° in the diaphysis, and 120° distally (see **chapter 3.3.3**). For transfixation, only thin (1.8–2 mm) wires that can be placed in a wider range should be used.

4.2 Preoperative planning

The main purpose of external fixation is to provide stable conditions for safe soft-tissue healing, and wound control on a temporary basis. The construct of the frame should therefore be as simple as possible, allowing full access to the wound, including the possibility of secondary soft-tissue procedures such as grafts, flaps, and free tissue transfer, as well as definitive internal fixation if desired.

To save time it may be advisable to preassemble the different components of the frame before its application.

4.3 Reduction techniques

The external fixator can be applied after reduction of a fracture, as described for plating or nailing. The external fixator can also be used as a reduction tool, especially if the tube-to-tube principle is applied (**Fig. 4.8.2-14**) (see **chapter 3.3.3**).

4.4 Choice of implant

In most situations the unilateral half pin frame will be the best choice for diaphyseal fractures. Circular frames with tensioned thin wires, including the hybrid frame, are useful in fractures that involve the proximal and distal tibia, as they allow stable fixation close to a joint without impairing joint movement. If the use of an intramedullary nail is planned at a later stage, it may be possible to apply a pinless fixator as a temporary device—see **chapter 3.3.3**.

External fixation is useful in severe open fractures or polytrauma.

With external fixation, the surgeon can build a custom-made device almost without limits. To increase stability there are several options, such as:

- spreading the pins as far apart as possible,
- increasing the number of pins,
- decreasing the distance between bar and bone,
- adding a second bar,
- adding a second frame to build a V-construct.

Too much rigidity may delay fracture healing due to a lack of loading at the fracture site.

4.5   **Tricks and hints**

For detailed instructions on application of the external fixator, see **chapter** 3.3.3.

In case of severe soft-tissue compromise it will be helpful to add a pin in the first metatarsal with the foot at a 90° angle, to prevent plantar flexion contracture (**Fig. 4.8.2-15**). As an alternative a footplate can be attached to the frame to hold the foot in neutral position.

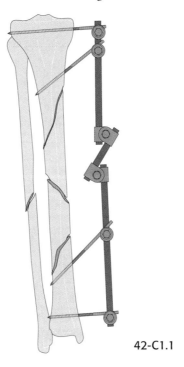

42-C1.1

Fig. 4.8.2-14: Example of a 42-C1.1 fracture stabilized by external fixator with tube-to-tube clamps.

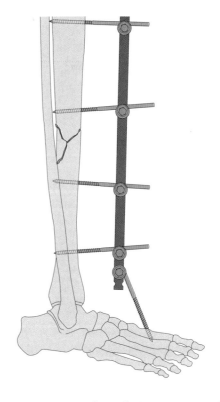

Fig. 4.8.2-15: To prevent plantar-flexion contracture of the foot, a pin may be placed in the first metatarsal and connected to main frame by a single bar.

4.6 Postoperative care

This will vary considerably, depending on the treatment plan and the soft-tissue conditions. If external fixation is considered as the definitive device, weight bearing starting at 10–15 kg should be encouraged early, as in plate fixation. As soon as callus formation is visible and once there are no clinical signs of instability, the patient can start to bear full weight. After removal of the external fixator, it may be prudent to protect the leg temporarily in a splint or brace.

When, as more frequently happens, the plan is to replace external by internal fixation, the timing of the second surgery becomes important, especially if intramedullary nailing is being considered. The interval between initial application of the fixator and the nailing should not be any longer than 14 days because the danger of pin-track infection appears to increase considerably after that time. Any signs of pin track irritation should preclude replacement of the fixator by a nail or even a plate.

The patient has to be shown how to take care of the pin sites by regular cleaning and the application of sterile dressings.

4.7 Pitfalls and complications

As already mentioned, pin site infection and pin loosening are the problems most frequently encountered with external fixation. The two are usually related and either can give rise to the other. Almost always they indicate instability of the entire construct. Loose or infected pins must therefore be repositioned and oral antibiotics may sometimes be required.

External fixation constructions that are too rigid can lead to delayed union, as the necessary loading of the fracture is missing. Therefore, sequential reduction of the rigidity of a frame, equivalent to dynamization of a nail, may be advisable.

5 Conclusions

In diaphyseal fractures of the tibia there are different, well-established treatment modalities [13]. Each one has its special indications, advantages, and disadvantages, and each technique must be correctly applied to obtain success. Although the intramedullary nail has gained much popularity, not least thanks to the smaller solid nails inserted without reaming, the pendulum presently seems to be swinging back in favor of the plate, especially in the proximal and distal third of the bone, where more "biological" approaches are applied. Now, more than ever, the state of the soft-tissue cover governs which fixation device should be used.

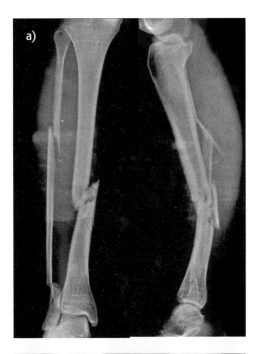

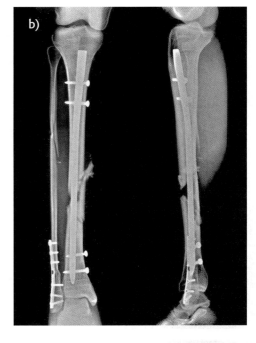

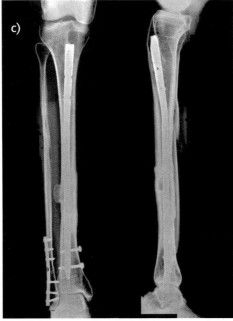

Fig. 4.8.2-16:
a) Complex fracture of tibial diaphysis (42-C1.1)
with distal fracture of fibula.
b) Postoperative view after fixation of the fibula
with one-third tubular plate and of the tibia with a
statically locked 8 mm solid tibial nail (UTN).
c) One-year follow-up.

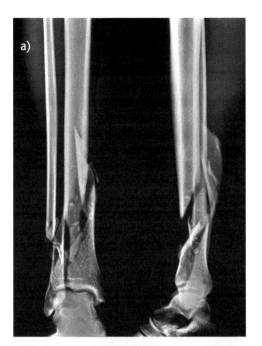

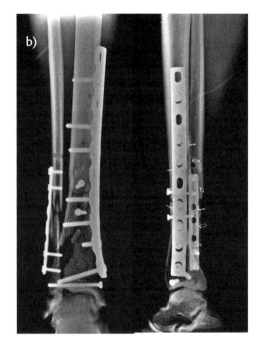

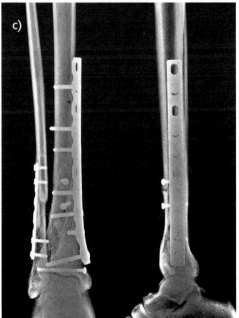

Fig. 4.8.2-17:
a) Complex fracture of distal segment of the tibia (42-C1.3) not readily amenable to intramedullary nailing.
b) Postoperative view after plating with narrow LC-DCP 4.5 of the tibia and one-third tubular plate of the fibula.
c) One-year follow-up with good functional result.

6 Bibliography

1. **Lang GJ, Cohen BE, Bosse MJ, et al.**
    (1995) Proximal third tibial shaft
    fractures. Should they be nailed?
    Clin Orthop; (315):64–74.

2. **Brunner C, Weber B** (1982) "Biologic"
    fixation of the fractured tibia. *Special
    Techniques in Internal Fixation.* Berlin
    Heidelberg New York: Springer-Verlag:
    160–161.

3. **Mast J, Jakob R, et al.** (1989) *Planning
    and Reduction Techniques in Fracture Surgery.*
    Berlin Heidelberg New York: Springer-
    Verlag.

4. **Matter P, Schultz M, Bühler M, et al.**
    (1994) [Clinical results with the limited
    contact DCP plate of titanium—a
    prospective study of 504 cases].
    Z Unfallchir Versicherungsmed; 87 (1):6–13.

5. **Rüedi T, Webb JK, Allgöwer M** (1976)
    Experience with the dynamic
    compression plate (DCP) in 418 recent
    fractures of the tibial shaft. *Injury;*
    7 (4):252–257.

6. **Krettek C** (1997) Concepts of minimally
    invasive plate osteosynthesis. *Injury;*
    28 (Suppl 1):805–809.

7. **Alho A, Ekeland A, Strømsøe K, et al.**
    (1990) Locked intramedullary nailing for
    displaced tibial shaft fractures [published
    erratum appears in (1991) *J Bone Joint
    Surg [Br];* 73 (1):181]. *J Bone Joint Surg [Br];*
    72 (5):805–809.

8. **Court-Brown CM, Christie J,
    McQueen MM** (1990) Closed
    intramedullary tibial nailing. Its use in
    closed and type I open fractures.
    J Bone Joint Surg [Br]; 72 (4):605–611.

9. **Bone LB, Sucato D, Stegemann PM,
    et al.** (1997) Displaced isolated fractures
    of the tibial shaft treated with either a
    cast or intramedullary nailing. An
    outcome analysis of matched pairs of
    patients. *J Bone Joint Surg [Am];*
    79 (9):1336–1341.

10. **Keating JF, O'Brien PJ, Blachut PA,
    et al.** (1997) Locking intramedullary
    nailing with and without reaming for
    open fractures of the tibial shaft. A
    prospective, randomized study.
    J Bone Joint Surg [Am]; 79 (3):334–341.

11. **Schweighofer F, Fellinger M,
    Wildburger R** (1992) [Combined tibial
    and ankle joint fractures]. *Unfallchirurg;*
    95 (1):47–49.

12. **Behrens F, Searls K** (1986) External
    fixation of the tibia. Basic concepts and
    prospective evaluation.
    J Bone Joint Surg [Br]; 68 (2):246–254.

13. **Szyszkowitz R** (1992) *Tibia shaft
    fractures.* Berlin Heidelberg New York:
    Springer-Verlag: 574–576.

7 Updates

Updates and additional references for this chapter
are available online at:
http://www.aopublishing.org/PFxM/482.htm

4.8.3 Tibia: distal (pilon)

Christoph Sommer & Thomas P. Rüedi

1 Assessment of fractures and soft tissues

1.1 Diagnosis

1.1.1 History and clinical examination

The **outcome of pilon fractures depends on the quality of reconstruction of the joint** [1] and on **how well the soft tissues recover.** Knowledge of the mechanism of injury is most important. Low-energy trauma (e.g., skiing) usually leads to simpler fracture patterns with minimal soft-tissue injury, while high-energy trauma with axial compression (fall from height, road traffic accident) produces complex intra-articular fractures with metaphyseal impaction and bone loss [2]. There may be contused or crushed soft tissues or an open injury. The clinical assessment has to include the state of the soft parts as well as the sensory and motor function of the foot structures [3]. Special attention has to be given to the early signs of a compartment syndrome. Grossly displaced or dislocated fractures must be reduced immediately.

1.1.2 X-ray examination/classification

Standard antero-posterior and lateral x-rays are taken, but in complex fractures more information about the tibio-talar joint is necessary. Conventional tomography in two planes or a CT scan with 3-D reconstruction may be used. MRI-studies are rarely required at this stage; later, they may be informative about vascularity of the bone and vitality of the cartilage. All fractures are classified according to the Müller AO Classification (**Fig. 4.8.3-1**).

2 Surgical anatomy

2.1 Bone structures and ligaments

The ankle joint, formed by the distal ends of tibia and fibula, as well as the talus, including joint-capsule and ligaments, is considered a functional entity (**Fig. 4.8.3-2**). Any incongruency between components (length, axis, and

Outcome depends on quality of articular reconstruction and on soft-tissue conditions.

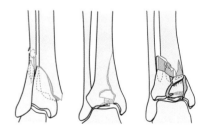

43-A1   43-B2   43-C3

Fig. 4.8.3-1: Müller AO Classification

rotation) or an unduly broad ankle mortise will lead to local overload, frequently resulting in cartilage degeneration and posttraumatic osteo-arthritis [4–9].

The distal fibula, as the most important structure of the ankle joint, is held in the notch of the tibia by the interosseous membrane and the anterior and posterior tibiofibular ligaments. In pilon fractures involving both bones, the syndesmotic ligaments per se are usually intact [1, 10], but often avulsed from the tibia with minor or major tibial fragments (Tilleaux-Chaput tubercle). However, the fibulotalar ligaments may be torn, especially in that type of varus injury where the fibula remains intact. The deltoid ligaments are nearly always intact, permitting indirect reduction by ligamentotaxis in selected cases.

Complex fractures require open reduction.

Soft-tissue conditions govern choice of procedure.

2.2 Blood supply

The distal fibula is supplied by branches of the peroneal artery, the distal tibia by branches of the anterior and posterior tibial arteries. **Too extensive a surgical exposure may endanger the anteromedial portion of the tibia**; and in the older age group with vulnerable blood vessels, the injury itself may already have put the local vascularity at risk.

An excessive surgical exposure may endanger the vascularity of the distal tibia.

3 Preoperative planning

3.1 General remarks and indication for surgery

As is the case with most displaced articular fractures, exact reconstruction of the distal end of the tibia is best achieved by open reduction and internal fixation (ORIF). While simple fracture patterns might be managed non-operatively or by minimally invasive procedures, **complex fractures almost always require open surgery**. From a technical point of view, the majority of displaced pilon fractures are salvageable by ORIF [2]. Exceptions are severely shattered fractures, where the only solution may be a (preferably) secondary fusion [11]. **The soft-tissue conditions usually determine the choice of procedure**, which is based on the individual situation and not necessarily on general principles [12, 13]. One of the more important factors for success appears to be the experience of the surgeon.

3.2 Choice of procedure

Reconstruction may be achieved by a one-stage open procedure, embracing the traditional four principles [1] (**Fig. 4.8.3-3**):

1. Reconstruction of the fibula.
2. Reconstruction of the tibial joint surface.
3. Autogenous cancellous or cortico-cancellous bone graft.
4. Support by buttress plate (medial/anterior—see **section 4**).

Fig. 4.8.3-2: Surgical anatomy and standard approaches.

a)

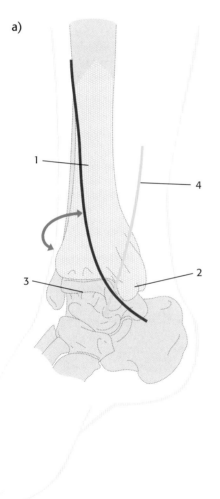

b)

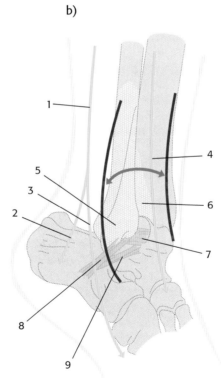

a) Antero-medial incision for tibia.
1   Anterior border of tibia
2   Medial malleolus
3   Ankle joint (talocrural joint)
4   Saphenous nerve

b) Postero-lateral incision for fibula.
1   Peroneal nerve
2   Lateral calcaneal branches of
     peroneal nerve
3   Lateral dorsal cutaneous nerve
4   Intermediate dorsal cutaneous
     nerve
5   Lateral malleolus
6   "Tubercle of Chaput"
7   Anterior talofibular ligament
8   Calcaneofibular ligament
9   Lateral talocalcaneal ligament

Between the two incisions a
broad bridge of healthy tissue
must be preserved.

With critical soft-tissue conditions, staged surgery may be advisable.

In **cases with critical soft-tissue injuries** as well as in open fractures, it may be advisable to **proceed in sequential steps** with several options [11–15] (**Fig. 4.8.3-4**):

First stage options:
- temporary joint bridging external fixator (tibia to talus/calcaneus),
- fibular reconstruction and bridging external fixator,
- fibular reconstruction and hybrid ring fixator,
- combination of K-wires/cannulated screws and external fixator.

Second stage:
- completion by ORIF.

In case of a large soft-tissue defect the plastic surgeons must be involved as early as possible. In very complex fractures with extensive damage to metaphyseal bone as well as to soft tissue, primary shortening may, exceptionally, be an alternative to salvage. This will then require secondary lengthening (e.g., proximal distraction) later [13].

Fig 4.8.3-3: Standard reconstruction of a 43-C3.1 fracture respecting the four traditional principles (see text). In most cases, the standard procedure is used with:
- reconstruction of the fibula (4-hole or 5-hole one-third tubular plate),
- reconstruction of the tibial joint surface,
- autogenous cancellous bone graft and buttress plate for the tibia (cloverleaf plate 3.5 medially).

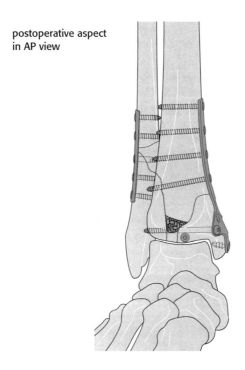

postoperative aspect in AP view

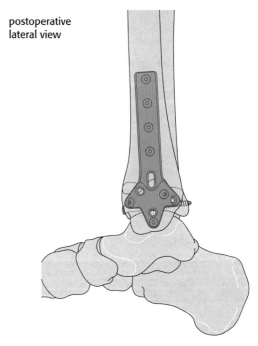

postoperative lateral view

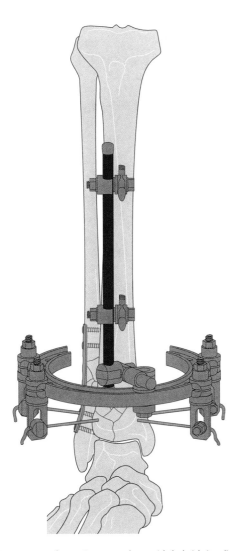

Fig. 4.8.3-4: Alternative procedure with hybrid ring fixator: In cases with severe soft-tissue injuries as well as open fractures, a hybrid ring fixator for the tibia may be used in combination with standard plating of the fibula. As definitive treatment, this technique is only suitable for simple articular fractures, which can be reduced anatomically by indirect reduction techniques and fixed by percutaneous lag screws. In complex fractures an anatomical and stable reconstruction of the articular bloc usually requires ORIF.

3.3 Timing of surgery

The best time for surgery is determined by the soft-tissue conditions. They must permit 2–3 hours of surgery. Only simple fractures with minimal soft-tissue injury may be definitively stabilized within the first 6–8 hours [3, 10].

For open fractures, the general principles require initial wound débridement, usually combined with some sort of preliminary external fixation as already mentioned, while definitive reconstruction of bone and soft tissue (see below) follows at a later date [13, 14].

For all other fractures we prefer to delay surgery for 7–10 days [3]. Until the soft-tissue edema is gone and the skin begins to wrinkle, calcaneal traction or a joint bridging external fixator should be used with limb elevated. This also allows for a detailed radiological assessment (tomography or CT scan) and careful preoperative planning on paper.

Soft-tissue conditions dictate timing and type of surgery.

3.4 Planning of reduction techniques

Preoperative planning is an essential part of the treatment of pilon fractures [3]. It consists of careful study of the x-rays, drawings both of the fracture fragments and the desired end result, consideration of intraoperative reduction techniques, as well as the choice of implants (see **chapter 2.4**). Once we have drawn and outlined all the fragments of the fibula and tibia in two planes, the following questions have to be answered:

1. Can we follow the classical principles or not?
2. **Do we need a bone graft:** cancellous, corticocancellous, etc.?

Careful planning is mandatory.

80% of type C fractures require a bone graft.

3. Is there a lateral key fragment in conjunction with the anterior syndesmosis that should be fixed separately (percutaneous cannulated screw)?
4. Are screws alone sufficient or do we need buttressing? If so, which size plate and in which position?

Finally, we draw the reconstructed distal tibia and fibula with the implants and define the sequence of the different steps of the operation.

3.5 Positioning

For surgery, the patient lies supine on a radiolucent table. After preparation of the entire limb including the ipsilateral iliac crest, the leg is placed on a pad. This permits rotation for better access both to the medial and lateral sides. A sterile tourniquet is applied to the thigh, but inflated only if necessary.

3.6 Approaches

> The cloverleaf plate is the standard implant for the tibia. One or two one-third tubular plates or LC-DCP 3.5 are often preferable.

We approach the fibula by a straight or slightly curved incision posterior to the fibular crest (**Fig. 4.8.3-2b**). Care must be taken not to damage the superficial peroneal nerve.

In the tibia we use the standard approach [10] (**Fig. 4.8.3-2a**) for all type A, B, and C fractures with an anteromedial fracture localization: The incision runs initially in a straight line lateral to the tibial crest, curving medially over the ankle joint in the direction of the tip of the medial malleolus. Between the postero-lateral incision over the fibula and the anterior one for

the tibia there should be a distance of at least 6–7 cm to preserve the vascularity of the anterior skin bridge. The incision should go straight down to the bone to avoid superficial skin flaps. Minimal exposure and careful handling of the periosteum are essential to avoid further vascular damage of the bone fragments. The tibiotalar joint is opened in the same vertical (sagittal) direction. A transverse incision of the anterior capsule to expose the joint creates the risk of devascularization of the anterior fragments (e.g., branches of the anterior tibial artery).

3.7 Choice of implants

The standard implant for the fibula is the one-third tubular plate, which can be applied either on the lateral aspect or on the posterior crest of the fibula in an antiglide position. A complex fracture may warrant the stronger LC-DCP 3.5. In the rare situation of severe lateral soft-tissue damage, an intramedullary pin, inserted from the tip of the fibula, may be a useful option, but it does not control rotation [10].

For the tibia, the standard implant is the cloverleaf plate, which is placed on the medial or anterior aspect of the distal tibia in buttress mode. An alternative choice is to use one or two one-third tubular plates or LC-DCP 3.5 anteriorly and medially, which allow a more individual indirect reduction, for example, push-pull technique in different planes (**Fig. 4.8.3-6a/b**). Plate-independent screws, (3.5 or 4.5 mm) regular or cannulated, are often required for additional fixation of the tibial joint bloc.

4 Surgical treatment— tricks and hints

4.1 Standard technique in four steps

4.1.1 Fibula

A simple fracture of the fibula is reduced directly with reduction forceps and is stabilized by a 4-hole or 5-hole one-third tubular plate in a lateral (**Video AO20160a**) or dorsal antiglide position (**Fig. 4.8.3-5a/b**). This first step usually reduces the lateral "key fragment" of the tibia automatically to its correct position and length.

A complex fracture is reduced indirectly by the push-pull technique or with the small distractor. It is essential to achieve the correct length, rotation, and axis. For stabilization we advocate long bridging plates.

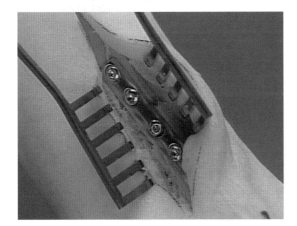

Video AO20160a

Fig. 4.8.3-5a–e: Illustration of the different operative steps.

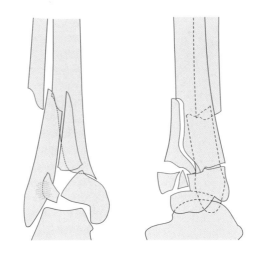

a) Preoperative situation: Fracture type 43-C2.

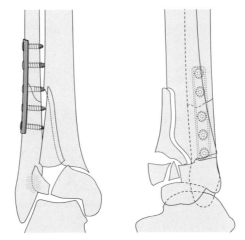

b) After anatomical reduction of the fibula using a 5-hole one-third tubular plate, correct length and position of the lateral "key" fragment of the tibia are obtained.

The four principles
1 Reconstruction of fibula
2 Reconstruction of articular surface of tibia
3 Bone autograft
4 Buttressing with plate(s)

4.1.2   Tibial articular surface

In complex cases with several articular fragments and considerable metaphyseal impaction, it may be helpful to apply an external joint-bridging distraction device (small distractor, external fixator) medially to get a preliminary indirect reduction of length and axis. Alternatively a transverse Schanz screw through the talus or calcaneus can help the reduction maneuver.

Temporary K-wires keep the fragments aligned.

Following the standard anteromedial approach (**Fig. 4.8.3-2a**), the tibial articular bloc is reduced by a combination of direct and indirect techniques. Anterior and medial fragments may be retracted by a pointed hook or a small bone spreader in order to obtain a view into the joint. This brings the central and posterior fragments clearly into view. The posterior fragment, often a key to reduction, may need to be derotated, something best done by a K-wire used as a "joystick". An impactor or elevator reduces impacted fragments. **All articular fragments are lined up one after the other using the talus as a mold to restore anatomical congruence**. Once aligned, the fragments are held in position by a pointed reduction forceps and/or preliminary K-wires (**Video AO20160b**), preferably those compatible with cannulated screws. These K-wires must be inserted parallel to the joint surface so as to allow subsequent interfragmentary compression without creating articular steps (**Fig. 4.8.3-5c**). Another key fragment, the anterolateral edge of the tibia, which is usually joined by the intact anterior syndesmotic ligament, must be perfectly aligned (**Fig. 4.8.3-5b/c**). Ideally this is done through a separate stab incision avoiding the anterior tibial artery. The preliminary reduction must be checked by x-ray or image intensifier before

Use talus as mold to restore anatomical congruence of articular fragments.

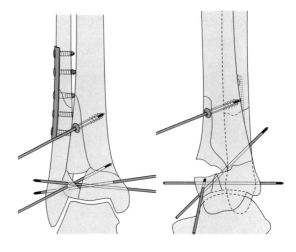

Fig. 4.8.3-5c/d: c) Reduction of the articular bloc and preliminary fixation with 1.2 mm K-wires which, if required, can be replaced by 3.5 mm cannulated screws.

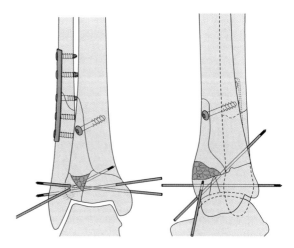

d) A bicorticocancellous bone graft fills the metaphyseal bone defect. Alternatively autogenous cancellous graft (or bone substitutes) may be used.

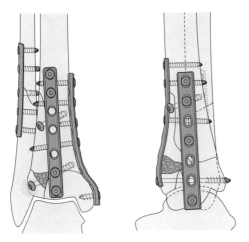

Fig. 4.8.3-5e: Tibial stabilization by an anterior as well as a medial LC-DCP 3.5 in buttress function. In addition, a lag screw was used to fix the anterolateral fragment, which is connected to the anterior syndesmosis.

definitive stabilization is started. Wherever possible, anatomical reconstruction and stable fixation by interfragmentary lag screws should be achieved, thus permitting early motion and good outcome.

4.1.3 Bone grafting

In all cases with articular impaction and/or a metaphyseal bone defect (B2, B3, C2, C3 fractures) the latter **has to be filled up, preferably by an autogenous bone graft or bone substitute**. Usually the graft is applied prior to the buttress plate, which will then be placed over this zone. Sometimes it is easier to fix the plate first to keep the main fragments in an anatomically reduced position and only then fill the defect. In cases with a marked loss of substance or loss of support a bicortico-cancellous bone bloc can be used as a strut (**Fig. 4.8.3-5d**).

4.1.4 Medial buttressing

The plate(s), precisely contoured, should be placed on the medial and/or anterior aspect of the tibia in buttress function depending on the site of the main impaction zone, as well as the soft-tissue conditions. The cloverleaf plate (**Video AO20160c**) is usually placed medially

Bone graft all metaphyseal defects.

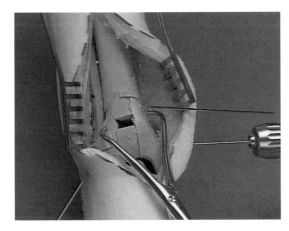

 Video AO20160b

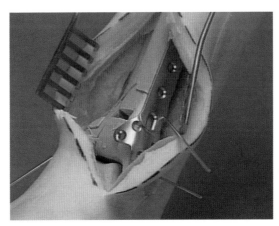

 Video AO20160c

Tricks for indirect reduction
with push-pull technique.

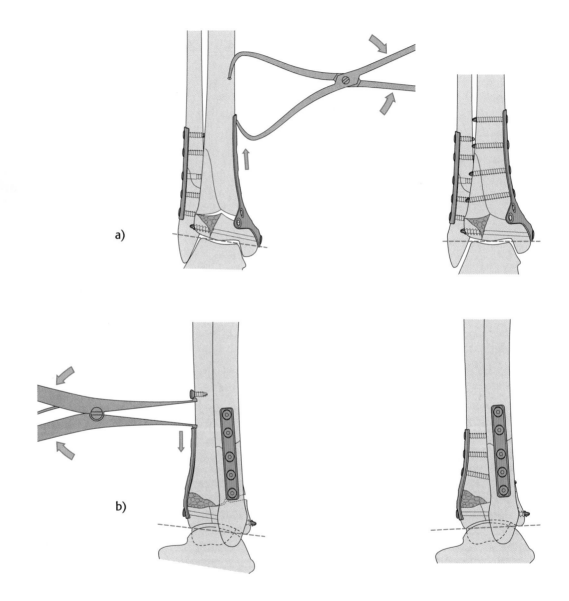

a)

b)

Fig. 4.8.3-6: Push-pull technique by one-third tubular plate(s). Axial deviations can
be corrected indirectly by either a "pull" (a) or a "push" (b) technique using a
pointed reduction forceps for compression or a small bone spreader for distraction.

(**Fig. 4.8.3-3**), where it should be well covered by a healthy soft-tissue flap. If placed anteriorly, the distal middle tab of this plate can be cut off with a strong cutting forceps. **Fig. 4.8.3-5e** illustrates the position of two LC-DCPs 3.5 on the medial and anterior aspects of the tibia respectively.

4.1.5 Wound closure

Before wound closure radiological confirmation of joint congruency, length, and axial alignment is mandatory. The anterior joint capsule is closed, but the anterior tibial fascia is left open to prevent a postoperative compartment syndrome. Suction drains are placed medially and laterally close to the fracture lines. **Finally, the skin is sutured paying great attention to an atraumatic technique**. Should a tension-free skin closure not be possible, the lateral incision may be left open and covered after some days by a split skin graft [10].

4.2 Alternative procedures

In cases with severe bone and soft-tissue injuries, it may be inadvisable or even impossible to achieve an anatomical and safe reconstruction by the standard procedure described. Alternative methods must therefore be considered. Selection of the best procedure has to be made on an individual basis [13]. Although there are other possibilities, temporary joint bridging by external fixation or the application of a hybrid ring fixator [16] (**Fig. 4.8.3-4**) are probably the most reliable as already mentioned above. As these alternative procedures are usually applied in the emergency situation as a first step, definitive surgery may be planned subsequently.

5 Postoperative treatment

With the patient still anaesthetized, a below-knee plaster splint is applied in 90° dorsiflexion to prevent an equinus position. The injured leg is elevated, with physical therapy starting on day 1 after removal of the suction drains. After 5–7 days ambulation is started on two crutches, allowing toe-touch partial weight bearing (10–15 kg), depending on the quality of fixation and reconstruction, as well as on patient compliance. A removable patellar-tendon-bearing (PTB) walking caliper may be adopted after the swelling has completely subsided (after 2–3 weeks) and is to be used for 2–3 months [1]. Full weight bearing may be started after 8–10 weeks, depending on radiological fracture consolidation, as well as on the clinical follow-up. In cases with extensive articular comminution or needing large bone grafts, definitive consolidation may take up to 4–5 months.

Atraumatic skin closure is crucial. Any tension is to be avoided.

6 Pitfalls and complications

6.1 Pitfalls

The most important steps to prevent pitfalls and complications are careful preoperative planning, including correct timing of the operation, and the perioperative handling of the soft tissue. Many of these factors are hard to describe and are mostly a question of personal experience. **Complex pilon fractures should therefore be treated by the most experienced surgeons and are not the domain of junior staff**.

Planning, timing, and careful soft-tissue handling are essential to prevent complications.

The more complex the fracture, the greater the need for an experienced surgeon.

6.2   Complications

Most complications stem from soft-tissue problems.

Many complications can follow operative treatment of pilon injuries [16, 17]. **Most stem from soft-tissue problems** such as wound dehiscence and skin necrosis with superficial infection. The literature reports ranges of between 10–35%. There is also a strong correlation with the mechanism and energy of the injury (extent of soft-tissue damage), as well as the surgeon's experience. If management is not timely and adequate (wound revision, antibiotics, free tissue transfer), the early complications (osteitis, septic arthritis) can become disastrous with deep infection (2–30%) resulting in early arthrodesis or even amputation.

Delayed and/or non-unions occur in 0–22% of cases and are strongly dependent upon fracture pattern and the stability achieved. The greater the comminution and impaction, the higher the risk of non-union [10]. An adequate primary bone graft in the defect can prevent some of the metaphyseal delayed unions, but other non-unions, especially of borderline articular fragments, are due to a vascular deficiency resulting from the trauma itself or too wide a surgical exposure (**Table 4.8.3-1**).

Table 4.8.3-1: Main pitfalls and the resulting complications in operated pilon fractures.

Pitfalls	Complications
Correct preoperative planning, but not strictly adhered to during surgery.	Incorrect reconstruction with deformity, non-union, osteoarthritis.
Wrong timing: operation too soon after trauma.	Wound-healing problems (skin necrosis and/or infection).
Incorrect reconstruction of fibula (too short, malrotation, axial deviation).	Deformity (valgus, varus), prevention of correct tibial reduction.
Persistent intra-articular dislocations (gaps > 2 mm, steps > 1 mm).	Articular incongruency with posttraumatic osteoarthritis.
Anterolateral tibial key fragment not anatomically reduced and fixed.	Too wide ankle mortise with posttraumatic osteoarthritis.
Insufficient bone graft in metaphyseal defect.	Secondary collapse of articular surface, delayed union.
Too early partial or full weight bearing, poor patient compliance.	Implant loosening and/or failure with deformity and/or non-union.

Table 4.8.3-2: Complications following the operative treatment of intra-articular pilon fractures (some selected publications).

Author	Publ. year	No. of cases	ORIF	MIO	Wound healing problems*	Deep infection	Delayed non-union
Rüedi, Allgöwer [1]	1969	82 (B-/C-Fx)	78		10 (12%)	4 (4.8%)	1
Heim [9]	1991	187 (B-Fx) 167 (C1/2-Fx) 311				21 (6.7%)	1 14 (8.4%)
Beck [18]	1993	380	most			9 (2.5%)	6 (1.6%)
Muhr, Breitfuss [17]	1993	229	182	47		13% 4.8%	
Nast-Kolb, et al. [19]	1993	54	11	43	3 (27%) 6 (14%)	5%	2 (3.6%)
Tornetta, et al. [20]	1993	17 (B-/C-Fx)		17	1	1	0
Rommens, et al. [11]	1994	45 (–STI)* 36 (+STI)*	44 22	1 14	5 (11%) 5 (14%)	3 (6.7%) 8 (22.2%)	4 (9%) 9 (25%)
Bastian, et al. [21]	1995	51 (B-/C-Fx)	15	36	5 (33%) 8 (22%)	5 (10%)	
Sommer, Rüedi [8]	1999	112 (B-/C-Fx)	106	6	1 (1%)	0	4 (3.6%)

* Wound-healing problems = wound dehiscence, skin necrosis, superficial infection.
–STI = without soft-tissue injury.
+STI = with soft-tissue injury.
MIO = Minimally Invasive Osteosynthesis.

7 Results

There is a strong correlation between anatomical reconstruction and functional outcome.

Three main factors influence results after pilon fractures:

- the impact (energy) of injury reflected in the fracture and soft-tissue classification [12, 15],
- the surgeon's abilities and experience,
- the patient (compliance, general condition, vascular status, etc.).

It is very difficult to compare results from different publications. The patient groups vary greatly (rate and grade of soft-tissue injury, percentage of complex fractures) as do the operative procedures between the traditional ORIF, purely percutaneous techniques, and combinations of both.

As in other articular fractures, good functional results can be observed in 60–80% of patients [1, 12, 18, 20–22]. **Furthermore, there seems to be a direct correlation between a correct anatomical reconstruction of the ankle joint and a good outcome even over a prolonged period of time [7–9].** On the other hand, radiological appearance does not necessarily reflect the clinical and functional results. Ankle fusions are seldom necessary (3–27%) and are mostly related to cases with osteitis/arthritis [14] (**Table 4.8.3-2**). The best functional results can be achieved in patients with high compliance, more often seen in self-employed, sport-active, and socially integrated people (**Table 4.8.3-3**). In our consecutive series of 112 patients the functional result after 1 year was good in 74.5% and improved after an average of 10 years (80.9%), although the degree of radiographic osteoarthritis increased [8].

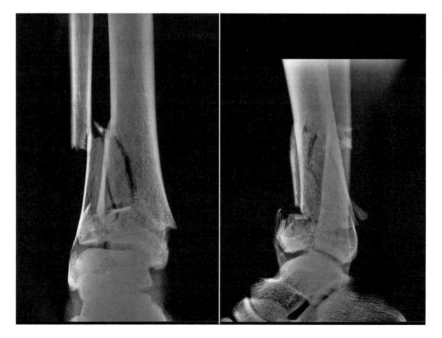

Fig. 4.8.3-7a:
Male, 30 years of age.
43-C2 fracture, AP and lateral view.

Table 4.8.3-3: Late results in operatively treated intra-articular pilon fractures.

Author	Publ. year	ORIF/ MIO	No. of cases	No. of follow-up cases	Follow-up time (years)	Severe osteo-arthritis	Arthro-desis	Good/ very good results
Rüedi, Allgöwer [1]	1969	ORIF	82	78	1		4 (4%)	59 (70%)
Rüedi [5]	1973	ORIF	82	54	9		7 (13%)	46 (85%)
Heim [9]	1991	mostly ORIF	289 (B-Fx)	187	1	30 (10.4%)	1	
			391 (C-Fx)	213	1	82 (20.9%)	6 (3%)	
Beck [18]	1993		380	256	7.5		1	209 (82%)
Muhr, Breitfuss [17]	1993	ORIF		182	5		34 (18%)	
		MIO		47	2		3 (6%)	
Nast-Kolb, et al. [19]	1993	ORIF		14	1–4	6 (43%)		71.7%
		MIO		28		5 (18%)		
Tornetta, et al. [20]	1993	MIO		17	1–3.5			12 (70%)
Helfet, et al. [23]	1994	ORIF		28	1.4			21 (62%)
		MIO		6				
Rommens, et al. [11]	1994		81	64	1		2 (3%)	41 (64%)
Bastian, et al. [21]	1995	ORIF	71	15	1.3	3 (4.2%)	4 (27%)	
		MIO		36		7 (19.1%)	8 (22%)	
Sommer, Rüedi [8]	1999	ORIF	77	13 (B-Fx)	10	2 (15.4%)	0	11 (84.6%)
				34 (C-Fx)		3 (8.8%)	1 (3%)	27 (79.4%)

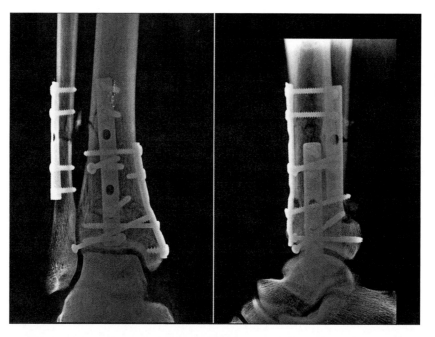

Fig. 4.8.3-7b:
Postoperative view after fixation of fibula by a one-third tubular plate and of the tibia by two DCPs 3.5, AP and lateral.

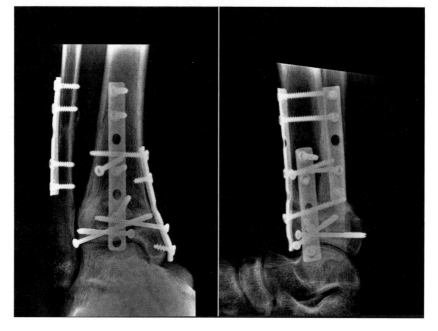

Fig. 4.8.3-7c:
One-year follow-up with good functional result, AP and lateral.

8 Bibliography

1. **Rüedi T, Allgöwer M** (1969) Fractures of the lower end of the tibia into the ankle joint. *Injury*; 1:92–99.

2. **Heim U** (1993) Morphological features for evaluation and classification of pilon tibial fractures. In: Tscherne H, Schatzker J, editors. *Major Fractures of the Pilon, the Talus, and the Calcaneus*. Berlin Heidelberg New York: Springer-Verlag, 29–41.

3. **Mast J** (1993) Pilon fractures of the distal tibia: a test of surgical judgment. In: Tscherne H, Schatzker J, editors. *Major Fractures of the Pilon, the Talus, and the Calcaneus*. Berlin Heidelberg New York: Springer-Verlag, 7–27.

4. **Heim U, Naser M** (1976) [Operative treatment of distal tibial fractures. Technique of osteosynthesis and results in 128 patients (author's transl)]. *Arch Orthop Unfallchir*; 86 (3):341–356.

5. **Rüedi T** (1973) Fractures of the lower end of the tibia into the ankle joint: results 9 years after ORIF. *Injury*; 5 (2):130–134.

6. **Resch H, Pechlaner S, Benedetto KP** (1986) [Long-term results after conservative and surgical treatment of fractures of the distal end of the tibia]. *Aktuelle Traumatol*; 16 (3):117–123.

7. **Resch H, Benedetto KP, Pechlaner S** (1986) [Development of posttraumatic arthrosis following pilon tibial fractures]. *Unfallchirurg*; 89 (1):8–15.

8. **Sommer C, Rüedi T** (1999) Late results after operative treatment of intra-articular pilon fractures. (in preparation).

9. **Heim U** (1991) *The pilon tibial fracture: classification, surgical techniques, results*. 1st ed. Berlin Heidelberg New York: Springer-Verlag.

10. **Bonar SK, Marsh JL** (1993) Unilateral external fixation for severe pilon fractures. *Foot Ankle*; 14 (2):57–64.

11. **Rommens PM, Claes P, De Boodt P, et al.** (1994) [Therapeutic procedure and long-term results in tibial pilon fracture in relation to primary soft-tissue damage]. *Unfallchirug*; 97 (1):39–46.

12. **Trentz O, Friedl HP** (1993) Critical soft-tissue conditions in pilon fractures. In: Tscherne H, Schatzker J, editors. *Major Fractures of the Pilon, the Talus, and the Calcaneus*. Berlin Heidelberg New York: Springer-Verlag, 59–64.

13. **Bone L, Stegemann P, McNamara K, et al.** (1993) External fixation of severely comminuted and open tibial pilon fractures. *Clin Orthop*; (292):101–107.

14. **Crutchfield EH, Seligson D, Henry SL, et al.** (1995) Tibial pilon fractures: a comparative clinical study of management techniques and results. *Orthopedics*; 18 (7):613–617.

15. **McDonald MG, Burgess RC, Bolano LE, et al.** (1996) Ilizarov treatment of pilon fractures. *Clin Orthop*; (325):232–238.

16. **McFerran MA, Smith SW, Boulas HJ, et al.** (1992) Complications encountered in the treatment of pilon fractures. *J Orthop Trauma*; 6 (2):195–200.

17. **Muhr G, Breitfuss H** (1993) Complications after pilon fractures. In: Tscherne H, Schatzker J, editors. *Major Fractures of the Pilon, the Talus, and the Calcaneus*. Berlin Heidelberg NewYork: Springer-Verlag, 65–67.

18. **Beck E** (1993) Results of operative treatment of pilon fractures. In: Tscherne H, Schatzker J, editors. *Major Fractures of the Pilon, the Talus, and the Calcaneus.* Berlin Heidelberg New York: Springer-Verlag, 49–51.

19. **Nast-Kolb D, Betz A, Rodel C, et al.** (1993) [Minimal osteosynthesis of tibial pilon fracture. *Unfallchirurg;* 96 (10):517–523.

20. **Tornetta P, Weiner L, Bergman M, et al.** (1993) Pilon fractures: treatment with combined internal and external fixation. *J Orthop Trauma;* 7 (6):489–496.

21. **Bastian L, Blauth M, Thermann H, et al.** (1995) [Various therapy concepts in severe fractures of the tibial pilon (type C injuries). A comparative study]. *Unfallchirurg;* 98 (11):551–558.

22. **Waddell JP** (1993) Tibial plafond fractures. In: Tscherne H, Schatzker J, editors. *Major Fractures of the Pilon, the Talus, and the Calcaneus.* Berlin Heidelberg New York: Springer-Verlag, 43–48.

23. **Helfet DL, Koval K, Pappas J, et al.** (1994) Intra-articular "pilon" fracture of the tibia. *Clin Orthop;* (298):221–228.

9 Updates

Updates and additional references for this chapter are available online at:
http://www.aopublishing.org/PFxM/483.htm

4.9 Malleolar fractures

David M. Hahn & Chris L. Colton

1 Introduction

The ankle joint may be damaged either by direct or, more commonly, by indirect rotational, translational, and axial forces. These result in subluxation or dislocation of the talus out of the ankle mortise, usually associated with a fracture complex.

Malleolar injuries are articular fractures. The treatment aims at restoring normal joint anatomy and providing sufficient stability for early movement. While stable undisplaced fracture patterns can be treated by closed methods, anatomical restoration and stable fixation of the unstable displaced fracture is best achieved by open reduction and internal fixation.

The decision to operate is not based on the fracture pattern alone. The ankle joint is substantially subcutaneous and so the condition of the soft-tissue envelope is of paramount importance. Patient factors such as age, diabetes, and osteoporosis may alter the indications and fixation techniques for this fracture.

2 Functional anatomy and biomechanics

Stability of the osseoligamentous mortise relies both on the bony configuration and on the osseoligamentous system. The bony mortise consists of the articulation of three bones: the distal aspect of the tibia, the distal aspect of the fibula, and the talus. The main articulation is between the saddle-shaped dome of the talus and the tibial plafond. The talus also has important medial and lateral facets, which articulate with the respective malleoli.

The bony components of the ankle are stabilized by two ligamentous complexes:

1) Inferior tibiofibular complex ("syndesmosis")
The distal tibia and fibula are held together to provide a tight elastic ankle mortise and this syndesmotic bond consists of three elements:
- The anterior syndesmotic (anterior tibiofibular) ligament joins the anterior tibial tubercle (tubercle of Tillaux-Chaput) to the lateral malleolus (**Fig. 4.9-1a**).
- The posterior syndesmotic (posterior tibiofibular) ligament is stronger and joins the lateral malleolus to the posterior tibial tubercle (**Fig. 4.9-1b**).

Most malleolar fractures result from indirect forces.

- The interosseous ligament binds the tibia to the fibula in the incisura fibularis, and is continuous with the interosseous membrane proximal to the syndesmotic ligaments.

2) The collateral ligaments prevent varus-valgus tilting of the talus in the ankle mortise and include the following:

The lateral ligament complex which has three distinct elements:

- The anterior talofibular ligament originates from the anterior border of the fibula and inserts onto the lateral aspect of the talar head and neck.
- The calcaneofibular ligament originates at the tip of the fibula and runs posteriorly and distally deep to the peroneal tendons to insert onto the calcaneus.
- The posterior talofibular ligament originates from the posterior aspect of the distal fibula and inserts posteriorly onto the talus (**Fig. 4.9-2a**).

The medial collateral ligament complex, or deltoid ligament, has two portions:

- the superficial, fan-shaped tibio-calcaneal ligament, and
- the deep anterior and posterior talotibial ligaments (**Fig.4.9-2b**).

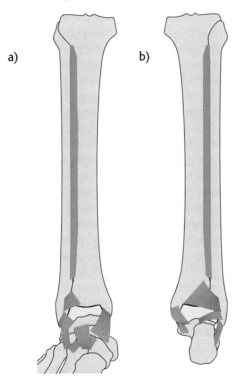

Fig. 4.9-1: The anatomy of the tibiofibular ligaments.
a) Anterior view showing the anterior tibiofibular ligament and the anterior tibial tubercle of Tillaux-Chaput.
b) Posterior view showing the posterior tibiofibular ligament.

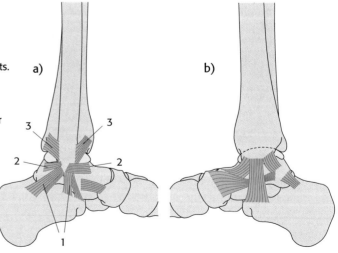

Fig. 4.9-2: The collateral ligaments.
a) The lateral ligament complex:
 1) calcaneofibular,
 2) anterior and posterior talofibular,
 3) anterior and posterior syndesmotic.
b) The medial ligament complex or deltoid ligament.

2.1 Mortise congruity

The talus remains in close contact with the entire articular surface of the mortise in all positions of dorsiflexion and plantar flexion. This intimate contact is important for even distribution of the load at the ankle [1] and must be restored after injury. Biomechanical studies have shown that ankle congruity is maintained not by movement as a hinge but by a combination of sliding and rotating of the talus, coupled with translational movement of the fibula, in all positions of dorsiflexion and plantar flexion [2, 3].

Plantar flexion of the ankle is accompanied by internal rotation of the talus; dorsiflexion results in external rotation of the talus and combined posterolateral translation and external rotation of the fibula. This fibular motion at the syndesmosis is an essential part of the normal ankle function.

The total congruity of the articulation is the most important element in protecting the thin articular cartilage of the ankle from high mean stress and secondary degeneration. **Small disturbances of this congruity reduce the contact area and thereby overload the articular cartilage** [4, 5].

3 Pathogenesis/ mechanism of injury: the basis of classification

The position of the foot and the direction of the deforming force dictate the pattern of failure of the osseoligamentous mortise. The position of the foot determines which structures are tight at the onset of the deformation, and therefore

most likely to fail first. If the foot is supinated (inverted), the lateral structures are tight and the medial structures relaxed. By contrast, in pronation (eversion), the medial structures are tight and fail first. The deforming force can be rotational, usually external, or translational in abduction or adduction. The resulting specific fracture patterns of the lateral malleolus form the basis for the classification (**Fig. 4.9-3**).

3.1 The infrasyndesmotic injury (type A)

(see **Fig. 4.9-9**)

With the foot supinated and an adduction deforming force applied to the talus, the first injury will occur on the lateral side, which is under tension. This may be either rupture of the lateral ligament, osseoligamentous avulsion or **transverse fracture of the lateral malleolus, at or just below the level of the tibial plafond** (**Fig. 4.9-4a**). If the deforming force then continues, the talus tilts and this causes a shearing compression fracture of the medial malleolus (**Fig. 4.9-4b**).

3.2 The transsyndesmotic injury (type B)

(see **Fig. 4.9-10**)

The commonest pattern of injury occurs with axial loading of a supinated foot. By virtue of the obliquity of the axis, about which subtalar movement occurs, inversion results in external rotation of the talus (**Fig. 4.9-5**). Firstly, the fibula fails producing an oblique fracture,

The talus remains in contact throughout the range of ankle movement.

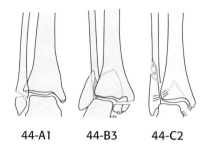

44-A1   44-B3   44-C2

Fig. 4.9-3: Müller AO Classification

Type A fractures:
Transverse fracture of the lateral malleolus, at or just below the level of the ankle joint.

Small disturbances of congruity overload articular cartilage.

Type B fractures:
The commonest pattern of injury occurs with axial loading of the supinated foot.

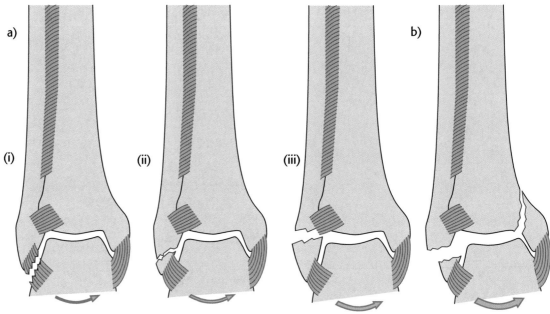

Fig. 4.9-4: Sequence of morphological changes giving rise to type A fractures.

a) Failure in tension of the lateral side with the foot supinated and an adduction force applied:
  (i)   rupture of the lateral ligament
  (ii) osseoligamentous avulsion
  (iii) transverse fibular fracture

b) Medial injury resulting from forced talar adduction. With failure of the lateral side plus vertical axial load, the talus tilts causing a shearing, compression fracture of the medial malleolus.

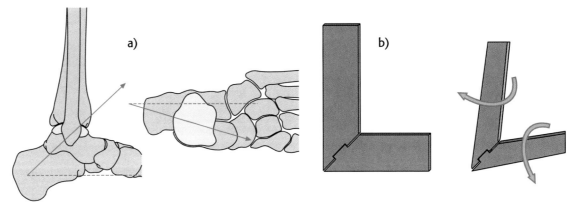

Fig. 4.9-5: a) The axis about which movement takes place at the subtalar joint, is angled an average 42° above the horizontal and 16° medially.

b) This causes the subtalar joint to act as a torque converter, similar to an angled hinge, so that as the os calcis inverts, the talus is caused to rotate externally.

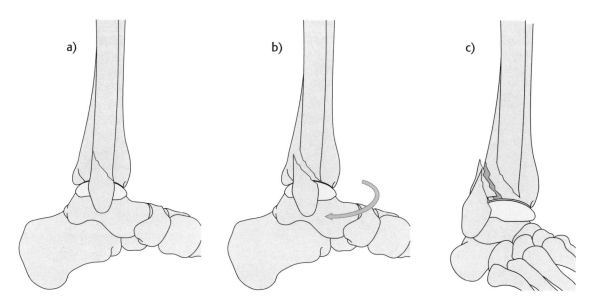

a)

b)

c)

Fig. 4.9-6: Sequence of morphological changes giving rise to type B fractures. Failure of lateral side with foot in supination, resulting in violent talar external rotation.
a) The first injury is an oblique fracture of the fibula starting at the level of the ankle joint and passing posteriorly. This may be a non-displaced crack fracture if the deforming force ceases at this point.
b) Progressive talar rotation causes posterior displacement of the fibular fracture.

c) Further talar rotation results in a fracture of the posterior articular lip of the tibia (Volkmann's fracture) and as the talus leaves the mortise posteriorly, medial failure (malleolar fracture or deltoid ligament rupture) occurs as the final event of the sequence.

3.3 The suprasyndesmotic injury (type C)

(see **Fig. 4.9-11**)

starting at the level of the ankle joint and extending proximally from anterior to posterior (**Fig.4.9-6a**). Progressive talar external rotation causes posterior displacement resulting in either an injury to the posterior syndesmotic ligament or fracture of the posterior malleolus. Finally, as the talus subluxates posteriorly, the medial complex fails either by rupture of the deltoid ligament or by a transverse fracture of the medial malleolus (**Fig. 4.9-6c**).

A third type of injury occurs when the foot is in pronation, the medial structures are under tension (**Fig. 4.9-7**), and an external rotation force is applied. The first injury will occur on the tensioned medial side in the form of a deltoid ligament rupture or a medial malleolar avulsion fracture. This allows the medial side of the talus to translate anteriorly. As the talus rotates externally, it forces the fibula to twist about its vertical axis. This results a rupture of

Fig. 4.9-7: Sequence of morphological changes giving rise to type C fractures. Mechanism of failure with the foot in pronation and external rotation force applied.
a) The first injury is failure of the medial side with deltoid ligament rupture or medial malleolar fracture. This allows the talus to move anteriorly as it laterally rotates.

b) The fibula is caused to rotate and to translate laterally, causing failure of the syndesmotic ligaments.

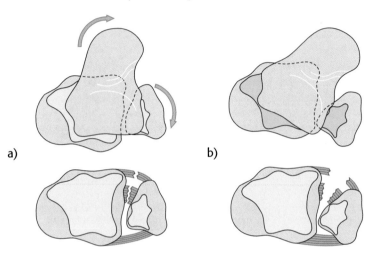

a)   b)

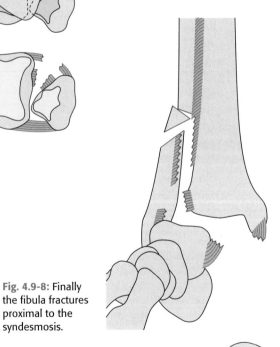

Fig. 4.9-8: Finally the fibula fractures proximal to the syndesmosis.

the anterior syndesmotic ligament and then of the interosseous ligament. At this point the tibia dislocates medially off the rotating talus, forcing separation (diastasis) of the fibula from the tibia. This causes failure of the posterior syndesmotic ligament (or rarely, avulsion of the posterior malleolus), and finally an indirect fracture of the shaft of the fibula, the level of which depends on how far proximally the interosseous membrane ruptures (**Fig. 4.9-8**).

The Müller AO Classification is based on the ability to recognize and describe the x-ray appearance of the fracture pattern. Obviously, ligament complexes are not seen on x-rays, and so to understand fully the anatomy of the injury, **one needs to be able to infer the ligamentous injuries from the fracture pattern.**

Ligamentous injuries can be inferred from the fracture pattern.

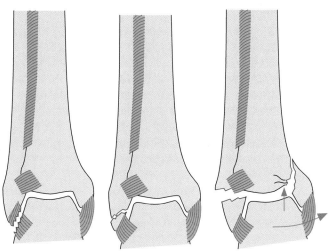

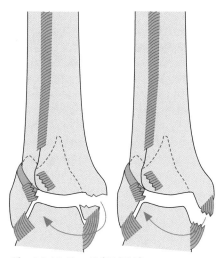

Fig. 4.9-9: Type A (44-A1.3)
Transverse avulsion fracture of the fibula at or below the level of the ankle joint can be associated with a shear fracture of the medial malleolus and impaction of tibial plafond medially.

Fig. 4.9-10: Type B (44-B1.3)
Oblique fracture of the distal fibula passing upwards and backwards from the level of the tibial plafond. As the talus continues to rotate, the fibular fracture displaces posteriorly. The posterolateral corner of the tibia may fracture (Volkmann's triangle). The medial side may be either intact or a rupture of the deltoid ligament, or a transverse fracture of the medial malleolus is present.

Fig. 4.9-11: Type C (44-C1.3)
Medial failure occurs first, either as a deltoid ligament rupture or an avulsion fracture of the medial malleolus.
The inferior tibiofibular ligaments tear as the syndesmosis opens up from anteriorly, due to the external rotation and lateral translation of the fibula. Indirect fibular fracture then occurs above the syndesmosis.
a) The anterior syndesmotic ligament may fail by avulsion either of the anterior tibial tubercle (of Tillaux-Chaput), or
b) of its fibular attachment.
c) Rarely does a posterior tibial lip fracture accompany this injury complex.

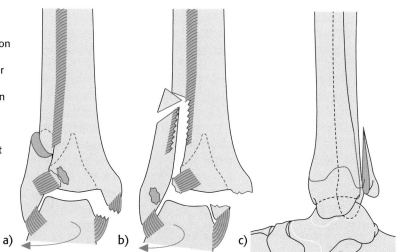

a)   b)   c)

Malleolar fractures have a special segment code in the Müller AO Classification.

A transverse fibular fracture below the level of the ankle joint implies an adduction injury with the syndesmotic ligament remaining intact. With foot supination and talar external rotation, the fibular fracture is oblique and starts anteriorly at the level of the ankle joint with possible partial disruption of the anterior syndesmotic complex (**Fig. 4.9-10**). The interosseous membrane, as a rule, remains intact. The posterior syndesmotic complex is either intact or detached in continuity with a fracture of the posterior tibial lip (Volkmann's triangle).

An indirect fibular shaft fracture, not extending below the syndesmotic ligaments, implies that both the medial and syndesmotic complexes have been disrupted and there is likely to be major instability. The interosseous membrane, from the ankle joint proximally to at least the level of the fibular fracture, and the syndesmotic ligaments are ruptured through their substance or avulsed with their bony attachments. Although this is the common and potentially more serious implication of this pattern, a suprasyndesmotic spiral fracture may occur from a purely external rotation of the fibula. This will disrupt only the anterior tibiofibular ligament, resulting in a more stable pattern as the fibula rotates externally on the intact interosseous membrane and posterior tibiofibular ligament.

On this basis, the three main types of ankle fractures described may be classified according to the level of the fibular fracture as A, B, and C with increasing instability of the mortise. This is the basis of the Müller AO Classification of malleolar fractures.

The unique nature of the complexity of malleolar fractures and their necessary distinction from vertical compression injuries

of the tibial pilon require the allocation to them of a special code. As an exception to the rest of the Müller AO Classification, a regional code 4 is used. Malleolar fractures are therefore categorized as 44.**

For deeper levels of the malleolar classification, refer to "The Comprehensive Classification of Fractures of Long Bones" [6] and/or "Müller AO Electronic Long Bone Fracture Classification" [7].

4   Fracture assessment and decision making

Three radiographic views of the ankle are required. These are the anterioposterior view, the AP view obtained in 20° of internal rotation to bring the transmalleolar axis parallel to the plate (mortise view) and the lateral view. Shortening of the fibula is best appreciated by a step in the alignment of the subchondral plates of the tibial plafond and the lateral malleolus (**Fig. 4.9-12a/a'**). The talocrural angle is 83° ± 4° and if greater or lesser indicates instability or displacement of the mortise. The joint space between the talus and plafond should equal the space between the medial malleolus and medial talus. **Widening of the medial space is indicative of mortise displacement.** The lateral view demonstrates the pattern of fibular fracture and any anterior or posterior translation of the talus.

CT scanning is rarely required for malleolar fractures.

Stress films or views are only useful in the fully anesthetized patient and when compared to the normal side (**Fig. 4.9-12b/c**).

Widening of the medial joint space indicates instability of the mortise.

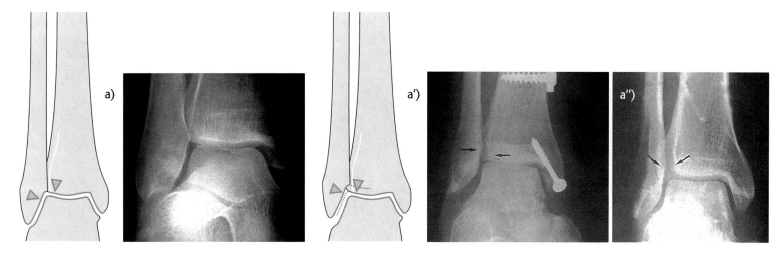

Fig. 4.9-12: Evaluation of the x-rays.
a) The normal ankle articulation with the foot in 20° of internal rotation: the joint space is of equal width throughout. The line of the subchondral plate of the tibial plafond, projected over the gap, is continuous with that of the lateral malleolus without a step.
a') Even the slightest shortening of the fibula can be recognized radiologically as a step in the alignment of the subchondral plates of the tibial plafond and the lateral malleolus. Lateral shift of the talus and consequent widening of the medial joint space are seen.
a") Same case as a') after lengthening osteotomy of the fibula, the joint congruency is re-established.

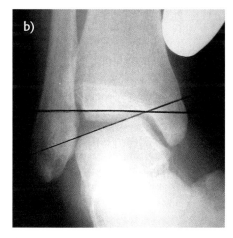

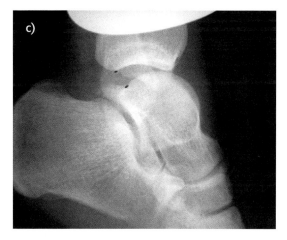

b) AP stress x-ray of the ankle joint. Note the 10° varus tilt of the talus. This denotes that the important calcaneofibular ligament is injured, in addition to the anterior talofibular ligament.

c) Anterior subluxation of the talus seen on lateral view with anterior stress applied to the hindfoot. A difference between the injured and uninjured ankles of 3 mm or more in the height of the joint space is pathognomonic of an injury of the anterior talofibular ligament.

4.1 Operative vs. non-operative treatment

Ankle mortise incongruity is poorly tolerated and causes abnormal loads on cartilage.

The decision whether an ankle fracture requires open reduction and internal fixation should be based on how best the normal anatomy can be restored and stability maintained. **Ankle mortise incongruity is poorly tolerated and leads to abnormal loads on the articular cartilage.**

Isolated infrasyndesmotic (type A) fractures of the distal fibula that do not involve the medial side may well be stable and capable of being treated non-operatively.

Isolated non-displaced transsyndesmotic (type B) fractures of the lateral malleolus that do not involve the medial side can be treated non-operatively, provided that the ankle mortise remains congruent [8, 9]. The determination of whether the deltoid ligament has been disrupted relies upon clinical findings of tenderness on the medial side. If this is associated with evidence of a displaced mortise, then treatment should be operative stabilization of the fibula. All displaced ankle injuries are likely to be unstable and accurate anatomical reduction can usually only be secured by open reduction and stable internal fixation.

4.2 Preoperative planning

The discipline of preoperative planning for any fracture involves consideration of the timing of surgery, the choice of incision, and the selection of implants. It may involve graphic planning with the use of implant templates from a preoperative planning kit. The standard implants required for the vast majority of malleolar fractures are in the small fragment set. A tension band wiring set should also be available.

Tracing out of fracture fragments and their reduction, using the techniques illustrated in the planning chapter, is often extremely useful when dealing with malleolar fractures. The length of the fibular plate and placement of lag screws can be planned preoperatively and their availability ensured before starting the operation.

4.3 Timing of surgery

Timing of surgery is dictated by the state of the soft tissues.

The ideal time for surgery to the ankle is before any true swelling or fracture blisters have developed. The initial swelling is due to hematoma formation and not to edema. The techniques of open reduction and internal fixation often release this hematoma and allow primary closure without tension of the surgical wound. However, it is accepted that in many situations it is not always possible to operate before soft tissues become compromised. **Timing of surgery is then dictated by the state of the soft tissues.** In the presence of intradermal edema (peau d'orange), marked subcutaneous edema, or fracture blisters it is strongly advisable that surgery be delayed until the soft-tissue condition has improved. In this event, the fracture is reduced by gentle manipulation and immobilized in a well-padded plaster splint with the leg then elevated. Surgery is postponed until the soft-tissue injury has resolved. This is evidenced by resolution of fracture blisters, epithelialization of abrasions, and the presence of the wrinkle sign at the operative site (skin wrinkles normally if ankle is inverted or everted).

5 Surgical techniques

5.1 Patient position

The patient is positioned supine with a sandbag underneath the buttock of the affected side. This allows the foot to lie in neutral position and prevents the normal external rotation of the leg in the anesthetized patient. The lower leg can then be placed on a foam block with the knee flexed to 30°. This allows ease of simultaneous access to both the medial and lateral sides. The use of a tourniquet is advised, unless otherwise contra-indicated.

For ease of access to the posteromedial aspect of the distal tibia it is sometimes helpful to place a sandbag beneath the opposite buttock and to rest the injured ankle on the opposite shin (with appropriate padding) in the figure-4 position.

Occasionally the prone position on bolsters will allow access by the posterior approach to the posterior malleolus, particularly if it is a large fragment or comminuted and requiring buttressing. The approach to the medial malleolus is more difficult in this position but can be done safely.

5.2 Choice of incision

(see **Fig. 4.9-13**)

5.2.1 Posterior approach

The incision is between the Achilles tendon and the peroneal tendons. The sural nerve must be avoided. Dissection is continued through the posterior fat pad and on to the posterior aspect of the tibia. Flexor hallucis longus is medial and protects the posterior tibial artery and nerve. The fracture is easily identified and reduced. By internally rotating the leg and using a posteriomedial incision, the medial malleolus is exposed.

5.2.2 Lateral side

The skin incision on the lateral side is placed so that the minimum of soft-tissue dissection needs to be carried out to obtain reduction and fixation. If a lateral plate is required for the fibula, then the surgical incision may be placed slightly anteriorly so that on skin closure the plate does not lie immediately beneath it. Care should be taken not to damage the superficial fibular nerve that runs anteriorly to the fibula (**Fig. 4.9-13a**). A more posterior incision can be used either if a posterior plate is to be placed on the fibula or if access is required to the posterolateral corner of the tibia. Such an incision must avoid damage to the sural nerve.

5.2.3 Medial side

The standard medial incision runs either posterior or anterior to the malleolus. The saphenous vein and nerve should be protected (**Fig. 4.9-13b**).

6 Steps in open reduction and internal fixation

In most instances the first step in fixation is reconstruction of the fibula. Soft-tissue dissection should be kept to a minimum, but in simple fractures minimal exposure of the fracture lines is necessary to allow anatomical reduction and provisional stabilization with pointed reduction forceps or K-wires. Occasionally the medial side must be exposed prior to definitive stabilization because the deltoid ligament or an osteochondral fragment may be interposed, preventing full reduction. Inability to reduce the fibula is a clue to the need to open the medial side.

If fixation has been delayed for reasons of soft-tissue recovery, the fracture planes must be meticulously cleared of organized blood clot prior to reduction.

6.1   Infrasyndesmotic fibular fractures: type 44-A1.3 malleolar fractures

Where the whole lateral malleolus is avulsed with a transverse fracture line, it is reduced and

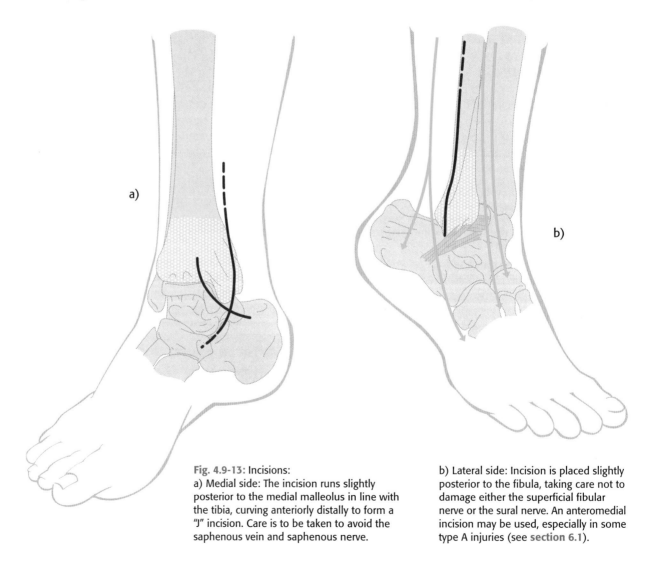

Fig. 4.9-13: Incisions:
a) Medial side: The incision runs slightly posterior to the medial malleolus in line with the tibia, curving anteriorly distally to form a "J" incision. Care is to be taken to avoid the saphenous vein and saphenous nerve.

b) Lateral side: Incision is placed slightly posterior to the fibula, taking care not to damage either the superficial fibular nerve or the sural nerve. An anteromedial incision may be used, especially in some type A injuries (see **section 6.1**).

may be stabilized by a one-third tubular plate functioning as a tension band (**Fig. 4.9-14a**). A tension band wiring technique or a retrograde screw, inserted up the fibular medullary canal, may also be used when the lateral failure is of the osseoligamentous type. With avulsion of only the tip of the lateral malleolus, tension band wiring is used (**Video AO00068a**), supplemented by ligamentous suture where appropriate (**Fig. 4.9-14b**).

If the lateral injury is a rupture of the lateral ligament complex, this should be sutured only if the ankle is unstable and a reduction cannot be maintained (**Fig. 4.9-14c**).

The next step is to expose the medial malleolus from anteromedially and clear

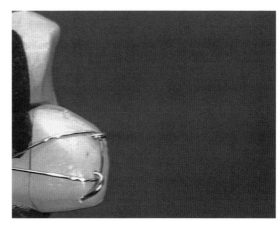

 Video AO00068a

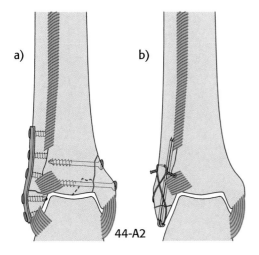

44-A2

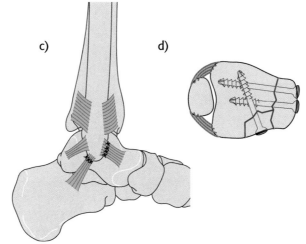

a) b) c) d)

Fig. 4.9-14: Type A fracture—typical internal fixation:
a) Where the bone is of good quality, a large lateral malleolar fragment may be fixed with a well-contoured one-third tubular plate under slight compression, functioning as a tension band.
b) An avulsion fragment of the lateral malleolus is first stabilized with two K-wires and then fixed under compression by means of a tension band wire loop.

c) A rupture of the lateral collateral ligament complex may be sutured.
d) Posteromedial fragments associated with type A3 fractures are rare. They always lie next to the medial malleolar fragment. Such fragments may be exposed, reduced, and fixed with small cancellous bone screws from a posteromedial direction.

any entrapped periosteum from between the fracture surfaces. The anterior capsule is often torn and this permits an excellent view of the intra-articular portion of the fracture. Small bone fragments can be removed, but larger fragments should be preserved. The surface of the tibial plafond at the medial corner should be inspected by hinging open the fracture plane anteriorly. Any impaction fracture is reduced and bone grafted.

In an adduction fracture the main fracture line of the medial malleolus is often vertical or oblique and is on the compression side of the injury (the tension being on the lateral side). Tension band wiring techniques are not suitable for these compression fractures.

Once reduction is complete and held provisionally with K-wires, definitive fixation is achieved by lag screws placed perpendicular to the main fracture plane. Application of a buttressing washer or a short (two or three holes) one-third tubular plate at the apex of this fracture will improve the stability of the construct.

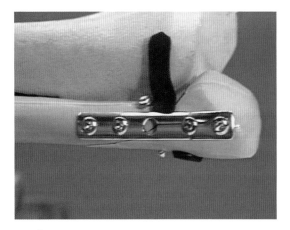

 Video AO00069a

6.2 Transsyndesmotic fibular fractures: type 44-B1.3 malleolar fractures

The fibular fracture is usually oblique, running from distal anterior to proximal posterior. The lateral malleolus is usually shifted proximally, displaced posteriorly, and externally rotated. Inspection of the dome of the talus may be possible through the fracture itself and any loose chondral flakes can be removed manually or by irrigation. Dissection of the distal lateral malleolus is kept to a minimum. Reduction of the simple, short oblique fracture of the lateral malleolus is best achieved with gentle traction and internal rotation of the foot. Pointed reduction forceps can then be applied across the fracture for temporary stabilization.

If reduction is difficult, it may occasionally be because the tip of the proximal fibular fragment can fracture and swing, on a pedicle of fibers of the anterior tibiofibular ligament, into the fracture gap. This is not always obvious and must be sought and extracted before the reduction is completed.

The accuracy of reduction can be assessed by inspecting the anterior edge of the fibula at the level of the anterior syndesmosis. To achieve definitive fixation, 3.5 mm cortex lag screws are placed from anterior to posterior. A one-third tubular plate contoured to the lateral aspect of the fibula acts as a neutralization plate (**Video AO00069a**). Care must be taken when placing the screws in the distal lateral malleolus to ensure that the articular surface is not penetrated. The metaphyseal bone of the lateral malleolus is often quite soft and better purchase of the screws can be achieved either by inserting cortex screws without tapping or by the use of untapped fully threaded cancellous bone screws (**Fig. 4.9-15a**).

6.3 Posterior "anti-glide" plate

(**Fig. 4.9-15b**)

The main deformity of the lateral malleolus with a type B fracture is of external rotation, posterior displacement, and proximal shift. Reduction of this fragment is often maintained by pushing the distal fragment from posteriorly, while at the same time reducing the external rotation deformity. If the fracture of the lateral malleolus is not simple and does not lend itself to stabilization with lag screws, a one-third tubular plate can be placed posteriorly on the fibula as a buttress, resisting the posterior displacement [10]. Occasionally, a lag screw can be incorporated through the plate. If this technique is to be used, the incision should be placed more posteriorly to allow access to the posterior edge of the fibula. Usually a 5-hole or 6-hole one-third tubular plate is applied to the posterior aspect of the fibular so that it covers the proximal apex of the fracture. The plate is straight and either clamped to the fibula proximally or attached with a screw through the most proximal hole. The screw just proximal to the fracture is now inserted and this forces the straight plate to push the distal fragment along the oblique fracture surface, effecting a reduction and stability. A reduction forceps on the tip of the fibula is helpful in controlling rotation during plate application. The remaining screws are then inserted and a lag screw can be inserted through the plate (**Video AO00069b**).

6.4 Medial side

Injuries of the deltoid ligament do not require routine exploration. However, if after reduction of the fibular fracture the intraoperative films or x-rays show that the medial joint space remains widened, or if there are difficulties with accurate reduction of the fibular fracture, the medial side should be explored. On occasions, the medial ligament or an osteochondral fragment will have become trapped into the medial joint space and must be lifted out. The deltoid ligament can then be repaired, largely in order to prevent its reinterposition postoperatively during joint mobilization (**Fig. 4.9-15g**).

Very rarely, a block to reduction can arise from the entrapment of the tibialis posterior tendon within the ankle joint after a severely displaced fracture-dislocation.

Injuries of the medial malleolus in type B fractures are usually avulsion fractures caused when the talus displaces posteriorly out of the mortise. They may extend posteromedially and are of variable size. Exposure of the fracture is

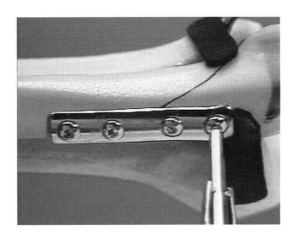

 Video AO00069b

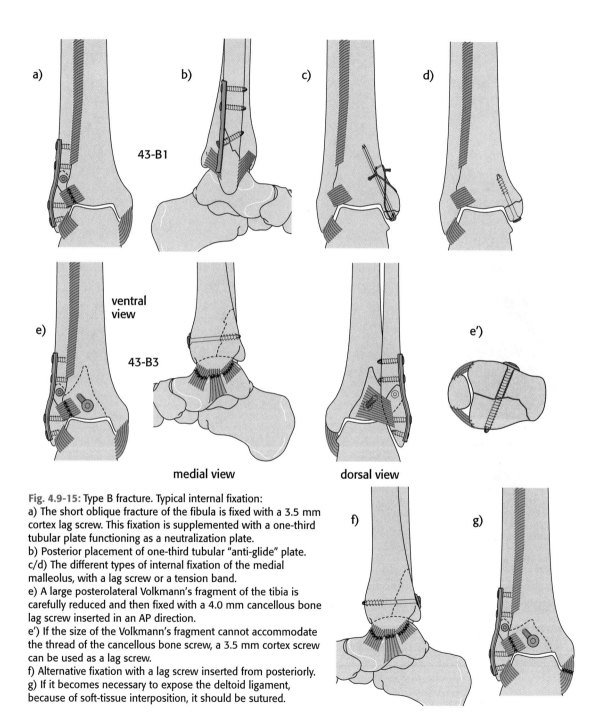

43-B1

ventral view

43-B3

medial view

dorsal view

e)

e')

f)

g)

Fig. 4.9-15: Type B fracture. Typical internal fixation:
a) The short oblique fracture of the fibula is fixed with a 3.5 mm cortex lag screw. This fixation is supplemented with a one-third tubular plate functioning as a neutralization plate.
b) Posterior placement of one-third tubular "anti-glide" plate.
c/d) The different types of internal fixation of the medial malleolus, with a lag screw or a tension band.
e) A large posterolateral Volkmann's fragment of the tibia is carefully reduced and then fixed with a 4.0 mm cancellous bone lag screw inserted in an AP direction.
e') If the size of the Volkmann's fragment cannot accommodate the thread of the cancellous bone screw, a 3.5 mm cortex screw can be used as a lag screw.
f) Alternative fixation with a lag screw inserted from posteriorly.
g) If it becomes necessary to expose the deltoid ligament, because of soft-tissue interposition, it should be sutured.

achieved by a standard medial incision and any interposed periosteum is removed from the fracture gap to allow accurate reduction. A small pointed reduction forceps to grasp the medial malleolus and hold it reduced is helpful. Temporary stabilization with K-wires is followed by definitive stabilization, achieved with a 4.00 mm partially threaded cancellous bone lag screw (**Fig. 4.9-15c**). If the fragment is large enough, two

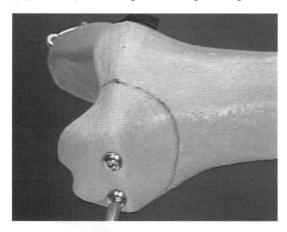

Video AO00068b

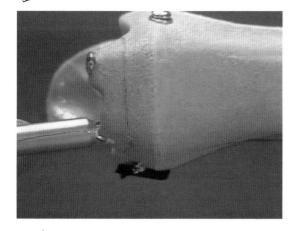

Video AO00070a

parallel screws can be used (**Video AO00068b**). With smaller fragments, one screw can be combined with a K-wire (**Video AO00070a**). The screws should only be long enough to allow the thread to pass fully beyond the fracture plane. Screws of excessive length in the distal tibia gain poor purchase in the often sparse cancellous bone of the metaphysis, especially in the older patient or if fixation is delayed.

An alternative technique is to use two parallel K-wires and a tension band wire (**Fig. 4.9-15d**).

6.5 Posterolateral fragments or posterior malleolar fractures

The posterolateral corner (Volkmann's) fragment in type B or rarely C fractures is often displaced along with the lateral malleolus, being bound to it by the posterior syndesmotic ligament. Accurate reduction of the fibular fracture will have reduced some of the upward displacement of the posterior fragment, but the fracture gap may still remain open. Fragments of less than 25% of the articular surface on the lateral view need not be stabilized unless there is a tendency for the talus to sublux posteriorly. Larger fragments can be fixed either by the placement of a lag screw through a stab incision from anterior to posterior (**Fig. 4.9-15e**) (**Video AO00070b**) or by direct exposure of the posterior fragment through the posterolateral incision and insertion of a lag screw from posterior to anterior (**Fig. 4.9-15f**). The latter technique requires more dissection but often gives a more accurate placement of the screw. When using the percutaneous anterior to posterior technique, it should be remembered

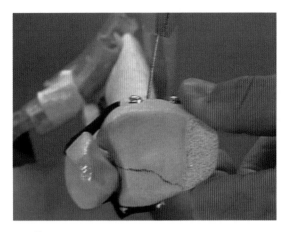

 Video AO00070b

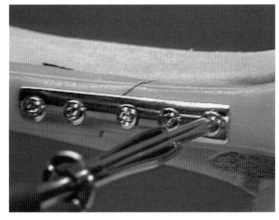

Video AO00070c

that the fragment in a type B fracture will lie at the posterolateral corner of the tibia and therefore the screw must be directed appropriately (**Fig. 4.9-15e**).

6.6 Suprasyndesmotic fibular fracture: type 44-C1.3 malleolar fractures

(**Fig. 4.9-16**)

As in the case of the type A and B fractures, the first step in dealing with type C fractures is to approach the fibula. The key to successful fixation is to restore the length and rotation of the fibula. If the fibular fracture is short oblique, or spiral, then the fracture can be exposed, accurately reduced with the use of reduction forceps, and fixed using lag screws and a one-third tubular plate (**Video AO00070c**). If the

fibular fracture, however, is multifragmentary, then techniques of indirect reduction should be used. There, the best technique is to use the plate as a reduction tool. The lateral malleolus and fibular shaft distal to the fracture, and the proximal fibula above the fracture zone, are exposed, but no dissection is carried out around the area of comminution. A one-third tubular plate is then contoured, remembering that on reduction the fibula will effectively be lengthened and therefore a long enough plate must be chosen. It is advisable to plan this graphically before operation. The plate is anchored to the distal fibula, spanning the comminuted area. A screw is then placed in the fibular shaft proximal to the upper end of the plate and the proximal end of the plate is secured lightly to the fibula with a plate-holding clamp. Using a laminar spreader against the screw, the plate is pushed distally, thereby lengthening the fibula.

X-rays are taken to check the accuracy of the reduction determined by the correspondence of the subchondral plateau of the tibial plafond and the lateral malleolus. A preoperative plan of the uninjured ankle serves as an intraoperative reference.

The plate can then be anchored proximally, with fibular length and orientation restored and with the multiple intermediate fragments indirectly reduced.

Proximal fractures, occurring through the fibular neck, need not as a rule be exposed, but the fibula must be reduced down into its normal position in the incisura fibularis by traction, using a towel clip or pointed reduction forceps. Reduction can then be temporarily held with one or two K-wires passed through the fibula into the tibia, later to be replaced by definitive positioning screw fixation (see below).

The medial malleolar fractures are reduced and fixed using the techniques described above for type B fractures.

6.7 Fibulotibial "syndesmotic" positioning screw

The decision as to whether any further fixation is necessary depends on the stability of the syndesmosis once the fibular length has been restored, the fibula fixed, and the medial side reconstructed. The anterior syndesmosis can be exposed via the lateral incision. If avulsed with the anterior tibial tubercle (Tillaux-Chaput) or from the fibula, it can be reduced and fixed with a small lag screw. If the anterior syndesmotic ligament is torn within its substance it may be repaired with sutures.

Whether any further fibular stabilization is then necessary can be determined by the use of the hooktest, in which the fibula is grasped with bone forceps, or a bone hook, and pulled gently laterally to reveal any significant residual fibulotibial instability. In addition, stress views in external rotation must be taken intraoperatively. Widening of the medial joint space by more than 2 mm suggests syndesmotic instability.

If the syndesmosis is unstable, a positioning screw should be placed from the fibula into the tibia. This screw is introduced obliquely from posterior to anterior at an angle of 25–30° and parallel to the tibial plafond. It is placed just proximal to the fibulotibial joint. As this screw is not intended to act as a compressive lag screw, the fibula and tibia should both be fully tapped and a 3.5 mm cortex screw inserted, while the fibula is held, without compression, in its anatomical relationship to the tibia.

During the procedure, the foot should be maintained in slight dorsiflexion. In this position the wider anterior part of the talar body is engaged in the mortise to prevent narrowing, which can often lead to permanent loss of dorsiflexion, even after screw removal (see below).

There is no clear agreement on whether one or both tibial cortices should be engaged by the positioning screw threads. Certainly, if the fibular fracture is so high that its direct fixation is not possible (as in the Maisonneuve injury), then both tibial cortices should be used. Occasionally, two positioning screws may be needed in these circumstances. A further advantage of engaging both tibial cortices is that, should a positioning screw break in a non-compliant patient, the thread fragment can easily be removed via a small window in the medial tibial cortex.

Intraoperative check x-rays or image intensification to confirm the position of the screw are advised.

Stability of the syndesmosis determines whether a positioning screw is used.

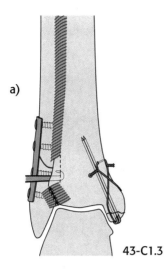

a)

43-C1.3

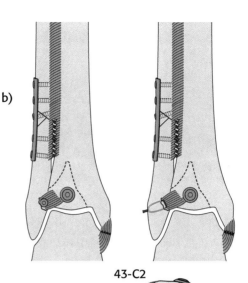

b)

43-C2

b')

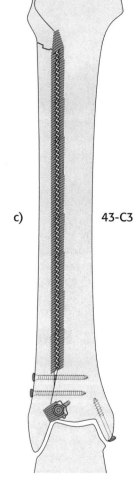

c)

43-C3

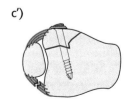

c')

Fig. 4.9-16: Typical internal fixation for type C fracture.
a) The fibular shaft fracture is reduced and stabilized with a one-third tubular plate. The small avulsion fracture of the medial malleolus is fixed with two K-wires and a tension band wire loop. The torn anterior syndesmotic ligament is then tested with a small hook.

b/b') A fracture of the midshaft of the fibula is fixed with a plate. The anterior syndesmosis has been avulsed from its attachment to the lateral malleolus. This is reduced and fixed with either a small cancellous bone screw or a transosseous wire suture. The ruptured deltoid ligament may be sutured. A large posterolateral fragment is rare in this injury, but if present is carefully reduced and then fixed with a cancellous bone lag screw. This restores stability of the ankle mortise.

c/c') Not infrequently, a very proximal fibular fracture is not shortened and does not need open reduction. It is most important, however, to check very carefully for any shortening on an AP of the ankle. Look for any step in the alignment of the subchondral plates of the tibial plafond and the lateral malleolus. Any shortening must be corrected. A small avulsion fracture of the anterior syndesmotic ligament from the tibia is reduced and fixed with a small cancellous bone lag screw.
Since this injury involves almost the full extent of the interosseous membrane, the fixation of the anterior syndesmotic origin may not provide sufficient stability to the ankle mortise and a positioning screw is necessary. This will be revealed by the hook test. Two screws should be introduced obliquely from back to front at an angle of 25–30°, the thread being tapped into both the fibula and the tibia. The avulsion fracture of the medial malleolus is fixed under compression, using one or two 4 mm cancellous bone lag screws. Positioning screws should be removed at 6–8 weeks.

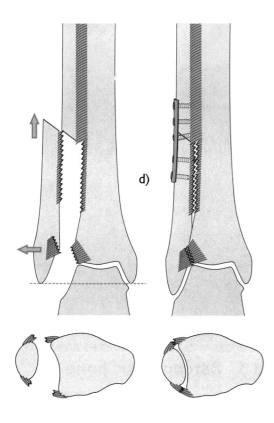

Fig. 4.9-16: Type C fracture (cont.)
d) Exact anatomical reduction of the fibula into the fibular notch of the tibia (incisura fibularis) guarantees a normal ankle mortise. Imperfect reduction with shortening or rotation of the fibula leads to widening of the ankle mortise and valgus tilt of the talus. Even small degrees of malreduction are likely to lead to posttraumatic degenerative arthritis (see **Fig. 4.9-12**). On the left the fibula is shortened and externally rotated, resulting in syndesmotic incongruity and secondary ankle instability. On the right after anatomical reduction of the fibula the fibulotibial relationship is again normal.

7 Postoperative management

Both medial and lateral wounds are closed using fine sutures without tension. The use of suction drainage on the lateral side is recommended. The ankle is rested in a plaster of Paris back slab with the foot at 90° to prevent an equinus deformity. Where an anatomical reduction of the fibular fracture may not have been possible, it is wise to obtain a CT scan of the syndesmosis in the early postoperative period to exclude malrotation of the fibula [11]. The patient is encouraged to start early active movement of the toes and, if the wounds are satisfactory at 24–48 hours, then active mobilization of the ankle can be started under skilled supervision. The decision as to whether, once active dorsiflexion has been achieved, the patient can be left free, or protected in a cast, depends on a number of factors. These include the stability of fixation achieved by the surgeon, the general mobility of the patient, and the prospect of compliance with the chosen postoperative regime. Studies [12, 13] have shown that the long-term outcome is similar, whether the ankle is immobilized or free during 6 postoperative weeks. A decision regarding weight bearing, either in or out of a cast, also largely depends on the stability of fixation achieved and the cooperation of the patient. No problems have been experienced by the authors using a regime of progressive, light weight bearing in a cast for 6 weeks, although the return to full activity is more rapid in the early mobilization-group. At the end of this period, active mobilization and full weight bearing can be allowed.

If a syndesmotic screw has been used and the patient left free, then it is recommended that weight bearing be protected for the first 6–8 weeks.

Light weight bearing in a protective cast is permissible.

Controversy exists over syndesmotic screw removal. The syndesmotic screw may be removed at 6–8 weeks, before return to full normal activity. In cases where both the medial and syndesmotic failures have been exclusively ligamentous, it is advisable to retain the positioning screw and restrict full activity for 10–12 weeks.

If the positioning screw is not removed, it will either erode a wider track through the fibula as normal fibulotibial motion occurs, or it will break. These possibilities are explained to the patients so that they are well aware of the postoperative course.

8   Pitfalls and complications

8.1   Soft-tissue problems

Ankle fractures can swell dramatically within hours of injury. If surgery can be performed within 6–8 hours, the swelling is almost always hematoma and not edema within the tissues. Primary closure of the surgical wounds can usually be achieved in these instances. If, however, this can only be achieved with tension, the wound should be left open, absorbent sterile dressings applied, and the foot elevated. Careful preoperative planning of the placement of the incisions should take this possibility into account and avoid leaving the implants exposed. At 48 hours the wounds can be reinspected and very often can be closed at that time.

If edema and blisters have developed, it is highly recommended that surgery be delayed for up to 4–6 days until the soft tissues are recovering.

8.2   Open fractures

The soft-tissue wounds in open fractures of the ankle should be dealt with according to the surgical principles outlined for all open fractures [14] (**chapter 5.1**). The most common wound in open ankle fracture-dislocations is a medial transverse laceration. Anatomical reduction and stable fixation of the ankle mortise should still be achieved in most cases once débridement of all open wounds has taken place. Soft-tissue wounds should then be left open, although the surgical extensions of the débridement may be closed primarily, provided all tension is avoided. A well-padded, non-adherent, and absorbent dressing is applied, followed by limb elevation and then a "second look" at 48–72 hours. Definitive wound closure decisions will take account of the principles referred to above.

8.3   Osteoporotic bone

Where the bone is osteoporotic, techniques already described for the lateral side include the use of the anti-glide plate and indirect reduction techniques for restoration of the fibular length. The use of closed reduction and intramedullary fibular fixation in fracture patterns that are axially stable may be another alternative for osteoporotic bone, in particular if there are compromised soft-tissue conditions. On the medial side the medial fragment cannot withstand the use of a cancellous bone lag screw and therefore K-wire stabilization and tension band wiring may be more useful in the B and C injuries.

9 Bibliography

1. **Calhoun JH, Li F, Ledbetter BR, et al.** (1994) A comprehensive study of pressure distribution in the ankle joint with inversion and eversion. *Foot Ankle Int;* 15 (3):125–133.

2. **Lundberg A, Goldie I, Kalin B, et al.** (1989) Kinematics of the ankle/foot complex: plantarflexion and dorsiflexion. *Foot Ankle;* 9 (4):194–200.

3. **Michelson JD** (1995) Fractures about the ankle. *J Bone Joint Surg [Am];* 77 (1):142–152.

4. **Ramsey PL, Hamilton W** (1976) Changes in tibiotalar area of contact caused by lateral talar shift. *J Bone Joint Surg [Am];* 58 (3):356–357.

5. **Riede UN, Schenk RK, Willenegger H** (1971) [Joint mechanical studies on post-traumatic arthrosas in the ankle joint. I. The intra-articular model fracture]. *Langenbecks Arch Chir;* 328 (3):258–271.

6. **Müller ME, Nazarian S, Koch P, et al.** (1990) *The Comprehensive Classification of Fractures of Long Bones.* Berlin Heidelberg New York: Springer-Verlag.

7. *Müller AO Electronic Long Bone Fracture Classification.* (2002) AO Publishing/ Thieme. (in preparation).

8. **Bauer M, Bergstrom B, Hemborg A, et al.** (1985) Malleolar fractures: nonoperative versus operative treatment. A controlled study. *Clin Orthop;* (199):17–27.

9. **Kristensen KD, Hansen T** (1985) Closed treatment of ankle fractures. Stage II supination-eversion fractures followed for 20 years. *Acta Orthop Scand;* 56 (2):107–109.

10. **Brunner CF, Weber BG** (1982) *Special Techniques in Internal Fixation.* Berlin Heidelberg New York: Springer-Verlag.

11. **Wanders L, Oliver CW** (1998) Fibular malreduction in AO/Weber type C ankle fractures. *Injury;* 29 (2):144–146.

12. **Stuart PR, Brumby C, Smith SR** (1989) Comparative study of functional bracing and plaster cast treatment of stable lateral malleolar fractures. *Injury;* 20 (6):323–326.

13. **Hedstrom M, Ahl T, Dalen N** (1994) Early postoperative ankle exercise. A study of postoperative lateral malleolar fractures. *Clin Orthop;* (300):193–196.

14. **Wiss DA, Gilbert P, Merritt PO, et al.** (1988) Immediate internal fixation of open ankle fractures. *J Orthop Trauma;* 2 (4):265–271.

10 Updates

Updates and additional references for this chapter are available online at:
http://www.aopublishing.org/PFxM/49.htm

4.10 Foot (calcaneus/talus/metatarsus): decision making

Deborah M. Eastwood

1 Introduction

Displaced fractures of the foot can cause significant disability if their severity is not appreciated and the injury treated inappropriately [1]. The hindfoot is a complex structure where bones, joints, and soft tissues interrelate to provide a solid foundation for weight bearing. Accordingly, the hindfoot, consisting of talus and calcaneus, must be correctly aligned with the weight bearing forces and be strong enough and high enough to withstand applied loads. Since the hindfoot converts rotary tibial forces into foot pronation, normal gait depends on normal function of the tarsometatarsal and metatarsophalangeal joints and the relationship of individual bones to each other.

2 Fractures of the calcaneus

2.1 Assessment of fractures and soft tissues

The calcaneus is the most frequently injured tarsal bone and most fractures are intra-articular and due to high-velocity injury. The bony anat-

omy of the calcaneus is complex. There are four articular facets supported by a corticocancellous structure. The posterior part, containing the posterior facet of the subtalar joint and the middle facet of the sustentaculum tali, is separated from the anterior portion of the calcaneus by the sinus tarsi and tarsal canal. The anterior portion contains the small anterior facet of the subtalar joint and a saddle-shaped articular surface for the calcaneocuboid joint.

The calcaneus has an unusual and complex shape, the three dimensions of which may be difficult to appreciate on 2-D images. Lateral and axial plain x-rays are of limited use. The lateral view defines Essex-Lopresti joint depression and tongue-type injuries. Measurement of Bohler's angle may indicate that significant displacement has occurred. The axial view, particularly in the injured foot, is unlikely to demonstrate the subtalar joint properly.

The lateral oblique view shows the anterior facet and helps identify any other tarsal bone fractures. **Computed tomographic images are essential.** Imaging can be performed in various planes and the nomenclature of these has not been consistent in the literature. True coronal views are difficult to obtain and thus,

Displaced fractures of the foot can cause significant disability.

CT scan images are essential.

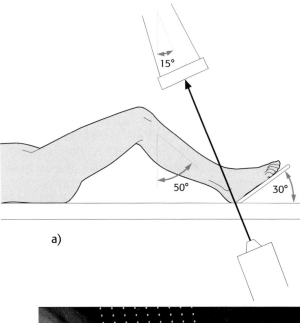

in most cases, oblique coronal views are obtained but the position of both the patient and the gantry are important (**Fig. 4.10-1**). Coronal scans provide information about both the articular and non-articular aspects of the fracture. Thus, lateral shift, angulation, and impaction of the tuberosity fragment at the medial wall fracture site can be gauged, as can disruption of the posterior facet articular surface (**Fig. 4.10-2**). Axial scans parallel to the sole of the foot add information concerning the calcaneocuboid joint, fracture displacement and comminution. A three-dimensional appreciation of fracture anatomy can be achieved by viewing these

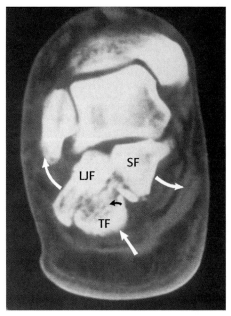

Fig. 4.10-1:
a) Position of foot, ankle, and the gantry for coronal CT scans of the calcaneum.
b) Plane of imaging for coronal CT scans of the calcaneum.

Fig. 4.10-2: Coronal CT scan of a fracture of the calcaneum identifying the lateral joint fragment (LJF), the sustentacular fragment (SF), and the tuberosity or body fragment (TF). There is considerable lateral shift, impaction, and angulation at the medial wall fracture site and displacement at the articular surface.

scans. Formal 3-D reconstructions are not, however, particularly useful [2]. In all, five major fragments involving two major joints may be identified (**Fig. 4.10-3**) and this is the basis of the presently available classification system (OTA) (**Fig. 4.10-4**) [3].

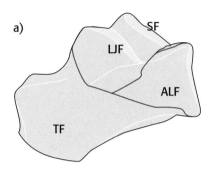

Fig. 4.10-3:
a) Lateral view of a calcaneum showing lateral joint fragment (LJF), sustentacular fragment (SF), and tuberosity or body fragment (TF) in the posterior portion of the bone, and the anterolateral (ALF) and anteromedial (AMF) fragments anteriorly. The fracture lines define an Essex-Lopresti joint depression type injury.

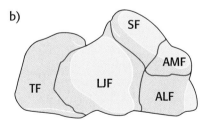

b) Superior view of the same calcaneum showing lateral joint fragment (LJF), sustentacular fragment (SF), and tuberosity or body fragment (TF) in the posterior portion of the bone, and the anterolateral (ALF) and anteromedial (AMF) fragments anteriorly. The fracture lines define an Essex-Lopresti joint depression type injury.

The forces that fracture the calcaneus also damage the soft tissues. The medial structures are submitted to shear and stretch while the plantar surface is compressed. The lateral structures are often least damaged. Thus, fracture blisters occur most frequently on the medial side and initially, at least, bruising is most apparent on the sole of the foot. In cases of calcaneal fractures, compartment syndromes are often missed; the diagnosis must be considered in all cases of foot injury [4].

2.2 Surgical anatomy

In fractures of the calcaneus there are two components to consider. One is the intra-articular displacement, particularly at the posterior facet of the subtalar joint, but also anteriorly. The other is the non-articular component which considers the degree of displacement at the medial wall fracture site in terms of loss of height, loss of length, and increase in width of the calcaneus as well as of varus/valgus angulation. **Strong ligaments attach the sustentaculum tali to the talus, and thus the sustentacular fragment is often in a relatively normal position. This is the key to reduction and stable internal fixation of displaced intra-articular fractures of the calcaneus**. If the fragment is comminuted, stable fixation is difficult to achieve by standard methods. The neurovascular bundle runs close to the medial wall fracture site and entrapment of the bundle and/or the tendon of flexor hallucis longus may occur at the time of injury or upon reduction. If such displacement or angulation is not reduced, there will be a major change in the weight bearing alignment of the lower limb.

Soft-tissue injury is always considerable.

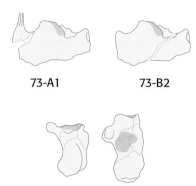

73-A1   73-B2

73-C2

Fig. 4.10-4: OTA Classification[1]

Sustentaculum tali is the key to reduction and fixation.

---

[1] An AO classification of foot fractures prepared by the AO Foot and Ankle Expert Group is in its final stages of evaluation as this volume goes to press.

2.3 Preoperative planning

Management of displaced intra-articular injuries of the calcaneus has been controversial but now that the pathological anatomy is better understood, operative treatment is more widespread and more successful. As with all other severe injuries of weight bearing joints, there is an argument for considering operative reduction and internal fixation within the first few hours of fracture. However, such swift access to the appropriate imaging is presently only possible in some centers. Once imaging has been obtained, **the timing of any surgical intervention depends on the degree of swelling and the state of the soft tissues.** Longer delays between injury and operation mean more extensive soft-tissue dissection around the displaced fragments and greater difficulties with wound closure.

For unilateral fractures a full lateral position is used with the injured foot uppermost. In patients with bilateral fractures who have sufficient external rotation of the hips, a prone position is used with the feet lying in external rotation. Good quality x-ray screening facilities are essential (see **Fig. 4.10-8**).

The basic requirements include a small fragment screw set, K-wires, and a choice of plates, one-third tubular, reconstruction 3.5, H-plate, or new calcaneal plates. The cannulated screw system is helpful. If distraction is required, a Steinmann pin or Schanz screw and/or a distractor unit may be useful.

2.4 Surgical treatment— tricks and hints

A lateral incision is preferred and its siting is crucial for wound healing (**Fig. 4.10-5**). The distal limb of the L-shaped incision is placed

> Timing of surgery depends on the soft tissues.

> The lateral full-thickness flap must be treated gently!

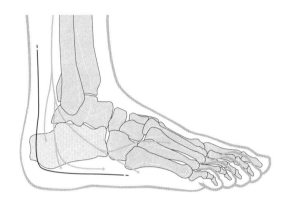

Fig. 4.10-5: Extended lateral incision.
The approach begins in the midline posteriorly some 7 cm proximal to the tip of the fibula. It passes distally and slightly anteriorly so that at the level of the tip of the fibula it lies just in front of the Achilles tendon. At the point of the heel it turns 90° and passes forward along the lateral border of the heel as far as the base of the fifth metatarsal. In its distal limb, the incision lies below the line of demarcation between the bruised area around the lateral hindfoot and the unbruised skin on the sole of the foot.

parallel to the sole of the foot in unbruised skin. For the junction between the proximal and distal limbs a right angle is recommended by some, others prefer a curve [2] (**Video AO24018a**). A full-thickness soft-tissue flap is raised which will include the peroneal tendons in their sheath and possibly small cortical bone fragments. The entire lateral wall of the calcaneus should be exposed up to the calcaneocuboid joint, taking care not to damage the tendon of the peroneus longus as it enters the sole of the foot, or the sural nerve at either extreme of the exposure. **The flap must be treated gently to preserve its vascularity.** It may be secured in its raised position by placing K-wires into the talar neck. Depending on the configuration of the

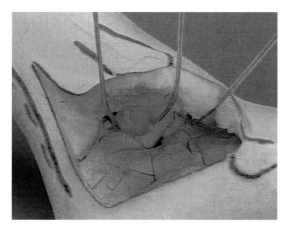

Video AO24018a

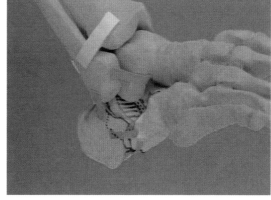

Video 4.10-1

lateral wall of the calcaneus in the region of the subtalar joint, the calcaneofibular ligament may be readily visible. If not, it is likely that the cortical shell of bone obscuring the lateral joint fragment will need to be reflected distally (Fig. 4.10-6) [2]. The calcaneofibular ligament must be divided to allow access to the posterior facet of the subtalar joint. The key to reduction of the calcaneal fracture is the reduction and axial alignment of the tuberosity fragment to the sustentaculum/medial wall fragment. It is often necessary to dislocate the lateral joint fragment on its posterosuperior soft-tissue hinge so that the medial wall fracture site and the subtalar joint can be seen. A Schanz screw inserted into the tuberosity will aid distraction while a bone lever may be inserted through the fracture to the medial wall in order to reduce and realign the fragments (Fig. 4.10-7) (Video 4.10-1).

Once the medial wall fracture site has been reduced, its position is held with K-wires. The articular surface is now reconstituted by replacement of the lateral fragment, and held

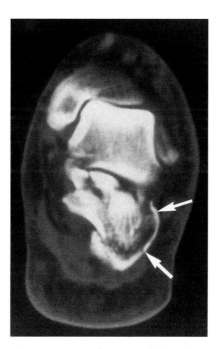

Fig. 4.10-6: Coronal CT scan. The lateral cortex of the tuberosity fragment "hides" the lateral joint fragment. To expose the lateral joint fragment and allow reduction of the fracture, the lateral cortex must be reflected.

Reduction must be checked
by x-ray.

a)

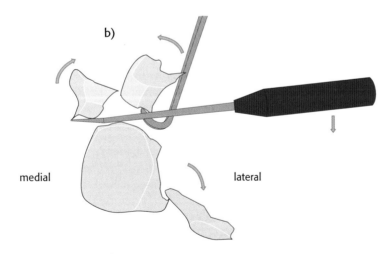

with a K-wire while **the reduction is checked with lateral and axial x-rays**. Positioning of surgeon, patient, and image intensifier is important (**Fig. 4.10-8**). A large bony defect should be filled with cancellous autograft.

Attention is now turned to the anterior part of the calcaneus. The anterolateral fragment often lies in the sinus tarsi and if operative treatment has been delayed, its reduction can be difficult without an extensive soft-tissue release. This fragment forms the distal half of Gissane's angle and is stabilized with a temporary K-wire. If the preoperative images suggest significant involvement of the calcaneocuboid joint, this must now be inspected and a congruent surface restored whenever possible. If the reduction is complete and satisfactory on lateral, axial, and oblique views, definitive fixation can be com-

b)

medial   lateral

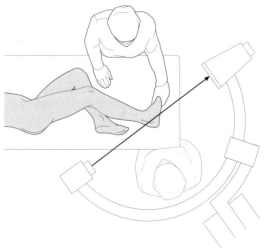

Fig. 4.10-7:
a) Diagram showing insertion of a Schanz screw into the tuberosity fragment for distraction of the fracture.
b) The insertion of a periosteal elevator across the fracture to the medial wall may allow disimpaction and realignment of the fracture fragments. The lateral joint fragment has been rotated out of the subtalar joint on its soft-tissue hinge.

Fig. 4.10-8: Diagram to show the position of patient, surgeon, and image intensifier for perioperative views of the calcaneum and subtalar joint.

menced. A 3.5 mm cortex lag screw is inserted across the subchondral bone of the posterior facet: cannulated screws are easier to insert. The screw must be within and not inferior to the sustentaculum tali if damage to the delicate structures in that region is to be avoided. Once the joint reduction is secured, a plate is contoured to conform to the shape of the lateral wall while screws through the plate are used to stabilize the remaining fracture fragments. **The choice of plate depends on the fracture pattern**. Fully threaded cancellous bone screws are used posteriorly, while cortex screws are preferable anteriorly (**Fig. 4.10-9**) (**Video AO24018b/4.10-2**). The reduction is again checked in both the lateral and axial planes to ensure that no angulation into varus has occurred at the medial wall fracture site. Careful wound closure over a suction drain is performed.

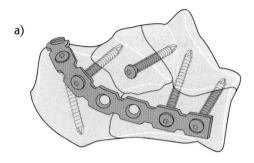

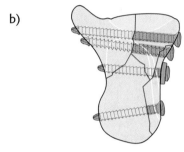

Choice of plate depends on fracture pattern.

Fig. 4.10-9: Lateral and axial diagrams of the reduction and fixation of a calcaneal fracture with a reconstruction plate 3.5.

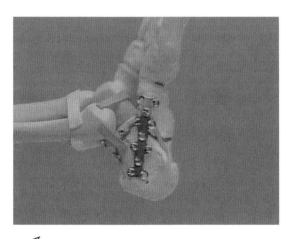

Video AO24018b/4.10-2

Extra-articular fractures of the tuberosity

These fractures are considered to be avulsion injuries and often occur in more osteoporotic elderly patients. If significantly displaced, reduction and fixation are required to restore normal function of the Achilles tendon. While some surgeons favor a percutaneous method of reduction and screw fixation, most prefer a formal posterolateral approach (the proximal limb of the extended lateral incision). A bone hook aids reduction, and fixation may be either with two cancellous bone screws (4.0 or 6.5 mm) or by a cerclage wire placed around the fragment and through a transverse drill hole in the main tuberosity of the calcaneus. All such cases require a below knee cast with the foot in 10° of equinus and a toe-touching gait.

2.5   Postoperative treatment: articular fractures

Wound healing is a major consideration and the limb must rest in the elevated position for much of the first 5–7 days. The limb may be supported in a well-padded removable plaster splint with the foot at 90°. Providing the wound is satisfactory, joint mobilization can be commenced at 24–48 hours. The patient then mobilizes non-weight bearing either without a cast so that joint movements can continue, or in a below knee cast, depending on patient compliance. In most cases, weight bearing can commence at 4–6 weeks post fixation if clinical and radiographic union is evident.

2.6   Pitfalls and complications

Wound healing

Wound edge necrosis and subsequent infection are still the major concern following operative management of a calcaneal fracture. Attention to detail in planning and performing the incision and closure is important. If the wound is sited correctly, it will not overlie any of the fixation devices and thus, even if complete wound closure is not possible, the wound edges may be approximated and the wound heals by secondary intention.

Malunion

The other major pitfall is a failure to reduce and hold the fracture adequately. Large bony defects may be due to incomplete reduction or also a result of severe comminution. In this situation a cancellous autograft is recommended. A thorough understanding of fracture anatomy is essential before operative treatment, and high-quality image intensification is most helpful. If there is considerable comminution extending into the calcaneocuboid joint, it may be preferable to extend the plate fixation across the joint to increase stability.

2.7   Results

Assessment of hindfoot function is difficult and debate continues as to whether emphasis should be given preferentially to radiographic features or to clinical symptoms. After operative reduction and internal fixation, the subtalar joint is invariably rather stiff compared to the non-injured side, but what movement is present is usually comfortable and the patient can wear normal shoes. Thus, many patients do retain some ability to cope with uneven ground, ladders, steps, and even rock climbing. In general, results worsen with increasing comminution and chondral damage [2, 3, 5]. **In cases of painful osteoarthritis of the subtalar joint, secondary fusion is much simpler than if the hindfoot is already well aligned compared to cases of a non-operatively treated, impacted, and widened calcaneus**. It would appear that the best results are achieved when there is anatomical reduction of both the articular and non-articular components of the fracture [5].

Disturbed wound healing remains a big concern.

Secondary subtalar fusion is simpler after ORIF than after non-operative treatment.

3 Fractures of the talus

3.1 Assessment of fractures and soft tissues

Talar fractures are uncommon and the outcome may be poor, with disability due to malunion or the development of avascular necrosis. Management depends entirely on whether or not the fracture is displaced and therefore a thorough assessment is essential. Standard x-ray views of the hindfoot including an AP, a lateral and two oblique films are supplemented by more specialized views of the talar neck or computed tomography. Most significant fractures of the talus affect the neck and the classification system most commonly used is shown in **Table 4.10-1**.

The soft tissues of the hindfoot are vulnerable to injury and must be assessed carefully,as damage is likely to affect the timing of surgery and the choice of incision.

Table 4.10-1:

Classification of fractures of the talus [6]

Type 1	Non-displaced vertical fracture of the talar neck.
Type 2	Displaced fracture of the talar neck with subluxation or dislocation of the subtalar joint.
Type 3	Displaced fracture of the talar neck with the dislocation of the body from both the subtalar and ankle joints.

3.2 Surgical anatomy

The talus is unique in having no muscular attachments; 60% of its surface is covered by articular cartilage. The vascular supply is via the posterior and anterior tibial arteries and the peroneal artery, but the area available for its entry to the bone is small. There is an anastomosis between branches from all three of these vessels in the tarsal canal inferior to the talar neck. The major blood supply thus enters the talus posterior to the neck, so isolated neck fractures are unlikely to lead to vascular damage. The body itself has a rich blood supply. An important vessel lies on the inner surface of the deltoid ligament, and in many cases of fracture it is this artery which maintains viability of the talar body. In such instances, the surgical incision must not damage the blood supply further, keeping the deep fibers of the deltoid ligament intact.

The talus has no muscle origins, and 60% articular cartilage coverage resulting in a circumscribed blood supply.

In talar fractures, outcome may be poor due to malunion or avascular necrosis.

3.3 Preoperative planning

Fractures of the talus are either displaced or not. **All displaced fractures must be reduced anatomically and stabilized as early as possible.** Even moderate displacement may be associated with considerable pressure on the soft tissues and if skin necrosis and vascular damage are to be avoided, prompt reduction by either closed or open means is essential. Such cases represent surgical emergencies, as do many Hawkins type 3 fractures that are open and where prompt, adequate wound débridement is an essential first step.

Hawkins type 2 fractures may respond to closed reduction techniques, but type 3 fractures rarely do. Closed reduction must not cause further damage to the soft tissues. Under general

Displaced fractures must be reduced and stabilized as an emergency.

or regional anesthesia with the patient supine, traction is applied to the hindfoot and the forefoot is flexed to realign the fracture fragments. An image intensifier is essential. If an anatomical reduction is obtained, fixation may be achieved via open or percutaneous insertion of screws through the posterior approach. Temporary fixation can be achieved with K-wires but for permanent fixation screws are required.

If closed reduction is unsuccessful, open reduction must be performed. The choice of incision is influenced by the presence of a wound, by a medial malleolar fracture and by the degree of displacement of the fracture fragments. The two most popular incisions are the anteromedial and the anterolateral.

3.4 Surgical treatment— tricks and hints

The anterolateral incision minimizes the risk of further damage to the talar blood supply. The approach is simple and direct. The extensor tendons and the neurovascular bundle are reflected medially. The capsule of the ankle joint has usually been torn and the talar neck is readily visible. If further access is needed to view the talar body, a transverse fibular osteotomy (at the level of the ankle mortise) can be performed.

The anteromedial incision is useful when the body of the talus is dislocated posteriorly or if there is a medial malleolar fracture. If the medial malleolus is intact, an osteotomy is performed, but great care must be taken to ensure that the deep fibers of the deltoid ligament are not damaged when the malleolus is reflected distally. A Steinmann pin inserted into the cal-

caneus allows traction to be applied to the hindfoot, thus facilitating reduction of the talar body. Nevertheless, reduction may take time and patience.

Once reduction has been achieved, careful assessment of the subtalar joint must be performed either under direct vision, or radiographically, to ensure that the reduction is anatomical. K-wires may be used for provisional fixation, but only in comminuted fractures are they suitable for definitive fixation. **Compression of the fracture by the insertion of two lag screws enhances fracture healing.** Screws may be either 4.0 or 6.5 mm cancellous bone screws or 3.5 mm cortex lag screws. If 6.5 mm screws are used, a 4.5 mm drill bit for the gliding hole may be recommended. The screws should be placed perpendicular to the fracture planes and the heads must be countersunk to avoid impingement on any articular surface (**Fig. 4.10-10**). Biomechanically, screws inserted from posteriorly offer better stability [7].

Temporary K-wire fixation must hold the fracture in the reduced position without interfering with the definitive fixation. In this respect the cannulated screw system is of considerable benefit, facilitating the procedure.

If the medial side is comminuted, the insertion of a compression screw carries the risks of placing the fracture into varus—a common finding in cases of malunion. It is therefore essential that good quality x-rays or a CT scan be taken after both temporary and definitive fracture fixations to confirm the correct reduction.

Malleolar osteotomies or fractures must be reduced anatomically and fixed by standard means to ensure joint congruity for an optimal outcome.

If closed reduction is not successfull, open reduction and internal fixation is mandatory.

Interfragmentary lag screws are the method of choice.

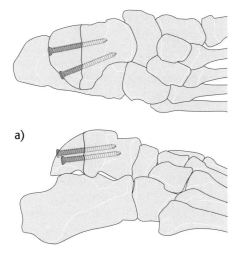
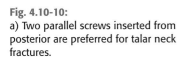
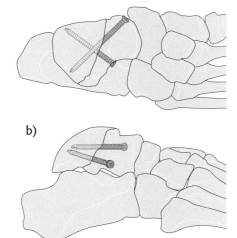
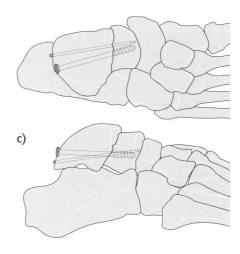

Fig. 4.10-10:
a) Two parallel screws inserted from posterior are preferred for talar neck fractures.

b) Anteriorly placed screws may cross each other. The entry point is determined by the fracture configuration and the articular surfaces.

c) Occasionally, one screw and one K-wire is the most appropriate method of gaining reduction and stable fixation.

Wounds must never be closed under tension, although it is preferable to cover joints and tendons. If this is not possible, they may remain uncovered until definitive plastic surgical procedures can be performed. A delayed primary wound closure at 5 days is often required.

Fractures of the talar body and head

These injuries are less common, but they should, whenever possible, be treated similarly to the neck fractures by anatomical reduction and stable internal fixation to retain congruity of the peritalar joints.

3.5 Postoperative treatment

The limb is rested in a well-padded plaster splint with the foot at 90°. If fixation is satisfactory and the joint stable, early motion must be encouraged. In unstable cases, a below-knee cast is applied for 6–12 weeks. Weight bearing may be commenced in type 2 injuries within 2–4 weeks. Alternatively, a patellar-tendon-bearing walking caliper may be applied. Union may be delayed due to the relatively tenuous blood supply.

3.6   Pitfalls and complications

Wound breakdown

The skin of the foot and ankle region is not supported by much subcutaneous tissue and wound infection and skin necrosis do occur. Wounds must be observed closely until healing is assured.

Avascular necrosis

Technetium bone scans and MRI may help identify those fractures in which there is change in vascularity. The treatment of a fracture with avascular changes is controversial but may include protected weight bearing for up to 2 years in an attempt to prevent collapse during renewed vascularization.

3.7   Results

A poor outcome is related directly to the degree of initial displacement, but even fractures with less severe displacement may do surprisingly badly. Although all reports endorse the philosophy of prompt anatomical reduction and stable fixation of the fracture, it is important to recognize that the outcome also depends on the degree of soft-tissue and cartilage damage incurred at the time of injury [8, 9].

Delayed union is common but non-union is rare. Malunion in varus may occur in up to 50% of Hawkins type 2 injuries leading to abnormal weight-bearing patterns and strain of the subtalar joint. Salvage surgery is successful in most cases [8].

Injuries to the tarsometatarsal joint are most painful and prone to later disability. Be aware of a compartment syndrome.

4   Tarsometatarsal joint injuries

4.1   Assessment of fractures and soft tissues

With any injury to the foot, even the seemingly trivial accidental slip, damage to the tarsometatarsal (or Lisfranc) joint must be suspected. **Injuries at this level are renowned not only for the immediate, often disabling, pain and swelling (compartment syndrome) with which they are associated, but also for later problems due to alteration in foot mechanics and degenerative change. Anatomical reduction with stable fixation of the fractures and joint subluxations or dislocations is advised.**

Clinically, these feet are usually very swollen and painful and the deformity associated with any subluxation or dislocation may be hidden (**Fig. 4.10-11**) [10]. A compartment syndrome should always be considered.

Plain x-rays in the AP, lateral and lateral oblique planes are essential for full assessment of these injuries. The radiological features may be subtle and easily overlooked, particularly in cases where the subluxation has spontaneously reduced and in patients who have more obvious injuries that distract attention. Features which must be looked for include avulsion fractures at the level of the tarsometatarsal joint (the fleck sign), and two straight unbroken lines: the line which runs along the medial edge of the 2nd metatarsal base and on to the medial edge of the intermediate cuneiform and another which follows the medial aspect of the base of the 4th metatarsal to the medial edge of the articular surface of the cuboid (**Fig. 4.10-12**) [11].

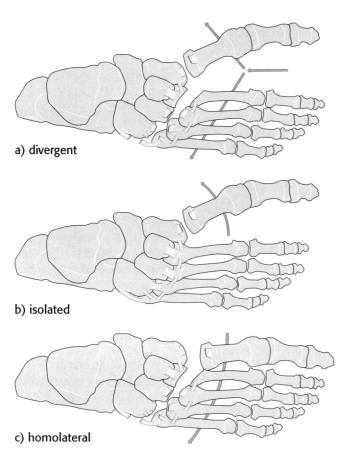

a) divergent

b) isolated

c) homolateral

Fig. 4.10-11: Descriptive classification of tarsometatarsal injuries.

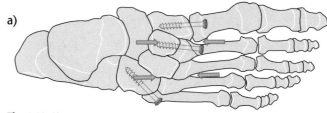

Fig. 4.10-12:
a) Diagram which shows the unbroken lines (arrows) of alignment which must be looked for on x-rays of suspected tarsometatarsal joint injuries and which are shown in this example of a reconstituted fracture.

Unstable injuries with considerable displacement should be treated surgically.

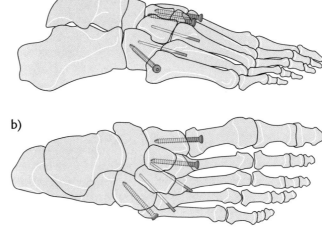

b) Diagram illustrating common patterns of fracture fixation with 3.5 mm cortex screws. K-wires may be used for the 3rd and 4th metatarsals.

4.2 Surgical anatomy

The intrinsic stability of this region, which is crucial to foot function, is provided primarily by the bony Roman arch whose features include the trapezoidal shape of the 2nd, 3rd, and 4th metatarsal bases (when seen in transverse section) and by the fact that the base of the 2nd metatarsal is recessed between the medial and lateral cuneiforms. The surrounding soft tissues such as the joint capsules, the plantar ligaments, the plantar fascia, and the tendon of peroneus longus all enhance the stability of this region. There is a relative weakness dorsally, particularly between the 1st and 2nd metatarsals, which helps to explain the direction of displacement in cases of injury. At this same point, the dorsalis pedis artery enters the sole of the foot and damage to this vessel is not uncommon in injuries around the tarsometatarsal joint.

4.3 Preoperative planning

When possible, early treatment is favored to reduce the stretching and compression forces on the vessels and the soft tissues. If the injury presents late, the limb must be elevated until the swelling diminishes and the tissues have stabilized. An anatomical reduction may be obtained by closed means under a general or spinal anesthetic. The patient is positioned supine with a sandbag under the affected buttock to place the foot in neutral rotation. Wire toe traps are used to suspend the toes with countertraction applied through the hindfoot and additional gentle manipulation at the fracture site as necessary. Reduction is confirmed on x-ray and the position then held with either percutaneous K-wires or screws. If there is a displacement greater than 2 mm or a talometatarsal angle of more than 15°, the position is unacceptable and an open reduction must be performed [12]. A set of small fragment screws (cannulated if possible) and K-wires are required.

4.4 Surgical treatment—tricks and hints

Either one or several longitudinal dorsal incisions are used depending on the location and number of metatarsals involved, the site of any wounds, and the presence of a compartment syndrome. The incision should be centered just distal to the tarsometatarsal joint line and measure 5–6 cm. **Entrapment of bony fragments or soft tissues within the joint commonly obstructs closed reduction.** Once these blocks have been removed and an anatomical reduction achieved it may be held with temporary K-wires. The unstable metatarsals are

Entrapment of bony fragments or ligaments within the joints obstructs closed reduction.

then fixed to the midfoot with 4.0 mm cancellous bone or 3.5 mm cortex lag screws placed through a notch on the dorsal surface of the bone approximately 1.5 cm distal to the joint (**Fig. 4.10-13**) and cannulation can again be advantageous. The screw should be perpendicular to the joint and care should be taken not to split the base of the metatarsal. K-wires may be used as definitive fixation for the 3rd/4th metatarsals if necessary (see **Fig. 4.10-12**).

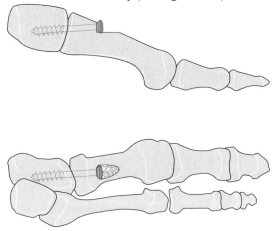

Fig. 4.10-13: A dorsal notch in the metatarsal shaft will prevent the dorsal cortex from splitting on screw insertion and will reduce the prominence of the screw head. The drill hole should be placed in the top of the notch.

4.5 Postoperative treatment

The foot should be immobilized in a well-molded and well-padded splint and the neurovascular status observed. Once the swelling has diminished, a below-knee cast is applied. The patient remains non-weight bearing for 6 weeks. The

K-wires are then removed. Progressive weight bearing with aggressive physiotherapy may then commence. Opinions vary as to the need to remove the screws: those who favor their removal do so at 12 weeks.

4.6 Results

Anatomical reduction combined with stable fixation appears to provide the best results, although other factors, such as chondral damage and soft-tissue injury, may significantly affect the outcome [12].

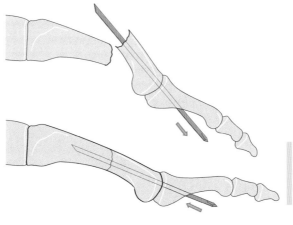

Anatomical reduction and stable fixation provide the best results!

Fig. 4.10-14: Metatarsal alignment with K-wires to prevent dorsal displacement or angulation of the distal fragment. The wire must transfix the metatarsophalangeal joint to allow for correct alignment of the metatarsal.

5 Metatarsal fractures

Metatarsal fractures are common and, although significant displacement is rare, malunion is a cause of considerable disability. **Shortening of the first metatarsal must be avoided,** so such fractures may require open reduction via a dorsal incision and internal fixation with either the plate 2.7 system or a one-third tubular plate and 3.5 mm screws. Intra-articular extensions at the proximal and distal ends of the first metatarsal must also be treated aggressively with a small lag screw when possible.

Dorsal angulation of the distal fragments must also be avoided with metatarsal shaft and neck fractures. They should be reduced and the position maintained with intramedullary K-wires, a mini fragment plate, or K-wire transfixion to a neighboring bone (**Fig. 4.10-14**).

With these more severe injuries, a non-weight bearing below-knee cast is used initially and the wires removed at 4–6 weeks.

Fractures of the proximal fifth metatarsal

The proximal portion of the fifth metatarsal has been divided into three zones (**Fig. 4.10-15**). Zone 1 injuries represent avulsion fractures and usually no operative treatment is required. Injuries in zone 2 are often more painful, but operative treatment is only required if displacement exceeds 5 mm. Zone 3 fractures occur in the proximal metaphysis and are often stress fractures. They usually need stable fixation, particularly if a prompt return to full function is required. Acute fractures in this region are usually managed non-operatively with cast immobilization and protected weight bearing for 6–8 weeks and then increasing to full function. Fixation methods include the use of two small lag screws or a wire tension band [13, 14].

Shortening of the first metatarsal must be avoided.

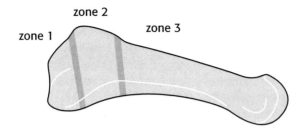

Fig. 4.10-15: The three zones of injuy in proximal fractures of the 5th metatarsal.

6 Navicular and cuboid fractures

Tarsal navicular fractures

Displaced fractures of the navicular should be treated operatively.

The navicular is one of the midfoot tarsal bones and part of Chopart's joint. It is also part of the medial arch of the foot and articulates with the talar head proximally, the three cuneiforms distally, and the cuboid laterally. The medial and plantar aspects of the navicular are supported by soft tissues, especially the insertion of the tibialis posterior tendon. This tendon can become entrapped in fracture dislocations involving the navicular, making reduction difficult. Because of its important position in the foot, injuries to the navicular are usually associated with other joint injuries and these must be excluded by clinical and radiographical examination.

There are three types of injury: cortical avulsions, fractures of the tuberosity, and fractures of the body. A stress fracture is occasionally seen.

Cortical avulsion fractures are a result of a twisting injury rupturing the talonavicular capsule and the most anterior fibres of the deltoid ligament; a piece of bone is also avulsed. Treatment is in a short leg walking cast for 6 weeks. If the fragment includes more than 20–30% of the articular surface, it should be stabilized with a wire or small screw.

Tuberosity fractures are caused by an eversion injury, with the tibialis posterior tendon pulled off the navicular tuberosity. If seen with a crush fracture of the cuboid, this injury may indicate an occult dislocation or subluxation of the midtarsal joint. Treatment is usually in a short leg walking cast for 6 weeks, unless proximal displacement is greater than 1 cm. Then it is reduced and stabilized with a screw or suture.

Body fractures are associated with other midtarsal injuries which must be diagnosed and treated. Undisplaced fractures are treated in a well moulded short leg cast for 6 weeks. **Displaced fractures are treated operatively with screws and sometimes a temporary small external fixator.** Bony defects should be filled with an autograft.

Fractures of the cuboid

The most common significant injury to the cuboid bone occurs as a result of the "nutcracker" effect described by Hermel and Gershon-Cohen [14]. If there is minimal impaction, conservative management with a below-knee cast would be appropriate. However, if there is significant loss of length or alignment on the lateral column of the foot, it is likely that the long term outcome will be associated with pain and dysfunction around the calcaneocuboid joint and the peroneus longus tendon. Initial management might therefore include a restoration of length with ORIF or primary arthrodesis of the calcaneocuboid joint [15].

Compression fractures of the cuboid bone are a rare but well recognized cause of foot pain and a reluctance to walk in children. Stress fractures may also occur in this area.

7 Bibliography

1. **Zwipp H** (1994) *Chirurgie des Fusses.* Berlin: Springer-Verlag.
2. **Eastwood DM, Phipp L** (1997) Intra-articular fractures of the calcaneum: why such controversy? *Injury*; 28 (4):247–259.
3. **Zwipp H, Tscherne H, Thermann H, et al.** (1993) Osteosynthesis of displaced intraarticular fractures of the calcaneus. Results in 123 cases. *Clin Orthop*; (290):76–86.
4. **Myerson M** (1990) Diagnosis and treatment of compartment syndrome of the foot. *Orthopedics*; 13 (7):711–717.
5. **Sanders R, Fortin P, DiPasquale T, et al.** (1993) Operative treatment in 120 displaced intraarticular calcaneal fractures. Results using a prognostic computed tomography scan classification. *Clin Orthop*; (290):87–95.
6. **Hawkins LG** (1970) Fractures of the neck of the talus. *J Bone Joint Surg [Am]*; 52 (5):991–1002.
7. **Swanson TV, Bray TJ, Holmes GB, Jr.** (1992) Fractures of the talar neck. A mechanical study of fixation. *J Bone Joint Surg [Am]*; 74 (4):544–551.
8. **Canale ST, Kelly FB, Jr.** (1978) Fractures of the neck of the talus. Long-term evaluation of seventy-one cases. *J Bone Joint Surg [Am]*; 60 (2):143–156.
9. **Kenwright J, Taylor RG** (1970) Major injuries of the talus. *J Bone Joint Surg [Br]*; 52 (1):36–48.
10. **Hardcastle PH, Reschauer R, Kutscha-Lissberg E, et al.** (1982) Injuries to the tarsometatarsal joint. Incidence, classification and treatment. *J Bone Joint Surg [Br]*; 64 (3):349–356.
11. **Arntz CT, Hansen ST, Jr.** (1987) Dislocations and fracture dislocations of the tarsometatarsal joints. *Orthop Clin North Am*; 18 (1):105–114.
12. **Myerson MS, Fisher RT, Burgess AR, et al.** (1986) Fracture dislocations of the tarsometatarsal joints: end results correlated with pathology and treatment. *Foot Ankle*; 6 (5):225–242.
13. **Dameron TB** (1995) Fractures of the proximal fifth metatarsal: selecting the best treatment option. *J Am Acad Orthop Surg*; 3(2):110–114.
14. **Smith JW, Arnoczky SP, Hersh A** (1992) The intraosseous blood supply of the fifth metatarsal: implications for proximal fracture healing. *Foot Ankle*; 13 (3):143–152.
15. **Hermel MB, Gershon-Cohen J** (1953) The nutcracker of the cuboid by indirect violence. *Radiology*; 60:850.

8 Updates

Updates and additional references for this chapter are available online at:
http://www.aopublishing.org/PFxM/410.htm

4.11 Spine

John O'Dowd

1 Introduction

The management of spinal trauma, either in isolation or as part of the management of the polytraumatized patient, is difficult because of the number of potential pitfalls awaiting the general trauma surgeon faced with such injuries.

The general principles of resuscitation apply. Although the majority of injured patients should be assumed to have an unstable spinal injury until a full evaluation has been completed, certain patient groups are particularly at risk. Those who

- are complaining of axial pain,
- have suffered polytrauma,
- have any head injury,
- have facial injuries,
- are unconscious or obtunded,
- are road traffic accident victims.

In these patients, the cervical spine should be controlled with a firm collar, or two sandbags (or infusion packs) and forehead tape (**Fig. 4.11-1**). The thoracolumbar spine should be protected by the use of a spine board and thereafter only by log rolling the supine patient.

The orthopedic assessment of the spine should include evaluation of both the skeletal and neurological injuries, and a careful search for associated spinal and non-spinal injuries. Identification of instability and potential instability, classification of the injury, and a complete management plan are essential.

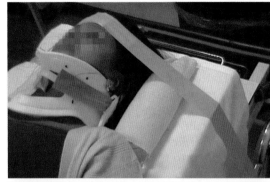
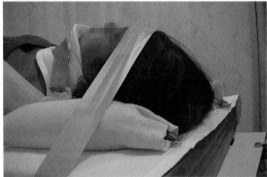
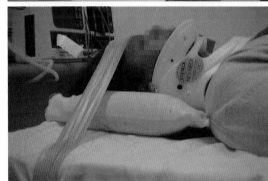

Fig. 4.11-1:
Patient positioned with tape, sandbags, and collar.

Orthopedic assessment of the spine should include evaluation of skeletal and neurosurgical injuries and a careful search for associated spinal and non-spinal injuries.

Rectal examination is mandatory if there is any suspicion of neurological injury, and anal tone, sensation, and the bulbocavernosus reflex tested.

The spine must be inspected and palpated from occiput to coccyx.

2 Clinical evaluation

A description of the exact mechanism of injury from the patient, any eyewitnesses and emergency service personnel is important. In addition, any reported transient or persistent neurological symptoms might indicate significant spinal instability.

The spine must be inspected and palpated from occiput to coccyx and the presence of the following signs indicates significant injury:
- Pain with movement.
- Tenderness.
- Gap or step.
- Edema or bruising.
- Spasm of associated muscles.

Neurological assessment must be comprehensive. All muscle groups should be evaluated and graded on a dedicated neurology chart. Weakness should be graded according to the Medical Research Council (MRC) method (**Table 4.11-1**)[1]. Sensation should be tested, including light touch, pinprick, proprioception, and vibration. All dermatomes should be examined bilaterally. Reflexes should be documented. Any sensory and motor level should

be recorded. **Rectal examination is mandatory if there is any suspicion of neurological injury, and anal tone, sensation, and the bulbocavernosus reflex tested.** In the patient with spinal cord injury, vital signs including pulse, blood pressure, and respiratory rate should be monitored continuously.

3 Radiological evaluation

3.1 Cervical spine

All patients with a suspected spinal cord or column injury should be further investigated. The primary survey will have included a cross table lateral film of the cervical spine. The definitive radiological assessment of any patient with spinal injury will include further plain x-rays, as well as CT scanning and MRI scanning.

In the cervical spine the lateral film should show the spine from the occiput to the C7/T1 disc and if this has not been achieved, special views, such as the "swimmers view" will be required (**Fig. 4.11-2**). With a lateral film alone the false negative diagnosis rate is up to 15%. A through-the-mouth odontoid peg view and an AP x-ray of the cervical spine must always be taken.

Table 4.11-1: Standard grades of muscle power.

Grade	Testing parameter
0	Total paralysis
1	Barely detectable contracture
2	Not enough power to act against gravity
3	Strong enough to act against gravity
4	Still stronger but less than normal
5	Full power

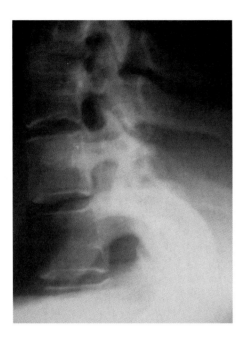

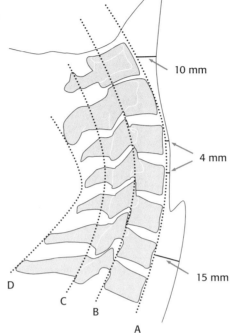

Fig. 4.11-2:
Swimmers view

10 mm

4 mm

15 mm

D

C

B

A

Fig. 4.11-3:
Line diagram of four cervical lines (A-D)
and soft-tissue width (in mm).

In the cervical spine the following abnormalities should be specifically sought:

- Loss of normal cervical lordosis.
- Increased anterior soft-tissue width (normal prevertebral shadow is less than 4 mm at C4 and less than 15 mm at C6) (**Fig. 4.11-3**).
- Increased interspinous distance posteriorly (**Fig. 4.11-4**).
- Loss of spinous process alignment and/ or increased interspinous distance on AP x-ray.
- Fractures of the body, lateral mass, pedicle, spinous process.
- Fractures of the odontoid peg or the ring of atlas.
- Any loss of alignment indicating subluxation or dislocation (**Fig. 4.11-5a**).
- More than 11° angulation or 3 mm translation at any level (**Fig. 4.11-5b**).

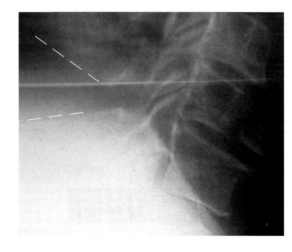

Fig. 4.11-4: Lateral x-ray with interspinous widening.

Fig. 4.11-5:
Unifacet dislocation

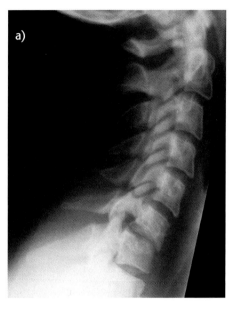

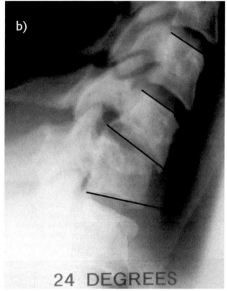

24 DEGREES

3.2 **Thoracolumbar spine**

In the thoracolumbar spine high-quality AP and lateral x-rays are required. The following abnormalities may be seen:

- Loss of vertebral alignment on AP or lateral x-rays (**Fig. 4.11-6**).
- Fractures of vertebral body, or posterior, spinous or transverse processes elements.
- Widening of interspinous distance.
- Abnormal pedicle separation on AP x-ray (**Fig. 4.11-7**).
- Loss of vertebral body height, vertebral wedging, and kyphosis.

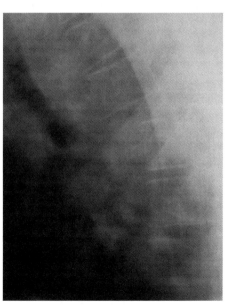

Fig. 4.11-6:
Lateral x-ray of thoracolumbar dislocation.

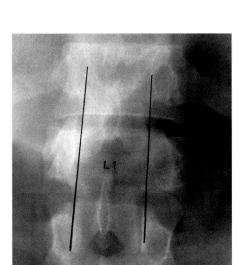

Fig. 4.11-7:
AP view of x-ray thoracolumbar spine showing pedicle separation.

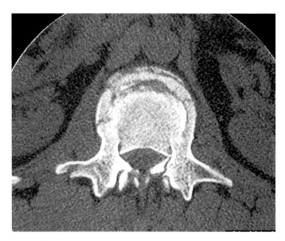

Fig. 4.11-8:
CT scan of burst fracture with posterior element fracture.

3.3 Further steps

A standardized approach to further imaging should be adopted. **The incidence of a second spinal injury is up to 20%, so if a significant spinal injury has been identified at one level, the rest of the spine should be re-examined clinically as well as by plain AP and lateral x-rays of every level.**

If any fractures other than minor process fractures are identified on x-ray, cross sectional imaging with CT scanning should be obtained (**Fig. 4.11-8**). The complete fracture configuration is rarely identified on x-rays alone. 3-D reconstructions aid comprehension and surgical planning, but do not enhance the accuracy of the CT data. CT scans may also be indicated in

the following areas if injury is suspected, when adequate x-rays cannot be obtained:
• Occipitocervical junction.
• C1/C2 injuries.
• Cervicothoracic junction.
• Sacroiliac region.

MRI scanning will demonstrate soft-tissue injury to posterior ligamentous structures and intervertebral discs. If available, its use is mandatory in single or bilateral facet cervical dislocations before reduction, in order to avoid spinal cord injury from the possible concomitant disc protrusion. The precise nature of any spinal cord injury can also be identified on MRI sequences.

The incidence of a second spinal injury is up to 20%, so if a significant spinal injury has been identified at one level, the rest of the spine should be re-examined clinically as well as by plain AP and lateral x-rays of every level.

3.4 Dynamic radiography

Dynamic radiography, such as flexion/extension, or traction lateral, cervical x-rays, is inappropriate if an unstable spinal injury is diagnosed. Flexion/extension x-rays or fluoroscopy of the cervical spine must be personally supervised by a trauma specialist. It must be recognized that these measures may not be adequate to determine spinal stability and are potentially dangerous. Longitudinal sagittal scanning with MRI, or spiral CT, will provide additional information and the former allows imaging of the entire neuraxis. However, few patients are stable enough for MRI scanning, and MRI compatible anesthetic equipment is not commonly available. The safest policy is to continue to protect the spinal column until the patient can cooperate with dynamic imaging without reporting significant pain.

3.4.1 Conscious patient

In a conscious and cooperative patient with persistent neck pain and no radiographic evidence of fracture or dislocation, supervised flexion/extension x-rays are taken and will exclude significant instability. However, these should be delayed until paravertebral spasm has settled, so that flexion and extension movements actually occur. Until this stage is reached, possibly some weeks after injury, the patient should be treated in a firm orthosis.

3.4.2 Unconscious patient

In the obtunded patient spinal column assessment must be meticulous. The standard clinical and radiological investigations are undertaken. The fracture surgeon is often asked to make a judgment on spinal stability when the plain x-rays and, sometimes, CT scans at selected levels appear to be normal. The safest policy is to assume an unstable injury, to log roll the patient and to use a firm cervical orthosis until the protocol in section 3 can be completed. Spinal cord injury in an unconscious patient should be suspected if any combination of the following is present:

- Flaccid areflexia.
- Diaphragmatic breathing.
- Pain response above, but not below the clavicle.
- Bradycardia and hypotension.
- Priapism.

4 Spinal instability

The term instability is used to describe a wide variety of spinal conditions, including clinical, radiological and biomechanical abnormalities. The most widely used general definition is that of White and Panjabe [2] and states that: "The loss of the ability of the spine under physiological loads to maintain its pattern of displacement so that there is no initial or additional neurological deficit, no major deformity, and no incapacitating pain". **Instability missed during the initial management phase may produce or exacerbate a spinal cord injury or permit displacement of fractures or dislocations**, thereby precipitating the need for more invasive interventions. In the long term it can lead to chronic instability, pain on movement, and a higher risk of degenerative changes, particularly if overall sagittal alignment is lost. The assessing clinician should make use of all of the clinical and radiological signs which have been described to judge the stability of the spinal column.

Instability missed during the initial management phase may produce or exacerbate a spinal cord injury or permit displacement of fractures or dislocations.

In the obtunded patient spinal column assessment must be meticulous.

Fig. 4.11-9:
Diagram of the two
spinal columns.

posterior   anterior

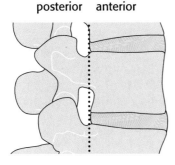

Since descriptions of spinal injuries were first reported, authors have considered the spine in conceptual divisions or columns. The work of Denis [3] has popularized the idea of three spinal columns. There is an increasing realization, however, that the use of a two column (**Fig. 4.11-9**) description simplifies understanding of the injury and has facilitated the process of applying AO classification principles to the spine. Following an injury, the presence of an intact anterior, or posterior, column will usually exclude the problems associated with instability. Careful assessment of both columns is essential, as the combination of clinical and radiological investigations may reveal significant injury to both. For example, what may appear to be an isolated compression fracture of the anterior column, may have an associated ligamentous posterior column injury diagnosed only by clinical examination, or MRI scanning.

5 Classification–skeletal injury

The AO classification is now widely used for the thoracolumbar and subaxial cervical spine. C1 and C2 level injuries are still classified differently.

Atlanto-occipital fracture dislocations are extremely uncommon and usually prove fatal. In the rare survivors they may only be diagnosed on sagittal CT reconstructions.

C1 level

The classical C1 fracture is the Jefferson fracture [4] (**Fig. 4.11-10a**), which is a burst fracture of the ring of C1. Stability is assessed by measuring the atlanto-dens interval on a lateral x-ray (normal < 4 mm), and by the lateral mass spread on the AP odontoid peg view (normal < 8 mm) (**Fig. 4.11-10b**). Other injuries of C1 include isolated lateral mass and anterior or posterior arch injuries.

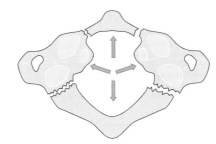

Fig. 4.11-10:
a) Diagram of Jefferson fracture.

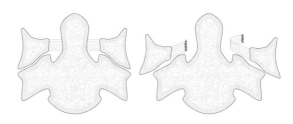

b) Diagram of lateral mass excursion.

C1/2 level

Atlanto-axial rotary subluxation of C1/C2 was described by Fielding and Hawkins [5]. This injury is characterized by fixed rotary subluxation of the joint and was subdivided into four types:

I	Rotary fixation, no displacement.
II	Rotary fixation, unilateral anterior displacement.
II	Rotary fixation, bilateral anterior displacement.
IV	Rotary fixation, posterior displacement.

The possibility of atlanto-axial disturbance should be considered where there is unexplained posttraumatic neck pain and torticollis.

Diagnosis can be very difficult but should be considered whenever there is unexplained posttraumatic neck pain and torticollis. Careful inspection of the x-rays and CT scans will normally demonstrate the lesion.

C2/odontoid

Odontoid peg fractures were classified by Anderson and D'Alonzo according to the level of the fracture [6] (**Fig. 4.11-11**). Type I fractures are at the tip of the odontoid process, and represent ligamentous avulsion which may rarely produce instability. Type II fractures are transverse or oblique fractures through the base of the odontoid process. Type III fractures are

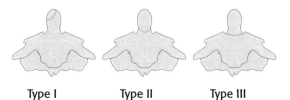

Type I   Type II   Type III

Fig. 4.11-11: Diagram of the three odontoid fracture types.
Type I   Sometimes as a ligamentous avulsion. Seldom causes instability.
Type II   These basal fractures may be transverse or oblique.
Type III These fractures pass through cancellous bone in the body of C2 close to the base of the odontoid.

through the cancellous bone of the body of C2 adjacent to the odontoid process.

Levine and Edwards have best classified traumatic spondylolisthesis of C2, the so-called hangman's fracture [7]. Type I injury is a neural arch fracture of C2, with no angulation and less than 3 mm displacement of C2 on C3. Type II injuries are displaced, with more than 5° of angulation and more than 3 mm of displacement (**Fig. 4.11-12**). Type IIA injuries are characterized by significant angulation, but no displacement, and by the observation that traction causes widening of the C2/3 disc space. Type III injuries have severe angulation and displacement and single or bilateral C2/3 facet dislocation.

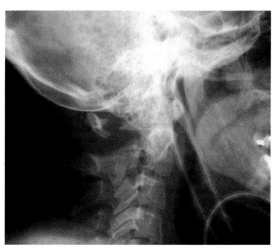

Fig. 4.11-12: X-ray of type II hangman's fracture.

Lower cervical, thoracic, and lumbar spine

Subaxial cervical and thoracolumbar fractures are classified according to Magerl et al. [8]. The AO group and the Orthopaedic Trauma Association have adopted this classification [9] (**Fig. 4.11-13**).

Type A

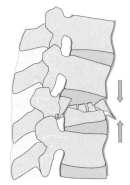

Type B

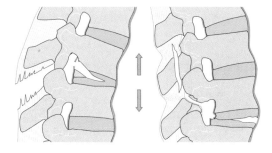

Type C

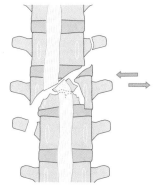

Fig. 4.11-13: Müller AO Classification

Type A   Compression injury of the anterior column.
Type B   Two-column injury with either posterior or
          anterior transverse distraction.
Type C   Two-column injury with rotation.

The spine, which is bone group 5, is divided into three sections:

Cervical	51
Thoracic	52
Lumbar	53

There are three basic injury patterns:

A	Compression injuries of the vertebral body.
B	Distraction injuries of the anterior and/or posterior elements.
C	Type A or type B injuries with rotation, and complex fractures and dislocations.

In the lower cervical spine distraction injuries are more severe than rotational, and so are classified in type C, with rotational injuries in type B.

6 Classification– neurological injuries

Cervical cord injury leads to tetraplegia and thoracic and lumbar injuries to paraplegia. **Neurological injuries are described as complete if there is no recovery of distal neurological function once the stage of spinal shock has passed, for example, when the bulbocavernosus reflex returns.** The American Spinal Injury Association (ASIA) and the International Medical Society of Paraplegia have refined the original Frankel [10] functional classification.

ASIA Impairment Scale

A	Complete lesion.
B	Incomplete sensory preservation.
C	Incomplete motor preservation < MRC grade 3.
D	Incomplete motor preservation > MRC grade 3.
E	Normal neurological function.

Neurological injuries are described as complete if there is no recovery of distal neuro-logical function once the stage of spinal shock has passed, e.g., when the bulbocavernosus reflex returns.

Incomplete lesions can fit into the following clinical syndromes:

- **Brown Sequard syndrome:** Ipsilateral motor and proprioceptive loss and contralateral pinprick and temperature loss.
- **Central cord syndrome:** Cervical cord lesion with severe tetraparesis, upper limbs worse than lower limbs and sacral sparing.
- **Anterior cord syndrome:** Most of the spinal cord affected with dorsal column sparing only.
- **Conus lesion:** This will produce a mixed picture of sacral cord and lumbar root injuries, with areflexic bowel and bladder.
- **Cauda equina lesion:** This produces nerve root injury with areflexic bowel and bladder.

7 Initial management

Controlling the spine and preventing further injury are the guiding principles during the evaluation period.

The patient with a spinal cord injury may be considered for a high dosage methylprednisolone protocol as soon as diagnosis is made. The 2nd National Acute Spinal Injury Study [1], a randomized, multi-center, doubleblind trial of methylprednisolone, established that early administration of very high doses led to better motor and sensory scores 6 months following injury. The initial dose is a bolus of 30 mg/kg body weight, followed by 5.4 mg/kg/hour for 23 hours. The proven improvement in recovery is, however, marginal and many of the patients in the original study also had early

surgery, which is a confounding factor. Although systemic complications were not reported from this protocol, there was a delay in wound healing in the surgical patients. A thorough study and understanding of these results are suggested before a patient can be advised that this protocol is functionallly effective and without major complications

Non-displaced cervical injuries

Non-displaced cervical injuries, whether stable or potentially unstable, can be controlled with a firm orthosis during the initial phase.

Displaced and unstable injures

Displaced and unstable injuries to the cervical spine should be managed with the use of halo traction. The admitting trauma surgeon or musculoskeletal specialist should apply this device under local anesthesia. A halo is preferable to tongs, or calipers, because of superior head and neck control, and because modern haloes are both MRI compatible and can be attached to a molded jacket as definitive treatment.

The anterior pins are placed in the supraorbital ridge, lateral to the supraorbital notch, with the patient's eyes tightly closed during insertion. The halo ring should lie so that it is 1 cm higher than the superior tip of the pinna. Local anesthetic is inserted, the pins are positioned and gently tightened, following which diagonally opposite screws are tightened simultaneously. A torque wrench should be used so that all screws are tightened to 6 in/lb (**Fig. 4.11-14**).

Non-displaced cervical injuries, whether stable or potentially unstable, can be controlled with a firm orthosis during the initial phase.

Controlling the spine and preventing further injury are the guiding principles during the evaluation period.

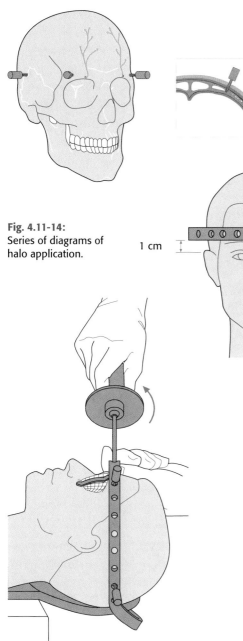

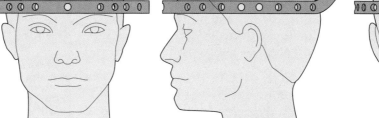

Initially, 2.5–4.5 kg longitudinal traction is applied and a lateral check x-ray is obtained. In a type IIA hangman's fracture, traction may cause segmental distraction, and should this occur, the traction should be removed, a halo jacket applied in the best obtainable position, and the patient transferred urgently to a specialist spinal unit.

Fig. 4.11-14:
Series of diagrams of halo application.

1 cm

Other displaced cervical injuries

All other displaced cervical injuries should reduce with traction increasing incrementally every 15 minutes or so and monitored by neurological examination and lateral x-ray. As a rule of thumb, the weight should be about 2.5 kg plus 2.5 kg for each level from C1/C2 down. Displaced Jefferson fractures, hangman's fractures, odontoid fractures (types II and III), displaced subaxial fractures, and dislocations can all be treated in this fashion in the first instance. Reduction can also be maintained by traction until a definitive management program is determined.

Some authors describe the necessity for traction forces over 50 kg for facet dislocations, although usually much less weight is required. Reduction of cervical spine injuries in the presence of spinal cord injury is equally urgent.

Thoracolumbar fractures

Patients with non-displaced stable or potentially unstable thoracolumbar fractures should be nursed supine, with intensive pressure area care during this phase. Most of those with significant spinal injuries will require urethral catheterization, and **patients with complete spinal cord injuries will need physiological optimization in an intensive care unit, so as to maintain spinal cord perfusion and oxygenation**.

8 Definitive management

The definitive treatment of spinal injuries may be surgical or non-surgical. In the age of surgical subspecialization, **much of the decision making and surgical intervention should be performed in dedicated spinal surgical units**, by a team consisting of orthopedic surgeon, neurosurgeon, and, if appropriate, a spinal cord injury rehabilitation physician.

Many believe that the only indication for early surgical intervention is a deteriorating neurological situation persisting despite appropriate non-surgical management, together with a demonstrable bony or disc compressive lesion on imaging. This combination often requires an anterior vertebrectomy and decompression, a dangerous undertaking in the acute situation, especially when there is concomitant visceral trauma. Such patients must always be transferred to a specialist unit.

Unstable spinal column injuries

Unstable spinal column injuries, with or without neurological injury, will often need surgical stabilization after reduction. However, in the absence of spinal cord injury some injuries may be managed in a halo jacket or rigid orthosis. Displaced Jefferson fractures, hangman's fractures, type III odontoid fractures, and subaxial fractures may all be treated in a halo jacket for 6–8 weeks after reduction, with frequent x-ray monitoring. Such injuries should then be treated in a rigid orthosis until 3 months post injury.

Odontoid fractures–type II

Type II odontoid fractures, displaced more than 25% on original x-ray (**Fig. 4.11-15**) even after reduction, or undergoing recurrent displacement, have a high risk of proceeding to non-union and will need surgical fixation. These too should be transferred to a specialist spinal unit.

Soft-tissue subaxial cervical disruptions

Significant soft-tissue subaxial cervical disruptions, particularly after reduction of facet dislocations, will need surgical stabilization with an anterior plate system. Irreducible facet dislocations will need posterior open reduction, stabilization, and fusion. Cord compression from either bone or disc mandates an anterior approach, decompression, often including vertebrectomy, and fusion with plate stabilization.

Non-displaced and stable cervical injuries

Non-displaced and stable cervical injuries should be treated in an appropriate firm orthosis.

Patients with complete spinal cord injuries will need physiological optimization in an intensive care unit, so as to maintain spinal cord perfusion and oxygenation.

Much of the decision making and surgical intervention should be performed in dedicated spinal surgical units.

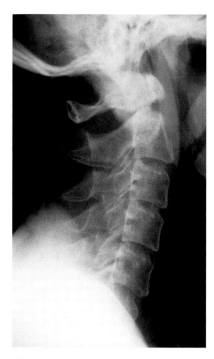

60492- D006
5-5mm
24NOV92
13:05
:355mm 6.0
9
TILT:
+9.0
R
I
G
H
T
0
Linear
PICKER INTL 1200

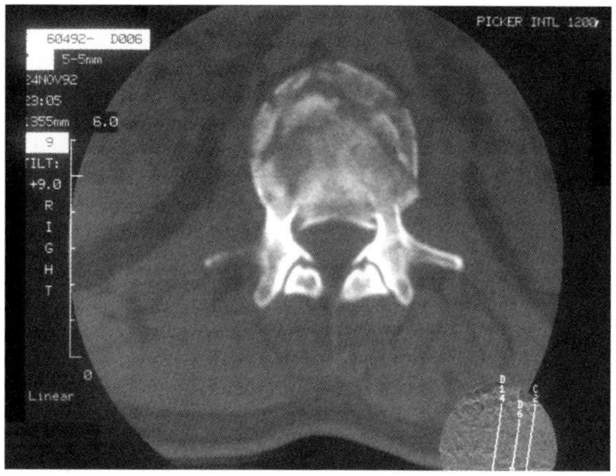

Fig. 4.11-16:
CT scan of high-grade thoracolumbar burst fracture.

stabilization (**Fig. 4.11-16**). There is some evidence that cord recovery is enhanced by such early intervention, but to minimize the mortality and morbidity the procedure should only be performed by a spinal surgeon with experience of this approach.

Fig. 4.11-15:
Displaced type II odontoid fracture.

Thoracolumbar dislocations

Thoracolumbar dislocations, with or without neurological compression, need open reduction and stabilization through a posterior approach and, with partial or complete neurological injuries where spinal shock is still present, this should be performed as soon as the patient's general condition allows.

Thoracolumbar burst fractures

Thoracolumbar burst fractures where there is partial, deteriorating, or complete neurological loss with persistent spinal shock should be considered for emergency decompression and

Unstable injuries

Unstable injuries where there is significant two-column disruption need surgical stabilization, using posterior stabilization systems.

Type A fractures in the thoracolumbar region

Type A fractures in the thoracolumbar region, with more than 50% loss of anterior body height and significant regional kyphosis, or wedging (> 30° at the thoracolumbar junction, or > 10° in lumbar spine), are best treated by posterior indirect reduction and posterior fusion (**Fig. 4.11-17**). Surgeons with experience of pedicle screw insertion in the thoracolumbar region should be able to manage most type A fractures requiring surgery using this method.

Most thoracolumbar fractures do not meet these indications and can be treated non-operatively. A TLSO (thoraco-lumbo-sacral orthosis) will aid pain control, but most stable injuries are sufficiently pain-free after the first 2 weeks not to require this. In addition, the predominant injuring force is axial compression, and external bracing will not control this.

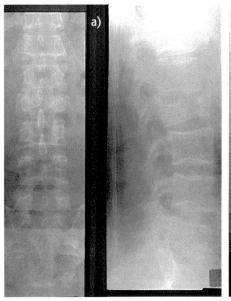
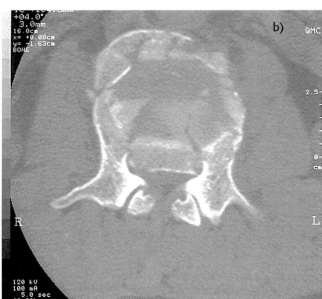
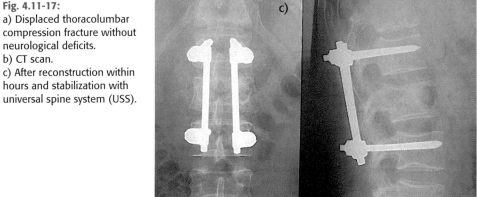

Fig. 4.11-17:
a) Displaced thoracolumbar compression fracture without neurological deficits.
b) CT scan.
c) After reconstruction within hours and stabilization with universal spine system (USS).

9 Bibliography

1. **Bracken MB, Shepard MJ, Collins WF, et al.** (1990) A randomized, controlled trial of methylprednisolone or naloxone in the treatment of acute spinal-cord injury. Results of the Second National Acute Spinal Cord Injury Study. *N Engl J Med;* 322 (20):1405–1411.

2. **White AA, Panjabe MM** (1990) *Clinical Biomechanics of the Spine.* Philadelphia: J.B. Lippincott Co.

3. **Denis F** (1984) Spinal instability as defined by the three-column spine concept in acute spinal trauma. *Clin Orthop;* (189):65–76.

4. **Jefferson G** (1920) Fracture of atlas vertebra: report of four cases, and a review of those previously recorded. *Br J Surg;* 7:407–422.

5. **Fielding JW, Hawkins RJ** (1977) Atlanto-axial rotatory subluxation. (Fixed rotatory subluxation of the atlanto-axial joint). *J Bone Joint Surg [Am];* 59 (1):37–44.

6. **Anderson L, D'Alonzo R** (1974) Fractures of the odontoid process of the axis. *J Bone Joint Surg [Am];* 56 (8):1663–1674.

7. **Levine AM, Edwards CC** (1985) The management of traumatic spondylo-listhesis of the axis. *J Bone Joint Surg [Am];* 67 (2):217–226.

8. **Magerl F, Aebi M, Gertzbein SD, et al.** (1994) A comprehensive classification of thoracic and lumbar injuries. *Europ Spine J;* 3 (4):184–201.

9. **Spiegel PG** (1996) Fracture and dislocation compendium. *J Orthop Trauma;* 10 (Suppl 1):151–153.

10. **Frankel HL, Hancock DO, Hyslop G, et al.** (1969) The value of postural reduction in the initial management of closed injuries of the spine with paraplegia and tetraplegia. *Paraplegia;* 7 (3):179–192.

Suggestions for further reading

1. **Aebi M, Thalgot JS, Webb JK** (1998) AO ASIF Principles in Spine Surgery. Berlin Heidelberg: Springer-Verlag.

2. **Tscherne H, Blauth M** (1998) *Tscherne Unfallchirurgie Wirbelsäule.* Berlin Heidelberg: Springer-Verlag.

10 Updates

Updates and additional references for this chapter are available online at:
http://www.aopublishing.org/PFxM/411.htm

5.1 Open fractures

R. Paul Clifford

1 Introduction

The term **"open" fracture indicates a communication between the fracture and the external environment** and inevitably involves injury to the soft tissues and skin near the fractured bone. Because these are frequently high-energy injuries, bone and soft-tissue damage can be severe. Such damaged and ischemic tissues, surrounded by hematoma and contaminated by bacteria, provide a poor environment for fracture and tissue healing and poor resistance to bacterial proliferation. As a result, the **risks of infection, delayed union and non-union are significantly increased** in proportion to the applied energy levels and the damage to bone and soft tissue.

2 History

A century ago, the high mortality rate following major long bone open fractures frequently left amputation as the treatment of choice to preserve life. Even by the start of World War I the mortality rate from open fractures of the femur remained over 70%. Major advances over the last 100 years have moved the focus of management of such injuries away from preservation

of life and limb to preservation of function and avoidance of complications. Nonetheless, there remains no place for complacency. In the **most severe open tibial fractures associated with vascular injury, the documented amputation rates remain in excess of 50%** [1].

3 Etiology and mechanism of injury

Open fractures characteristically tend to be caused by more severe violence than closed fractures. However, low-energy indirect torsional fractures may penetrate the skin from within, particularly where the bone lies just under the skin, unprotected by a muscular sleeve (**Fig. 5.1-1**). More severe open fractures usually occur as a result of direct high-energy trauma. The energy (E_k) dissipated at the time of injury is proportional to the mass (m) and the square of the velocity (v) according to the formula $E_k = mv^2/2$. Most high-energy open fractures seen in civilian hospitals today follow either road traffic accidents or falls from a height with the victim as a missile injured by

Open fracture indicates a communication between fracture and external environment.

Most severe open tibial fractures associated with vascular injury show documented amputation rates in excess of 50%.

Risks of infection, delayed union and non-union are high.

sudden deceleration at the time of impact. **The degree of trauma suffered is related to the impact energy** and degree of protection of the victim, accounting for the high incidence of severe open fractures of the lower legs in motorcyclists. These high-energy incidents frequently cause severe multiple injuries to the head, trunk, and limbs, whose management may take priority over the open fracture.

4 Epidemiology

The frequency of open fractures seen in individual hospitals varies according to geographic and socio-economic factors, population size, and trauma delivery systems. The incidence of open fractures in the Edinburgh Orthopaedic Trauma Unit in Scotland has been documented in detail [2]. This unit treats all fractures in a mixed urban and rural population of 750,000. Over a 75-month period between January 1988 and March 1994, 1,000 open fractures in 933 patients were reported, representing a frequency of 21.3 per hundred thousand population per year. The relative proportions of open to closed fractures for different anatomical regions is documented in **Table 5.1-1**. In the major long bones, open fractures were more common in diaphysis than in metaphysis (c.f. 15.3% diaphyseal vs 1.2% metaphyseal). The highest proportion of open major long bone diaphyseal fractures was seen in the tibia (21.6%) followed by the femur (12.1%), radius and ulna (9.3%), and humerus (5.7%). However, the virtual absence of gun shot injuries (one case) suggests these figures are unrepresentative of more violent communities elsewhere.

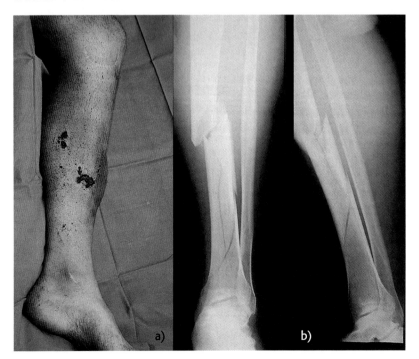

Fig. 5.1-1:
Open fracture after blunt, low-energy trauma.
a) Minor skin lacerations on medial aspect of lower leg, with rapidly developing compartment syndrome.
b) Complex fracture of tibia 42-C1.

Table 5.1-1: Relative frequencies of open fractures [2].

Location	Total fractures	Open fractures	% open fractures
Upper limb	15,406	503	3.3%
Lower limb	13,096	488	3.7%
Shoulder girdle	1,448	3	0.2%
Pelvis	942	6	0.6%
Spine	683	0	0.0%
Total	31,575	1,000	3.17%

5 Microbiology

Most open fractures are contaminated with bacteria, at or shortly after the time of injury, 60–70% showing positive wound cultures before treatment begins [3]. Fortunately, most of these bacteria are relatively innocuous skin and environmental contaminants, which rarely cause infection. However, the presence of pathogenic enteric gram negative bacilli or more virulent environmental contaminants such as *Clostridia* or *Pseudomonas* is more ominous and carries a significant risk of progression to infection. **Most commonly, infection follows contamination after arrival at hospital, with pathogenic *Staphylococcus aureus*,** *Enterococcus* or *Pseudomonas*. Small numbers of contaminating bacteria do not cause infection, but once the critical inoculum of 10^5 organisms per gram of tissue is reached, the immunological defense mechanisms become overwhelmed and the risk of infection becomes high.

6 Classification

In an attempt to document prognostic indicators and allow comparative studies, numerous classifications, based on injury severity, have been developed. Of these, the most widely used was initially described by Gustilo and Anderson in 1976 [3]. They divided open fractures into three types in ascending order of severity based on broad categories of skin and soft-tissue damage and fracture type (**Table 5.1-2**).

Table 5.1-2: Classification of open fractures [4].

Type	Description
I	• Skin wound less than 1 cm • Clean • No fracture comminution
II	• Skin wound more than 1 cm • Soft-tissue damage not extensive • No flaps or avulsions • No fracture comminution
III	• High-energy injury involving extensive soft-tissue damage • Or severe crushing injuries • Or vascular injury requiring repair • Or severe contamination including farmyard injuries • Or fracture comminution, segmental fractures or bone loss irrespective of size of skin wound

Most commonly, infection follows contamination after arrival at hospital, with pathogenic *Staphylococcus aureus*.

Gustilo and colleagues later modified the type III injuries with descriptions of three subtypes based on the degree of contamination, extent of periosteal stripping and bone exposure, and the presence of vascular injury (**Table 5.1-3**) [4] (**Fig. 5.1-2**).

This classification is relatively simple and remains a useful, if not entirely accurate, guide to prognosis. It has been validated in terms of time to union, incidence of non-union, and requirement for bone grafting [**5, 6**]. Unfortunately, its main pitfalls are an almost inevitable product of its simplicity. They relate to the high degree of inter-observer error arising from the subjective nature of the injury description and from the multiple non-exclusive variables described in each injury type.

The AO classification of soft-tissue injuries, described in **chapter 1.5**, is designed to be used in conjunction with the Müller AO Classification of fractures (**chapter 1.4**). It thus provides a very detailed classification of open fractures. Injuries to skin, muscle/tendon, and neurovascular structures are classified separately into four or five types. This enables each category to include objectively defined single variables only. When used in a large database, this classification permits more refined comparison of injury types and is thus extremely useful as a research tool. Unfortunately, its complexity makes it awkward for communication in everyday clinical practice. The same holds true for the Hannover Fracture Scale (HFS) originally described by Tscherne.

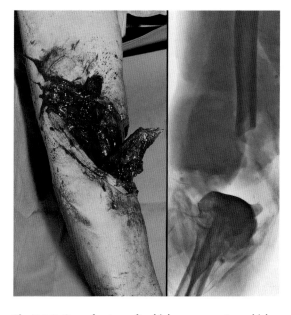

Fig. 5.1-2: Open fracture after high-energy motor vehicle accident. The right upper arm of the 57-year-old woman was entrapped, which resulted in a IIIC open humeral fracture (Müller AO Classification: 12-A3 IO4-MT4-NV4) with disruption of brachial artery and vein, neuropraxia of median and radial nerves.

Table 5.1-3: Classification of type III open fractures [4].

Type	Description
IIIA	• Adequate soft-tissue cover of bone despite extensive soft-tissue damage.
IIIB	• Extensive soft-tissue injury with periosteal stripping and bone exposure. • Major wound contamination.
IIIC	• Open fracture with arterial injury requiring repair.

7 Principles of management

The **ultimate goal in the management of the open fracture is the early return to normal function of the injured limb**. This is dependent on early wound healing with full soft-tissue recovery and fracture union with restoration of the anatomy and avoidance of complications. Infection is the single factor most likely to have a deleterious effect on outcome.

Principles of management

- Prevention of infection.
- Soft-tissue healing and bone union.
- Restoration of anatomy.
- Functional recovery.

8 Stages of care

The achievement of these goals requires a disciplined, logical, sequential management approach. This commences with good prehospital care and is followed by careful assessment and mature clinical judgement in the emergency and operating rooms. Primary surgical intervention focuses on the avoidance of infection by staged wound débridement and fracture stabilization. Secondary surgical procedures address the issues of early skin cover and soft-tissue reconstruction followed by bone reconstruction. Rehabilitation with early movement and mobilization commences as soon as possible as an integrated part of this staged management protocol.

Stages of care

- Initial assessment and accident room management.
- Primary operations
  - staged wound débridement,
  - fracture stabilization.
- Secondary operations
  - skin and soft-tissue reconstruction,
  - bone reconstruction.
- Rehabilitation.

9 Emergency room— initial assessment and management

The primary aims of assessment and management in the emergency room are:
- Resuscitation and assessment of priorities.
- Prevention of further wound contamination.
- Administration of antibiotics.
- Realignment and splintage of limb deformities.
- Clinical and radiological evaluation of individual injuries.

Management commences **at the accident site, where prehospital personnel should protect the wound with a sterile dressing.** Thereafter, to protect the wound from further bacterial contamination, the dressing should be disturbed as little as possible. Tscherne and colleagues demonstrated a four-fold reduction in infection rate by adhering to these policies [7].

In the emergency room, attention is first focused on the resuscitation of vital functions and the treatment of immediately life-threatening pathology. External hemorrhage from an open

Ultimate goal in the management of the open fracture is the early return to normal function of the injured limb.

At the accident site prehospital personnel should protect the wound with a sterile dressing.

fracture contributing to hemodynamic instability is managed by manual pressure over multiple layers of sterile dressings. Once resuscitative measures are well established and immediate threat to life has been addressed, attention can be turned to determining the history of the event and a careful clinical examination and evaluation of the whole patient.

For assessment of the injury the sterile dressing is disturbed once, at which time it is good practice to take a Polaroid photograph for future reference (**Fig. 5.1-3**). The size and depth of the wound and condition of the surrounding skin are noted. Major contaminating fragments of debris may be removed and severely soiled wounds may be lavaged with sterile fluid. Otherwise, wounds should not be probed and after redressing should remain undisturbed. The rest of the limb should be carefully examined, both proximal and, in particular, distal to the open fracture. Vascularity and circulation, neurological function, and musculotendinous continuity must all be assessed. Deformed limbs should be gently realigned and, if possible, obviously dislocated joints reduced. The limb should be splinted and x-rays taken to include the whole length of the fractured bone.

By this stage, the surgeon should be well informed about the history of the event, the overall status of the patient, the extent and basic characteristics of the open wound and surrounding skin, the extent and characteristics of the fracture, and the function of the vessels, nerves, muscles, and tendons traversing the zone of injury. Thus armed, he can formulate a provisional management. Surgery to preserve life and limb takes priority. Surgical débridement of the contaminated wound is urgent before bacterial proliferation approaches the critical inoculum, above which infection becomes highly likely. It has been suggested that

> Preoperative assessment of the wound may only be done once when taking a Polaroid photograph.

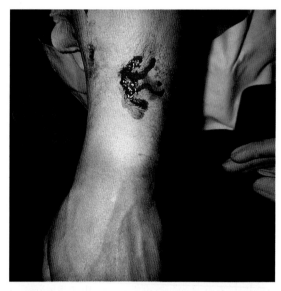
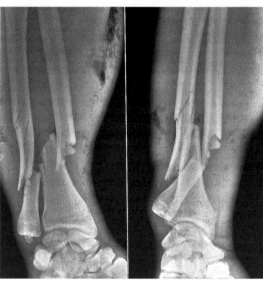

Fig. 5.1-3: Assessment of injury by Polaroid photography. Apparently minor skin lesion but ischemic hand after crush injury on distal forearm in a 30-year-old male. Associated both bone forearm fracture 22-C3.

this point is reached in six hours from the time of inoculation, but it is likely that many factors influence this, including the early administration of intravenous antibiotics.

10 Antibiotics

The choice of antibiotic is dictated by the potential bacterial contaminant. First or second-generation cephalosporins have a broad spectrum of activity and are suitable for most wounds. Major wounds, or those of the femur or pelvis at risk of fecal contamination, should have, in addition, an aminoglycoside or one of the newer betalactam penicillins. Farmyard injuries at risk of clostridial infection should be treated with high-dose penicillin. High serum antibiotic levels are achieved by intravenous administration, given as early as possible, and continued for 48 hours. **Prolonged antibiotic administration is not necessary** and risks the emergence of resistant strains of bacteria, although repeated short courses are advised as prophylaxis at the time of any subsequent surgical procedure. Antitetanus measures should be taken if necessary. Tetanus toxoid and tetanus immunoglobulin should be given if the patient has not received tetanus immunization in the previous ten years.

11 Operating room— primary operations

The aims of primary surgery are:
- Preservation of life and limb.
- Definitive injury assessment.
- Staged wound débridement.
- Fracture stabilization.

Initial priorities focus on lifesaving surgery to the trunk, pelvis, and head and on limb revascularization.

11.1 Definitive assessment

Definitive injury assessment in the operating room requires a full evaluation of the extent and degree of damage to individual anatomical structures. This is accomplished by an initial clinical re-examination of the whole limb and further x-rays as necessary. However, the assessment is not complete until the depths and extent of the wound have been surgically explored after cleansing and draping of the whole limb. **A tourniquet should be applied, but not inflated,** unless there is excessive hemorrhage. The wound should be thoroughly cleansed, including the bone ends, which, if necessary, should be delivered through the wound. Contaminating foreign material should be removed and the wound should be irrigated with large volumes of Hartman's or Ringer Lactate solution. Powered pulsed lavage (jet lavage) should be used with caution, since this may drive foreign debris deeper into the wound. It may be safer to use a gravity feed via a standard intravenous giving set.

The concept of "the zone of injury" is important (see **chapter 2.1, Fig. 2.1-3**). This delineates the true dimensions of the wound as opposed to **the skin wound, which is merely the "window" through which the true wound communicates with the exterior.** In many instances this window may be small while the underlying wound is large. This is particularly common in fractures well covered by muscle and distant from the skin, for example, the mid-shaft of the femur or humerus and the calf and posterior aspect of the tibia. Puncture

The choice of antibiotic is dictated by the potential bacterial contaminant.

A tourniquet should be applied, but not inflated.

Prolonged antibiotic administration is not necessary.

The concept of "the zone of injury" is important. The skin wound is merely the "window" through which the true wound communicates with the exterior.

Evaluation of the wound demands a detailed assessment of the true extent of the zone of injury.

wounds in these regions should never be interpreted as grade I open fractures, since significant underlying soft-tissue damage is almost inevitable. Full **evaluation of the wound demands a detailed assessment of the true extent of the zone of injury.** This usually requires enlargement of the window by surgical extension of the skin wound or occasionally another incision to create a second window. Such incisions must be carefully planned and sited. They must respect vascular territories, which may already be compromised by the injury. They must also take into account the planned position of any internal or external fixation device and the possible siting of a soft-tissue reconstruction flap. Management of these complex problems should, ideally, involve both an experienced plastic and orthopedic surgeon from the outset and be regarded as a joint venture. Following the definitive assessment of the patient and the injury, the decision can then be made to proceed with surgical débridement or, occasionally, to amputate.

ous viability can safely be left until the second look, when viability will be obvious. Damaged subcutaneous fat should be freely excised and fasciotomies performed liberally. The consequences of leaving devitalized muscle in the wound may be catastrophic even within a short time. Careful attention must thus be paid to muscle in the initial débridement. All muscle of dubious viability must be resected to pink bleeding edges, which contract when gently pinched. Intact tendon can be cleaned and re-examined at the second look. Bone ends should be scrupulously cleaned and the medullary cavity cleared of any foreign material or bone fragments. Detached, avascular bone fragments should be discarded. Major neuro-vascular structures should be preserved and repaired if necessary.

Surgical débridement remains an exacting surgical procedure and must be performed with diligence. Care must be taken to ensure complete removal of all non-viable tissues whilst at the same time preserving blood supply to the rest.

11.2 Staged surgical débridement

Surgical débridement demands meticulous excision of all dead and devitalized tissues.

Surgical débridement demands meticulous excision of all dead and devitalized tissues. It ranks as the most important single activity influencing outcome in the management of the open fracture. The cost of leaving dead, necrosing tissue in the wound is high and a **"second look" should be routinely performed after a delay of 48–72 hours.** Débridement should thus be regarded as a staged procedure.

Débridement commences at the outside working inwards. Skin which is manifestly dead and macerated should be excised. Skin of dubi-

A "second look" should be performed routinely after 48–72 hours.

Type II and type III open fractures are almost inevitably displaced and unstable. This usually dictates surgical fixation.

11.3 Fracture stabilization

The fracture in a type I injury may be treated in the same way as a comparable closed fracture. In many cases this will involve surgical fixation, but not necessarily so. The decision is based on the characteristics of the fracture and the condition of the patient rather than the complicating minor wound. The outcome in these injuries is similar to that of their closed counterparts [8].

Type II and type III open fractures are almost inevitably displaced and unstable. These characteristics usually dictate surgical fixation. The presence of a significant open wound with extensive soft-tissue damage is a major complicating factor, which increases the need for fracture stabilization. Restoration of the anatomy is one of the stated goals of management, upon which the ultimate aim of "return to normal function of the limb" depends. Restoration of length and correction of bony deformity facilitates anatomical alignment and tensioning of the soft-tissue structures, thereby reducing dead space and hematoma volume. Stability at the fracture site prevents further damage from mobile bone fragments. The inflammatory response is dampened, exudate and edema reduced, and tissue revascularization encouraged.

Furthermore, uncluttered stable fixation allows free access to the wound for soft-tissue surgical procedures and facilitates physiological mobilization of the injured limb. Overall, restoration of the anatomy and stabilization of the fracture provide the optimal environment and conditions for tissue repair and recovery. Theoretically, these factors should improve the host defense mechanisms against bacteria and reduce the risk of infections, although other variables make this difficult to confirm in clinical studies. **However, there is experimental evidence to suggest that fracture stability can be helpful in inhibiting bacterial proliferation** [9–10].

The value of stable fixation in open fractures is beyond dispute. However, the selection of the method remains contentious. Available techniques include internal fixation using plates or intramedullary nails, external fixation, or a combination of these. **The benefits of stable fixation must be balanced against the pitfalls of further damage to local blood supply and the risk of complications.** In practice, each case must be individually assessed. Factors to be considered include the anatomical site and characteristics of the fracture, the state of the surrounding skin and soft tissues, including the site and the size of the open wound, the degree of contamination, the presence of other injuries, and the overall condition of the patient.

Type I wounds need rarely influence the choice of method, which in the majority of cases can be the same as for comparable closed fractures. More serious wounds, however, may significantly affect the choice of fixation device. The general principles of anatomical reduction of joint surfaces (**chapter 2.3**) and restoration of length and alignment of diaphyseal and metaphyseal fractures (**chapter 2.2**) should be followed. The concepts and applications of absolute and relative stability should be carefully considered and adopted. The high-energy nature of these injuries, with fracture fragmentation and compromised soft tissues, renders them particularly amenable to relatively stable fixation and minimally invasive techniques. Respect for the soft tissues is paramount. Careful preoperative planning (**chapter 2.4**) is essential and should take into account the frequent need to position the implant or fixator in an unconventional site. **Implants should, wherever possible, be applied through the wound, while respecting the need to cover metal with soft tissue.** Additional, separate incisions are preferably avoided, but if absolutely necessary should be minimal and carefully sited to avoid devascularization of any intervening skin bridge. All surgical approaches, implants, and external fixators should be sited in such a way that they do not compromise further orthopedic or plastic surgical procedures.

Articular fractures should be fixed with judiciously placed screws, protected, if necessary, by an external ring fixator or occasionally a bridging transarticular external fixator.

Implants should, wherever possible, be applied through the wound, while respecting the need to cover metal with soft tissue.

There is experimental evidence to suggest that bacterial proliferation is influenced by fracture stability.

The benefits of stable fixation must be balanced against the pitfalls of further damage to local blood supply and the risk of complications.

Metaphyseal fractures can often be stabilized by a plate applied through the wound. If the wound is small or in an awkward site, the plate may be slid subcutaneously and held with percutaneous screws. Occasionally a metaphyseal fracture may be better managed by screw fixation protected by an external fixator.

Diaphyseal fractures are fixed by intramedullary nails, plates, or external fixators depending on the individual bone, the degree of periosteal stripping, and the nature of the soft-tissue sleeve.

Definitive fixation should not necessarily be regarded as a prerequisite in the initial operative intervention. It may be judicious to apply temporary stabilization using a spanning external fixator, if necessary bridging across a joint to maintain length and alignment and to revise to definitive fixation at a later date when swelling has settled and the full extent of the soft-tissue wound has been assessed and controlled. The pinless external fixator avoids penetration of the medullary cavity and is of particular value if intramedullary nailing is to be considered as the definitive fixation.

> It is not essential to achieve definitive fixation at the first intervention.

11.4 Plates

(see **chapters 3.2.2** and **3.3.2**)

Plates remain the definitive choice for fixation of open metaphyseal fractures (**Fig. 5.1-4**). They are also particularly useful in diaphyseal fractures of the forearm where the soft-tissue sleeve makes them relatively safe and where no other fixation device can provide the stability required to maintain the important anatomical relationship between radius and ulna (**Fig. 5.1-5**).

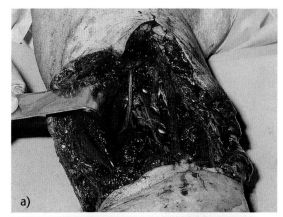
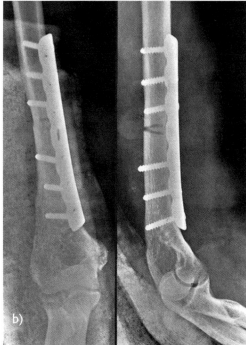

Fig. 5.1-4: Same case as **Fig. 5.1-2**:
a) After assessment of soft-tissue injuries, the humerus was osteotomized for shortening of 15 mm and then plated (LC-DCP) through the wound.
b) Postoperative x-ray with atypically located plate on ventral aspect of humerus; uneventful postoperative recovery with satisfactory function of arm and elbow.

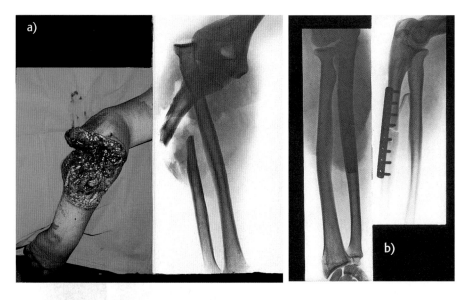

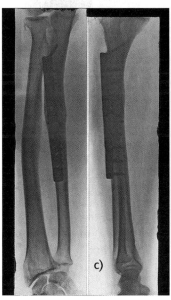

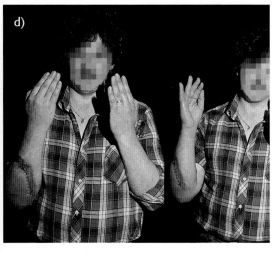

Fig. 5.1-5:
a) 29-year-old male: IIIA open Monteggia fracture of right arm, no major neurovascular deficit.
b) Emergency ORIF with 8-hole 3.5 DCP, wound débridement, and adaptation of transected muscles. Secondary skin closure.
c) 37 weeks post accident. Solid union and
d) good functional recovery with full working capacity as mason.

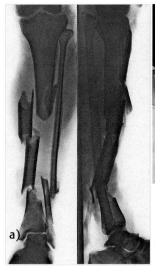
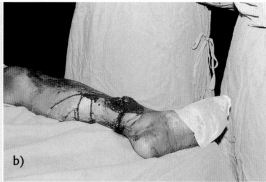
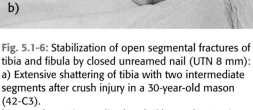
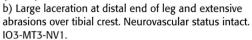

Fig. 5.1-6: Stabilization of open segmental fractures of tibia and fibula by closed unreamed nail (UTN 8 mm):
a) Extensive shattering of tibia with two intermediate segments after crush injury in a 30-year-old mason (42-C3).
b) Large laceration at distal end of leg and extensive abrasions over tibial crest. Neurovascular status intact. IO3-MT3-NV1.
c) Postoperative x-ray after stabilization of tibia with statically locked 8 mm UTN.

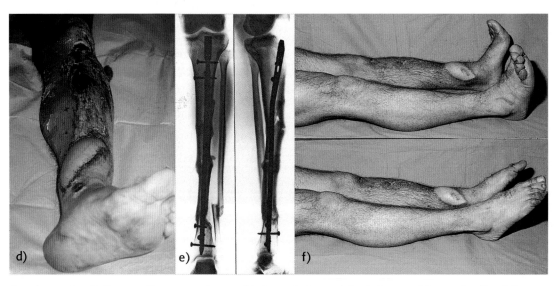

d) 36 hours after ORIF a cancellous autograft was added to the distal fracture focus while soft-tissue defect was covered by a free musculocutaneous flap.

e) Uneventful soft-tissue and fracture healing; follow-up x-rays at one year.
f) Excellent functional result, no disability.

11.5 Intramedullary nails

(see chapter 3.3.1)

Intramedullary nailing of open fractures has not been popular in the past because of the perceived concern about damage to the medullary blood supply and subsequent risk of catastrophic infection. The development of the locking nail has improved the stability of intramedullary devices and has extended the indications such that they are now the almost universal choice for the fixation of closed and type I open fractures of the femoral and tibial diaphysis and their use is becoming increasing popular in the humerus. Recently these indications have been further extended by enthusiasts to include all grades of open fractures of the femoral and tibial diaphysis. Initial results seem encouraging, with low infection rates in even type IIIb fractures [11–14].

The unreamed nail has been developed with the aim of reducing the disruption of medullary blood supply (**Fig. 5.1-6**). Experimental work demonstrating a reduction in cortical blood supply of 30%, compared to 70% after medullary reaming, suggests that these aims have been successfully achieved [15]. However, other experimental works suggest that reaming has a beneficial effect by stimulating periosteal blood flow and periosteal bone formation [16]. In clinical practice, the results in open tibial diaphyseal fractures are remarkably similar, whether the unreamed nail or the reamed nail is used, with the exception of a higher implant failure rate in the unreamed nail [17, 18].

The impressive results with intramedullary nailing in even the most severe open diaphyseal fractures should, however, be interpreted with caution. They originate from centers of excellence, where equally impressive simultaneous progress has been made in the surgical techniques of soft-tissue reconstruction. Until such facilities can be matched universally, external fixation may remain the safest option in the most severe open tibial fractures.

11.6 External fixation

(see chapter 3.3.3)

External fixation has the great advantage of providing relatively stable fracture fixation without violation of the zone of injury. **External fixators** are particularly useful when wounds and soft-tissue characteristics contraindicate direct surgical access to the fracture (**Fig. 5.1-7**). They are **usually the device of choice in severely soiled and contaminated wounds**, where metallic implants, with the risk of bacterial adherence, are best avoided. The development of ring fixators has extended the indications to include periarticular and intra-articular fractures (**Fig. 5.1-8**).

The main disadvantages of external fixators are poor patient tolerance and the significant risk of pin track infection, which is increased when the pins transfix muscle [5, 19]. Ideally, pins should be inserted outside the zone of injury in areas where the bone lies subcutaneously. External fixators are thus particularly useful in the tibia, but of less value in bones circumferentially surrounded by muscle, such as the femur and humerus. External fixation may be used as an initial, temporary method of fixation and revised at a later date. Conversion to an intramedullary nail should be performed early, since delays of over several weeks have been associated with high infection rates [20]. If such a conversion is planned from the outset, a pinless fixator may be a better option.

External fixators are the device of choice in severely soiled and contaminated wounds.

11.7 Summary

By the end of the initial operation, resuscitation should be complete and all injuries evaluated. The full extent of the open fracture should have been carefully assessed, the wound meticulously debrided and lavaged, and the fracture stabilized. Wound cultures should be taken at the end of the surgical procedure. The wound should be left open, although surgical extensions may be primarily closed, if this can be done without tension.

The initial surgical procedure is now complete, but débridement is not, since it should be considered as a staged procedure in which all but the most minor wounds are surgically re-explored within 48–72 hours. All the recesses of the wound should be fully revisited and hematoma and exudate should be removed by lavage. The state of tissues of previously dubious viability should now be obvious and further débridement performed as appropriate. If necessary,

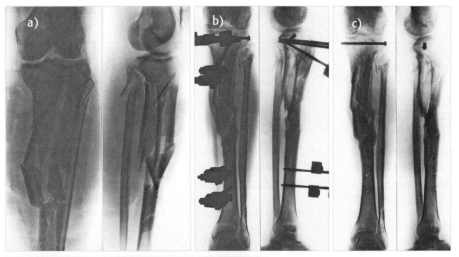

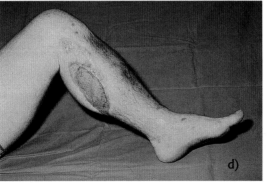

Fig. 5.1-7: Application of external fixator in a IIIa open tibial and fibular fracture involving the tibial plateau and most of the shaft.

a) Extensive multifragment fracture of proximal tibia and fibula extending into shaft in a 47-year-old male caught under a rock (41-B1/42-C2).

b) Lag screw fixation of articular fracture and unilateral external fixation, x-rays after 5 months and after removal of one bar.

c) Follow-up after removal of external fixator and well-consolidated fracture healing.

d) Clinical aspect 8 months after injury, good function, no disability.

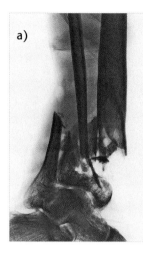

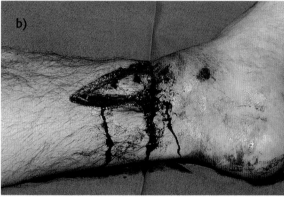

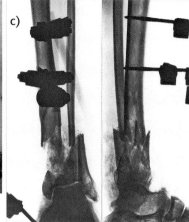

Fig. 5.1-8: Staged management of IIIa open fracture of distal end of tibia (pilon fracture):

a) 43-C2 fracture in 34-year-old male after motorcycle accident.

b) Tibial shaft penetrating on medial side of leg, neurovascular status intact (IO3-MT2-NV1).

c) As first step the wound was debrided and left open. A joint-bridging external fixator was applied.

d) With safe soft-tissue conditions the fibula was plated with 3.5 LC-DCP and the joint bridging fixator converted to a hybrid frame. Cancellous autograft for tibial defect.

e) Removal of hybrid fixator after 20 weeks. Follow-up at 2 years with good functional result and minimal posttraumatic arthrosis.

f) Clinical aspect and function of ankle joint. Soft-tissue healing occurred without any major plastic procedure.

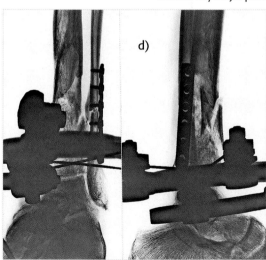

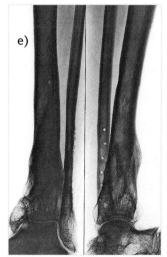

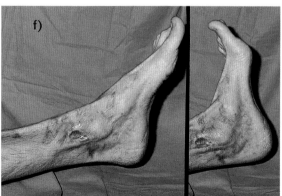

the débridement should be repeated at 48-hour intervals.

The goals of the primary surgical operations are to gain early control of the open fracture and its environment to allow progress to reconstructive procedures.

Delayed union and non-union occur more frequently after open fractures than in closed fractures.

12   Skin cover and soft-tissue reconstruction

(see **chapter 5.2**)

Skin cover and soft-tissue reconstruction procedures should be performed early. Leaving the wound open longer than 7 days increases the risk of infection. In practice, small type I wounds may be left open to granulate and heal quickly by second intention. Type II and type IIIa wounds may occasionally be closed by delayed primary suture, but care should be taken to avoid tension. A releasing incision may be considered but care should be taken to avoid ischemia of the intervening skin bridge. More frequently, these wounds are covered by split skin grafts. These are of particular value if the wound has a healthy soft-tissue floor but can occasionally be used to provide short-term cover of exposed periosteum. Meshing the skin reduces the risk of the graft being lifted off by hematoma and exudate and minimises the area of donor skin. By definition, type IIIb wounds leave bone exposed and usually require the transfer of soft tissues as well as skin to reconstruct the defect. Local fasciocutaneous flaps remain useful when the skin wound is relatively small and if the skin adjacent to the wound is in good condition. Muscle flaps have the great advantage of introducing a rich local blood supply to the wound and underlying damaged

Early fracture stabilization and soft-tissue reconstruction promote early movement.

bone. They can be turned as a composite myocutaneous flap including skin, but more usually as a muscle only flap, which is then covered by split skin graft. Large wounds and those unsuitable for a local flap are best covered by a free flap (**chapter 5.2**).

13   Bone reconstruction

Delayed union and non-union occur more frequently after open fractures than in closed fractures and in proportion to the severity of injury. In the more severe cases, particularly those with circumferential bone loss, non-union can be predicted. Surgical intervention to reconstruct bone defects and stimulate fracture healing should thus be performed relatively early. This may be combined with soft-tissue reconstruction or, more frequently, be delayed until after the soft tissues have healed. In most instances, a cancellous bone graft is used, but major segmental defects, in particular those greater than 6 cm, may require a free fibular graft, a free composite graft, or the use of bone transport techniques. Depending on the method used, any temporary fracture fixation may be revised at this time.

14   Rehabilitation

If the goals of "return to normal function" are to be achieved, the management of these injuries must not be regarded as a surgical exercise only. **The great benefit of an aggressive surgical approach involving early fracture stabilization and early tissue reconstruction is that joint and soft-tissue immobilization is avoided and early movement facilitated.** These advantages should be exploited by the patient and rehabilitation team and goals should be set to maximize the potential benefits. Nowhere is the long held concept of the AO "Life is movement: Movement is life" so important.

15 Pitfalls and complications

The management of severe open fractures is time-consuming and difficult. It involves staged, often technically demanding surgical procedures, the timing of which is crucial and requires close cooperation between the orthopedic surgeon and the plastic surgeon. Basic principles must be carefully followed, but ingenuity is required to deal with the complexities of each individual case. Experience, technical skill, and significant resources are required and this often means transferring the patient to a specialist center where these are freely available. The possible pitfalls along the way are numerous. **Infection remains the major risk and almost inevitably follows poor surgical technique, inadequate débridement, or a delay in achieving skin cover.** The risk of compartment syndrome is high and fasciotomies must be performed liberally. Inadequate or delayed soft-tissue and bone reconstruction will be followed by delayed or non-union. Prolonged immobilization and lack of appropriate rehabilitation result in poor function despite successful soft tissue and fracture healing.

16 Special situations

16.1 Vascular injuries

Open fractures associated with major vessel disruption are classified as type Gustillo IIIc by definition. They are frequently associated with devastating damage to bone, soft tissues, and neurological structures. Despite strict adherence to the principles and techniques already described, the outcome is disappointing with reported overall amputation rates in excess of 40% [21]. Type IIIc open fractures of the tibia carry a particularly poor prognosis, with amputation rates of over 50%, even if treated in the best of hands [1]. These injuries require extremely careful assessment. The decision on salvage or to primary amputation depends on sensible, rational, and mature judgement. **To persist with futile attempts at salvage in a situation clearly doomed to failure is ill-conceived.** It commits the patient to a long-term program of painful and psychologically distressing surgery and rehabilitation, only to end up with amputation (**Fig. 5.1-9**). The problem lies in determining which limbs are salvageable and which are better primarily amputated. Several authors have attempted to address this issue [22–25]. In tibial injuries the consensus of opinion is that disruption of the posterior tibial nerve with an insensitive sole of the foot or severe crush injury with a warm ischemia time of over six hours are absolute indications for primary amputation. Further relative indications include severe associated polytrauma or severe ipsilateral foot trauma with an anticipated protracted course to obtain soft-tissue cover and tibial fracture healing (**chapter 5.2**).

The management of severe open fractures is time-consuming and difficult.

Futile attempts at salvage in situations doomed to failure are ill-conceived.

Infection remains the major risk and follows poor surgical technique, inadequate débridement, or delay in skin cover.

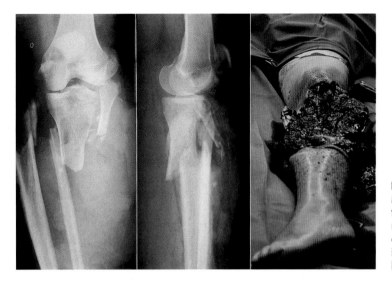

Fig. 5.1-9:
Mangled lower leg in a 19-year-old female polytraumatized after motorcycle accident. No circulation or sensory-motoractivity distal to injury (IO5-MT5-NV5). Situation before amputation.

16.2   Gunshot injuries

In cases amenable to attempted salvage, urgent revascularization is the immediate goal. In the lower limbs angiography is only necessary in situations where the level of vascular injury is unclear. Whenever possible, this should be performed on the operating table to avoid wasting valuable time in the angiography suite [21]. Rapid fracture fixation prior to the vascular repair provides protection to the anastomosis. The method of fixation is less important than the time needed to achieve it. Temporary vascular intraluminal shunts may provide valuable extra time. Fasciotomy is mandatory in anticipation of reperfusion swelling. Even in these carefully considered situations, secondary tibial amputation rates approach 50% and the final functional outcome in salvaged limbs is often disappointing.

As with blunt injuries, the severity of damage resulting from a gunshot injury is related to the amount of energy dissipated at the time of impact ($mv^2/2$). High velocity rifles (muzzle velocity > 600 m/sec) and close-range shotguns may cause devastating injuries because of the high energy of the impact, the secondary cavitation produced, and the secondary missile effects of shattered bone fragments (**Fig. 5.1-10**). Fortunately, most gunshot wounds encountered in civilian practice are caused by low velocity handguns (< 500 m/sec) and are less severe unless neuro-vascular structures are damaged. Cavitation is not significant and although bone fragmentation may be considerable, the secondary missile effects are minimal and bone fragments are rarely stripped off their soft-tissue attachments and blood supply.

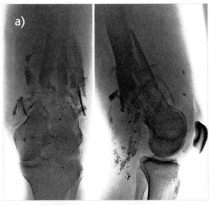

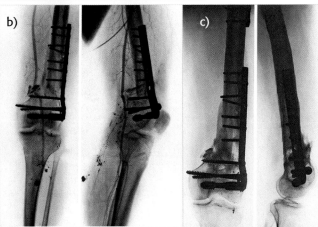

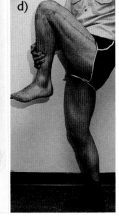

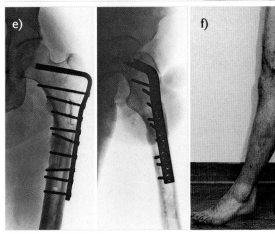

Fig. 5.1-10: Rifle injury to distal femur in 40-year-old male, disruption of popliteal artery and vein.
a) Close-range rifle injury shattering distal femur.
b) Final fixation, accepting 25 mm shortening with arteriogram showing good distal outflow following 3-stage procedure: i) provisional fixation, ii) vascular repair, iii) completion of fixation.
c) Distal femoral healing at one year.
d) With good recovery of knee function patient requested femoral lengthening.
e) Follow-up x-ray one year later.
f) Final length with full return to employment as a laborer.

High velocity weapons and close-range shotguns produce severely contaminated type III open fractures which should be surgically managed according to the principles and techniques already outlined for high-energy blunt injuries. Low velocity weapons may produce significant fracture comminution, but since soft-tissue attachments are not disrupted, these fractures behave in a relatively benign way. Soft-tissue wounds are not severe and skin wounds are small. Widespread experience in violent communities has shown that these wounds can be managed by minor débridement and virtually ignored in relation to the fracture, which should be treated on its individual merits. However, careful neurovascular assessment is essential and caution should be employed in the case of the tibia and in close-range injuries. Bullets lodged in joints should be removed to avoid lead arthropathy and systemic lead poisoning.

17 Summary

An open fracture is defined as one which communicates with the surrounding external environment. Open fractures represent approximately 3% of all limb fractures and most frequently occur as a result of high-energy trauma. Co-existing multiple injuries are common. The severity of injury can be classified and is the most important factor affecting outcome. The ultimate goal is the early return of normal function of the limb and is dependent on the adherence to the basic principles of prevention of infection, early soft-tissue and fracture healing, restoration of the anatomy, and functional recovery. Management protocols should follow the sequential steps of careful initial assessment, staged meticulous wound débridement, fracture stabilization, soft-tissue and bone reconstruction, and rehabilitation. The surgical techniques are demanding and are dependent on the availability of appropriate resources, including orthopedic, plastic, and microvascular surgical expertise. The possible pitfalls are many and may lead to disastrous complications. However, in the majority of cases these pitfalls can be avoided by careful attention to detail and the application of rational and mature clinical judgement.

18 Bibliography

1. **Lange RH, Bach AW, Hansen ST, Jr., et al.** (1985) Open tibial fractures with associated vascular injuries: prognosis for limb salvage. *J Trauma*; 25 (3):203–208.
2. **Court-Brown CM, Brewster N** (1996) Epidemiology of Open Fractures. In: Court-Brown CM, McQueen MM, Quaba AA, editors. *Management of Open Fractures.* London: Martin Dunitz: 25–35.
3. **Gustilo RB, Anderson JT** (1976) Prevention of infection in the treatment of one thousand and twenty-five open fractures of long bones: retrospective and prospective analyses. *J Bone Joint Surg [Am]*; 58 (4):453–458.
4. **Gustilo RB, Mendoza RM, Williams DN** (1984) Problems in the management of type III (severe) open fractures: a new classification of type III open fractures. *J Trauma*; 24 (8):742–746.
5. **Court-Brown CM, Wheelwright EF, Christie J, et al.** (1990) External fixation for type III open tibial fractures. *J Bone Joint Surg [Br]*; 72 (5):801–804.

6. **Court-Brown CM, McQueen MM, Quaba AA, et al.** (1991) Locked intramedullary nailing of open tibial fractures. *J Bone Joint Surg [Br];* 73 (6):959–964.

7. **Tscherne H, Oestern HJ, Sturm J** (1983) Osteosynthesis of major fractures in polytrauma. *World J Surg;* 7 (1):80–87.

8. **Court-Brown CM, Christie J, McQueen MM** (1990) Closed intramedullary tibial nailing. Its use in closed and type I open fractures. *J Bone Joint Surg [Br];* 72 (4):605–611.

9. **Rittmann WW, Perren SM** (1974) *Cortical Bone Healing After Internal Fixation and Infection.* Berlin Heidelberg New York: Springer-Verlag.

10. **Worlock P, Slack R, Harvey L, et al.** (1994) The prevention of infection in open fractures: an experimental study of the effect of fracture stability. *Injury;* 25 (1):31–38.

11. **Lhowe DW, Hansen ST** (1988) Immediate nailing of open fractures of the femoral shaft. *J Bone Joint Surg [Am];* 70 (6):812–820.

12. **Brumback RJ, Ellison PS, Jr., Poka A, et al.** (1989) Intramedullary nailing of open fractures of the femoral shaft. *J Bone Joint Surg [Am];* 71 (9):1324–1331.

13. **Rütter JE, de Vries LS, van der Werken C** (1994) Intramedullary nailing of open femoral shaft fractures. *Injury;* 25 (7):419–422.

14. **Court-Brown CM, Keating JF, McQueen MM** (1992) Infection after intramedullary nailing of the tibia. Incidence and protocol for management. *J Bone Joint Surg [Br];* 74 (5):770–774.

15. **Klein MP, Rahn BA, Frigg R, et al.** (1990) Reaming versus non-reaming in medullary nailing: interference with cortical circulation of the canine tibia. *Arch Orthop Trauma Surg;* 109 (6):314–316.

16. **Reichert IL, McCarthy ID, Hughes SP** (1995) The acute vascular response to intramedullary reaming. Microsphere estimation of blood flow in the intact ovine tibia. *J Bone Joint Surg [Br];* 77 (3):490–493.

17. **Sanders R, Jersinovich I, Anglen J, et al.** (1994) The Treatment of open tibial shaft fracture using an interlocked intramedullary nail without reaming. *J Orthop Trauma;* 8 (6):504–510.

18. **Keating JF, O'Brien P, Blachut P, et al.** (1995) Interlocking intramedullary nailing of open fractures of the tibia: a prospective randomised comparison of reamed and unreamed nails. *Bone Joint Surgery [Br];* 77 (Suppl 1):73.

19. **Clifford RP, Lyons TJ, Webb JK** (1987) Complications of external fixation of open fractures of the tibia. *Injury;* 18 (3):174–176.

20. **Blachut PA, Meek RN, O'Brien PJ** (1990) External fixation and delayed intramedullary nailing of open fractures of the tibial shaft. A sequential protocol. *J Bone Joint Surg [Am];* 72 (5):729–735.

21. **Seligson D, Ostermann PA, Henry SL, et al.** (1994) The management of open fractures associated with arterial injury requiring vascular repair. *J Trauma;* 37 (6):938–940.

22. **Gregory RT, Gould RJ, Peclet M, et al.**
(1985) The mangled extremity syndrome
(M.E.S.): a severity grading system for
multisystem injury of the extremity.
J Trauma; 25 (12):1147–1150.

23. **Howe HR, Jr., Poole GV, Jr., Hansen KJ,
et al.** (1987) Salvage of lower extremities
following combined orthopedic and
vascular trauma. A predictive salvage
index. *Am Surg;* 53 (4):205–208.

24. **Johansen K, Daines M, Howey T,
et al.** (1990) Objective criteria accurately
predict amputation following lower
extremity trauma. *J Trauma;*
30 (5):568–572; discussion 572–563.

25. **Russell WL, Sailors DM, Whittle TB,
et al.** (1991) Limb salvage versus
traumatic amputation. A decision based
on a seven-part predictive index.
Ann Surg; 213 (5):473–480;
discussion 480–471.

19 Updates

Updates and additional references for this chapter
are available online at:
http://www.aopublishing.org/PFxM/51.htm

5.2 Principles of management of soft-tissue loss

Alain C. Masquelet

1 Introduction

Over the last two decades, considerable advances have taken place in the management of high-energy extremity trauma. Several factors have contributed to this evolution:

- The increasing incidence of severe injuries.
- The concentration of clinical experience in trauma centers.
- The improvement in stabilization techniques and materials.
- And, most importantly, the enormous advances in the development of procedures for repairing soft-tissue defects.

Until recently, the fracture was seen as the dominant element of these injuries, probably because trauma and orthopedic training was, by tradition, centered on the care of bone and joint injuries.

Now, however, **injury to the soft tissues has been accepted by the orthopedic and trauma surgeon as being the most important component of high-energy trauma**, often dictating the initial, and sometimes the definitive, management of the injured extremity [1, 2].

This awareness of the importance of the soft-tissue injury to the final fate of the severely traumatized extremity has raised a series of theoretical and practical questions which impinge on the responsibilities of orthopedic and trauma surgeons.

Why, when, how? Who should close the wound?
What should be done in the emergency situation?
When should the soft tissue be repaired?
What procedures are available to perform the repair?
Who should perform the soft-tissue repair?

Crucial questions have emerged about the assessment of the lesion, the proposed classification schemes, the predictive indices, the stabilization of the fracture, and the management of a large initial bone defect. Definitive answers to these questions should promote an optimal combination of techniques for soft-tissue management and bone reconstruction.

Injury to the soft tissues is the most important component of high-energy trauma.

Since every injury is unique, it is difficult to devise any sort of standard decision-making algorithm.

A soft-tissue defect is a bowl, with the various layers as its walls and the exposed deep structures as its base.

The envelope is composed of the skin, subcutaneous tissue, and deep fascia.

Granulation tissue is at once the best thing and the worst thing.

Repair of the envelope is essential for fracture healing and restoration of active motion.

Nonetheless, the overwhelming variety of the lesions makes it **difficult to devise any sort of standard decision-making algorithm, since every injury is unique and requires its own specific solution [2, 3].**

Therefore, we are going to present only those principles which are valid for the majority of the cases.

The redefinition, in the last two decades, of the blood supply to the skin and muscles, with its clinical applications to wound coverage by the use of muscle or skin flaps, has revolutionized the treatment of complex musculoskeletal trauma.

2 Why close the wound?

This question may seem ridiculous, but we should first be absolutely clear about the necessity to repair soft-tissue defects, based on a correct concept of soft tissues and soft-tissue defects.

The soft tissues comprise several layers and components, including skin, subcutaneous tissue, fascia, muscle, periosteum, tendon units, and neurovascular bundles. **The envelope, which is of paramount importance, is composed of the skin, subcutaneous tissue, and deep fascia.**

Looking at the locomotor apparatus, the muscles, tendons, nerves, and vessels represent the motor "engine" which, in turn, drives the frame, constituted by the bones and joints. The closing of a wound, i.e., **the repair of the envelope, is essential for healing of the fracture and restoration of active motion,** implying healthy joints and functional musculotendinous and nerve units [1, 4, 5].

The two main possibilities for treating a soft-tissue defect are promotion of spontaneous healing and surgical procedures. The dilemma

is how to choose the optimal solution. This requires a good understanding of how soft tissues heal. The attitude of the surgeon is governed by assessment of the defect, the possibilities of a spontaneous healing, and the availability of surgical procedures for tissue repair. This assessment is crucial; it comprises two questions:

1) Which tissue is involved in the defect?
2) What deep structure is exposed?

If a soft-tissue defect is seen as a bowl, the various layers are its walls and the exposed deep structure its base. The possibility of spontaneous repair of the defect by ingrowth of granulation tissue, which implies coverage of the deep structure, should be assessed as follows:

a) Are the surrounding tissues (walls of the bowl) well enough vascularized to generate granulation?
b) Is the exposed structure (bottom of the bowl) likely to produce granulation?
c) And—an essential question—is it, in fact, desirable for this deep structure to be covered by granulation.

It is important to understand that in this situation **granulation tissue is at once the best thing and the worst thing;** the best because it means a good capacity for the tissue to repair spontaneously by fibroblastic proliferation, and the worst because such tissue is always inflammatory and infected, and the healing leads to fibrous tissue. Thus, repair of the defect by granulation tissue implies two risks: an immediate risk of infection of the deep structure and, in the longer term, a retractile scar impeding the normal excursion of the underlying mobile structures.

One can ask what kind of tissue can repair by granulation:

- Subcutaneous tissue: This is composed of grease and is poorly vascularized, especially when it is thick. This, when exposed, produces poor granulation and tends to evolve into an eschar. Most of the time it proves preferable, after a short period, to excise the layer of grease in order to apply a split-thickness skin graft on well-vascularized fascia or muscles.
- Fascia: Fascia on its superficial aspect is well vascularized by a fine areolar tissue which granulates very well. However, in a degloving injury produced by shear forces, this layer, with its blood supply, is destroyed and is no longer suitable for granulation or for accepting a graft. Excision is therefore indicated.
- Muscles: Muscular bellies are well vascularized and certainly the best tissue at providing a plane of granulation to be covered by skin graft.
- Tendons: Tendons are normally covered with a thin, well-vascularized tissue (e.g., the extensor tendons on the dorsum of the hand). This tissue has both protective and vascular roles and provides a good bed for applying a skin graft or producing granulation. However, fibrous scar tissue or adhesion to the skin graft can restrict tendon excursion. For that reason, tendons should be covered by flaps. A fasciocutaneous flap is preferable to a muscle flap, since its deep aspect provides a gliding surface over the course of the tendons.

2.1 Nerves and vessels

Nerves cannot remain exposed for long without definitive damage to their blood supply, and should therefore be quickly covered by a flap. On the other hand, a vascular bundle, comprising artery, venae comitantes, and a cuff of surrounding vascularized tissue, can remain exposed since the protective tissue provides good granulation. However, any vein graft to restore the continuity of the interrupted vascular axis should be covered in some way by a surgical procedure.

Nerves cannot remain exposed for long without definitive damage to their blood supply.

2.2 Bone and joints

High-energy trauma often implies exposure of the skeletal frame. **An exposed joint must be covered quickly to avoid infection.** Fasciocutaneous flaps are preferable. They provide a supple tissue which is likely to preserve the motion of the joint, especially at the upper extremity. An exposed long bone requires precise assessment. If the vascularized periosteum is intact, without underlying fracture, as happens in a degloving injury, granulation tissue will provide excellent coverage. However, granulation tissue does not proliferate on denuded cortical bone unless the area exposed is quite small, when the defect is repaired from the surrounding tissues.

If there is a fracture, the problem is quite different and repair of soft-tissue defect by granulation is inappropriate. Granulation tissue is inflammatory and contaminated and leads to infection of the medullary canal through the fracture site [5]. One should remember that uninterrupted cortical bone, even without periosteum, can remain uncovered for a long time without being infected, unless the medullary

An exposed joint must be covered quickly to avoid infection.

canal is exposed. When it is, infection is very swiftly acquired, so an open fracture should be rapidly covered using a surgical procedure, while a segment of healthy bone, with intact periosteum, can safely await coverage with granulation tissue.

It follows from these considerations that **assessment of the tissue defect is crucial in selecting the repair procedure.** Numerous factors should be taken into account, including the size of the defect, the nature of the surrounding tissues, their viability, the severity of any infection, the nature of the structure exposed, and the evaluation of how spontaneous repair of the defects might turn out. Successful wound closure implies removal of necrotic tissue, control of any infection, and the assurance of a good blood supply. Once decided, the management of tissue granulation is both technically demanding and time-consuming. Alternate dressings with pro-inflammatory and anti-inflammatory products are mandatory. Recent studies have confirmed the possibilities of using vacuum-assisted closure [6]. There is considerable evidence that this principle works! There should be strict immobilization of the bone and joint frame to promote the granulation process, although trophicity and stiffness are often the price to be paid. **Ultimately, in the majority of cases, repair of a soft-tissue defect will be quickly obtained by a surgical procedure, using a flap.**

Assessment of the tissue defect is crucial in selecting the repair procedure.

The urge to classify is inherent in the human spirit.

Ultimately, the repair of any soft-tissue defect is best obtained surgically.

3 The problem of the classification of the lesions[1] [2, 3, 7–9]

The urge to classify is inherent in the human spirit. It facilitates the transmission of the knowledge and experience and it provides a basis for determining the treatment and estimating the prognosis. Moreover, it constitutes a tool for comparison of results. Despite many attempts over the years, progress in this field has, for several reasons, been disappointing. Some classifications of open fractures do not take account of the severity of multiple lesions of the various soft-tissue components. The schemes of Cauchoix and Duparc [7] refer only to the external envelope without considering the deep lesions. Gustilo and Anderson [8] include the possibility of adequate bone coverage but do not detail the injuries to the soft tissues.

More recent attempts have sought to address in more detail the assessment of the soft-tissue injury. Tscherne's classification [9] refers to the overall severity of the soft-tissue lesion, whereas the AO scheme [9] seems to be the most accomplished attempt so far to evaluate soft-tissue injuries in specific terms. Each component of the soft-tissue envelope is graded separately on a scale, including the skin, muscles, tendons, and the neurovascular bundles. However, the progressive complexity of these classifications serves only to confirm that each major injury

---

[1] Editors' note: We feel that the views expressed in this chapter are most valid for the more experienced trauma surgeon. For an alternative approach please see **chapter 1.5**.

has its own specificity and that **the initial major task for the surgeon is not so much to classify the injury but to describe as well as possible all of its components,** bone and soft tissue alike, without forgetting the periosteum. Fitting this description into a classification should be, in our opinion, a secondary task to facilitate computer entry or other documentation. The difficulty with classification is bound up with the subjectivity of the assessment and in this context a recent study [10] has pointed to poor interobserver reliability between trauma or orthopedic surgeons, despite their expertise. Moreover, the assessment of, in particular, soft-tissue lesions requires continual re-evaluation. The initial assessment is seldom sufficient because, in complex trauma, it is impossible to define the lesions before the débridement has revealed their extent. Therefore, the initial energy of the trauma, the various degrees of damage to each tissue component, and successive débridements all combine to constitute the personality of the injury, which is more that the sum of its component lesions [2]. This personality, in keeping with the definition of the word, is, of necessity, unique and is consequently difficult to fit in to a system of classification, especially at the outset.

4 The assessment of the patient and the problem of an early amputation
[11, 12]

In complex injuries, one should determine whether limb salvage is possible and desirable. Certain very severe lesions must be specifically assessed and accurately documented,

such as the loss of sensitivity of the weight-bearing area of the foot or the possible existence of a compartment syndrome. **An open fracture, however severe, does not exclude a compartment syndrome in a deep or localized compartment** which has not been laid open by the initial trauma.

The general status of the patient is assessed: the presence of shock or significant blood loss will influence the viability of the soft tissues. Any underlying medical problems, diabetes, neurological disorders, or peripheral vascular disease should be taken into account before undertaking reconstruction. The challenging problem is that the treatment should be precisely appropriate for the individual patient, following a rigorous analysis; this demands great experience on the part of the surgeon.

Sometimes in extremely severe crushing trauma, bone and soft-tissue reconstruction is obviously not feasible. In some other difficult situations, the physician estimates that salvage is possible, but not desirable for the patient because the final functional outcome will be very poor. This usually happens in the elderly or in patients with a large nerve defect involving the posterior tibial nerve, associated with considerable loss of muscle.

Generally speaking, in the upper limb, there is no indication for amputation when reconstruction is feasible. Any function of the upper limb, however poor, is always preferable to a prosthesis. The dilemmas of amputation largely concern the lower extremity, since a well-fitted prosthesis below the knee should be seen as an excellent alternative option [12]. On the other hand, amputation at the level of the thigh should only be considered when the salvage is impossible. Nonetheless, we think that even where limb salvage is possible, though perhaps

The initial major task for the surgeon is to describe as well as possible all the components of the injury.

An open fracture does not exclude a deep compartment syndrome.

In complex injuries, one should determine whether limb salvage is possible and desirable.

not desirable, amputation should, as a rule, not be performed in the emergency situation. It must be discussed with the patient at the first opportunity, before setting out on the complex prolonged and hazardous path of reconstruction. **In any event, an amputation, immediate or secondary, must imply the possibility of using the sacrificed part for vascularized or conventional transplants of tendon, bone, skin or muscle flap, nerve graft,** etc.

From a practical point of view, predictive **indices to identify high-energy extremity injuries which are beyond salvage are no substitute for clinical judgement, since every case is specific.** The problems of predictive indices are similar to the problems of classification [2, 13]. An important decision such as an amputation cannot be taken solely on the basis of a numbered scale. The only two elements which must be consistently and accurately assessed in decision making are the posterior tibial nerve deficit, providing sensibility to the plantar aspect of the foot, and the degree of muscle damage. These two factors correlate best with the outcome in terms of initial healing and ultimate function.

5   Bone stabilization

Bone stabilization cannot be considered separately from soft-tissue reconstruction procedures, even if the latter are not to be performed immediately. Internal fixation, whether by intramedullary nail or screws and plates, will, after the débridement, require either a viable soft-tissue envelope or immediate coverage. If wound closure is not possible without using a flap, coverage and fixation should be undertaken in the same operation as this will ensure an excellent and definitive débridment and the certitude that the surgical procedure employed will be viable [3].

It is of paramount importance to understand that there is a high risk of infection in leaving any fracture exposed after it has been stabilized by an internal fixation procedure, because this makes it difficult to carry out repeated débridement and cleaning of the fracture site.

In most situations, plating is recognized as inappropriate because it further damages the periosteum, and the additional volume of material makes closure more difficult. Intramedullary nailing combined with immediate wound closure now represents a widely accepted protocol in open fractures. But if the surgeon decides not to close the wound immediately because of infection, uncertain quality of débridement, or lack of expertise in flap procedures, he should apply an external fixator. This represents a safe, reliable, and reasonable solution which will provide effective stabilization of the fracture with easy access to the soft tissues.

The unilateral frame is generally preferred to the circular frame which is difficult to apply in the emergency situation and makes access to surrounding tissue difficult.

The conditions for the use of an external device are as follows (see **chapter 3.3.3**):

- Emergency placement should be easy and quick.
- Pins and frame should not obstruct access to the envelope. In the leg, medial and lateral aspects should be kept free to allow mobilization of flaps from the posterior compartment.
- The frame must be easily loosened to facilitate repeated débridement and the cleaning of bone extremities.

Placement of the pins of the fixator must not impede the rotation of flaps, so the surgeons should calculate the main possibilities of coverage before placement of the pins [14]. This consideration must be strongly emphasized during specialist training and during the integration of multispecialist teams.

Fixation of the fibula considerably improves the rigidity of the skeletal frame and contributes to the stability of the soft-tissue envelope. In our opinion, a segmental fracture of the fibula should always be stabilized at both levels.

6 Emergency management

After initial assessment, which must continually be reviewed, the goal of treatment is to prevent infection, to restore, if needed, the blood supply to the extremity, and to preserve function. The main steps of the surgical management are:

- Débridement
- Vascular repair
- Bone stabilization
- Wound closure

6.1 Débridement

This stage is of crucial importance to obtain a clean wound. The principle is to evacuate the hematoma and to excise all non-viable tissue. Even in stage I and II of Cauchoix classification, the skin wound should be widely extended to permit exploration of the deep-tissue planes

and the removal of non-viable muscle segments.

The current trend is to be less aggressive in skin excision and more aggressive in excising non-viable deep tissue [2].

Initial excision can be done under a tourniquet which should then be deflated for the more detailed final stages. Extensive fasciotomies should be performed prophylactically, to prevent compartment syndrome.

Cleaning of the bone ends is essential to prevent medullary infection. A large completely detached bone fragment should not be routinely discarded. If the wound is not obviously and massively infected, it is worth keeping the fragment and fixing it by a minimal internal fixation, to improve the reduction and the stability of the fracture. Nonetheless, we emphasize that, if this is to be done, immediate wound closure must be possible and this is not always the case.

It is acknowledged that irrigation lowers the risk of infection. However, we do not advocate pulsatile irrigation techniques. These may provoke additional trauma to soft tissue and instead of removing deeper particulate foreign matter, may drive it further in.

6.2 Revascularization

If there has been **prolonged ischemia it is advisable to revascularize the extremity as soon as possible.** Before stabilization of the bone, a temporary shunt is employed to restore continuity of the main vascular axis and to supply the distal extremity. Then, after stabilization of the skeleton, vascular repair by a graft is usually carried out.

In external fixation pin placement is crucial for later reconstructive procedures.

Be less aggressive in skin excision and more aggressive in excising non-viable deep tissue.

Fixation of the fibula considerably improves the rigidity of the skeletal frame.

Irrigation lowers the risk of infection, but pulsatile irrigation is not advocated.

Revascularization should be undertaken as soon as possible.

6.3 Bone stabilization

To restate the principles:

- If closure is delayed, an external device is mandatory. Fixation of the fibula in severe trauma to the lower leg improves the stability of the skeletal frame and of the soft-tissue envelope.
- In case of circumferential bone loss a cement spacer or antibiotic-impregnated PMMA beads may be placed into the bone defect at the same time as closure. Major bone reconstruction is not advocated as an emergency procedure. The cement spacer will preserve space for secondary reconstruction [1, 3]. Moreover, the bone membrane induced by the foreign body promotes corticalization of a later cancellous bone autograft [3].

6.4 Wound closure

When should it be done?

After thorough débridement, followed by vascular repair and bone stabilization, the problem is to get the wound closed. If vital structures, such as nerve and vascular grafts, have not been left exposed and the bone was stabilized by an external fixator, coverage can be delayed for 3–5 days. Godina [15] has shown that coverage within 72 hours is effective and safe and decreases infection rates. Coverage should be done in the acute phase— the first 5 days according to Byrd et al. [16] and the first 17 days according to Yaremchuk et al. [17]. Most authors [4, 14, 18, 19] agree that **coverage is required before the end of the first week.**

Wound coverage should be done before the end of the first week.

The routine of performing immediate coverage in all cases [20] is not, in our opinion, a safe approach because of the difficulty and uncertainty of evaluating the tissue viability in the emergency situation.

6.5 Schematically, one can consider several situations

Skin closure is achieved at the outset. Indeed, this is the ideal solution, which corresponds to stages I and II of most classifications.

Skin closure is not possible, but coverage of the vital underlying structures, tendons, neurovascular bundles, and fracture remains feasible by suturing vascularized subcutaneous tissue or muscle to the edges of the surrounding skin without using a flap.

Some components remain exposed but they are covered with some well-vascularized tissue. Granulation tissue will proliferate, but one should try to foresee the final functional outcome in order to estimate whether or not this process is desirable. As an example, intact bone and tendons on the dorsum of the foot can, in functional terms, tolerate coverage by granulation tissue.

Wound closure is impossible to do as a primary procedure. At the end of the débridement and stabilization, the fracture site remains exposed. Clinical assessment of tissue viability of the wound is crucial in determining which kind of surgical procedure is needed to cover it. Here again, different scenarios must be considered:

- The débridement performed is judged as definitive: the remaining tissues are obviously healthy, well supplied, and non-infected, and a local rotational pedicle flap is feasible. Coverage must to be done immediately **because rotating a local flap will be more difficult a few days later, due to edema and the development of an inflammatory reaction** which can impair the mobilization of the flap and its arc of rotation. When conditions for coverage are ideal but when a local flap is not possible, one can perform a free flap immediately, but it requires a very specialized environment and facilities.

- Débridement is uncertain, tissue viability is not well defined, and the wound is massively infected. Immediate coverage does not seem a reasonable option. All viable tissues should be retained and reassessed 1 day later. **Repeated débridement is required until the wound is finally clean.** Between surgical débridements a temporary dressing should be applied and left in place. Dressings must avoid desiccation and infarction of vital exposed structures (nerves, arteries, tendons, and bones); so instead of packing the wound with wet gauze which dries in a few hours, an antibiotic bead pouch can be applied to maintain a physiologically moist environment. The dressing should promote neither the desiccation of the structures exposed nor the granulation process which means the development of the infection. Proinflammatory dressings are contraindicated.

- The very similar wounds resulting from barnyard injuries, high-velocity gunshot injuries, or electrical injuries should be debrided a number of times before the definitive closure. It is important that delayed coverage be performed no more than 10 days after the initial injury, and preferably before the end of the first week. It must be done, in any event, before the development of granulation, which will affect all the tissues and particularly the venous return from the injured area.

- Delayed definitive coverage allows a good assessment of the tissue by means of repeated débridement and gives time for arteriography, to help in planning the coverage procedure. Indeed this situation demands a coordinated plan for fracture stabilization and soft-tissue repair. At the time of coverage the final débridement must be performed at the site of the fracture. The fracture must be inspected, the medullary canals of the two bone ends must be washed and cleared of hematoma and small particulate matter. This presumes the use of a very versatile external fixator which allows opening of the fracture itself and immediate retrieval of the reduction by locking the device.

Delayed rotation of a local flap may be difficult due to edema.

If in doubt, repeated débridement is required.

7 Soft-tissue repair: how to do it [21]

7.1 Principles

Soft-tissue repair should be conceived as a reconstructive ladder escalating from the simplest procedure to the most sophisticated. Each procedure has its own indication according the size and the depth of the defect, the structures exposed, and local considerations such as vascular status and availability of regional flaps. In many cases different solutions are theoretically possible but are restricted by the local conditions to a single procedure.

Table 5.2-1 gives a suggested sequence of surgical procedures.

When a simple solution is not indicated (skin graft or rotation flap) we use, as far as possible, an island pedicled flap. This is a safe, reliable, and quick procedure if the vascular conditions have been well assessed. Exposed bone is covered by muscle flaps, whereas tendons are covered with fasciocutaneous flaps.

Distant pedicled flaps such as the groin flap for upper limb reconstruction and cross leg flap for the lower limb are not advocated for emergency use, especially if there is an underlying fracture. They are not closed procedures and always lead to a local area of inflammation or infection. **The immobilization of the limb required by these procedures generates edema and stiffness** and one should remember the high risk of venous thrombosis asso-

ciated with the cross leg flap. Moreover, the blood supply of these flaps will depend on the vascular conditions at the recipient site. For these reasons groin and cross leg flaps should be reserved as secondary resurfacing procedures. Nonetheless, despite its numerous drawbacks, the pedicled groin flap remains a reliable procedure for reconstructive surgery of the hand. It now remains to explore the main possibilities of coverage by flap procedures according the site of the posttraumatic defect.

7.2   Upper limb

Three areas should be differentiated: the upper arm, the forearm, and the hand and wrist.

7.2.1   Upper arm

The upper arm includes the shoulder girdle and the elbow; there is no indication for a free flap at this level. Open fractures of the shoulder girdle, including the head of humerus, the acromioclavicular joint, and the clavicle can be covered to a limited extent by pedicled flaps of

Immobilization of the entire limb generates edema and stiffness.

Table 5.2-1:

The ladder of soft-tissue reconstructive procedures

1. Spontaneous healing or vacuum-assisted closure.
2. Local plasties (rhomboid flaps).
3. Skin graft.
4. Local skin flap "at random" (rotation, translation, or advancement).
5. Local rotational axial skin flap (peninsular flaps).
6. Rotational muscle flaps.
7. Local island pedicled skin or muscle flap.
8. Distant pedicled flap (groin flaps or cross leg flap).
9. Free skin or muscle flap with vascular anastomosis in situ.
10. Free skin or muscle flaps revascularized by vascular grafts.

pectoralis minor muscle. Huge defects of the arm and the elbow can be safely reconstructed by the latissimus dorsi pedicled flap (**Fig. 5.2-1** and **Fig. 5.2.-2**). Very large soft-tissue defects which could compromise flexion of the elbow are repaired by functional transfer of the latissimus dorsi according to the Zancolli technique.

A latissimus dorsi muscle flap, later supplemented by a distal skin paddle, is a suitable and reliable technique for repairing open fractures of the elbow which can encompass the distal humerus or proximal forearm.

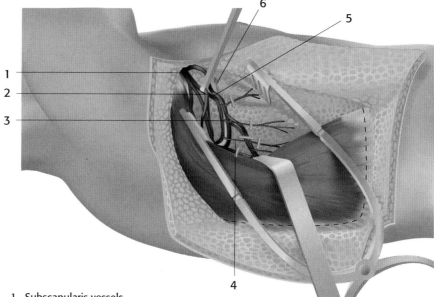

Fig. 5.2-1: The dissection of the latissimus dorsi muscle flap.
The totality of the muscle flap can be raised on a patient lying supine with a carefully positioned sand bag.
The anterior border of the muscle is slightly retracted in order to expose the vascular supply. The thoracic vessels should be ligated and divided to permit mobilization of the muscle.

1 Subscapularis vessels
2 Circumflex scapular vessels
3 Neurovascular pedicle
4 Vascular pedicle to serratus anterior
5 Thoracodorsal vessels
6 Motor nerve to latissimus dorsi
Arrows indicate ligation of vessels needed to mobilize the muscle on its main proximal pedicle.

Fig. 5.2-2: Area of coverage of the pedicled latissimus dorsi flap.
a) Anterior aspect
b) Posterior aspect
Note that the muscle can cover the posterior aspect of the elbow.

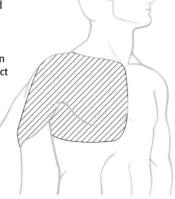
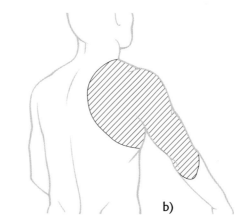

a)

b)

Open injury of the proximal third of the arm, with associated soft-tissue and bone defects, can be treated in a one-stage reconstructive procedure by using a composite transfer which includes the latissimus dorsi muscle flap and a vascularized segment of the 9th or 10th rib.

7.2.2   Forearm

In the forearm, a fracture of the bone frame with a soft-tissue defect compromising the function of the hand is a "no go area" for pedicle flap procedures. **A distant flap from the groin is always possible but its drawbacks are well known; the major risk is an infection** of the fracture which must remain partially exposed. More frequently, large defects of the forearm require a free flap. **Primary repair of the envelope is of crucial importance,** since reconstruction of tendon and bones can be performed in secondary procedures. Available flaps are latissimus dorsi, serratus anterior, and scapular muscle flaps. The so-called "Chinese" flap raised on the contralateral radial artery can be a good solution to restore, at the same time, a tissue defect and the continuity of an interrupted artery giving rise to hand ischemia.

7.2.3   Hand and wrist

The increasing number of pedicled flaps raised from the forearm has correspondingly reduced the indications for a free flap at this level. A Chinese flap, interosseous posterior flap, or a pedicled fascial flap from the distal radial side or ulnar side of the wrist can solve practically all the problems. All of these generally require viable anastomoses between the vascular system at the palm or the dorsum of the wrist,

since they are based on a distal pivot point and a retrograde arterial blood flow.

When no distally-based pedicle flap is available, a free flap can come from serratus anterior (coverage of the palm of the hand), or from temporalis or dorsalis pedis fascia or lateral brachial skin area for the dorsum of the hand.

7.3   Lower limb

Three areas should be differentiated: pelvic ring and thigh, knee and leg, ankle, and foot. In fact, most open fractures occur in the lower limb including knee, leg, ankle and foot.

7.3.1   Pelvic ring and thigh

Indications for soft-tissue repair following injury are very rare at the pelvic girdle and thigh. Limited defects exposing the anterior iliac crest are well covered by a pedicled rectus abdominis muscle flap distally based on the epigastric artery. Defects of the posterior aspect of the pelvis (posterior iliac crest, sacrum) can be covered with the gluteus maximus muscle flap. Combined trauma of the anterior part of the pelvic ring is a good indication for a proximally-based pedicled vastus lateralis muscle flap.

7.3.2   Knee and proximal third of the leg

The two heads of gastrocnemius are suitable for covering the knee or proximal third of the leg. The area of coverage at the knee can be considerably increased by a large skin paddle overlapping one and half times the area of the muscle. A skin paddle supported by the distal

A groin flap is possible but may become infected.

In open forearm fractures primary repair of the envelope takes precedence over reconstructive procedures.

The two heads of gastrocnemius are suitable for covering the knee or proximal third of the leg.

a)

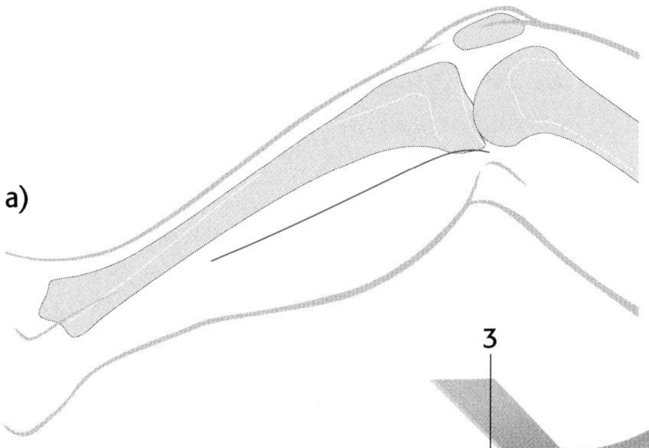

Fig. 5.2-3: The distally-based hemisoleus flap for covering the distal third of the leg. The flap is supplied by the midpoint branch that issues from the posterior tibial artery.
a) Incision

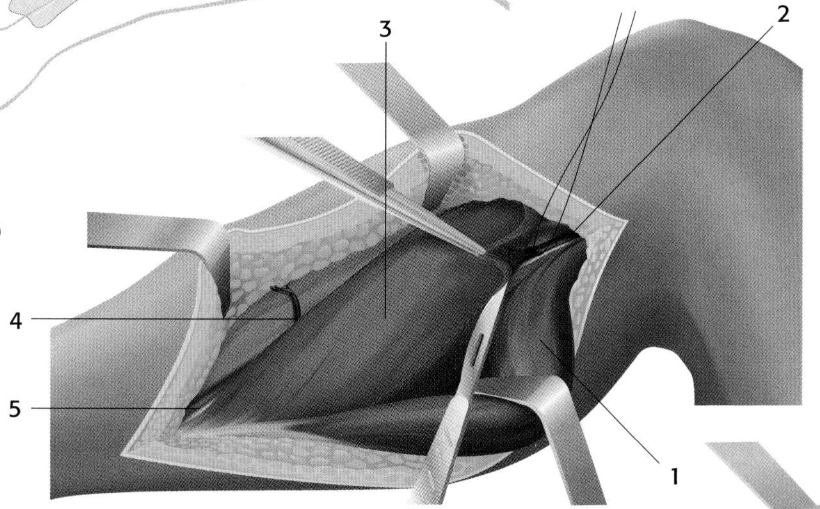

b) The medial head of the gastroc-nemius is retracted to expose the superficial aspect of the soleus. The proximal attachments are ligated and divided. The muscle is split according a vertical midline.

1 Medial head of gastrocnemius
2 Posterior tibial artery
3 Medial hemisoleus
4 Vascular pedicle that constitutes the pivot point of the flap
5 Neurovascular axis in deep posterior compartment

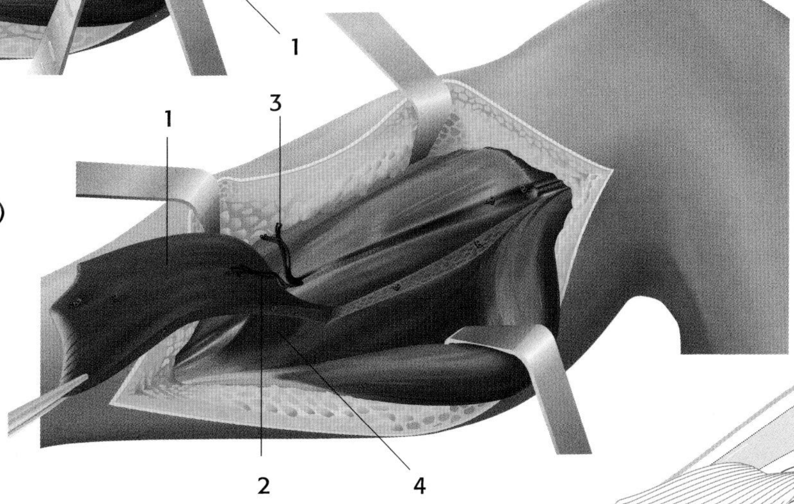

c) The medial hemisoleus is released as far as the secondary attachment, which constitutes the pivot point of the flap.

1 Hemisoleus
2 Vascular pedicle arising from the posterior tibial artery
3 Vascular bundle to the skin
4 A distal hinge with the lateral portion of the muscle is spared.

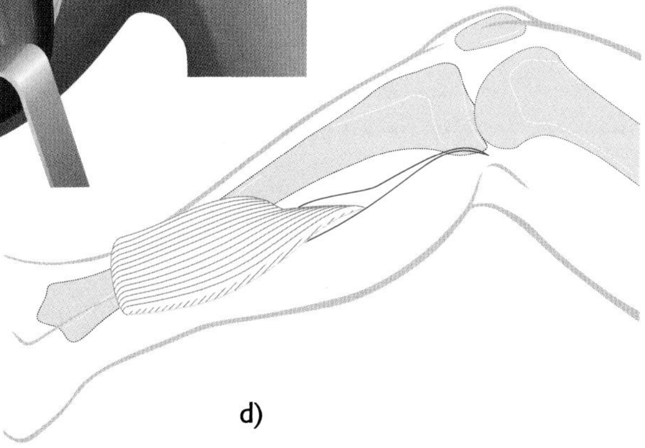

d) The muscle flap is rotated on its hinge. The flap is supplied by an arterial pedicle that is not located in the injured area.

Combination of flaps may allow coverage of larger areas.

part of the medial head of the gastrocnemius permits coverage of defects at the junction of the proximal and middle thirds of the leg.

7.3.3 Middle third of the leg

This is the territory to be covered by the soleus muscle. Before using this muscle one should assess the volume and the length of its muscle belly, which varies according to the size of the patient.

Wide short defects of the middle third are indications for a proximally-based soleus muscle flap. Long and narrow defects over the medial or the anterior aspect of the tibia require a proximally-based medial hemisoleus flap, which is more adaptable than when the whole muscle is used.

7.3.4 Distal third of the leg

Until recently, the distal third of the leg was a true "no go area" for local flaps. New advances have broadened the indications for a pedicled flap at this level.

- Small defects of the distal quarter of the leg are repaired by flexors of toes.
- The proximally-based soleus flap generally covers the proximal part of the distal third. The area that can be covered depends on the morphology of the muscle.
- The distally-based medial hemisoleus pedicled flap can cover practically the entire distal third of the leg except for the supra malleolar region. Pivot point and blood supply are provided by a constant branch from the tibialis posterior artery at the middle of the leg (**Fig. 5.2-3**).

- **Association of flaps can be an interesting procedure**: proximally-based soleus flaps and flaps from the flexors of the toes or soleus can be combined with a subcutaneous fascial supra malleolar flap.
- The supra malleolar flap is a very quick and reliable procedure to repair a defect of the distal quarter of the leg (see **Fig. 5.2-5d**).
- The sural flap based on the vascular network of the sural nerve can also be used for the distal third.
- The indications for flaps according to the level of the defect are summarized in **Fig. 5.2-4**.

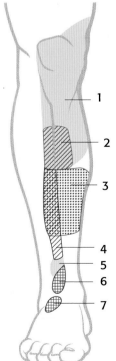

Fig. 5.2-4: Areas of coverage of pedicled flaps raised from the lower limb.
Note that the areas of coverage of the soleus muscle and medial hemisoleus muscle are different.

1 Medial head of gastrocnemius
2 Proximally-based hemisoleus (proximal third)
3 Soleus
4 Distally-based hemisoleus (distal third)
5 Flexor digitorum longus
6 Flexor hallucis longus
7 Extensor digitorum brevis pedicled on the lateral tarsal artery (without interrupting the continuity of the dorsalis pedis artery)

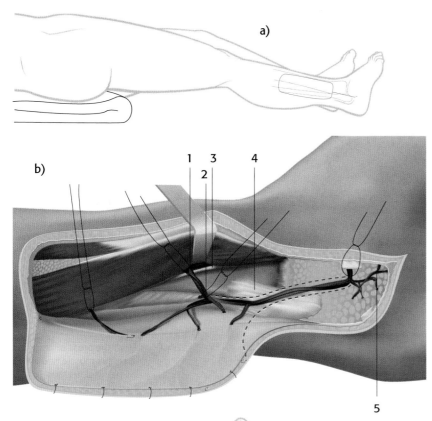

a)

b)

1 3 4
2

5

Fig. 5.2-5: The lateral supra malleolar flap is a very useful procedure for coverage of the distal quarter of the leg, the ankle, and foot. Nonetheless, it requires a good assessment of the vascular conditions of the injured area and a special expertise in dissection.

a) Design of the flap. It includes the depression in the lower part of the tibiofibular space where the perforating branch of the peroneal artery pierces the interosseous membrane.

b) Dissection of the flap. A posterior cutaneous hinge is maintained. Vascular pattern is identified to determine the pivot point of the flap which is the sinus tarsi. At this point the perforating branch of the peroneal artery anastomoses with the lateral tarsal artery. The flap is supplied by one or two cutaneous branches that issue from the perforating branch very close to the inter-osseous membrane.

  1 Ligature of the anterior malleolar artery
  2 Anterior tibial artery
  3 Deep peroneal nerve
  4 Inferior tibiofibular ligament
  5 Anastomosis with the lateral tarsal artery

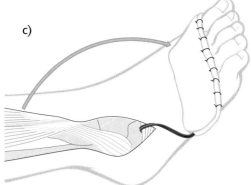

c)

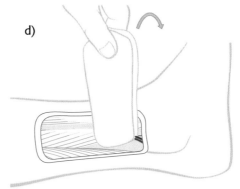

d)

c) The pedicle has been isolated and raised as far as the sinus tarsi. The arc of rotation provided by the pedicle allows cover of all the areas of the dorsal aspect of the foot.

d) The lateral supra malleolar flap can be used as a rotational flap to cover the distal quarter of the medial aspect of the tibia.

7.3.5   **Ankle and foot**

Soft-tissue defects of the foot are always a special challenge.

Soft-tissue defects of the foot are always challenging problems and we will give only the principles and the main procedures.

- Small defects of the hind foot may be covered by flaps from abductor hallucis muscle on the medial side and from abductor digiti quinti on the lateral side. These procedures are rarely used in fresh fractures and should be reserved for secondary procedures.
- The extensor brevis muscle pedicled on its supplying lateral tarsal artery is suitable for covering a limited defect of the lateral aspect of the ankle. Continuity of the dorsalis pedis artery is not compromised (**Fig. 5.2-4**).
- The dorsum of the foot can be covered by a lateral supramalleolar flap (**Fig. 5.2-5**) and a distally-based sural flap. Selection of the pivot point of the lateral supra malleolar flap is subject to a viable anastomosis. Fractures of the calcaneum rendered secondarily open by skin necrosis on the lateral aspect of the hind foot represent a good indication for a sural flap.

- Coverage of the heel: The posterior aspect of the heel, including the distal insertion of an Achilles tendon, can be covered by supramalleolar or sural flaps (**Fig. 5.2-6** and **Fig. 5.2-7**). Large compound defects of the weight-bearing area of the heel remain an unsolved problem; repair usually requires a free flap, and muscle flaps covered with skin are preferable as they are more adherent than a fasciocutaneous flap. Composite flaps including a piece of vascularized bone are difficult to match the defect. Reconstruction of the bone is best performed secondarily, either by a bone graft or by a progressive bone transport.

The very last question is the most important of all: Who should perform the soft-tissue repair?

The author believes that a perfect cooperation between plastic and trauma or orthopedic teams is not always easy to achieve, even in highly specialized centers, and he remains convinced that the best answer to the question lies in the training of specialized reconstructive surgeons capable of conceiving a coherent strategy of treatment and of performing all the procedures including bone stabilization, soft-tissue repair, and later, secondary procedures such as bone grafting. **The complexity of the lesions produced by high-energy trauma requires an holistic point of view** and not an aggregation of surgical procedures performed by various separate teams.

The complex lesions of high-energy trauma require a holistic approach to management.

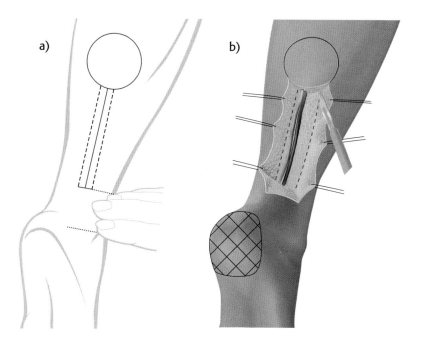

a)

b)

Fig. 5.2-6: The distally-based neurocutaneous sural flap. The flap is supplied by the vascular axis of the sural nerve. The pivot point of the pedicle corresponds to a huge anastomosis of the vascular axis of the nerve with the peroneal artery.
a) Design of the flap. The pivot point of the pedicle is three finger's breadth proximal to the tip of the lateral malleolus.
b) Isolation of the subcutaneous fascial pedicle.
c) The flap and the pedicle are raised, fascia (1) included.
d) Arc of rotation allows coverage of the heel.

Fig. 5.2-7: Indications of flaps for coverage of the hind foot.
1 Flexor hallucis longus
2 Medialis pedis flap
3 Medial plantar flap
4 Lateral supramalleolar flap and distally-based sural flap
5 Peroneus brevis.

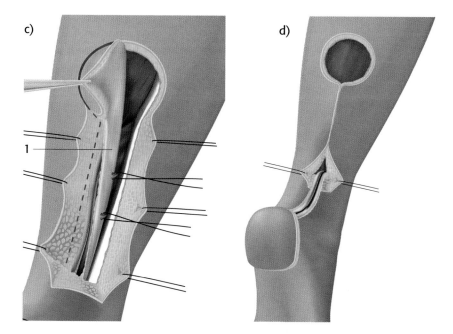

c)

1

d)

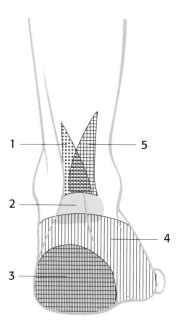

1   5

2

4

3

8 Bibliography

1. **Levin LS** (1993) The reconstructive ladder. An orthoplastic approach. *Orthop Clin North Am;* 24 (3):393–409.

2. **Norris BL, Kellam JF** (1997) Soft-tissue injuries associated with high-energy extremity trauma: principles of management. *J Am Acad Orthop Surg;* 5 (1):37–46.

3. **Masquelet AC, Begue T, Court C** (1995) *Fractures ouvertes de jambe.* Paris: Elsevier.

4. **Francel TJ, Vander Kolk CA, Hoopes JE, et al.** (1992) Microvascular soft-tissue transplantation for reconstruction of acute open tibial fractures: timing of coverage and long-term functional results. *Plast Reconstr Surg;* 89 (3):478–487; discussion 488–497.

5. **Holden CE** (1972) The role of blood supply to soft tissue in the healing of diaphyseal fractures. An experimental study. *J Bone Joint Surg [Am];* 54 (5):993-1000.

6. **Argenta LC, Morykwas MJ** (1997) Vacuum-assisted closure: a new method for wound control and treatment: clinical experience. *Ann Plast Surg;* 38 (6):563–576; discussion 577.

7. **Cauchoix J, Duparc J, Ducourtiaux JC** (1957) Traitement des fractures ouvertes de jambe. *Mem Acad Chir;* 83:811.

8. **Gustilo RB, Mendoza RM, Williams DN** (1984) Problems in the management of type III (severe) open fractures: a new classification of type III open fractures. *J Trauma;* 24 (8):742–746.

9. **Müller ME, Allgöwer M, Schneider R** (1991) *Manual of Internal Fixation.* Berlin Heidelberg New York: Springer-Verlag.

10. **Brumback RJ, Jones AL** (1994) Interobserver agreement in the classification of open fractures of the tibia. The results of a survey of two hundred and forty-five orthopaedic surgeons. *J Bone Joint Surg [Am];* 76 (8):1162–1166.

11. **Hansen ST, Jr.** (1987) The type-IIIC tibial fracture. Salvage or amputation [editorial]. *J Bone Joint Surg [Am];* 69 (6):799–800.

12. **Georgiadis GM, Behrens FF, Joyce MJ, et al.** (1993) Open tibial fractures with severe soft-tissue loss. Limb salvage compared with below-the-knee amputation. *J Bone Joint Surg [Am];* 75 (10):1431–1441.

13. **Bonanni F, Rhodes M, Lucke JF** (1993) The futility of predictive scoring of mangled lower extremities. *J Trauma;* 34 (1):99–104.

14. **Gorman PW, Barnes CL, Fischer TJ, et al.** (1989) Soft-tissue reconstruction in severe lower extremity trauma. A review. *Clin Orthop;* (243):57–64.

15. **Godina M** (1986) Early microsurgical reconstruction of complex trauma of the extremities. *Plast Reconstr Surg;* 78 (3):285–292.

16. **Byrd HS, Spicer TE, Cierney G** (1985) Management of open tibial fractures. *Plast Reconstr Surg;* 76 (5):719–730.

17. **Yaremchuk MJ, Brumback RJ, Manson PN, et al.** (1987) Acute and definitive management of traumatic osteocutaneous defects of the lower extremity. *Plast Reconstr Surg;* 80 (1):1–14.

18. **Sanders R, Swiontkowski M, Nunley J, et al.** (1993) The management of fractures with soft-tissue disruptions. *J Bone Joint Surg [Am];* 75 (5):778–789.

19. **Small JO, Mollan RA** (1992)
Management of the soft tissues in open
tibial fractures. *Br J Plast Surg;*
45 (8):571–577.
20. **Najean D, Tropet Y, Brientini JM,
et al.** (1994) [Emergency cover of open
fractures of the leg. Apropos of a series of
24 clinical cases]. *Ann Chir Plast Esthet;*
39 (4):473–479; discussion 480–471.
21. **Masquelet AC, Gilbert A** (1995) *An
atlas of flaps in limb reconstruction.* London:
Martin Dunitz.

9 Updates

Updates and additional references for this chapter
are available online at:
http://www.aopublishing.org/PFxM/52.htm

5.3 Polytrauma: pathophysiology, priorities, and management

Otmar L. Trentz

1 Definition

The term polytrauma means a syndrome of multiple injuries exceeding a defined severity (ISS > 17) with sequential systemic traumatic reactions which may lead to dysfunction or failure of remote organs and vital systems, which had not themselves been directly injured.

2 Importance of fractures

Fractures are frequently components of polytrauma patterns. They must be considered as wounds of bone and soft tissue, giving rise to stress, pain, and hemorrhage. They can be contaminated and cause compartment syndromes with ischemia-reperfusion injury.

The instability of the skeleton renders the patient immobile and abolishes the option to select the nursing position most suitable for intensive care of brain and chest injuries.

3 Pathophysiological background

The wound around a fracture is an inflammatory focus, consisting of dead tissue in an ischemic or marginally perfused, hypoxic zone. This focus behaves like an endocrine organ, releasing mediators and cytokines locally to tissue macrophages, as well as into the circulation, thus causing systemic reactions.

By releasing these substances a cascade of local and systemic defense mechanisms is activated and immuno-competent cells are attracted to control, debride, and repair the tissue defects.

Stress and pain are potent stimuli [1] for neuroendocrine, neuroimmunological, and metabolic responses (**Table 5.3-1**). If, in addition, hemorrhage, contamination, and ischemia-reperfusion injury complicate fractures or if these are caused by associated injuries, **systemic reactions to trauma produce a whole-body inflammation [2] or a Systemic Inflammatory Response Syndrome (SIRS)**. SIRS is associated with a general capillary leak syndrome and high energy consumption demanding a hyperdynamic hemodynamic state (flow-phase) and an increased availability of oxygen (**Table 5.3-2**). This flow-phase generates

Systemic reactions to trauma produce a whole-body inflammation or a Systemic Inflammatory Response Syndrome (SIRS).

Table 5.3-1: "Afferent input" in trauma and resulting reflex responses.

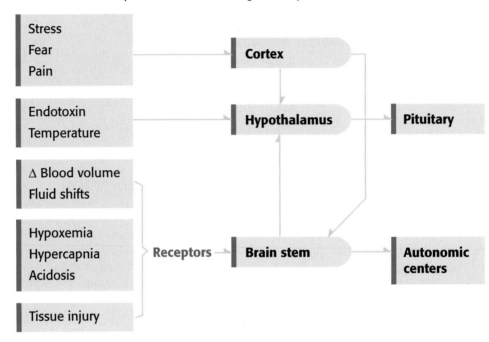

Table 5.3-2: Parameters to calculate oxygen availability (cardiac output, arterial oxygen saturation, concentration of hemoglobin) and estimated oxygen requirements in rest and severe trauma. A moderate, simultaneous decrease of these parameters in trauma induces oxygen debt and acidosis.

Available oxygen in hypovolemic shock:
(**Nunn, Freeman** (1964) *Anaesthesia;* 19:206)

$$O_2 \text{ av} = CO \times S_aO_2 \times Hb \text{ (g\%)} \times 1.34$$

250 ml/min: resting state
1,000 ml/min: shock, trauma

1,000 = 5,250 x 0.95 x 0.15 x 1.24
300 = 3,500 x 0.64 x 0.10 x 1.34

---

an intense metabolic load with significant muscle wasting, nitrogen loss, and accelerated protein breakdown. This hypermetabolic state is accompanied by an increase in core body temperature and by thermal dysregulation.

If adequate and timely resuscitation is neither permitted by the severity of trauma nor provided by the quality of care, the high energy consumption will lead to a "burn out".

This process moves from depletion of immuno-competent cells and acute-phase proteins to critical immuno-suppression and sepsis, then onward, via increased cell damage, to a Multiple Organ Dysfunction Syndrome (MODS) and ultimately lethal Multiple Organ Failure (MOF) [3–5].

4 Timing and priorities of surgery

(Table 5.3-3)

The primary objective in the initial care of poly-traumatized patients is survival with normal cognitive functions. The first priority is resuscitation to ensure adequate perfusion and oxygenation of all vital organs. This can be usually accomplished by conservative means such as intubation, ventilation, and volume replacement according to the ATLS® protocol. If the response to such measures is not successful, immediate life-saving surgery is necessary:

- Decompression of body cavities (tension pneumothorax, cardiac tamponade, epidural hematoma).
- Control of exsanguinating hemorrhage (massive hemothorax or hemoperitoneum, crushed pelvis, whole limb amputation, "mangled extremity").

If there are special circumstances which preclude immediate definitive surgery, the concept of damage control [6] applies. Control of hemorrhage and contamination, irrigation, packing, provisional closure of the wound or abdominal cavity, and stabilization of the physiological systems in the intensive care unit (ICU) may be followed by definitive surgery after 6–12 hours.

Table 5.3-3: Algorithm for initial assessment, life support, and day-1-surgery.

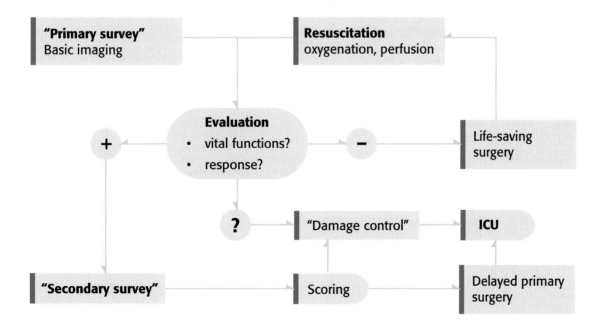

Within the locomotor system treat with high priority:
- Limb-threatening and disabling injuries.
- Long bone fractures, unstable pelvic injuries, highly unstable large joints, and spinal injuries—they require at least provisional reduction and fixation.

During this 5–10-day window of opportunity, scheduled, definitive surgery of long bone fractures—shaft and articular—can be performed in relative safety.

Early fracture fixation in polytrauma is beneficial in terms of mortality and morbidity.

If there is a positive response to resuscitation, the phase of delayed primary surgery can start. **Within the locomotor system** the following conditions should be treated with **high priority**:

- **Limb-threatening and disabling injuries** (including open fractures) require at least "damage control": débridement, fasciotomies, reduction, fixation, and revascularization [7].
- **Long bone fractures** (especially femoral shaft fractures), **unstable pelvic injuries, highly unstable large joints, and spinal injuries** require at least **provisional reduction and fixation.** Definitive fixation may need to wait and the better option might be temporary stabilization by means of an external fixator followed by a scheduled, definitive osteosynthesis (intramedullary nailing) during a window of opportunity between days 5 and 10 [7, 8].

There is a convincing body of evidence, from clinical experience as well as in the literature, that **early fracture fixation in polytrauma is beneficial in terms of mortality and morbidity** [9–14].

The arguments and experience in favor of early fixation of femoral fractures and unstable pelvic ring injuries are:

- Reduction of the incidence of ARDS, of fat embolism and pneumonia, of MODS, sepsis, and of thromboembolic complications.
- Facilitation of nursing and intensive care: upright chest position, early mobilization, use of less analgesia.

Definitive osteosynthesis as "day-1-surgery" is advisable only when all the endpoints of resuscitation [15, 16] have been accomplished (**Tables 5.3-4** and **5.3-5**).

Between the fifth and tenth day post trauma there exists an immunological window of opportunity when the phase of hyperinflammation is followed by a period of immunosuppression and when new cell-recruitment and synthesis *de novo* of acute-phase proteins is taking place.

During this window of opportunity, scheduled, definitive surgery of long bone fractures—shaft and articular—can be performed in relative safety.

This period of immunosuppression lasts for about 2 weeks, so that secondary reconstructive procedures can be planned for the third week post trauma.

Table 5.3-4: Parameters and criteria which indicate a successful resuscitation.

"Endpoints of resusciation"

- Stable hemodynamics
- No hypoxemia, no hypercapnia
- Lactate < 2 mmol/L
- Normal coagulation
- Normothermia
- Urinary output > 1 mL/kg/hour
- No need for vasoactive or inotropic stimulation

Table 5.3-5: Priorities and timing of surgery depending on the physiological status.

Physiological status	Surgical intervention	Timing
Response to resuscitation: −	Life-saving surgery	
?	"Damage control"	Day 1
+	Delayed primary surgery	
Hyper-inflammation	"Second look", only!	Day 2–3
"Window of opportunity"	Scheduled definitive surgery	Day 5–10
Immunosuppression	**No surgery!**	
Recovery	Secondary reconstructive surgery	Week 3

5 General aims and scopes of fracture management in polytrauma

Fractures may have an important impact on the severity of systemic traumatic reactions due to:
- Hemorrhage:
  Prolonged states of shock as well as exsanguinating hemorrhage are frequently associated with open or highly unstable pelvic ring injuries or femoral shaft fractures.
- Contamination:
  Open fractures must always be considered as contaminated. If a wound can only be debrided after some delay or if débridement is not radical enough, bacterial nutrients will develop in the wound. A second or even third débridement is therefore mandatory.
- Dead, ischemic tissue with a marginally perfused hypoxic zone:
  In unstable, displaced fractures, especially after high-energy impact, a radical soft-tissue débridement is necessary as soon as possible in order to control the source of the inflammatory reaction.
- Ischemia-reperfusion injury:
  (Table 5.3-6) Prolonged hypovolemic shock and compartment syndromes related to fractures without or with vascular injuries are prone to ischemia-reperfusion injury with microvascular damage due to oxygen radicals. Blunt tissue contusions may activate xanthine oxidase, ischemia will produce the substrate xanthine/hypoxanthine, and reperfusion will add the co-substrate oxygen. A dangerous triad is thus established.

Aims and scopes for fracture
management are:
- control of hemorrhage,
- control of sources of
  contamination, removal of
  dead tissue, prevention of
  ischemia-reperfusion injury,
- pain relief,
- facilitation of intensive care.

- Stress and pain:
  Unstable fractures cause pain and stress
  which, via "afferent input" [1] to the
  CNS, stimulate a neuroendocrine,
  neuroimmunological, and metabolic
  reflex arc (see **Table 5.3-1**).
- Interference with intensive care:
  Unstable fractures prevent effective
  patient postures (upright chest), and
  pain-free handling in intensive care.

The general aims and scopes for fracture management are therefore:
- **control of hemorrhage,**
- **control of sources of contamination, removal of dead tissue,
  prevention of ischemia-reperfusion
  injury,**
- **pain relief,**
- **facilitation of intensive care.**

These concepts can be realized by hemostasis,
débridement, fasciotomy, fracture fixation, and
tension-free wound coverage.

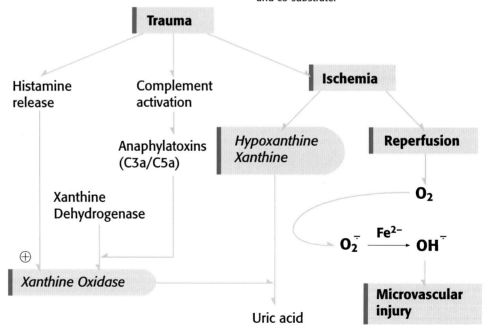

Table 5.3-6: Mechanism of ischemia-reperfusion injury:
"unhappy triad" of providing activated enzyme, substrate,
and co-substrate.

For stabilization of long bones, external and internal fixation, as well as plates and nails, are options depending on the circumstances.

6 Pros and cons of different fixation methods

Nailing is, from the biomechanical point of view, the method of choice for shaft fractures of femur and tibia. **However, femoral nailing, reamed as well as unreamed, has an adverse effect due to pulmonary embolization [17]**. The main reason is probably that manipulation of the content of the medullary canal by opening, insertion of guide-wire, reaming, and insertion of a nail increases the intramedullary pressure, so that emboli of bone marrow content, fibrin clots, and debris are introduced into the pulmonary circulation. In addition, this embolization causes activation of the coagulation and other cascade systems.

It may happen that the immense clearing capacity of the pulmonary endothelium is already compromised by a lung contusion, a massive transfusion of allogenic blood, a spill over of cytokines and mediators from large wound with dead tissues, or an incomplete resuscitation from shock. In this situation, the additional insult arising from iatrogenic embolization can crucially damage pulmonary function. Furthermore, it is important to realize that **simple fracture types (transverse and short oblique) in a young patient with a narrow medullary canal and a well-developed muscle envelope, are much more prone to pulmonary embolization** following nailing than complex fractures with extensive fragmentation of the femoral shaft, or fractures in elderly individuals with poorer muscles and a wide medullary canal. There is presently no evidence that nailing without reaming is less dangerous than nailing after reaming.

Plating requires a major surgical access and is usually technically more demanding. On the other hand, it allows better bleeding control and permits simultaneous débridement and fasciotomies.

External fixation minimizes additional surgical trauma. It is a fast and forgiving procedure and allows temporary shortening to avoid compartment syndromes. The drawbacks are insufficient stability for definitive treatment, pin-track infections, and limitation of escape-routes for plastic soft-tissue procedures.

In summary, every fixation method has its biological advantages and disadvantages. **Rigid protocols related to "timing and choice of implant" should therefore be avoided**.

7 Fracture management under specific conditions

7.1 Massive hemorrhage due to a crushed or disrupted pelvis [18–20]

Open or closed crush or disruption of the pelvic ring ("open book", "vertical shear" injuries) can produce exsanguinating hemorrhage into the retroperitoneum, the peritoneal cavity, or to an open or closed (semi-)circular degloving injury (Morel-Lavalle syndrome). Besides aggressive

External fixation minimizes additional surgical trauma.

Femoral nailing has an adverse effect due to pulmonary embolization.

Rigid protocols related to timing and choice of implant should be avoided.

Simple fracture types in a young patient with a narrow medullary canal are more prone to pulmonary embolization.

Massive pelvic hemorrhage requires immediate reduction and fixation of the pelvic ring by external fixator or C-clamp.

fluid replacement these patients require **immediate reduction and fixation of the pelvic ring by an external fixator** or a pelvic compression clamp (C-clamp). If the hemodynamic response is good, the diagnostic work-up can be completed and pelvic reconstruction be done as staged surgery (see **chapter 4.5**).

However, if the patient remains unstable, emergency laparotomy is mandatory to stop the bleeding. In these circumstances the pelvic ring must be stabilized by external or internal fixation, followed by surgical hemostasis, tight pelvic packing, and provisional closure of the abdomen. The possibility of abdominal compartment syndrome must be kept in mind [21, 22]. After recovery in the ICU, one or two "second-look procedures" are mandatory, followed by definitive stabilization of the pelvis and closure of the abdominal wall.

7.2 Early fracture fixation in patients with severe brain injury

In traumatic brain injury (TBI) it is of paramount importance, both to prevent secondary brain damage [23, 24] due to hypotension (**Table 5.3-7**) and hypoxemia, and to maintain optimal cerebral perfusion. Epidural or acute subdural hematomas require urgent surgical evacuation and hemostasis. Patients with TBI and Glasgow Coma Scale (GCS) < 9 or after craniotomy need ICP (intracranial pressure) monitoring immediately after life-saving surgery [25]. Given a good response to resuscitation (stable hemodynamics and adequate oxygenation), early fracture fixation has a positive effect [26] in brain-injured patients, by facilitating nursing care, by reducing painful

Table 5.3-7: Influence of hypotension on outcome after traumatic brain injury.

Traumatic Coma Database:
Influence of systemic hypotension on the outcome after severe traumatic brain injury
(**Chesnut** et al. (1993) *Acta Neurochir;* 59:121–125)

	n =	Death or vegetative state (GOS[1] 1–2) [%]	Favorable outcome (GOS[1] 4–5) [%]
No hypotension	307	17	64
Early hypotension[2] (from injury through resuscitation)	248	55	40
Late hypotension[2] (in the ICU)	117	66	20
Early and late hypotension[2]	39	77	15

[1] GOS = Glasgow Outcome Scale

[2] Systemic blood pressure < 90 mmHg

stimuli (afferent input), and by less need for sedation and analgesia.

Concerns that early fixation of major fractures in TBI patients, under the circumstances just described, may have a negative effect on mortality rates are not evidence-based. Lengthy and time-consuming fracture reconstructions should, however, be postponed to the fifth to seventh day during the window of opportunity following initial damage control with some type of external fixation.

7.3 Early fixation of femoral shaft fractures in severe polytrauma or polytrauma patients with chest injury

Several studies have well documented the advantages of early fixation of long bone fractures—especially of femoral shaft—in polytrauma. These advantages include facilitation of nursing care, early mobilization with improved pulmonary function, shorter time on the ventilator, and reduced morbidity and mortality [9–14, 27, 28].

Locked intramedullary nailing has become the standard method in closed and open femoral shaft fractures. However, there is abundant experimental and clinical evidence of a considerable increase in intramedullary pressure during the nailing procedure, especially in "simple" type A and B fractures. This leads to a significant release of mediators, as well as the passage of configured emboli into the lung. The latter can be demonstrated by transesophageal echocardiography [17]. While these side effects of nailing can be disregarded in patients with isolated fractures, they are likely to cause rapid

pulmonary deterioration in the multiply injured when the procedure is started [29, 30].

Other stabilization procedures, such as plating or application of an external fixator, can also initiate mediator release, but to a much lesser extent. In order to protect pulmonary function, one should refrain from using the biomechanically better method in favor of a more biological technique as being less distressing to already compromised endogenous defense systems and the pulmonary endothelium.

Primary intramedullary nailing of the femur (especially type A and B fractures) can only be recommended for polytraumatized patients **without significant chest injury**, respectively an **ISS < 25 points**. If the **ISS exceeds 40 points, primary stabilization is still essential, but should be done with external fixators only [8].**

Plating may be a good alternative for ISS values between these limits, especially if the soft-tissue conditions require débridement, fasciotomy, and active control of hemorrhage. Seriously compromised soft tissues may respond to additional distraction with a further reduction of perfusion, enhancing the possibility of a compartment syndrome. In such situations a temporary shortening of a limb has occasionally to be accepted.

In complex type C fractures with extensive comminution, the range of indications for nailing can be extended, because no substantial pressure increase can occur. As clinical and experimental data indicate that the application of solid nails with smaller diameters, for example, the solid femoral nail (UFN), may also cause relevant pulmonary impairment, their use has no significant advantage over conventional nails.

Primary intramedullary nailing only in patients with no significant chest injury or ISS < 25.

ISS > 40: primary stabilization is essential, but with external fixators.

Advantages include facilitation of nursing care, early mobilization with improved pulmonary function, shorter time on the ventilator, and reduced morbidity and mortalitiy.

Polytrauma must be considered as a systemic surgical disease.

Staged surgery in a subset of patients in critical conditions is generally accepted by most authors in Central Europe, but not in North America, where primary nailing is preferred in this situation.

Solid nails should therefore predominantly be used for open fractures (no dead space) and are especially recommended if a scheduled definitive change from external to internal fixation is intended. Any switch to a biomechanically better procedure should be performed early, ideally between the fifth and the tenth day after trauma (see **Table 5.3-5**).

This **concept of staged surgery in a subset of patients in critical conditions** appears to be **generally accepted by most authors in Central Europe**. In contrast, a variety of investigations from **North America** continue to argue that all femoral shaft fractures should be submitted to **primary nailing** regardless of the patient's clinical status [10, 31–33]. These retrospective studies, however, have a variety of inconsistencies regarding patient selection and comparability of study groups. A prospective randomized trial has not been conducted.

7.4 Limb salvage vs. amputation

The development of microsurgical techniques for free vascularized tissue transfer has increased the chances of saving mangled extremities and amputated or nearly amputated limbs [34]. In polytrauma, however, such salvage procedures are mostly not indicated, because, by their very nature, they increase the systemic inflammatory load. The Mangled Extremity Severity Score can assist in decision making [35]. There are only rare indications for heroic salvage attempts. These require a multi-stage concept with initial débridement, revascularization, fasciotomies, and fracture fixation, followed by repeated débridements and early soft-tissue reconstruction during a "window of opportunity".

When the decision is to amputate, this should be performed at a "safe" level with a "Guillotin" technique, combined with primary open wound management.

Summary

Polytrauma must be considered as a systemic surgical disease. Successful management requires a sound understanding of pathophysiology, complete resuscitation, correct triage and timing, and well-orchestrated plans of care.

Algorithms are meant to optimize the physiological state of patients prior to non-life-saving surgery and to provide procedures which are safe, simple, quick, and well executed.

The primary objective is survival of the patient. Early fixation of major fractures—performed with the right concept—has proved to be an important tool to obtain this primary objective.

8 Bibliography

1. **Gann DS, Lilly MP** (1984) The endocrine response to injury. *Prog Crit Care Med*; 1:15–47.
2. **Ertel W, Keel M, Marty D, et al.** (1998) [Significance of systemic inflammation in 1,278 trauma patients]. *Unfallchirurg*; 101 (7):520–526.
3. **Bone RC** (1996) Immunologic dissonance: a continuing evolution in our understanding of the systemic inflammatory response syndrome (SIRS) and the multiple organ dysfunction syndrome (MODS). *Ann Intern Med*; 125 (8):680–687.

4. **Ertel W, Keel M, Bonaccio M, et al.** (1995) Release of anti-inflammatory mediators after mechanical trauma correlates with severity of injury and clinical outcome. *J Trauma*; 39 (5):879–885; discussion 885–887.

5. **Goris RJ, te Boekhorst TP, Nuytinck JK, et al.** (1985) Multiple-organ failure. Generalized autodestructive inflammation? *Arch Surg*; 120 (10):1109–1115.

6. **Rotondo MF, Schwab CW, McGonigal MD, et al.** (1993) Damage control: an approach for improved survival in exsanguinating penetrating abdominal injury. *J Trauma*; 35 (3):375–382; discussion 382–373.

7. **Colton C, Trentz O** (1998) Severe limb injuries. *Acta Orthop Scand Suppl*; 281:47–53.

8. **Friedl HP, Stocker R, Czermak B, et al.** (1996) Primary fixation and delayed nailing of long bone fractures in severe trauma. *Techniques in Orthopaedics*; 11:59–66.

9. **Behrman SW, Fabian TC, Kudsk KA, et al.** (1990) Improved outcome with femur fractures: early vs. delayed fixation. *J Trauma*; 30 (7):792–797; discussion 797–798.

10. **Bone LB, Johnson KD, Weigelt J, et al.** (1989) Early versus delayed stabilization of femoral fractures. A prospective randomized study. *J Bone Joint Surg [Am]*; 71 (3):336–340.

11. **Goris RJ, Gimbrere JS, van Niekerk JL, et al.** (1982) Early osteosynthesis and prophylactic mechanical ventilation in the multitrauma patient. *J Trauma*; 22 (11):895–903.

12. **Johnson KD, Cadambi A, Seibert GB** (1985) Incidence of adult respiratory distress syndrome in patients with multiple musculoskeletal injuries: effect of early operative stabilization of fractures. *J Trauma*; 25 (5):375–384.

13. **Riska EB, von Bonsdorff H, Hakkinen S, et al.** (1976) Prevention of fat embolism by early internal fixation of fractures in patients with multiple injuries. *Injury*; 8 (2):110–116.

14. **Rüedi T, Wolff G** (1975) [Prevention of post-traumatic complications through immediate therapy in patients with multiple injuries and fractures]. *Helv Chir Acta*; 42 (4):507–512.

15. **Sturm JA, Lewis FR, Jr., Trentz O, et al.** (1979) Cardiopulmonary parameters and prognosis after severe multiple trauma. *J Trauma*; 19 (5):305–318.

16. **Vincent JL, Manikis P** (1995) End-points of resuscitation. In: Goris RJA, Trentz O, editors. *The integrated approach to trauma care*. Berlin Heidelberg New York: Springer-Verlag: 98–105.

17. **Wenda K, Runkel M, Degreif J, et al.** (1993) Pathogenesis and clinical relevance of bone marrow embolism in medullary nailing-demonstrated by intraoperative echocardiography. *Injury*; 24 (Suppl 3):73–81.

18. **Ertel W, Keel M, Eid K, et al.** (1999) Therapeutical strategies and outcome of polytraumatized patients with pelvic injuries—a six-year experience. *J Trauma*; (in press).

19. **Trentz O, Bühren V, Friedl HP** (1989) [Pelvic injuries]. *Chirurg*; 60 (10):639–648.

20. **Trentz O, Friedl HP** (1995) Therapeutic sequences in the acute period in unstable patients. In: Goris RJA, Trentz O, editors. *The integrated approach to trauma care.* Berlin Heidelberg New York: Springer-Verlag: 172–178.

21. **Ertel W, Oberholzer A, Platz A, et al.** (2000) Incidence and clinical pattern of the abdominal compartment syndrome after "damage control" laparotomy in 311 patients with severe abdominal and/or pelvic trauma. *Crit Care Med;* 28 (6):1747–1753.

22. **Saggi BH, Sugerman HJ, Ivatury RR, et al.** (1998) Abdominal compartment syndrome. *J Trauma;* 45 (3):597–609.

23. **Chesnut RM, Marshall LF, Klauber MR, et al.** (1993) The role of secondary brain injury in determining outcome from severe head injury. *J Trauma;* 34 (2):216–222.

24. **Chesnut RM, Marshall SB, Piek J, et al.** (1993) Early and late systemic hypotension as a frequent and fundamental source of cerebral ischemia following severe brain injury in the Traumatic Coma Data Bank. *Acta Neurochir Suppl;* 59:121–125.

25. **Stocker R, Bernays R, Kossmann T, et al.** (1995) Monitoring and treatment of acute head injury. In: Goris RJA, Trentz O, editors. *The integrated approach to trauma care.* Berlin Heidelberg New York: Springer-Verlag: 196–210.

26. **Hofman PA, Goris RJ** (1991) Timing of osteosynthesis of major fractures in patients with severe brain injury. *J Trauma;* 31 (2):261–263.

27. **Charash WE, Fabian TC, Croce MA** (1994) Delayed surgical fixation of femur fractures is a risk factor for pulmonary failure independent of thoracic trauma. *J Trauma;* 37 (4):667–672.

28. **Regel G, Lobenhoffer P, Grotz M, et al.** (1995) Treatment results of patients with multiple trauma: an analysis of 3,406 cases treated between 1972 and 1991 at a German Level I Trauma Center. *J Trauma;* 38 (1):70–78.

29. **Pape HC, Auf'm'Kolk M, Paffrath T, et al.** (1993) Primary intramedullary femur fixation in multiple trauma patients with associated lung contusion— a cause of posttraumatic ARDS? *J Trauma;* 34 (4):540–547; discussion 547–548.

30. **Pape HC, Regel G, Dwenger A, et al.** (1993) Influences of different methods of intramedullary femoral nailing on lung function in patients with multiple trauma. *J Trauma;* 35 (5):709–716.

31. **Bosse MJ, MacKenzie EJ, Riemer BL, et al.** (1997) Adult respiratory distress syndrome, pneumonia, and mortality following thoracic injury and a femoral fracture treated either with intramedullary nailing with reaming or with a plate. A comparative study. *J Bone Joint Surg [Am];* 79 (6):799–809.

32. **Boulanger BR, Stephen D, Brenneman FD** (1997) Thoracic trauma and early intramedullary nailing of femur fractures: are we doing harm? *J Trauma;* 43 (1):24–28.

33. **Reynolds MA, Richardson JD, Spain DA, et al.** (1995) Is the timing of fracture fixation important for the patient with multiple trauma? *Ann Surg;* 222 (4):470–481; discussion 478-481.

34. **Levin LS** (1993) The reconstructive ladder. An orthoplastic approach. *Orthop Clin North Am*; 24 (3):393–409.
35. **Johansen K, Daines M, Howey T, et al.** (1990) Objective criteria accurately predict amputation following lower extremity trauma. *J Trauma*; 30 (5):568–572; discussion 572–573.

9 Updates

Updates and additional references for this chapter are available online at:
http://www.aopublishing.org/PFxM/53.htm

Jorge E. Alonso

5.4 Children's fractures

1 General principles

The immature skeleton differs from that of the adult in both the normal and pathological states. Children's bones are capable of considerable plastic deformation before they fail. Comminuted fractures are rare and the presence of the growth plate presents challenges to the surgeon treating these injuries. **Failure of union is rare. Only relatively few fractures require operative treatment.**

1.1 Development and growth

In the past few years, interest in the morphology and physiology of bone has increased, with special research in the genetic aspects of development and growth of immature cellular tissues.

The immature bone is more capable of reaction and adaptation, but also more vulnerable, than the mature bone. A fracture in an immature bone can cause growth to speed up or slow down, superimposing the problems of deformity on the complications of the fracture itself. On the other hand, **children's fractures heal very rapidly and, depending on the age of the child and direction of the deformity, can remodel with correction of most angular malunion.**

It is evident that the special properties of growing skeleton play a role in the general physiological processes as well as carrying implications for the assessment of injury and the choice of treatment. This applies especially to the responses of those cell populations in the periosteum, the endosteum, and the cortex that participate in bone growth and remodeling.

The most important area of injury in the skeletally immature is the growth plate or physis, whose complex structure serves a balanced interplay between a number of physiological processes.

1.2 Regulation of epiphyseal growth

The physis is the primary center for growth in most bones and may be divided into two zones. The zone of functional growth and the zone of matrix formation. **The zone of growth is involved with both longitudinal and circumferential growth of bone.** The zone of matrix

Children's fractures heal rapidly and can, depending on age, correct most angular malunions.

Failure of union is rare. Only relatively few fractures require operative treatment.

Zone of growth involves longitudinal as well as circumferential growth.

formation is itself subdivided into several zones that reflect the different changes necessary for eventual ossification.

According to Ogden there are four functional zones [1]:

- growth,
- matrix,
- transformation, and
- remodeling.

For details of the morphometric structure and function of the physis, the reader is referred to the work of Hunziker and Schenk [2].

The physis is capable of responding to different stimuli, either compression or tension (distraction). Any increase in pressure along the axis of the bone, parallel to the direction of growth, will inhibit longitudinal growth. If traction is exerted in the same axis, growth can be accelerated.

Other stimuli to growth are insults which can come from foreign material, fracture, infection, or repeated attempts at reduction. All are capable of producing an acceleration of growth by increasing the local blood supply [1–4].

The physis responds to compression as well as to distraction.

1.3 Growth and remodeling of the metaphyseal bone

The metaphysis is the site of the most rapid changes in bone structures as the deeper physeal zones mature and the physis produces primary trabeculae. This bone is laid down on the surfaces of the calcified longitudinal matrix between the cell columns (interterritorial matrix); it is then rapidly remodeled and replaced by secondary trabeculae and later by more mature bone. The metaphysis can be regarded as the zone of transition between the physis and the diaphysis.

1.4 Growth patterns in the diaphysis

Circumferential growth of the diaphysis is a function of appositional bone formation by the periosteum, together with osteoclastic resorption by the endosteum so as to enlarge the medullary cavity [3]. Shaping of the diaphyseal area is accompanied by localized differences in the process of balanced remodeling along the periosteum and endosteum. Such growth in a bone that is bowed requires a change in the radius of curvature. This is achieved by a phenomenon of cortical drift during growth and remodeling (**Fig. 5.4-1**).

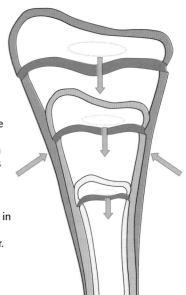

Fig. 5.4-1: As the diaphysis of a bone that is curved (and most are) grows in length, the curve is preserved by remodeling of the endosteal and periosteal surfaces in a controlled and differential manner. The resulting phenomenon of cortical drift is illustrated.

As growth continues, the bone is capable of reducing, or even correcting, angular deformity by selective resorption and apposition, possibly driven by compression and tension forces.

1.5 Incidence of fracture type

Mann et al. [5] reported that of 2,650 long bone fractures in children, 30% involved the physis. In other reports on physeal injuries about 50% occur in the distal radius. The second most commonly injured area is the distal humerus. The incidence of fracture types also depends on the child's activities; those involved in sports will have an increased incidence of long bone diaphyseal fractures and growth-plate injuries. **High-energy trauma is the most common cause of death in children** and ranks second to acute infections as a leading cause of morbidity. Musculoskeletal injuries are second only to injury to the central nervous system as the most frequent traumatic cause of permanent pediatric disability.

Surgeons have long expounded that pediatric fractures have no significant sequelae, but these data belie such orthodoxy.

1.6 Clinical examination of the injured child

1.6.1 Examination of the spine

After evaluation of all vital signs according to the ATLS schema, the spine should be examined next. Spinal column injuries are infrequent in the pediatric patient and represent only about 3% of all the pediatric injuries. However, in postmortem studies it is shown that the incidence of spinal fractures is about 12% in children below the age of 16 who have died from high-energy trauma [5].

The upper cervical spine is the most commonly injured vertebral zone in children. Pain, torticollis, limitation of motion, and muscle spasm should raise suspicion of an injury to the neck. Flexion forces tend to produce more severe spinal cord injuries than extension forces.

"Spinal shock" may follow a severe spinal cord injury. This presents as a flaccid paralysis with complete loss of all reflexes. This condition can last from 8 hours to several days. The earliest evidence of recovery of cord function is the appearance of the "anal wink" (perianal sphincter) reflex, or the bulbocavernosus reflex.

1.6.2 Examination of the pelvis

In the traumatized child the pelvic ring is assessed after the spine has been evaluated. Most pediatric pelvic fractures are stable. Adequate x-rays should be obtained and CT scans may be needed to complete the evaluation.

Acetabular fractures represent approximately 6% of pelvic fractures. It is of particular importance to evaluate injury to the triradiate cartilage, as this can produce a central growth arrest resulting in acetabular dysplasia with lateral subluxation of the femoral head.

1.6.3 Examination of the extremities

The extremities must be examined systematically, one at a time, from distal to proximal. All joints are tested for a full range of motion. The bones are examined for the clinical signs

High-energy trauma is the most common cause of death in children.

In children articular and periarticular fractures always involve the physis.

Comparable x-rays of the uninjured side help to evaluate growth-plate injuries.

of a fresh fracture, which include swelling, deformity, tenderness, and abnormal motion. Care must be taken not to focus on a single obvious injury, thereby omitting the rest of the examination. Soft-tissue injuries are noted, and vascular and neurological examinations are performed. Some fractures can be present in a child with no external evidence of injury. If the child complains of pain, a fracture should be assumed and adequate splintage applied before the child is taken to the x-ray suite.

1.7　X-ray examination and other imaging

X-ray evaluation of each suspected injury must include at least two views taken at 90° to each other. Anteroposterior and lateral projections should each include both the joint above and the joint below the suspected fracture area. **Suspected non-displaced growth-plate injuries should be evaluated with comparable views of the uninjured extremity** and also "stress" x-rays under narcosis to evaluate displacement. Computed tomography is important in evaluating spine, pelvic, and some intra-articular fractures. Other studies, such as arthrograms, might be used in evaluation of growth-plate injuries, especially in the very young with unossified epiphyses. Other diagnostic methods like ultrasound, have been used for the evaluation of stress fractures, and arteriograms assist in the assessment of vascular injury if the physical examination is equivocal. The role of magnetic resonance imaging (MRI) in the care of pediatric fractures is yet clearly to be defined. It certainly has a place in the evaluation of possible avascular necrosis. For this reason, fixations in vulnerable areas, such as the proximal radius and proximal femur, should preferably make use of titanium implants, which cause less artifactual distortion on MRI.

2　Periarticular and articular fractures— general principles and classification[1]

Articular and periarticular fractures in children are injuries that inevitably involve the physis. Both the treatment and prognosis for physeal injuries depend on the pattern of the injury, for example, whether the injury involves only the physis, the physis and the metaphysis, or the physis and the epiphysis.

The most frequently used classification of physeal injury is that of Salter and Harris [6] which describes five types. It fails, however, to recognize the injuries to the zone of Ranvier at the periphery of the physis, both the ligamentous avulsion type and those caused by open abrasive trauma: Rang later proposed that these be included retrospectively in the Salter-Harris classification as type VI.

Müller has proposed a classification based upon three major divisions according to whether the physis is damaged by shearing, by fracture perpendicular to the physeal plane, or by crushing.

Both these classifications are summarized in **Fig. 5.4-2**.

A new classification for children's fractures has been proposed especially for prospective clinical studies [7]. This takes into account the possibility that displacements may be corrected as growth progresses.

[1] Presently there are other groups working on a comprehensive classification for all fractures in children.

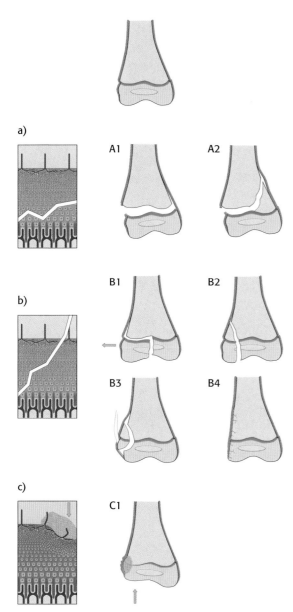

Fig. 5.4-2: Müller AO Classification of articular and periarticular fractures in children with involvement of the physeal plate; three main groups:

a) The fracture passes through the junction of the zones of hypertrophy and provisional ossification. The fracture line does not involve the growth zones. Growth disturbance is unlikely (except at the proximal femur and proximal radius), even with incomplete reduction. Deformity in the plane of motion is likely to remodel as long as growth continues.
A1: (Salter-Harris type I) This is a pure shearing injury of the physeal plate and usually results from a rotational force.
A2: (Salter-Harris type II) This is partly a shear injury of the physis and partly a metaphyseal fracture (Thurston-Holland fragment). 70% of physeal injuries are type A2.

b) The fracture line traverses the epiphysis and some, or all, of the layers of the physis. If reduction is not anatomically perfect, growth disturbance is highly likely.
B1: (Salter-Harris type III) Partial physeal separation with an intra-articular epiphyseal fracture. Open reduction with screw fixation is strongly indicated. The screw must not penetrate the physeal plate.
B2: (Salter-Harris type IV) The fracture plane passes from the joint surface through all layers of the physis and through the metaphysis. As in type B1, screw fixation is strongly indicated, using one screw in the epiphysis and one in the metaphysis, with neither crossing the growth plate.
B3: (termed by Rang the "type VI") Avulsion fracture of an insertion of a ligament, taking with it a portion of the perichondrial ring (zone of Ranvier). Accurate reduction and fixation are required, but growth disturbance can still follow.
B4 is an open abrasive injury of the periphery of the growth plate—this too often causes physeal bridging.

c) (Salter-Harris type V) There is compression of the articular surface and impaction of epiphyseal bone into metaphyseal bone, with consequent disorganization of part of the physeal cartilage. Partial growth arrest is to be expected and reconstructive procedures, such as those of Langenskiöld and Oesterman [8], are necessary later.
C1: Different degrees of impaction.

2.1   Type A
(Salter-Harris types I & II)

The fracture line does not involve the germinal zone of the physeal plate. If a proper reduction is carried out, no growth disturbance is to be anticipated, although exceptions exist.

2.2   Type B
(Salter-Harris types III & IV)

The fracture line crosses the epiphysis and the germinal zone of the physeal plate. An absolutely accurate, "watertight" reduction must be achieved, otherwise partial closure, with resultant eccentric growth disturbance, is to be anticipated. In addition, these injuries involve the articular surface and malunion can produce later joint degeneration.

At the distal femur, ligamentous avulsion of an osteochondral block spanning the edge of the physis may occur: growth arrest is likely unless perfect reduction is achieved. Open abrasive injury of the periphery of the physis, resulting in destruction of the zone of Ranvier [9], usually results in local growth arrest.

2.3   Type C
(Salter-Harris type V)

Compression of the physeal cartilage with impaction of epiphyseal bone into the metaphysis results in severe damage to the growth area and partial, or complete, closure of the epiphyseal plate with consequent growth disturbance is to be anticipated.

Ogden has proposed a most detailed and comprehensive classification, but in some ways this is not necessarily prospective, in as much as the assignment of some injuries to certain groups requires observation of the behavior of the physis over a period of time after injury.

For this reason, and because of its complexity, it has not been widely received as a "working" classification, but perhaps more as a research tool.

3   Treatment of fractures in children

3.1   Closed treatment

The majority of fractures in children and adolescents will be treated by closed reduction and casting or traction. The only way to splint and hold reduction is by applying a well-molded cast. Most fractures heal in a few weeks, and since children cannot be relied on to tell the doctor about pain, sensory alteration, circulatory disturbances, or other signs of impending complications, regular and competent clinical observation is required.

The cast should be applied only when the fracture has been satisfactorily reduced. The well-padded circular cast with three point moulding is the only splintage that is safe enough for the treatment of fractures in children. **The circulation and neurological status distal to the fracture must be checked frequently and thoroughly.**

The majority of fractures in children and adolescents will be treated by closed reduction and casting or traction.

Regular clinical checking of circulation, pain, and neurological status is mandatory after cast application.

3.2 Open treatment

Indications for surgical treatment of fractures in children include:

- Open fractures.
- Polytrauma.
- Patients with head injuries.
- Femoral fractures in adolescents.
- Femoral neck fractures.
- Certain types of forearm fractures.
- Certain types of physeal injuries.
- Fractures associated with burns.

3.3 Aims of surgical treatment

As in the adult, open fractures are surgical emergencies and must be treated aggressively to prevent infection and possible permanent disability. Tscherne and Gotzen [10] divided the management of open fractures into four priorities:

1) life preservation
2) limb preservation
3) avoidance of infection
4) preservation of function.

There are various soft-tissue classifications applicable to open fractures; please refer to **chapter 1.4** and **chapter 5.2** as well as **section 2** in this chapter.

In severe fractures the first decision is to determine whether the limb is salvageable. Grade IIIC open injuries are associated with a high amputation rate and limb salvage is often impractical in the adult. **In children, however, all efforts should be made to salvage limbs, unless all of the major nerves to the extremity are irreparably damaged.**

A thorough and aggressive débridement, comprising excision of all damaged and devitalized tissue (muscle, skin, bone, etc.) is mandatory. The wound should be irrigated copiously with Ringer lactate or Hartmann's solution both before and after débridement. Pulse lavage systems should be used with care as they have been shown to be capable of driving contamination deep into healthy tissue recesses. Pressure lavage cannot be a substitute for meticulous surgical excision of the damaged and contaminated tissue. Normal saline should be avoided as it can be cytotoxic, especially to tissues of compromised viability.

4 Types of fixation

The aim of internal fixation in children is to obtain an anatomical reduction and to maintain it using a minimum amount of metal. External splintage can be used postoperatively without the risk of fracture disease.

3.5 mm cortex screws, 4.0 mm cancellous bone screws (exceptionally 6.5 mm), and cannulated screws have been used in the treatment of periarticular and articular fractures.

K-wire fixation of epiphyseal and metaphyseal fragments is often all that is necessary for internal fixation, as the hard cancellous bone in children affords excellent purchase. **Physeal plates may, if necessary, be crossed by K-wires, but never by lag screws unless growth is nearly complete.** Transphyseal wires should be non-threaded, inserted by hand and directed, as far as possible, perpendicular to the growth plate. K-wires can be used percutaneously to maintain a reduction that cannot be held by closed methods. Multiple drilling and insertion of several K-wires at the same point must be avoided. K-wires can be left

Open fractures in children are, as in adults, surgical emergencies.

Internal fixation is intended to maintain reduction with a minimum of implants.

Growth plates may be crossed by K-wires, but not by screws.

In children limb salvage should always be attempted.

In external fixation take care not to injure the growth plate.

protruding through the skin and removed at 2–3 weeks as the bone heals rapidly. Alternatively, interfragmentary screws can be used parallel to the physeal plate, either in the metaphysis or the epiphysis, or both. This method is recommended in severely displaced epiphyseal fractures (type B) as it produces a so-called "watertight" reduction [11]. The disadvantage of screw fixation is the necessity for a second operation to remove the metal. On the other hand, the drawback of using percutaneous wires is the increased risk of infection. If growth disturbance occurs as a result of a bony tether across the physis, resection and the interposition of fat, or cold-curing bone cement, may restore normal growth [8, 12].

There is no scientific proof, that anatomical reduction of shaft fractures results in overgrowth.

External fixation devices are the preferred method for patients with open fractures, polytrauma, and fractures associated with burns. The size of the child will determine whether the large or the small fixator is used. **In the application of the external fixator great care must be exercised not to damage the growth plate** (**Fig. 5.4-3**) [13].

One-third tubular plates 3.5, or dynamic compression plates 3.5 (DCPs and LC-DCPs) are used in the forearm, and straight or T-plates 4.5, in metaphyseal areas of the distal femur, the tibia, and the humerus.

Standard closed intramedullary nailing may be used in femoral shaft fractures in adolescents. In younger children the use of elastic titanium nails (TEN), as popularized by the French school [14], is gaining more and more consideration as it is minimally invasive but still provides good fixation.

Early removal of the implants is recommended after fracture healing. **Anatomical reduction of shaft fractures has been said to increase the risk of overgrowth; this has, however, never been scientifically substantiated [4].**

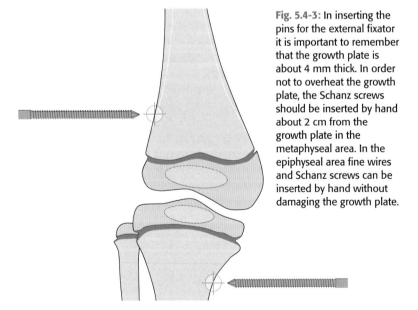

Fig. 5.4-3: In inserting the pins for the external fixator it is important to remember that the growth plate is about 4 mm thick. In order not to overheat the growth plate, the Schanz screws should be inserted by hand about 2 cm from the growth plate in the metaphyseal area. In the epiphyseal area fine wires and Schanz screws can be inserted by hand without damaging the growth plate.

5   Specific fractures

5.1   Fractures of the femur

5.1.1   Proximal femur

(Fig. 5.4-4)
Fractures of the femoral neck comprise an absolute indication for open reduction and stable internal fixation as an emergency. Immediately after the fracture, some of the retinacular vessels are usually still intact. Displacement of the fracture leads to kinking of these precious vessels, which predisposes to their occlusion and thrombosis. Additionally, the hemarthrosis may lead to a joint tamponade, which further threatens the epiphyseal vascularity.

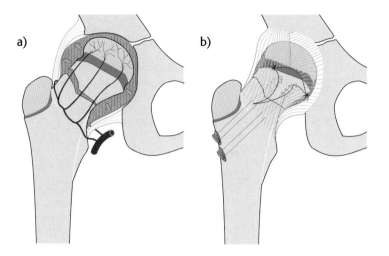

a)   b)

Fig. 5.4-4:
a) Intracapsular fractures of the neck in children result in an increase in intracapsular joint pressure ("joint tamponade") endangering any remaining blood supply to the proximal femoral epiphysis and physis. Emergency arthrotomy and open reduction are indicated.
b) Transcervical femoral fracture in a child. Two cancellous bone screws with 16 mm thread lengths (either 6.5 mm or 7.3 mm cannulated) are used. Make sure that the threads have passed fully across the fracture and that the screws do not penetrate the physis.

Femoral neck fractures require joint decompression and emergency ORIF with screws.

Stable internal fixation is achieved by inserting one or more 4.5, 6.5, or 7.0 mm (cannulated) cancellous bone screws, taking care not to cross the physis with a screw thread.

The hip capsule is exposed in the interval between the lesser glutei and tensor fasciae latae muscles and then opened by a T-shaped capsulotomy. The fracture is exposed with the aid of three small retractors. One is inserted over the anterior pelvic rim, the second very gently above the femoral neck and the third below it. Enormous care must be exercised in passing the retractors around the femoral neck, so as not to damage the retinacular vessels bound to the bone beneath the periosteum. Once reduced, the fracture is fixed temporarily with K-wires and the reduction checked, particularly at the level of the calcar, by flexing and rotating the hip. Definitive fixation is then carried out with two 4.5 or 6.5 mm cancellous bone screws, again taking care not to pierce the physis. The capsular incision is never fully closed, in order to avoid the danger of recurrent joint tamponade. The use of cannulated cancellous bone screws greatly facilitates this type of fixation. If possible, implants in the proximal femur

in children should be made of titanium, which will cause less MRI distortion than steel if avascular necrosis is to be investigated.

Nailing of these fractures is absolutely contraindicated. The cancellous bone is very hard, and in nailing, there is a great danger of driving the fragments apart and thereby tearing the retinacular vessels, which would also lead to avascular necrosis of the head.

5.1.2 Femoral shaft

In children below 6–8 years of age, fractures of the femoral shaft are usually treated non-operatively in skeletal traction. In older children femoral fractures, both diaphyseal and metaphyseal, can be treated by internal fixation with plates. This applies especially to subtrochanteric fractures (**Fig. 5.4-5**) and irreducible distal diaphyseal fractures with soft-tissue interposition, or "buttonholing" of the distal fragment through the lateral intermuscular septum [15]. Standard intramedullary nailing should be reserved for femoral shaft fractures in adolescents approaching appendicular skeletal maturity.

Nailing of femoral neck fractures is absolutely contraindicated because of the very dense cancellous bone.

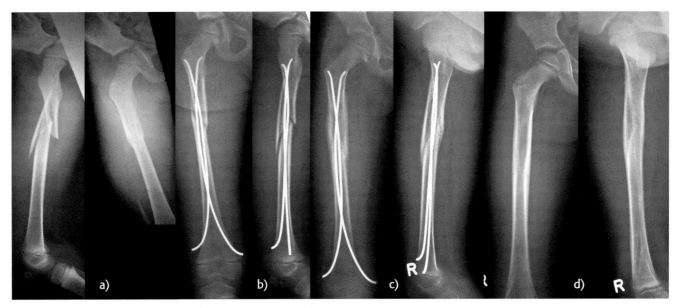

Fig. 5.4-5: a) Fully displaced, unstable, spiral, wedged subtrochanteric femoral fracture (32-B1.3) in a young adolescent. b) Treatment with elastic-stable-intramedullary nailing (ESIN): closed reduction on orthopedic table and stabilization with well prebent elastic titanium nail 3.5 (TEN). c) 8 weeks postoperative, full weight bearing after 6 weeks. d) X-ray at 6 months, after implant removal.

For the younger child, intramedullary elastic titanium nails (TENs) as described by the Nancy school [16] are available for shaft fractures. They can be inserted in a retrograde fashion from an entry point just above the distal growth plate in the distal femur. Usually two of these flexible nails can be inserted (**Fig. 5.4-6**).

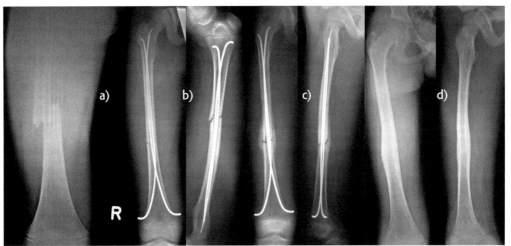

Fig. 5.4-6:
a) Displaced femoral fracture of the middle third (32-A3.2), classic indication for ESIN.
b) Postoperative x-ray after closed reduction and retrograde standard splinting.
c) 6-week follow-up with solid callus formation, full weight bearing allowed.
d) X-ray at 6 months, immediately after implant removal.

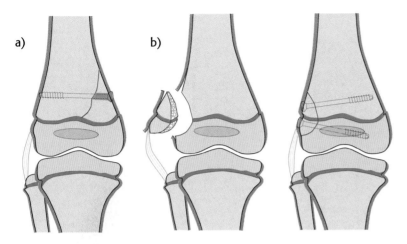

a)

b)

Fig. 5.4-7: Lag screw fixation in the distal femur with 4.5 or 7.3 mm cannulated screws.
a) Type A2 (Salter-Harris type II) fracture of the distal femur. If unstable, or irreducible, such fractures should be fixed, ensuring that the growth plate is not violated. Intraoperative image intensifier control should be used.
b) Type B3 avulsion fracture can be fixed by open reduction and internal fixation with one or two 4.0 mm cannulated lag screws if bony fragments are large enough for screw placement.

5.1.3 Distal Femur

Distal femoral fractures are mostly Salter-Harris type II (A2) separations of the epiphysis with a metaphyseal fragment. Here, satisfactory reduction is difficult both to achieve and to maintain. If the fractures cannot be reduced, or can be reduced but not retained, open reduction is needed and metaphyseal interfragmentary lag screw fixation is suggested (**Fig. 5.4-7a**). **Repeated attempts at closed reduction cause damage to the germinal cells of the growth plate, which may explain the unexpectedly high frequency of growth disturbance at the distal femur.**

Unrecognized ligament avulsion fractures may also be the cause of growth abnormalities after trauma. Avulsion fractures of the lateral collateral ligament that span the periphery of the physeal plate should be treated by means of open anatomical reduction and "watertight" internal fixation (**Fig. 5.4-7b**).

5.2 Fractures of the tibia

5.2.1 Proximal tibial growth-plate fractures

A displaced avulsion fracture of the tibial tuberosity should be treated by internal fixation. This injury usually occurs in adolescents when the physis is almost closed. Internal fixation is carried out with a tension band and/or interfragmentary cortex screws (**Fig. 5.4-8a**). If the child is young, then a wiring technique that respects the growth zone of the apophysis of the tibial tuberosity is preferred (**Fig. 5.4-8b**). **Premature growth arrest at the tibial tuberosity can cause serious, progressive genu recurvatum deformity.**

A displaced avulsion fracture of the tibial intercondylar eminence may exceptionally be treated closed by reduction in hyperextension. If perfect reduction fails, which is usually due

Repeated reduction maneuvers may explain the high incidence of growth disturbances at the distal femur.

Premature growth arrest at the tibial tuberosity can cause serious, progressive genu recurvatum deformity.

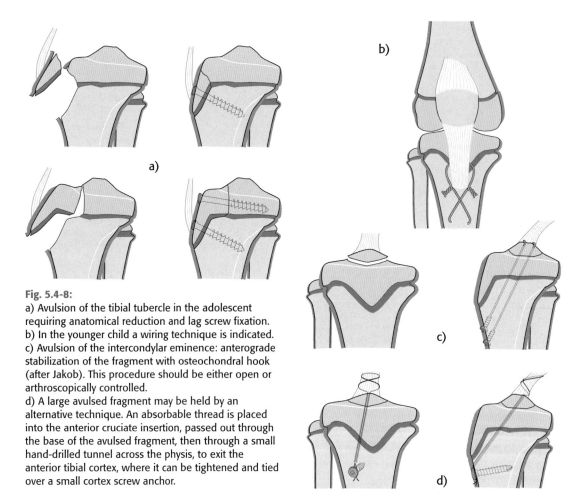

Fig. 5.4-8:
a) Avulsion of the tibial tubercle in the adolescent requiring anatomical reduction and lag screw fixation.
b) In the younger child a wiring technique is indicated.
c) Avulsion of the intercondylar eminence: anterograde stabilization of the fragment with osteochondral hook (after Jakob). This procedure should be either open or arthroscopically controlled.
d) A large avulsed fragment may be held by an alternative technique. An absorbable thread is placed into the anterior cruciate insertion, passed out through the base of the avulsed fragment, then through a small hand-drilled tunnel across the physis, to exit the anterior tibial cortex, where it can be tightened and tied over a small cortex screw anchor.

to interposition of the anterior horn of one of the menisci, there is a risk of permanent flexion deformity. Open reduction and internal fixation, using one, or even two, small cancellous bone screws, is mandatory. No screw should pierce the proximal tibial physis (**Fig. 5.4-8c**). If the avulsed fragment is thick and the intraepiphyseal screw would not gain purchase without transgressing the physis, the fragment may be held by an absorbable thread which is placed

into the anterior cruciate insertion and out through the base of the avulsed fragment. It is then passed through a small diameter tunnel drilled by hand through the bed of the fragment, across the physis, to exit the anterior tibial cortex, where it can be tightened and tied over a small cortex screw anchor. This holds the fragment in place to allow union, while the tethering suture absorbs and does not exert continued pressure across the physis (**Fig. 5.4-8d**) [1].

5.2.2 Tibial shaft fractures

The majority of fractures of the tibial shaft in children will be treated by closed means—namely reduction and casting, or traction. They can be expected to unite rapidly and so the timeframe for obtaining an acceptable position is limited.

Particular attention must be paid to the valgus fracture of the upper tibial metaphyseal area. The fracture gap is widened at the medial cortex and incomplete on the lateral side. Failure to obtain complete closure of the medial cortical gap indicates entrapment of soft tissue—periosteum, or fibers of the origin of the medial collateral ligament, and/or fibres of the pes anserinus. If any one of these is left in the fracture gap, there is a risk of progressive valgus deformity, the remodeling of which is variable and unpredictable. Through a very limited surgical exposure, entrapped tissue must be removed from the fracture gap. The reduction is completed and a suitably moulded long-leg cast is then applied [17, 18].

Under certain circumstances, surgical stabilization is required. **These indications include open fractures, closed fractures with major soft-tissue contusion and crushing, fractures associated with major vascular or nerve injury, where compartment syndrome has required fasciotomy, and uncontrollable displacement (especially shortening).**

In some fractures of the lower tibial shaft with an intact fibula, there is a marked tendency to varus malalignment. In case of failure to control this with closed reduction and casting, surgical fixation should be considered. One cause for the tendency to drift into varus is the positioning of the foot at a right angle, whereby the wider anterior portion of the talus is pressed against the medial malleolus and tilts the broken tibia into varus. The proposed solution is to cast the fracture with the foot in a slight equinus.

When the decision is made to surgically stabilize a child's tibial shaft fracture, the selection of technique is relatively straightforward. In open fractures, external fixation is the treatment of choice. In injuries where the fracture focus has to be surgically exposed—for example, with multiple fasciotomies, or where vessels need exploration, as well as in relatively distal or proximal fractures—plating is preferable. Whether plates 3.5 or 4.5 are used depends on the size of the bone.

Although standard intramedullary nailing is prohibited by the need to respect the proximal tibial growth zones, the use of elastic titanium rods [14] in fractures of the middle third of the diaphysis is a useful option in skilled hands with the appropriate resources.

5.2.3 Distal tibial growth-plate fractures

Displaced fractures of the type A2 (Salter-Harris type II) may be difficult to reduce closed as a periosteal flap may become entrapped in the metaphyseal fracture gap.

Open reduction with internal fixation is indicated when the fracture line crosses the epiphysis and the physeal plate, with or without fracture of the metaphysis, and remains displaced. Persisting articular incongruity is also an indication for surgery. For these fractures, interfragmentary lag screw fixation is preferable, rather than simple K-wire fixation, to achieve a perfect anatomical reduction of both the physeal lesion and the joint surface (**Fig. 5.4-9a–c**).

The triplane fracture (**Fig. 5.4-9d**) is unique to the ankle. This is a complex injury involving

Most closed tibial shaft fractures in children are the domain of non-operative treatment.

Exceptional indications for surgical stabilization in tibial fractures are:
- open fracture,
- severe closed soft-tissue injury,
- compartment syndrome,
- gross displacement/ shortening,
- varus malalignment.

Ankle fractures frequently require ORIF with small fragment implants to restore anatomy.

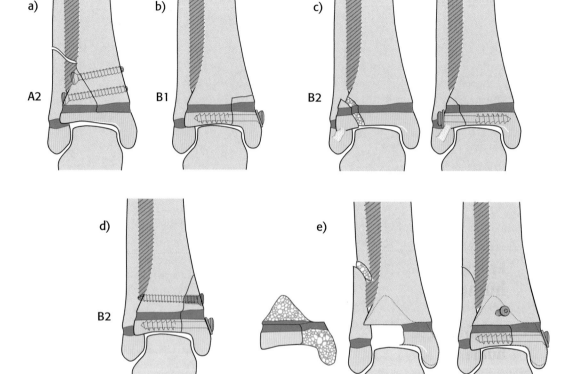

Fig. 5.4-9:
Ankle injuries.
a) Salter-Harris type II (A2) injury can be stabilized with one to two cannulated cancellous bone screws across the metaphyseal fracture.
b) Salter-Harris type III (B1) fracture of the medial malleolus after anatomical reduction and fixation with a 4.0 mm cancellous bone screw totally within the epiphysis.
c) Salter-Harris type IV (B2) of the tubercle of Tillaux fixed using intraepiphyseal lag screw. Type IV injuries are typically fixed, after open reduction, with a lag screw across the metaphyseal fracture and another in the epiphysis.
d) Type IV (B2) injury fixed using two screws, one each above and below the growth plate, for "watertight" adaptation.
e) The triplane fracture has a complex configuration and various forms. The lag screws, metaphyseal or epiphyseal, must be correctly placed, respecting the fracture planes. Additional stabilization of the fibula is usually not necessary in children.

the distal tibial epiphysis, physeal plate, and metaphysis. The most frequent variety consists of a vertical sagittal and coronal fracture plane through the epiphysis, a horizontal shear injury of the physeal plate, and a vertical coronal fracture plane separating a posterior metaphyseal fragment. This pattern, if displaced, will usually require open reduction and internal fixation to reconstruct the articular surface [19]. CT scanning with 3-D reconstruction has revolutionized the understanding of the pathoanatomy of these fractures and is essential for the careful preoperative planning that is needed.

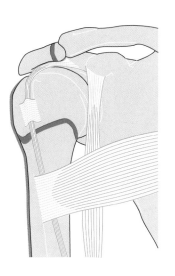 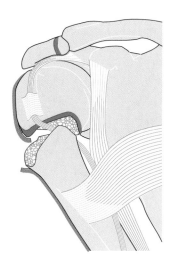 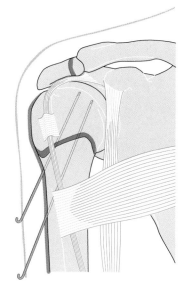

Fig. 5.4-10:
Proximal humeral physeal separation with deforming forces inducing adduction and extension.
Considerable deformity can be accepted, but in older children with soft-tissue interposition (biceps tendon) open reduction and transcutaneous K-wire fixation may be required.

5.3 Fractures of the humerus

5.3.1 Proximal humerus and humeral shaft

Malunion in relation to fractures involving the proximal humeral physis has a greater capacity to remodel with subsequent growth than at any other anatomical site. **Most fractures of the proximal humerus and of the humeral shaft can be treated non-operatively** in a sling or occasionally in skeletal traction for 2–3 weeks. Olecranon traction using a screw rather than a transolecranon pin, produces fewer complications (infection, early and late ulnar palsy, etc.). Occasionally, a proximal physeal plate separation has to be operated on because it cannot be reduced (e.g., due to interposition of the tendon of the long head of the biceps), or because a patient is close to skeletal maturity and the deformity cannot be expected to remodel (**Fig. 5.4-10**).

5.3.2 Distal humerus

In children's elbow fractures, comparative x-rays of both sides are necessary. Displaced supracondylar fractures of the humerus may be treated non-operatively by reduction under general anesthesia and immobilization in flexion in a cast. If after reduction stability of the fracture can only be achieved in extreme flexion (with the danger of ischemia and compartment syndrome), then either olecranon screw traction, or closed anatomical reduction followed by percutaneous or open K-wire fixation, is advisable, in order to maintain the reduction (**Fig. 5.4-11a**). Fractures which can only be partially reduced can alternatively be treated with overhead screw traction, applied just distal to the olecranon at the level of the coronoid process, for up to 10 days, until the

Most fractures of the proximal humerus and of the humeral shaft can be treated non-operatively.

Fig. 5.4-11:
a) Percutaneous K-wire fixation of supracondylar fracture of the humerus after closed reduction. Wires are removed after 2–3 weeks. Be aware of the ulnar nerve during percutaneous wire placement.

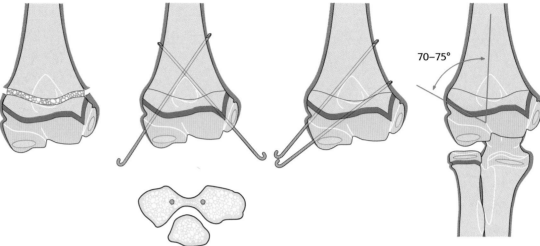

b) After reduction and fixation, Baumann's angle should be equal to that of the uninjured side (usually in the range 70–75°). Baumann's angle is the angle between the lateral condylar physis and the long axis of the humerus shaft. More than 75° usually denotes varus malposition. Correct rotational alignment is best judged on a lateral view.

c) Lateral condylar fracture of the distal humerus. If the metaphyseal fragment is large enough, a metaphyseal lag screw can be inserted via a posterolateral approach.

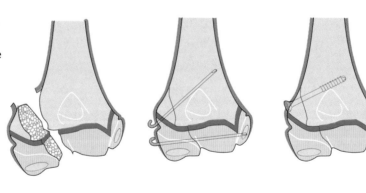

d) Apophyseal injury to the medial epicondyle of the distal humerus. K-wires or (less frequently) a figure-of-eight wire loop are used in younger children, but in the near mature child a screw should be used. Great care is needed to ensure a smooth surface over which the ulnar nerve will lie.

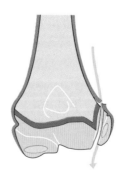
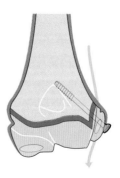
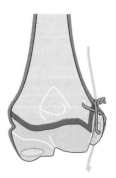

fracture site is no longer tender; a sling is then used for a further 2–3 weeks [20].

Open reduction is indicated only if the fracture is irreducible, implying soft-tissue interposition, or if it is associated with a vascular or nerve injury [21]. For open reduction, the surgical approach can be lateral, bilateral, or posterior, depending on the nature and site of any associated neurovascular lesion. If cubitus varus is to be avoided, particular attention must be paid to the restoration of the correct angle between the physeal plane of the lateral humeral condyle and the long axis of the shaft (Baumann's angle, **Fig. 5.4-11b**). This angle must be approximately 70–75° and should always be comparable to the angle on the uninjured side.

Displaced fractures of the lateral condyle are Salter-Harris type IV (B2) injuries. These intra-articular and epiphyseal fractures are usually treated by open reduction and screw, or K-wire, fixation: the wires should be removed after 2–3 weeks. Associated dislocation, or subluxation, of the elbow constitutes an absolute indication for surgical fixation, preferably with a screw (**Fig. 5.4-11c**). The easiest surgical approach for this procedure is from posterolateral, skirting the lateral border of the triceps tendon; this affords an excellent view of the joint fracture and direct access to the posterolateral metaphyseal fragment. This approach has been said to threaten the vascularity of the fragment, but as long as the metaphyseal fragment is not denuded of soft tissue, there is no risk.

Occasionally, cubitus varus can also result from capitellar overgrowth following this fracture, and cubitus valgus, with the danger of tardy ulnar palsy, may follow malreduction, or non-union.

Fractures of the medial condyle of the Salter-Harris type IV are less common than lateral condylar injuries. They are then associated with elbow instability. The principles of their management are the same as for the lateral injury.

Very occasionally a Y-shaped intercondylar fracture can occur in a child, which is analogous to the simultaneous occurrence of Salter-Harris type IV injuries of both medial and lateral condyles. **Perfect alignment of the physeal plate is absolutely essential** and may require compression screw fixation of the metaphyseal components, combined with K-wire stabilization of the epiphyseal mass. It is best dealt with via a posterior approach. This fracture carries a high risk of growth disturbance and should only be treated by those surgeons with great experience of complex physeal trauma.

Fragments of the apophysis of the medial epicondyle that have separated with valgus trauma to the elbow may become entrapped in the joint. Although this fracture may not be a true physeal injury, it does carry the risk of non-union, irritation of the ulnar nerve and instability. Tension band fixation, or screw fixation in the older child, is advised in place of K-wires alone (**Fig. 5.4-11d**). Union of such a fracture in malposition with distal displacement is usually associated with significant loss of elbow function, which can be permanent.

5.4 Fractures of the forearm

5.4.1 Proximal forearm, radial head, and neck

The epiphysis of the radial head is rarely fractured. If it is, then a B2 or Salter-Harris type IV injury has occurred and, if there is displacement, operative stabilization is mandatory to avoid premature growth arrest.

Perfect alignment of the physeal plate is absolutely essential, and may require operative stabilization.

Separation of the radial head, for example, radial neck injury, may be A1 or A2 (Salter-Harris type I or II), or a metaphyseal torus (wrinkle) fracture.

The vascular anatomy of the proximal radius sets it apart from other epiphyses (with the exception of the proximal femur), as it has no soft-tissue attachments and is totally covered by articular cartilage, receiving its blood supply from the metaphyseal circulation, via retinacular vessels tightly bound to the neck and the periphery of the physis by periosteum and perichondrium. In consequence, **a type A1 (Salter-Harris type I) separation carries a very high risk of premature physeal plate closure due to avascular necrosis of the epiphysis.** On the other hand, a type A2 (Salter-Harris type II) radial neck injury preserves those epiphyseal retinacular vessels associated with the attached metaphyseal fragment and, provided that the soft-tissue attachments of this fragment are preserved, normal growth can continue. The distinction between the two types is paramount in planning treatment and predicting the outcome.

In general, in children under the age of about 8 years, a radial head tilt (always into valgus) of up to 40° can be accepted, but above that age only tilting of 20° or less can be left unreduced.

One gentle attempt of closed manipulation is permitted. Failure to reduce to within the acceptable range is an indication for open reduction, which should be undertaken through an anterior Henry approach, not a lateral incision.

Fixation is provided by means of a K-wire inserted from below, supplemented by plaster splintage for 3 weeks (**Fig. 5.4-12**).

An alternative method of surgical reduction and fixation has been proposed by Métaizeau

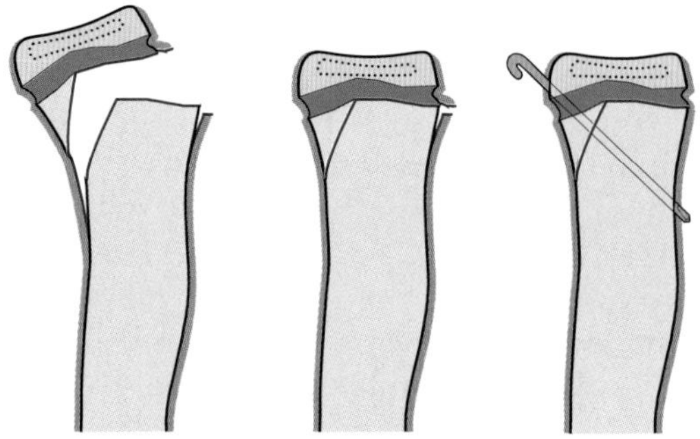

Due to the local vascular anatomy, an A1 injury to the radial head physis carries a high risk of avascular necrosis (AVN).

In Monteggia fractures anatomical reduction of the ulna usually reduces the radial head dislocation.

Fig. 5.4-12: Radial head and radial neck fractures
Angulation of the radial neck is acceptable up to 40° in the very young, up to 20° in children over 8 years of age. A gentle reduction by digital pressure is recommended, but if it fails, careful open reduction via a modified anterior Henry approach and K-wire fixation are indicated.

[22], whereby a blunt probe or elastic titanium nail (TEN) with a cranked tip is used percutaneously to nudge the radial head into an improved position by rotating the angled tip (**Fig. 5.4-13**).

5.4.2 Monteggia injuries

If in Monteggia fractures anatomical reduction of the ulna and radial head dislocation cannot be obtained or maintained by closed means, open reduction and internal fixation of the ulna becomes mandatory. Fixation by plate or nail of the ulnar fracture is recommended and leads to successful closed reduction of the radial head (**Fig. 5.4-14**). As the mechanism of this injury is one of hyperpronation of the forearm, the radial head is usually found to be stable in full supination, once the ulnar fracture has been fixed. The forearm should be immobilized in this position in a long-arm cast for 3–4 weeks.

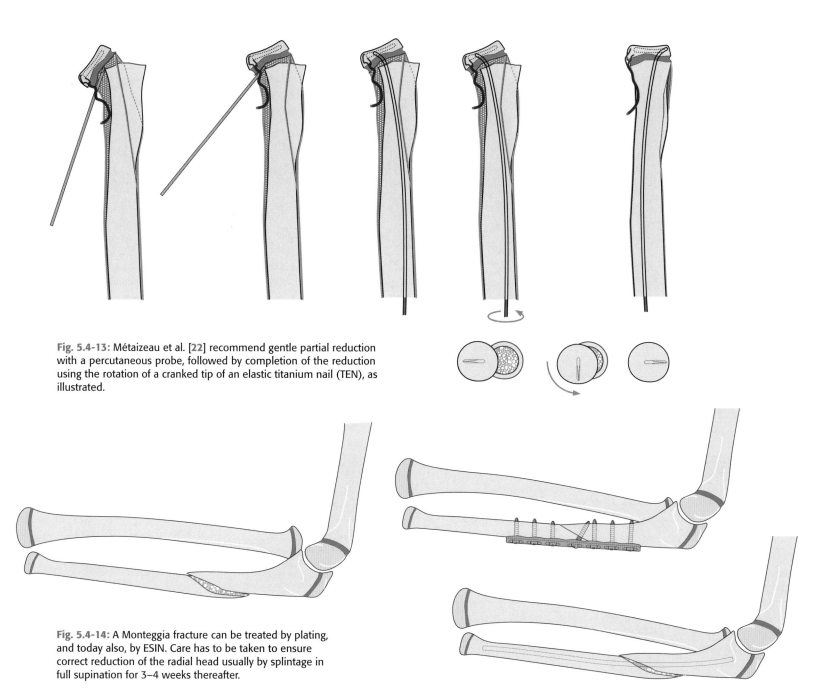

Fig. 5.4-13: Métaizeau et al. [22] recommend gentle partial reduction with a percutaneous probe, followed by completion of the reduction using the rotation of a cranked tip of an elastic titanium nail (TEN), as illustrated.

Fig. 5.4-14: A Monteggia fracture can be treated by plating, and today also, by ESIN. Care has to be taken to ensure correct reduction of the radial head usually by splintage in full supination for 3–4 weeks thereafter.

5.4.3   Forearm shaft fractures

Shaft fractures of the forearm bones in children under 10 years of age can almost always be treated non-operatively. The physiological bowing of the radius and ulna has to be restored to prevent limitation of pronation and supination. In the older child, poorly reduced forearm fractures are an indication for open reduction and plate fixation (**Fig. 5.4-15**) or the use of elastic medullary wiring [14]. In general, **displaced diaphyseal fractures of the forearm bones in children of 10 years of age or over, should be managed as in the adult by ORIF [23].**

Displaced forearm fractures in children over 10 years should be managed as in the adult by ORIF.

5.5   Multiple trauma in the injured child

Nearly 22 million children are injured every year in the United States, representing one out of every three children. Children with multiple trauma can rapidly decompensate and develop serious life-threatening complications. These patients should be transferred at an early stage to a pediatric facility capable of managing such injuries.

While open fractures and deformities might be more obvious, it must always be borne in

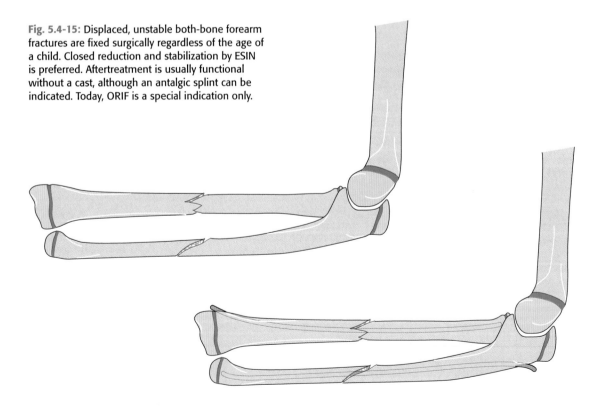

Fig. 5.4-15: Displaced, unstable both-bone forearm fractures are fixed surgically regardless of the age of a child. Closed reduction and stabilization by ESIN is preferred. Aftertreatment is usually functional without a cast, although an antalgic splint can be indicated. Today, ORIF is a special indication only.

mind that severe trauma often results in injury to areas other than the musculoskeletal system.

The priorities of assessment and management are the same as in the adult, securing the airway, breathing, and circulation, and reserving the musculoskeletal evaluation for the secondary survey, according to the ATLS principles.

Due to their size and shape, children require special consideration. When a child gets hurt, the energy imparted from fenders, bumpers, and the instant deceleration of falls results in a greater transmitted force per unit of body area than in the adult. This results in a high incidence of multiple organ injuries in the pediatric population.

In the management of fractures, early and accurate reduction with stable fixation is the "gold standard". **Many fractures that as single injuries would respond well to closed treatment, demand surgical fixation in polytrauma,** just as in the adult (see **chapter 5.3**). Marcus et al. **[24]** have demonstrated that early osteosynthesis of fractures in the child with multiple system injuries decreases hospital stay, intensive care time, and the period of ventilator dependency. It also greatly mitigates the distress felt not only by the child and its family, but also to those delivering the care.

The techniques employed are those used for single injuries, although external fixation may be preferable in certain instances by virtue of its speed of application and ease of later removal after fracture healing.

6 Bibliography

1. **Ogden JA** (1990) *Skeletal Injury in the Child*. Philadelphia: W.B. Saunders Co.
2. **Hunziker EB, Schenk RK** (1989) Physiological mechanisms adopted by chondrocytes in regulating longitudinal bone growth in rats. *J Physiol (Lond)*; 414:55–71.
3. **Weber BG, Brunner C, Frueler F** (1980) *Treatment of Fractures in Children and Adolescents*. Berlin Heidelberg New York: Springer-Verlag.
4. **von Laer L** (1991) *Frakturen und Luxationen im Wachstumsalter*. Stuttgart - New York: Georg Thieme Verlag.
5. **Mann CD, Rajimaira S** (1990) Distribution of physeal and nonphyseal fractures in 2,650 long-bone fractures in children aged 0–16 years. *J Pediatric Orthop*; 10 (6):713–716.
6. **Salter RB, Harris WR** (1963) Injuries involving the epipheal plate. *J Bone Joint Surg [Am]*; 45:857.
7. **von Laer L, Gruber R, Dallek M, et al.** (2000) Classification and Documentation of Children's Fractures. *Eur J Trauma;* 26 (1):2–14.
8. **Langenskiöld A, Oestermann K** (1983) Surgical Elimination of Posttraumatic Partial Fusion of the Growth Plate. In: Houton G, Thompson G, editors. *Problematic Musculoskeletal Injuries in Children*. London: Butterworth.
9. **Rang M** (1983) *Children's Fractures*. 2nd ed. Philadelphia: Lippincott – Raven.
10. **Tscherne H** (1984) In: Tscherne H, Gotzen L, editors. *Fractures with Soft Tissue Injuries*. Berlin: Springer-Verlag.

In multiple trauma the priorities of assessment and management are the same as in the adult, with special consideration of size and shape of the child.

In polytrauma most fractures should be stabilized surgically— preferably by external fixation.

11. **Gomes LS, Volpon JB** (1993)
    Experimental physeal fracture-
    separations treated with rigid internal
    fixation. *J Bone Joint Surg [Am]*;
    75 (12):1756–1764.

12. **Peterson HA** (1990) Loell and Winter's
    Pediatric Orthopaedics. In: Morrisy RT,
    editor. *Partial growth arrest*. 3rd ed.
    Philadelphia: Lippincott – Raven.

13. **Alonso JE, Horowitz M** (1987) Use of
    the AO/ASIF external fixator in children.
    J Pediatr Orthop; 7 (5):594–600.

14. **Prevot J, Lascombes P, Ligier JN**
    (1993) [The ECMES (Centro-Medullary
    Elastic Stabilising Wiring) osteosynthesis
    method in limb fractures in children.
    Principle, application on the femur.
    Apropos of 250 fractures followed-up
    since 1979]. *Chirurgie*; 119 (9):473–476.

15. **Foy MA, Colton CL** (1990)
    'Buttonholed' femoral shaft fracture in
    adolescents: an indication for internal
    fixation? *Injury*; 21 (6):382–384.

16. **Brouwer KJ** (1981) Torsional
    deformities after fractures of the femoral
    shaft in childhood. A retrospective study,
    27–32 years after trauma. *Acta Orthop
    Scand Suppl*; 195:1–167.

17. **Jordan SE, Alonso JE, Cook FF** (1987)
    The etiology of valgus angulation after
    metaphyseal fractures of the tibia in
    children. *J Pediatric Orthop*; 7 (4):450–457.

18. **Weber BG** (1977) Fibrous interposition
    causing valgus deformity after fracture of
    the upper tibial metaphysis in children.
    J Bone Joint Surg [Br]; 59 (3):290–292.

19. **Tinnemans JGM, Severijnen RS**
    (1975) The triplane fracture of the distal
    tibial epiphysis in children. *Injury*;
    12 (5):393–396.

20. **Worlock PH, Colton C** (1987) Severely
    displaced supracondylar fractures of the
    humerus in children: a simple method of
    treatment. *J Pediatr Orthop*; 7 (1):49–53.

21. **Broudy AS, Jupiter J, May JW, Jr.**
    (1979) Management of supracondylar
    fracture with brachial artery thrombosis
    in a child: case report and literature
    review. *J Trauma*; 19 (7):540–543.

22. **Métaizeau JP, Lascombes P, Lemelle JL,
    et al.** (1993) Reduction and fixation of
    displaced radial neck fractures by closed
    intramedullary pinning. *J Pediatr Orthop*;
    13 (3):355–360.

23. **Kay S, Smith C, Oppenheim WL**
    (1986) Both-bone midshaft forearm
    fractures in children. *J Pediatr Orthop*;
    6 (3):306–310.

24. **Marcus RE, Mius MF** (1983) Multiple
    injury in children.
    J Bone Joint Surg [Am]; 65 (9):1290–1294.

7 Updates

Updates and additional references for this chapter
are available online at:
http://www.aopublishing.org/PFxM/54.htm

5.5 Antibiotic prophylaxis

Werner Zimmerli

1 Introduction

Despite applying aseptic principles to the practice of surgery, surgical site infections still occur, not only after open fractures, but also after clean surgical procedures such as internal fixation of closed fractures or arthroplasties. **Antimicrobial prophylaxis is mainly indicated in procedures associated with a high rate of infection,** such as clean-contaminated or contaminated operations [1]. The criteria for a clean surgical wound include:
- The elective performance of the procedure (i.e., not emergency): Primary wound closure.
- The absence of acute inflammation.
- No break in aseptic technique.
- The absence of transection of colonized surfaces.

The infection rate of clean surgery among 47,000 procedures was shown to be 1.5% [2]. In such surgery, antibiotic prophylaxis is generally not indicated, because it is not cost-efficient. **However, perioperative prophylaxis has become standard practice in surgery using implants [3].**

The role of foreign material in potentiating wound infection was first demonstrated by Elek and Conen [4]. They demonstrated that in the presence of suture material a 10,000-fold lower innoculum of *Staphylococcus (S) aureus* led to skin abscesses in human volunteers. Zimmerli et al. [5, 6] confirmed the infection-potentiating effect of implant material in an animal model, and explained it as a locally acquired defect of granulocytes.

Prophylaxis of surgical site infection depends not only on appropriate antibiotic prophylaxis, but also on appropriate surgical management, proper awareness, and possible avoidance of the risk factors summarized in **Table 5.5-1**. **Antibiotic prophylaxis should not distract surgeons from careful aseptic surgery and avoidance of risk factors.** The quality standard for antimicrobial prophylaxis in surgical procedures has recently been published by an expert group from the US [7]. According to these experts, in orthopedic procedures with hardware insertion, parenteral antimicrobial prophylaxis should be administered.

Antimicrobial prophylaxis is mainly indicated in procedures associated with a high risk of infection.

Antibiotic prophylaxis is not a substitute for careful surgical technique.

Perioperative prophylaxis is standard for implant surgery.

Table 5.5-1: Risk factors for surgical site infections.

Host-related	Procedure-related
• High age	• Early preoperative hair removal
• Comorbidity (diabetes mellitus, obesity, inflammatory arthritis in joint replacement, malnutrition, malignoma)	• Shaving vs. hair clipping
• Drugs (steroids and other immunosuppressive or cytotoxic drugs, previous antibiotics)	• Lengthy surgical procedure
• Preoperative hospitalization	• Traumatic or unfamiliar surgical technique (hematoma, devitalized tissue, dead space, electrocautery, etc.)
• Remote infection	• Prolonged drainage
• Nasal carriage of *S aureus*	• Emergency procedure

The risk of infection varies according to the type of fracture and the surgical procedure. Patients undergoing joint replacement, or with closed fractures, have an infection rate between 0–5%. Those with open fractures have a rate between 5% (type 1) and > 50% (type 3A–C) [8]. In type 3 open fractures there is extensive soft-tissue damage. In this situation, surgery takes place in a heavily contaminated field. Therefore, short-term empirical treatment, and not prophylaxis, should be performed.

Staphylococci are the predominant infecting agents in implant surgery.

In fracture surgery, coagulase-negative staphylococci are less important than in joint replacement procedures.

2 Microbiology of bone-device-associated infections

The microbiology of prosthetic joint infections is well known. As in other types of device-associated infections, staphylococci are the predominating infecting agents. This is mainly due to two factors, namely (a) to their presence in the skin flora even at lower layers which are not reached by skin disinfection, and (b) to the host proteins, such as fibrin and fibronectin, which mediate adherence of staphylococci to foreign bodies [9]. In the series of 1,033 prosthetic joint infections from the Mayo Clinic, Steckelberg and Osmon [10] reported that:

- 25% were due to coagulase-negative staphylococci,
- 23% to *S aureus*,
- 11% to gram-negative bacilli,
- 8% to streptococci,
- 6% to anaerobes,
- 3% to enterococci, and
- 2% to other microorganisms.

Fourteen percent of the infections were polymicrobial, and in 8% no microorganism was detected.

In fracture surgery, coagulase-negative staphylococci are less important than in joint replacement procedures. *S aureus* largely predominates compared to other microorganisms. In the study of Boxma et al. [11], in the placebo group of patients with closed fracture, *S aureus* was found in 64%, coagulase-negative staphylococci in only 3%, streptococci in 8%, mixed gram-positive cocci in 5%, gram-negative bacilli in 6%, mixed gram-positive/gram-negative microorganisms in 8%, and mixed aerobic/anaerobic bacteria in 5% of the cases.

3 Selection of the appropriate antimicrobial drugs for prophylaxis

Various antimicrobial agents have been shown to be effective in perioperative prophylaxis. The drug should be active against the most common infecting agents involved in implant-associated bone infection. This spectrum is well known (as mentioned before); however, the susceptibility of these microorganisms may differ in various centers. Therefore, each hospital needs its up-to-date analysis of the resistance pattern of surgical site isolates. Another prerequisite for a drug used in antimicrobial prophylaxis is that its risk of toxic and allergic reactions should be minimal. Antimicrobial agents with a high potency to select resistant strains, such as cefoxitin or ceftazidim, which are strong β-lactam inducers, should be avoided. In case of otherwise identical quality of several substances, costs should also be considered in the choice of the prophylactic agents.

In fracture and orthopedic surgery, a rational choice is a first-generation or second-generation cephalosporin, such as cefazolin, cefamandole, or cefuroxime. If the patient is allergic to cephalosporins, or in settings with high prevalence of methicillin-resistant *S aureus*, vancomycin is an alternative option. In contrast, even in centres with high prevalence of methicillin-resistant coagulase-negative staphylococci, vancomycin should not be used. This is based on two arguments. First, cefamandole may be prophylactically active against methicillin-resistant coagulase-negative staphylococci [12]; and second, in the CDC recommendations for preventing the spread of vancomycin resistance, the use of glycopeptides in routine surgical prophylaxis is clearly discouraged [13].

4 Correct timing of prophylaxis

In order to get an optimal efficacy by the prophylactic agent, inhibitory antimicrobial tissue levels must be achieved at the time of incision and during the whole procedure. In the pioneer animal study of Burke [14], a very short period of prophylactic efficacy of 3 hours has been observed. **Even a 1 hour delay markedly decreased the efficacy of single-dose prophylaxis.** These animal data have been confirmed with a large retrospective clinical study [15]. In this study on 2,847 wounds, the risk of surgical site infection increased six-fold when prophylaxis was given either too early (> 2 hours before surgery) or too late (> 3 hours after surgery). Based on these studies, parenteral perioperative prophylaxis should be administered intravenously during the period beginning 60 minutes before incision [7]. **Administration up to the time of incision, or as close as possible to that time is to be preferred.**

When a tourniquet is used, antibiotic tissue levels are insufficient if the drug application is delayed to less than 5 minutes before inflation [16]. In another study the critical interval was

Various antimicrobial agents have been shown to be effective in perioperative prophylaxis.

Even a 1 hour delay markedly decreased the efficacy of single-dose prophylaxis.

Administration as close as possible to the time of incision is best.

Prophylactic antibiotics lower the incidence of infection in orthopedic surgery, if compared to placebo.

10 minutes and longer [17]. Consequently, for adequate prophylaxis antibiotics should be given at least 10 minutes before the tourniquet is inflated.

5 Review of controlled studies of prophylaxis in fracture and orthopedic surgery

There are only a few placebo-controlled studies dealing with antimicrobial prophylaxis of device-associated infections. Because each deep infection has devastating consequences, many studies have been ended prematurely. Nevertheless, the available information is clear enough to allow evaluation of the role of antibiotic prophylaxis in fracture and orthopedic surgery.

Table 5.5-2 summarizes the results of five placebo-controlled studies with a total of 4,728 patients [11, 18–21]. In four out of five studies **the infection rate of patients with antibiotics was significantly lower than in the placebo group,** whether the procedure was an arthroplasty or an internal fixation. The only study without a significant result was too small to show a significant difference [21]. The infection rates with a cephalosporin prophylaxis were 0.9–3.6%, as compared to 3.3–8.3% with placebo. According to these data, antibiotic prophylaxis is clearly indicated in fracture and orthopedic surgery.

In these studies, different regimens were used in the active arm, from first-generation to third-generation cephalosporins, and from single-dose to 5-day prophylaxis. Consequently, further studies were performed, comparing different antibiotics or different treatment

Table 5.5-2: Prospective, placebo-controlled trials of antimicrobial prophylaxis in fracture and orthopedic surgery.

Procedure	Infection rate		p-value	Reference
	Placebo	Active drug (duration)		
Hip replacement	35/1,067 = 3.3%	10/1,070 = 0.9% Cefazolin (5 days)	0.001	Hill et al. 1981 [18]
Different fixation devices	11/150 = 7.3%	2/134 = 1.5% Cefamandole (1 day)	< 0.05	Gatell et al. 1984 [19]
Dynamic hip screw	6/115 = 5%	1/124 = 1% Cefotiam (1 day)	< 0.05	Bodoky et al. 1993 [20]
Internal fixation of ankle fracture (with tourniquet)	3/62 = 4.8%	1/60 = 1.7% Cephalotin (1 day)	0.33	Paiement et al. 1994 [21]
Various internal fixation devices	79/956 = 8.3%	36/990 = 3.6% Ceftriaxone (single dose)	0.001	Boxma et al. 1996 [11]

duration. **Table 5.5-3** summarizes five controlled studies with a total of 4,918 patients comparing a short versus a long-duration regimen [22–26]. Prophylaxis beyond 1 day was not superior to the short course. However, in the study of Gatell et al. [23], a 1-day course of cefamandole resulted in a significantly lower infection rate than a single dose. In another study with cefuroxime, the 1-day prophylaxis resulted in a 46% reduction of joint infection compared to a single dose in a total of 2,651 patients [24]. Despite the large study population, this difference was not significant (p = 0.17) due to the low infection rate in both prophylaxis groups. From these studies, it can be concluded that **the duration of prophylaxis should not exceed 1 day, and that one-day prophylaxis should be preferred to a single dose in centers with high infection rates.**

In patients with open fractures, there are only a few controlled studies [27–29]. In these studies pre-emptive therapy, not prophylaxis, was performed, i.e., the duration of "prophylaxis" was 10 days. In the study of Patzakis et al. [27] the infection rate after open fractures was 11/79 (14%) in the control-arm, 9/91 (10%)

The duration of antibiotic prophylaxis should as a rule not exceed 1 day.

Table 5.5-3: Prospective trials of antimicrobial prophylaxis with active control in fracture and orthopedic surgery.

| Procedure | Infection rate | | Statistical analysis | Reference |
	Short regimen (duration)	Long regimen (duration)		
Hip and knee replacement, hip repair	Cefazolin (1 day) 3/186 = 1.6%	Cefazolin (7 days) 4/172 = 2.3%	NS*	Nelson et al. 1983 [22]
• Moore prosthesis • Other fixation devices	Cefamandole (single dose) 5/76 = 6.6% 15/306 = 5%	Cefamandole (1 day) 0/74 = 0% 3/261 = 1%	0.03 0.006	Gatell et al. 1987 [23]
Hip replacement	Cefuroxime (single dose) 11/1,327 = 0.83%	Cefuroxime (1 day) 6/1,324 = 0.45%	NS (p = 0.17)	Wymenga et al. 1992 [24]
• Hip replacement • Knee replacement	Cefuroxime (single dose) 1/187 = 0.5% 1/178 = 0.6%	Cefazolin (3 days) 2/168 = 1.2% 3/207 = 1.4%	NS NS	Mauerhan et al. 1994 [25]
Hip repair fixation devices	Cefuroxime (1 day) 6/210 = 3%	Cefadroxil (1 day p.os) 1/242 = 0.4%	NS (p = 0.07)	Nungu et al. 1995 [26]

* NS: not significant (p > 0.05)

in the penicillin/streptomycin-arm, and 2/84 (2%) in the cephalothin-arm. The reduction in the cephalothin-arm was significant (p < 0.03). However, in this study the overall infection rate was low with 9%, suggesting that only a few grade III open fractures were included. In all three studies a significant reduction of the infection rate was observed, indicating that in internal fixation of open fractures pre-emptive therapy with a first-generation or second-generation cephalosporin during 5–10 days is legitimate [27–29]. Unfortunately, there are no studies on the optimal duration of such a therapy. In addition, it is not clear whether a 1-day prophylaxis would be adequate for grade I and II open fractures. In our institution, a 5-day pre-emptive therapy with amoxicillin/clavulanic acid is only performed in patients with grade III open fractures, whereas a 1-day prophylaxis with cefuroxime is used in all other types of fracture surgery.

Quinolones should not be used in prophylaxis.

6 Controversial issues

There is little evidence to suggest that newer antimicrobial agents with a broader in-vitro antibacterial spectrum have any advantage compared to cephalosporins with narrower spectra. It should be the rule to choose as narrow a spectrum as possible. **Newer antibiotics should be reserved for treatment.** An excellent recent study by Boxma et al. [11] breaks this rule by using ceftriaxone, a third-generation cephalosporin. Compared to the different regimens with older cephalosporins, this agent has no advantage, except for the fact that it results in efficacious tissue levels during 24 hours, thus providing 1-day coverage as single dose. However, we prefer the use of a second-generation

Newer antibiotics should be reserved for treatment.

cephalosporin (e.g., cefuroxime or cefamandole), which can be given as single dose in centers with low infection rates and in three doses in centers with high or unknown rate of infection.

Up to now, quinolones have not been used in surgical prophylaxis. There is a danger that new quinolones with better activity against gram-positive cocci (e.g., sparfloxacin, trovafloxacin, levofloxacin) will be introduced in surgical prophylaxis. However, **quinolones should not be used in prophylaxis**, because of the rapid emergence of resistant staphylococci [30]. In addition, quinolones combined with rifampin are important drugs in the treatment of device-associated infection and should, therefore, be strictly avoided in prophylaxis [30].

Another controversial issue is the use of vancomycin in prophylaxis. For the reasons mentioned above (emergence of vancomycin-resistant enterococci), it should be strictly reserved for centers with a high prevalence of methicillin-resistant *S aureus* [13].

7 Guidelines for prophylaxis

From the different controlled studies, the following guidelines can be drawn.

Arthroplasty or internal fixation devices of closed fractures

In centers with infection rates < 5%:
*   Single dose of cefamandole (2 g i.v. 30 min before incision) or cefuroxime (1.5 g i.v. 30 min before incision).

In centers with unknown or high infection rates (> 5%) and in open fractures type 1 and type 2:

- Cefuroxime (1.5 g 30 min before incision, followed by 2 doses of 0.75 g every 8 hours), or
- Cefamandole (2 g i.v. 30 min before incision, followed by 4 doses of 1 g every 6 hours).

Internal fixation of grade III open fractures:

- Pre-emptive therapy with an anti-staphylococcal drug such as amoxicillin/clavulanic acid (2.2 g i.v. tid) or cefuroxime (1.5 g, followed by 0.75 g i.v. tid).

8 Bibliography

1. **Kaiser AB** (1986) Antimicrobial prophylaxis in surgery. *N Engl J Med;* 315 (18):1129–1138.
2. **Cruse PJ, Foord R** (1980) The epidemiology of wound infection. A 10-year prospective study of 62,939 wounds. *Surg Clin North Am;* 60 (1):27–40.
3. **Haas DW, Kaiser AB** (1994) Infections Associated with Indwelling Medical Devices. In: Bisno A, Waldvogel FA, editors. *Antimicrobial prophylaxis of infections associated with foreign bodies.* 2nd ed. Washington DC: American Society for Microbiology.
4. **Elek SD, Conen PE** (1957) The virulence of Staphylococcus pyrogenes for man: a study of the problem of wound infection. *Br J Exp Pathol;* 38:573–586.
5. **Zimmerli W, Waldvogel FA, Vaudaux P, et al.** (1982) Pathogenesis of foreign body infection: description and characteristics of an animal model. *J Infect Dis;* 146 (4):487–497.
6. **Zimmerli W, Lew PD, Waldvogel FA** (1984) Pathogenesis of foreign body infection. Evidence for a local granulocyte defect. *J Clin Invest;* 73 (4):1191–1200.
7. **Dellinger EP, Gross PA, Barrett TL, et al.** (1994) Quality standard for antimicrobial prophylaxis in surgical procedures. The Infectious Diseases Society of America. *Infect Control Hosp Epidemiol;* 15 (3):182–188.
8. **Gustilo RB, Mendoza RM, Williams DN** (1984) Problems in the management of type III (severe) open fractures: a new classification of type III open fractures. *J Trauma;* 24 (8):742–746.
9. **Greene C, McDevitt D, Francois P, et al.** (1995) Adhesion properties of mutants of Staphylococcus aureus defective in fibronectin-binding proteins and studies on the expression of fnb genes. *Mol Microbiol;* 17 (6):1143–1152.
10. **Steckelberg JM, Osmon DR** (1994) Infections associated with indwelling medical devices. In: Bisno AL, Waldvogel FA, editors. *Prosthetic joint infections.* Washington DC: ASM Press: 259–290l.
11. **Boxma H, Broekhuizen T, Patka P, et al.** (1996) Randomised controlled trial of single-dose antibiotic prophylaxis in surgical treatment of closed fractures: the Dutch Trauma Trial. *Lancet;* 347 (9009):1133–1137.
12. **Chin NX, Neu NM, Neu HC** (1990) Activity of cephalosporins against coagulase-negative staphylococci. *Diagn Microbiol Infect Dis;* 13(1):67–69.

13. **Tablan OC, Tenover FC, Martone WJ, et al.** (1995) Recommendations for preventing the spread of vancomycin resistance. Recommendations of the Hospital Infection Control Practices Advisory Committee (HICPAC). *MMWR Morb Mortal Wkly Rep;* 44 (RR-12):1–13.

14. **Burke JF** (1961) The effective period of preventive antibiotic action in experimental incisions and dermal lesions. *Surgery;* 50:1611–1168.

15. **Classen DC, Evans RS, Pestotnik SL, et al.** (1992) The timing of prophylactic administration of antibiotics and the risk of surgical-wound infection. *N Engl J Med;* 326 (5):281–286.

16. **Friedman RJ, Friedrich LV, White RL, et al.** (1990) Antibiotic prophylaxis and tourniquet inflation in total knee arthroplasty. *Clin Orthop;* (260):17–23.

17. **Oishi CS, Carrion WV, Hoaglund FT** (1993) Use of parenteral prophylactic antibiotics in clean orthopaedic surgery. A review of the literature. *Clin Orthop;* (296):249–255.

18. **Hill C, Flamant R, Mazas F, et al.** (1981) Prophylactic cefazolin versus placebo in total hip replacement. Report of a multicentre double-blind randomised trial. *Lancet;* 1 (8224):795–796.

19. **Gatell JM, Riba J, Lozano ML, et al.** (1984) Prophylactic cefamandole in orthopaedic surgery. *J Bone Joint Surg [Am];* 66 (8):1219–1222.

20. **Bodoky A, Neff U, Heberer M, et al.** (1993) Antibiotic prophylaxis with two doses of cephalosporin in patients managed with internal fixation for a fracture of the hip. *J Bone Joint Surg [Am];* 75 (1):61–65.

21. **Paiement GD, Renaud E, Dagenais G, et al.** (1994) Double-blind randomized prospective study of the efficacy of antibiotic prophylaxis for open reduction and internal fixation of closed ankle fractures. *J Orthop Trauma;* 8 (1):64–66.

22. **Nelson CL, Green TG, Porter RA, et al.** (1983) One day versus seven days of preventive antibiotic therapy in orthopedic surgery. *Clin Orthop;* (176):258–263.

23. **Gatell JM, Garcia S, Lozano L, et al.** (1987) Perioperative cefamandole prophylaxis against infections. *J Bone Joint Surg [Am];* 69 (8):1189–1193.

24. **Wymenga A, van Horn J, Theeuwes A, et al.** (1992) Cefuroxime for prevention of postoperative coxitis. One versus three doses tested in a randomized multicenter study of 2,651 arthroplasties. *Acta Orthop Scand;* 63 (1):19–24.

25. **Mauerhan DR, Nelson CL, Smith DL, et al.** (1994) Prophylaxis against infection in total joint arthroplasty. One day of cefuroxime compared with three days of cefazolin. *J Bone Joint Surg [Am];* 76 (1):39–45.

26. **Nungu KS, Olerud C, Rehnberg L, et al.** (1995) Prophylaxis with oral cefadroxil versus intravenous cefuroxime in trochanteric fracture surgery. A clinical multicentre study. *Arch Orthop Trauma Surg;* 114 (6):303–307.

27. **Patzakis MJ, Harvey JP, Jr., Ivler D** (1974) The role of antibiotics in the management of open fractures. *J Bone Joint Surg [Am];* 56 (3):532–541.

28. **Braun R, Enzler MA, Rittmann WW** (1987) A double-blind clinical trial of prophylactic cloxacillin in open fractures. *J Orthop Trauma;* 1 (1):12–17.

29. **Tscherne H, Oestern HJ, Sturm J**
(1983) Osteosynthesis of major fractures
in polytrauma. *World J Surg;* 7 (1):80–87.
30. **Zimmerli W, Widmer AF, Blatter M,
et al.** (1998) Role of rifampin for
treatment of orthopedic implant-related
staphylococcal infections: a randomized
controlled trial. Foreign-Body Infection
(FBI) Study Group [see comments].
JAMA; 279 (19):1537–1541.

9 Updates

Updates and additional references for this chapter
are available online at:
http://www.aopublishing.org/PFxM/55.htm

5.6 Thromboembolic prophylaxis

James B. Hunter & Ann E. Hunter

1 Thromboembolism: an issue in trauma surgery

Venous thromboembolism is a significant cause of mortality and morbidity in trauma and orthopedic practice. Despite the focus of research on elective orthopedics, particularly joint replacement, there is probably a greater problem in certain areas of trauma practice.

1.1 Clinically important outcomes

Sudden death

Fifty percent of those who die from a pulmonary embolism (PE) will die within 1 hour of the first symptom; the majority of those die almost immediately. Emergency surgery for PE is only realistically possible in the setting of a cardiothoracic unit. **Most of the patients who die will have had no symptoms of thrombosis prior to their PE.**

Symptomatic DVT or PE

Clinically evident non-fatal thromboembolism is relatively common in both trauma and elective practice. Serious sequelae are described particularly in general medical practice, such as chronic lung dysfunction following multiple PE's, but these are less common in orthopedic practice.

Postphlebitic limb

Occlusive proximal venous thrombosis in medical practice is frequently followed by chronic swelling, pigmentation, and ulceration of the leg. Despite the high rate of deep venous thrombosis (DVT) detected in orthopedic patients, the incidence of postphlebitic limb in follow-up studies has been low [1]. Plethysmographic studies have suggested flow problems in the medium term following DVT [2], but the rate of ulceration has not yet been shown to be increased in patients following major orthopedic surgery.

1.2 Surrogate outcomes and research interpretation

The interpretation of research findings in this field can be difficult. This is due to the volume of published literature and its contradictory nature. Clinical experiments in thrombosis are

Most of the patients who die will have had no symptoms of thrombosis prior to their PE.

not difficult to initiate, but are difficult to complete when restricted to useful clinical endpoints. Thus, many studies apply surrogate endpoints to achieve statistically significant outcomes of dubious clinical relevance. Confining one's reading to well-controlled studies with clinically relevant endpoints can drastically reduce the information overload available in this field.

Scanning the asymptomatic patient

The standard investigation for DVT or proximal venous thrombosis in the leg is the ascending venogram [3]. The investigation was devised to see if swelling and pain of a symptomatic leg could be explained by the presence of a thrombus. The investigation represents a snapshot of the leg at any particular time, and although a filling defect represents a thrombus whether or not the patient is symptomatic, one must remember that **thrombosis and fibrinolysis are a balanced, continuous homeostasis.** One cannot tell from a single venogram whether a thrombus is extending or resolving. The nature of venography makes repeat studies difficult, and it is thrombogenic in its own right. Doppler ultrasound has been used in various forms to investigate DVT. Simple flow "auscultation" at the femoral vein is ineffective. B-mode ultrasound is more effective and color-flow even more so. All ultrasound modalities are expensive, time-consuming, and operator dependent. They are less accurate than venography in the calf and above the inguinal ligament. Many other methods have been tried, such as liquid crystal thermography and plethysmography. Most have shown acceptable sensitivity and specificity in symptomatic patients but have been unsatisfactory for routine screening in an orthopedic setting [4, 5].

Thrombosis and fibrinolysis constitute a balanced, continuous homeostasis.

2 History and background

2.1 Virchow's triad

The pathophysiological background for thrombosis formation is attributed to Virchow. The "triad" of predisposing factors is:
- Damage to the vessel wall,
- Venous stasis,
- Hypercoagulable state.

It is clear that all three are present in orthopedic trauma and elective practice.

2.2 Charnley/Mayo experience with THR

Early reports from the originators of total hip replacement (THR) suggested that the incidence of fatal pulmonary embolism was extremely high, between 1–3%, and these figures were supported by venographic studies showing high rates of thrombosis following hip and knee replacement and hip fracture. More recent studies question the rate of fatal pulmonary embolism following joint replacement, suggesting the overall early mortality to be of the order of 1%, with PE accounting for between one half and one tenth of that [6]. The rate of fatal PE after a proximal femoral fracture has always been difficult to determine due to the patient population, lack of autopsy data, and a shortage of controlled trials.

2.3 Relationship of thromboembolism to fracture disease

Fracture disease as originally described is a syndrome of pain, swelling, and lack of function leading to fibrosis and stiffness. Although the mortality rate, particularly from peripheral fractures, has been low, the contribution of thrombosis to the condition was probably considerable.

3 Risk factors

3.1 General patient characteristics

Age

Age is a most important predictor of thromboembolism [7]. The risk increases with advancing age. The incidence in childhood is negligible. In adolescence other risk factors, such as oral contraception may be present. The majority of fracture patients are elderly, and doubly at risk.

Previous thromboembolism

Previous thromboembolism is an extremely important risk factor [7]. Many patients with recurrent thrombosis are now being found to have genetic and hematological risk factors, but even those without these are at great risk of a second episode. It is most important to seek a history of thromboembolism from patients, as this represents the only practical method of screening them for risk.

Genetic predisposition

Some families carry a genetic predisposition to thrombosis. In only 50 % of them a recognized abnormality may be detected. In the presence of antithrombin III, protein C or S deficiency there is a clear risk of thrombosis, particularly following surgery, immobilization, or trauma. Less clear is the role of Factor V Leiden. Five percent of the Caucasian population will inherit this trait, but only a small proportion will develop thrombosis. The presence of a family history of venoembolic disease in a first degree relative, especially at a young age, should alert the surgeon to the possible risk.

Pregnancy/oral contraception/HRT

Any patient who has an estrogen stress has an increased risk of thrombosis. This is exacerbated by any genetic predisposition. The risk increases as pregnancy progresses but is lower in patients taking oral contraception. There appears to be a small but finite risk of thrombosis in people taking hormone replacement therapy (HRT), but this is usually outweighed by the potential benefits. The incidence of thrombosis for those on HRT is 3 in 10,000 as against 1 in 10,000 in the general population.

3.2 Fractures and fracture surgery

Fractures and operations have an effect on all three elements of Virchow's triad. The surgical insult on top of the initial fracture doubles the risk.

Some families carry a genetic predisposition to thrombosis.

Thrombosis is probably a significant contributor to fracture disease.

The risk of thromboembolism increases with advancing age.

A history of previous thromboembolism is an extremely important risk factor.

Relative immobilization

All fracture management, however aggressive, contains an element of immobilization and in the affected limb this may be prolonged.

Lower limb surgery

Thrombosis of the upper limb is very unusual, even after surgery.

Fractures around the knee carry a particular risk.

Thrombosis of the upper limb is very unusual, even after surgery. The risk of thrombosis after lower limb fracture surgery increases from distal to proximal [8], with the worst risk following pelvic and acetabular fractures [9]. **Fractures around the knee carry a particular risk due to the proximity of the popliteal vein.** The tourniquet has paradoxical effects, on the one hand creating stasis, on the other, triggering fibrinolytic pathways. Its use in fracture surgery seems to be diminishing [10]. Pulmonary embolism can occur in those treated surgically for fractures distal to the hip but in general the embolism rate is low.

Influence of weight bearing

Delay in weight bearing is inevitable in most fractures. **Delayed mobilization is established as a cause of increased thrombosis in elective orthopedics** [11].

Delayed mobilization is an established cause of increased thrombosis.

Muscles pumps and venous return

Limited weight bearing influences thrombosis by increasing venous stasis. Muscle pumps that promote venous return exist both in the calf and the sole of the foot. The foot pump is probably the more important and is capacious. In normal walking it is activated by each step.

4   Prophylaxis

The rationale of prophylactic regimens for DVT is bewildering, as is their variety.

4.1   Strategies

Prophylaxis versus treatment

Prevention, rather than treatment of established disease, is the norm. Clinical diagnosis of DVT is so unreliable, even in patients without fractures, that it is not worth attempting. Conventional treatment of DVT does not dispel the thrombus, and thus lasting damage may be done to the vein, leading to recurrence. Pulmonary embolism normally occurs unheralded, and has considerable early mortality. Treatment by anticoagulation carries considerable morbidity in an orthopedic setting, and, following fracture, can promote a compartment syndrome. Thrombolysis is not an option following surgery. Filter placement in the vena cava will prevent recurrent emboli, but carries its own risks.

Surveillance

Surveillance by screening methods is commonly employed instead of, or as well as, prophylaxis. The deficiencies of most investigative methods of screening have been highlighted earlier. Screening by venography can be clinically effective but is probably not cost-effective.

4.2 Methods

4.2.1 Mechanical

Compressive stockings

It is slightly surprising that anyone ever thought of putting a compressive stocking on a limb insulted by trauma or surgery. Graduated compression stockings have been found to be effective thromboprophylaxis in abdominal surgery, but evidence for their preventative use in orthopedic and fracture surgery is poor and there have been some reports that found them to be positively detrimental [12]. Their only possible role in fracture surgery is after spinal fracture.

Mechanical pumps

Various compression devices exist to replace or enhance the natural muscle pump function. These range from simple inflatable boots that compress the calf to sequential compression devices that transport venous blood proximally. The latter are more effective. Devices that compress the sole of the foot to empty that plexus are relatively small and also effective, but not all patients can tolerate them. They carry the advantage of significantly reducing swelling and are also useful therapy for some fractures [13].

Vena cava filters

Filter placement is a strategy for prevention of PE in the face of known or likely thrombosis. Ideally, the patient will also be anticoagulated in order to prevent clotting around the filter itself. The risks and benefits of placing the filter prophylactically are not yet fully clear.

4.2.2 Chemical

Chemical agents have been the mainstay of thromboprophylaxis in most branches of surgery since the 1970s, as a result of their documented effectiveness. They have, however, never been popular with surgeons because of perceived bleeding complications and, certainly in the UK, their use amongst orthopedic surgeons is waning. This is surprising as more effective regimens and agents have become available.

Warfarin (coumadin)

Warfarin is a highly effective anticoagulant taken orally but is considerably bound by plasma proteins so that other agents (alcohol, antibiotics) have a major effect on its potency. There is a delay in the onset of anticoagulation so that initially other measures must be used. In fracture surgery warfarin is most commonly used for the treatment of an established DVT, and after pelvic and acetabular surgery. Its use must be monitored by blood test (INR, international normalized ratio, or prothrombin time ratio). In prophylaxis, an INR target value of 1.5 is frequently used, with higher values for treatment. Reversal of excessive INR values can be achieved with vitamin K, but high doses of this make the patient warfarin-resistant for days; so a dose of about 0.5–1.0 mg is sufficient for control. Warfarin is an effective prophylactic measure in hip fracture surgery.

Of the mechanical means for prophylaxis, the sequential compression boots appear to be the most effective.

Heparins

Heparins are naturally occurring anticoagulants. For clinical practice they are generally derived from pigs, which can lead to occasional allergic problems. Activity of unfractionated heparin is monitored using the APPT ratio (activated partial thromboplastin time). In full dose, this is the conventional drug to initiate anticoagulation. Full anticoagulation in the postoperative period has a high incidence of bleeding complications. The newer heparins are fractionated to contain more low molecular weight elements (hence, low molecular weight heparin, LMWH). They are supposed to allow antithrombotic rather than anticoagulant activity, thus reducing unwarranted bleeding; however, this theory is not strongly supported by clinical trials. Their action is best monitored using an assay of anti-Factor Xa action. Unfractionated heparin (UFH) in small doses was widely used for prophylaxis in trauma and orthopedic practice after its successful use in abdominal and elective orthopedic surgery. The evidence for its use, particularly in fracture surgery, was never especially strong. Even in meta-analysis it could not be demonstrated to save lives in the hip fracture population. **LMWH is more effective than UFH in clinical trials of prophylaxis in elective orthopedic surgery, and more effective than warfarin, though perhaps causing more bleeding [14]. LMWH has been used in several fracture trials and found to be effective, using venography as the endpoint.**

Aspirin

Aspirin is the oldest and cheapest chemical thromboprophylactic drug available. The mechanism of action is as an antiplatelet agent, and the meta-analysis conducted by the Antiplatelet Triallists' Collaboration has re-established its use [15]. In orthopedic trauma the reduction in DVT was from 42–36%, which seems modest; the PE rate, however, was more than halved, from 6.9–2.8%. Even in this large study of more than 8,000 patients no difference was observed in the overall death rate. A large multicenter prospective study of aspirin in patients with hip fractures is now underway in the UK to document the effect on the postoperative death rate. Low molecular weight heparinoid prevents more thromboses than aspirin [16], but aspirin may well have a beneficial effect against other causes of death [17].

5   Particular problems

5.1   The multiply-injured

In multiple injuries, coagulation mechanisms are severely disrupted. In the initial resuscitation phase with massive blood and fluid transfusion a clotting screen will demonstrate an hypocoagulable situation. **However, even at this stage, due to the influence of direct trauma, hypotension, and stasis, thrombosis may develop. Prophylaxis in this group is extremely difficult**. Low dose heparin is probably ineffective. Greater degrees of anticoagulation may be inappropriate due to other injuries. There is a trend, particularly in North America, towards the early placement of vena cava filters in the severely injured, and success is reported in comparisons with historical controls [18] by some though not by others [19]. A protocol for prophylaxis in multiple trauma that is sensitive to constraints of different injuries is invaluable.

In the multiply-injured thrombosis prophylaxis is difficult.

LMWH has been found to be effective in several trials.

5.2 Spinal injuries

Nowhere is there greater potential for disaster from bleeding complications, caused by chemical prophylaxis than in the spine. Spinal and cord injury carry a high incidence of DVT. Several small studies suggested that low-dose heparin was safe and effective in this situation—but there has been a steady stream of case reports of serious complications, and physical methods appear to be preferable.

5.3 Pelvis and acetabulum

These fractures, particularly if severe enough to warrant fixation, have a high incidence of proximal vein thrombosis (around 50%). This leads to a high rate of PE (2–10%) and fatality (0.5–2%) [9]. Diagnosis can be difficult, but is improved by magnetic resonance (MR) venography. Many use routine postoperative anticoagulation [20]; an alternative is an aggressive surveillance policy. Within this group there may be indications for filter placement, particularly for free-floating proximal thrombus and thrombosis occurring in the face of anticoagulation.

5.4 Hip fractures

Fracture of the proximal femur is associated with a high mortality. An audit of a single UK region showed the overall rate to be 18% at 90 days. Use of thromboprophylaxis was associated with a reduced death rate [21]. Studies are difficult to perform in this group, particularly if they involve invasive investigations. Meta-analysis in 1988 of studies involving UFH did not show an effect on the mortality rate. Reviews suggest the thrombosis rate in hip

fractures with LMWH prophylaxis remains very high [22]. Other factors affecting the mortality that the surgeon can influence are delay before surgery and early mobilization. Delay to surgery is a significant predictor of mortality [23].

5.5 Ambulant patients

The risk of DVT in outpatients is small but defined. Research has concentrated on two groups; patients who have been discharged to the community following major orthopedic surgery, and those receiving outpatient fracture treatment. PE does occur in those treated on plaster, but their risk compared to the general population is hard to assess. Careful venographic trials have shown reduced thrombosis rates in both postdischarge and ambulant fracture patients, but no trials have demonstrated an effect on a clinically important endpoint. In some countries the widespread use of prophylaxis in these clinical situations may be driven by medico-legal concerns.

Spinal and cord injuries carry a high incidence of DVT.

6   Bibliography

1.   **Francis CW, Ricotta JJ, Evarts CM, et al.** (1988) Long-term clinical observations and venous functional abnormalities after asymptomatic venous thrombosis following total hip or knee arthroplasty. *Clin Orthop;* (232):271–278.

2.   **McNally MA, Mollan RA** (1993) Total hip replacement, lower limb blood flow and venous thrombogenesis. *J Bone Joint Surg [Br];* 75 (4):640–644.

3.   **Rabinov K, Paulin S** (1972) Roentgen diagnosis of venous thrombosis in the leg. *Arch Surg;* 104 (2):134–144.

4.   **Magnusson M, Eriksson BI, Kalebo P, et al.** (1996) Is colour Doppler ultrasound a sensitive screening method in diagnosing deep vein thrombosis after hip surgery? *Thromb Haemost;* 75 (2):242–245.

5.   **Cruickshank MK, Levine MN, Hirsh J, et al.** (1989) An evaluation of impedance plethysmography and 125I-fibrinogen leg scanning in patients following hip surgery. *Thromb Haemost;* 62 (3):830–834.

6.   **Murray DW, Carr AJ, Bulstrode CJ** (1995) Pharmacological thromboprophylaxis and total hip replacement [editorial; comment]. *J Bone Joint Surg [Br];* 77 (1):3–5.

7.   **Lowe GDO, Greer IA, Cooke IA** (1992) Risk of and prophylaxis for venous thromboembolism in hospital patients. Thromboembolic Risk Factors (THRIFT) Consensus Group [see comments]. *BMJ;* 305 (6853):567–574.

8.   **Abelseth G, Buckley RE, Pineo GE, et al.** (1996) Incidence of deep-vein thrombosis in patients with fractures of the lower extremity distal to the hip. *J Orthop Trauma;* 10 (4):230–235.

9.   **Montgomery KD, Geerts WH, Potter HG, et al.** (1996) Thromboembolic complications in patients with pelvic trauma. *Clin Orthop;* (329):68–87.

10.   **Salam AA, Eyres KS, Cleary J, et al.** (1991) The use of a tourniquet when plating tibial fractures [see comments]. *J Bone Joint Surg [Br];* 73 (1):86–87.

11.   **Lassen MR, Borris LC, Christiansen HM** (1990) Mobilization—disregarded factor! Influence on postoperative thromboembolism. *Acta Orthop Scand;* 61 (Suppl 239):52.

12.   **Hui AC, Heras-Palou C, Dunn I, et al.** (1996) Graded compression stockings for prevention of deep-vein thrombosis after hip and knee replacement [see comments]. *J Bone Joint Surg [Br];* 78 (4):550–554.

13.   **Erdmann MW, Richardson J, Templeton J** (1992) Os calcis fractures: a randomized trial comparing conservative treatment with impulse compression of the foot. *Injury;* 23 (5):305–307.

14.   **Palmer AJ, Koppenhagen K, Kirchhof B, et al.** (1997) Efficacy and safety of low molecular weight heparin, unfractionated heparin and warfarin for thrombo-embolism prophylaxis in orthopaedic surgery: a meta-analysis of randomised clinical trials. *Haemostasis;* 27 (2):75–84.

15.   **Antiplatelet Trialists' Collaboration** (1994) Collaborative overview of randomised trials of antiplatelet therapy—III: Reduction in venous thrombosis and pulmonary embolism by antiplatelet prophylaxis among surgical and medical patients. *Brit Med J;* 308 (6923):235–246.

16. **Gent M, Hirsh J, Ginsberg JS, et al.**
(1996) Low-molecular-weight heparinoid
orgaran is more effective than aspirin in
the prevention of venous
thromboembolism after surgery for hip
fracture. *Circulation;* 93 (1):80–84.

17. **Nettleman MD, Alsip J, Schrader M,
et al.** (1996) Predictors of mortality after
acute hip fracture. *J Gen Intern Med;*
11 (12):765–767.

18. **Rogers FB, Shackford SR, Ricci MA,
et al.** (1995) Routine prophylactic vena
cava filter insertion in severely injured
trauma patients decreases the incidence
of pulmonary embolism [see comments].
J Am Coll Surg; 180 (6):641–647.

19. **Spain DA, Richardson JD, Polk HC, Jr.,
et al.** (1997) Venous thromboembolism
in the high-risk trauma patient: do risks
justify aggressive screening and
prophylaxis? *J Trauma;* 42 (3):463–467;
discussion 467–469.

20. **Fishmann AJ, Greeno RA, Brooks LR,
et al.** (1994) Prevention of deep vein
thrombosis and pulmonary embolism in
acetabular and pelvic fracture surgery.
Clin Orthop; (305):133–137.

21. **Todd CJ, Freeman CJ, Camilleri-
Ferrante C, et al.** (1995) Differences in
mortality after fracture of hip: the East
Anglian audit [see comments]. *BMJ;*
310 (6984):904–908.

22. **Green D, Hirsh J, Heit J, et al.** (1994)
Low molecular weight heparin: a critical
analysis of clinical trials. *Pharmacol Rev;*
46 (1):89–109.

23. **Perez JV, Warwick DJ, Case CP, et al.**
(1995) Death after proximal femoral
fracture—an autopsy study. *Injury;*
26 (4):237–240.

7 Updates

Updates and additional references for this chapter
are available online at:
http://www.aopublishing.org/PFxM/56.htm

5.7 Postoperative management: general considerations

Christian Ryf, Andy Weymann, Peter Matter

1 Introduction

The overall care plan for a trauma patient should cover the preoperative management, the treatment procedures, and the postoperative care.

All too often, it is during the period after the main intervention that vigilance is relaxed and complications may be permitted. These, at best, deprive the patient of the full benefit of whatever has been done and, at worst, may blight its outcome.

Postoperative management, therefore, must be directed to the patient in terms of the procedure, the effects of the injury, and the environment, not just in hospital, but at home and later at work and at leisure. To achieve this, three postoperative phases are recognized:
- In the first phase—immediately after surgery—emphasis is on mobilization, prophylaxis, and early recognition of complications.
- In the second phase—at the conclusion of hospitalization—attention is centered upon integration into the accustomed social environment.
- The final phase concludes treatment and returns the patient to his/her preoperative capabilities.

2 Immediate postoperative phase

2.1 Analgesics and dressings

The important role of analgesia for the patient in maintaining comfort and obtaining cooperation should be addressed from the outset. We recommend the following principles be followed regarding the treatment of pain:
- **Analgesics should begin early, before pain becomes unbearable.**
- Non-steroidal anti-inflammatory agents or paracetamol are ideal.
- If needed, morphine or morphine derivatives may be prescribed. In more extensive injuries where intense pain is to be expected, either a PCA pump (patient controlled analgesia) or an indwelling epidural catheter should be employed.
- The level of pain relief attained comforts the patient, and permits early postoperative mobilization.

So that the surgical wounds can dry as quickly as possible, they are covered in the operating room with sterile, absorbent gauze that allows

Treatment plan includes preoperative, perioperative, and postoperative management.

Give analgesics early before pain becomes unbearable.

for air circulation. When used, suction drainage remains in place for about 24 hours, with routine amounts of exudation. For larger amounts, as in pelvic or hip fractures, 48 hours may be required.

Articular fractures are a special case and should be drained for no more that 8–12 hours. Beyond these times, the risk of infection is increased.

If the wounds have bled a good deal, the first change of dressings takes place 24 hours after surgery (**Video 5.7-1**); otherwise they can remain in place 48 hours. Thereafter, the **dressings are changed daily in an effort to prevent the formation of any sort of a moist chamber.** Such changes are carried out under the strictest of hygienic conditions. Dilute iodine or chlorhexidine solutions are recommended for skin disinfection. Open wounds should be moistened with balanced electrolyte solution (e.g., lactated Ringer's) on a regular basis. Contaminated wounds are flushed with antiseptic solutions such as Lavasept® (see **chapter 6.1**). Such mechanical rinsing is particularly

Daily changes of dressing prevent moist chambers.

Elevation of the limb reduces postoperative swelling.

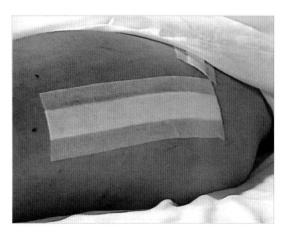

 Video 5.7-1

effective. As soon as bleeding or secretion ceases, the wound is left uncovered. Even with sutures in place, if the wound is temporarily protected by a watertight dressing (e.g., Op-Site Film®, Tegaderm®), the patient can bathe or undergo hydrotherapy.

2.2   Elevation and support of the injured limb

Many surgeons have their own preferred regimes, but the following guidelines are widely applicable. **Immediately after the operation, the treated extremity is positioned above the level of the heart to minimize swelling.**

Following osteosynthesis on the upper extremity, the limb is either placed on a cushion or elevated in a bag (**Fig. 5.7-1a**). When the latter is used, flexion of the elbow should not exceed 75°.

After any procedure, pressure, malpositioning, and deformity are to be prevented. In particular, the medial epicondyle of the elbow (ulnar nerve), and the head of the fibula (peroneal nerve) must be well padded. Removable plaster bandages or splints, if they are used, must not lead to malpositioning nor inhibit early postoperative mobilization and physical therapy. Splints on the forearm are placed in "intrinsic plus" position to prevent contracture of the muscles and joints of the hand.

In fractures near the hip, the affected extremity is placed in moderate abduction and held in that position between cushions or in a padded splint.

In distal and midshaft femur fractures, the lower leg is supported with the hip and knee joints each in 90° of flexion (**Fig. 5.7-1b**). An operated lower leg is similarly supported, but

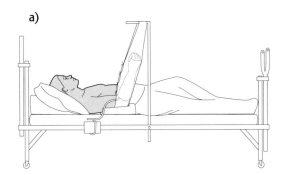

a)

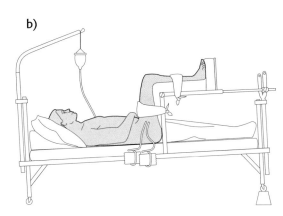

b)

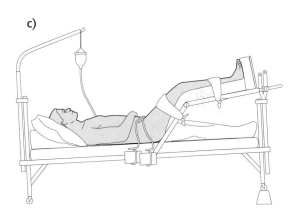

c)

Fig. 5.7-1: Positioning after operations. a) Upper extremity, b) distal/midshaft femur, c) lower leg.

it is sufficient to flex the knee and hip to 45° (**Fig. 5.7-1c**). **Articular fractures about the knee are best managed by continuous passive motion (CPM) (Fig. 5.7-2).** Such efforts to reduce swelling may be reinforced with cooling and/or non-steroidal anti-inflammatory drugs.

In patients with a tendency toward the equinus position, a U-bar is adapted to fit the limb. In the presence of articular fractures whose mobilization must begin gradually, or with associated ligamentous lesions, splints with limited mobility are helpful.

The combination of an operation and subsequent protracted immobilization is inappropriate, due to the increased rate of associated complications. External splintage

Articular fractures benefit from CPM.

Operation followed by plaster immobilization is a bad combination.

Fig. 5.7-2: In joint fractures the continuous passive motion splint is employed.

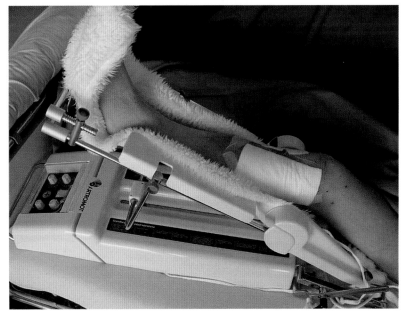

should only be used, when unavoidable, to prevent malpositioning, to ensure problem-free wound healing, or in connection with an additional injury.

2.3 Swelling and mobilization/prophylaxis of thrombosis

Eearly mobilization, and in certain circumstances elastic supports, can be very effective in preventing thrombosis. Medical prophylaxis against thrombosis [1] may be employed in addition, as described in **chapter 5.6**. Patients operated upon for injuries to the upper extremity can and should stand up on the day of their surgery. In the case of the lower extremity, ambulation is postponed until soft-tissue swelling has gone and the wound shows no signs of inflammation (**Video 5.7-2** and **Video AO40002a**). **How much weight may be taken depends upon the character of the fracture and the function of the implants employed, subject always to the prospects of patient com-**

pliance [2]. Although guidelines are helpful, the responsibility for deciding this must rest with the operating surgeon, who should be in the best position to know how reliable the fixation is. Care must be taken not to allow early mobilization to interfere with wound healing. If swelling occurs, elevation of the limb is resumed.

2.4 Antibiotics

The use of antibiotics prophylactically [3] and in the treatment of contaminated wounds is covered in **chapter 5.5**.

2.5 Activity and weight bearing

Postoperative physical therapy begins on the first postoperative day. In long bone injuries, the neighboring joints are immediately put through active and active-assisted movement (**Video 5.7-3**). Continuous passive motion may

Encourage early weight bearing in the compliant patient.

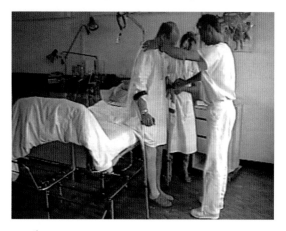

Video 5.7-2

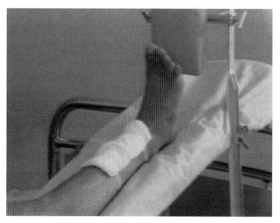

Video AO40002a

already be under way. At first, weight bearing—up to 15–20 kg—should take place with the assistance of crutches and walkers and only under the guidance of trained personnel [4]. Training in walking up and down stairs (**Video 5.7-4**) with canes is particularly difficult for patients, and should be carefully overseen. Hydrotherapy is an important means of providing weightless and pain-free mobilization for patients with fractures of the spine, shoulder area, pelvis, and hip; it also helps to build up confidence.

2.6 X-ray assessment

Postoperatively, and preferably following removal of the suction drains, x-rays are taken in at least two planes. These serve to document fracture reduction and fixation, record the orientation of implants, and provide a basis for the evaluation of how fracture healing is progressing.

2.7 Preparing for discharge

Throughout this first phase, the patient should be regularly and fully informed about the clinical state, the rate of progress, and what is to be expected in the timetable of recovery. The expectations of the patient and the family should be ascertained and appropriately influenced towards an understanding of the actual situation. All relevant support services should be brought in at this stage, in line with clinical progress.

Prior to discharge from the hospital the following points should be established between patient and staff:

- Wound free of inflammation.
- Postoperative x-rays taken.
- Instructions given for ambulation with crutches (including stairs), and for further mobilization (**Video AO40002b**).
- Information provided about symptoms and signs of possible complications.
- Instructions given to care-providers about aftercare.

Postoperative x-rays are mandatory.

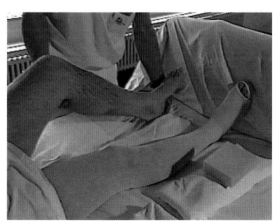

Video 5.7-3

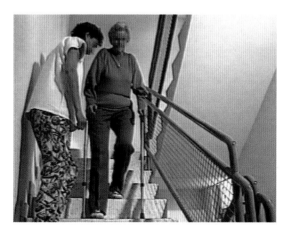

Video 5.7-4

3   The middle phase of fracture treatment

3.1   Clinical care outside hospital

Under normal conditions, the surgeon should ensure that a competent colleague will monitor the patient after discharge. He/she must be provided with sufficient information to be able to decide upon and carry out the next steps. **This physician must recognize irregularities in the healing process and prevent them from becoming serious complications.** The first postoperative consultation should take place 12–14 days postoperatively, conveniently at the time of suture removal. Despite certain injury-dependent restrictions, and given an appropriate profession, work can be resumed as early as 2 weeks after the operation if adequate arrangements for transportation can be made. However, a recovery period of 6–8 weeks is more usual [5–7].

Potential complications must be recognized and prevented.

Warning signs are local swelling, redness and tenderness, arrest or reversal of progress, and mobility.

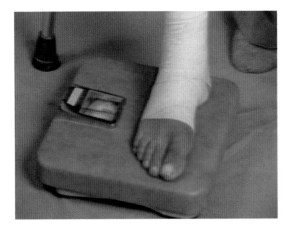

   Video AO40002b

3.2   Clinical and x-ray monitoring

The frequency and timing of return visits to a physician are largely a matter of local arrangement, but certain features are essential under any circumstances.

During periodic visits for monitoring, special attention should be given to specific questions regarding routine patient activities like: showering, bathing, sitting, lifting, work, and sport. These can be of great relevance to the patient's personal and professional life. The sooner any problems in these areas are resolved, the sooner the patient may again be assimilated into his/her accustomed environment. With good communication between patient and physician, this phase of fracture treatment can occur under conditions of optimal capabilities in work and sport.

Clinical features to be considered as **warnings are increased redness, swelling or local tenderness, arrest or reversal of progress, or mobility associated with pain.** Difficulty with activities, for example, weight bearing, which had previously been comfortable, is a valuable guide.

Radiographic monitoring at 4–6 week intervals must include views in two planes; in special cases additional views may be necessary. For fractures involving a joint surface in particular, tangential views may be essential in the evaluation of articular congruence. In long bone fractures, the neighboring joints should be included in the x-ray, which usually demands the use of a suitably long film.

Aims of radiographic monitoring: Evaluation of postoperative x-rays must be done based on the type of healing expected, the mode of fixation used, the underlying state of the bone, and the estimate made by the surgeon on completion of the fixation.

If direct healing is anticipated, the appearance of irritation callus or a widening of the fracture line may point to impending trouble and require modification of the management regime.

With indirect healing, timely development of callus surrounding the fracture site and steadily maturing is a welcome sight.

A careful watch is kept for secondary displacement, implant loosening (bone resorption), or failure and secondary displacement.

The surgeon should be sure at all time that union is progressing at a rate appropriate to the particular clinical situation, and be prepared to take action if not.

Given positive clinical and radiographic findings, weight bearing may be gradually increased. When joints are involved, a simultaneous decision is made regarding the allowable freedom of motion.

3.3 Implants—early removal

Implants that retard mobilization and fracture healing—such as positioning screws or external fixators—can, in general, be partially or completely removed after 6–8 weeks. This may enable the dynamizing of a medullary nail or a full range of motion—for example, following the removal of a positioning screw from the diastasis of a type C malleolar fracture.

It is just as important to listen to the patient as it is to look at the x-rays.

4 Third phase—conclusion of the fracture treatment

Fracture treatment is considered to be completed when the patient regains full capacity to work and to do sports. Should a new fracture occur, the surgeon must decide whether it is a "secondary fracture" or a "refracture" [8].

Definition of refracture

All five of the following criteria must be fulfilled, without exception:

1. The original fracture focus is involved.
2. Uncomplicated healing of a technically perfect osteosynthesis or appropriate conservative treatment.
3. Correct aftercare.
4. Appropriately timed removal of metal implants.
5. Absence of an adequate new trauma.

Definition of secondary fracture

At least one of the above criteria is invalid.

5 Implant removal— general comments

Implant removal represents the true completion of fracture treatment for many patients. **While giving due concern to the patient's own wishes, the expense, utility, and risks of removal of the implants must be weighed up.** When implant removal is appropriate, further x-rays should be taken and scrutinized both to ensure that fracture healing is complete and to provide current information documenting the condition and true location of the

In stable fixation the appearance of irritation callus or widening of the fracture suggests trouble!

The expense, benefits, and risks of removal of the implants must be weighed up.

It is just as important to listen to and to look at the patient as it is to study the x-rays.

The patient should be warned if the implant is likely to need removal.

In the upper extremity, implant removal is generally neither necessary nor recommended.

If removal of an implant carries a risk for the patient, it should be avoided.

implant(s). **It is always helpful if a patient has been given, at an early stage after surgery, a clear indication of the surgeon's opinion about the removal of implants in the particular situation.**

Indications for earlier removal may include inhibition of limb function or irritation of neighboring structures by the implant. Removal is more common among young patients and in lower limbs, since the risk of a new fracture in the area of the implant is higher and might be unnecessarily complicated by its continuing presence. **In the upper extremity, implant removal is generally neither necessary nor recommended.**

As a rule in older patients, implants may usually be left in place.

General health is also a factor. The risk and advantages of implant removal must be carefully considered in patients with immune deficiencies (e.g., HIV, hepatitis, tuberculosis) and with local circulatory disturbances (e.g., diabetes mellitus, peripheral arterial thrombosis). **Individual implants, and those lying in areas with an elevated risk of iatrogenic damage (e.g., forearm, shaft of the humerus, pelvis) are left in place.**

In case of probable contamination of the metal used in an osteosynthesis, the material should be removed following the completion of fracture healing. Allergic-type reactions can occur, but they are rare with stainless-steel implants and practically unknown with implants made of pure titanium (see **chapter 1.3**). The decision to remove the metal is made based upon the intensity of the reaction. External fixators and K-wires are always completely removed due to the danger of secondary displacement or migration, as well as pin-track infection.

When additional surgery is indicated (e.g., arthrolysis, tenolysis, neurolysis, scar revision), the implants may be removed at the same time if fracture healing is complete.

5.1   Timing of implant removal

When implant removal is indicated, timing is determined by the location of the fracture and the character of the implant(s) employed. The implants are usually left in place at least 1–2 years, during which time the progress of fracture healing is monitored on an ongoing basis. X-rays have to show complete fracture healing.

Following removal, given appropriate soft-tissue healing, full function and weight bearing may be resumed in a few days.

After removal of large plates, contact sports and heavy physical work should be postponed for at least 2–4 months. Thereafter and possibly after another x-ray control, fracture healing may be considered complete.

6 Bibliography

1. **Antiplatelet Trialists' Collaboration** (1994) Secondary prevention of vascular disease by prolonged antiplatelet treatment. *Brit Med J;* 308:81–106.

2. **Siebert W, Geyer M, Vahle A** (1993) Postoperative Teilbelastung—Was macht der Patient wirklich? *Orthop Praxis;* 3:196–202.

3. **Gillespie W, Walenkamp G, Hoffman C** (1997) Antibiotic prophylaxis in patients undergoing surgery femoral fracture. *The Cochrane Library.*

4. **Warren C, Lehmann J** (1975) Training procedures and biofeedback methods to achieve controlled partial weight bearing: an assessment. *Arch Phys Med Rehabil;* 56 (10):449–455.

5. **Ceder L, Thorngren K, Wallden B** (1980) Prognostic indicators and early home rehabilitation in elderly patients with hip fracture. *Clin Ortho;* (152):173–184.

6. **Cameron ID, Lyle DM, Quine S** (1994) Cost effectiveness of accelerated rehabilitation after proximal femoral fracture. *J Clin Epidemiology;* 47 (11):1307–1313.

7. **Galvard H, Samuelsson S** (1995) Orthopedic or geriatic rehabilitation of hip fracture patients: a prospective, randomized, clinically controlled study in Malmo, Sweden. *Aging (Milano);* 7 (1):11–16.

8. **Matter P, Weymann A, Egger P, et al.** (In prep.) Secondary fracture or refracture after removal of metal implants for primary internal fixation of shaft fractures. *J Ortho Trauma.*

7 Updates

Updates and additional references for this chapter are available online at:
http://www.aopublishing.org/PFxM/57.htm

6.1 Acute infection

Peter E. Ochsner & Urs Müller

1 Introduction

Acute infections after osteosynthesis are generally exogenous, i.e., infections due to a contamination with bacteria from outside the body. Contamination occurs from the trauma itself (open fracture), during osteosynthesis, or after osteosynthesis in case of disturbed wound healing. In theory, a hematogenous infection after ORIF is possible but probably very rare.

In contrast to the acute hematogenous osteomyelitis of adolescence, acute posttraumatic infection always involves an area already injured by trauma and/or an operation (**Fig. 6.1-1–3**). Once established in areas surrounding necrotic bone, the infection may become chronic. **The treatment of posttraumatic osteomyelitis must, therefore, always be operative and aggressive, with antibiotics playing an adjuvant role only.** The administration of antibiotics alone in the absence of a clear diagnosis will lead to chronic and neglected osteomyelitis.

2 Definitions

2.1 Early/delayed first manifestations of infection

The time of contamination can only be estimated, but the time of the first manifestation is ascertainable. This is the moment at which an infection is diagnosed on the basis of bacteriological and clinical or histological findings. Willenegger and Roth [1], therefore, classified posttraumatic infections as those which were early first manifestations (less than 2 weeks) and those which were delayed (more than 2 weeks). Late first manifestations, according to this definition, are infections appearing after the tenth week. They do not differ greatly in their prognosis from delayed manifestations and therefore will not be treated separately in this chapter. The term first manifestation does not define the time of contamination, which may precede the first manifestation by days, months, or even years. Not all early first manifestations present themselves as acute infections. Occasionally, progression is slow—chronic, one might say—from the outset.

Acute infections after osteosynthesis are generally exogenous, i.e., infections due to a contamination with bacteria from outside the body.

The treatment of posttraumatic osteomyelitis must always be operative and aggressive, with antibiotics playing an adjuvant role only.

2.2 Early first manifestations (less than 2 weeks)

Early first manifestation of an acute infection is characterized by clinical symptoms and pathological laboratory values within the first 2 weeks. Infection must, therefore, be clearly distinguished from disturbance of wound healing, necrosis of the wound edges, and post-traumatic/postoperative hematoma.

In delayed first manifestation, the outbreak is preceded by an insidious hidden infection, possibly masked by non-specific antibiotics.

- **Disturbance of wound healing:** Delayed wound closure generally goes hand-in-hand with local contamination. As long as the body is able to maintain its defense mechanisms, the clinical signs of infection, such as fever, swelling, and pain, will be absent and the laboratory values will remain normal (leukocytes, CRP). Healing may occur slowly with antiseptic dressing (**section 5.1.2**, **Fig. 6.1-6**) and without antibiotics.
- **Wound edge necrosis:** Devitalized wound edges become necrotic and as a rule local excision, antiseptic dressing, and depending on the extent, split skin grafting will bring about healing.
- **Wound hematoma:** Any localized hematoma provides a suitable medium for infection. If there is liquification or suture dehiscence, there is a risk of exogenous contamination. Painful or fluctuating hematomas require immediate operation with bacteriological investigation and thorough drainage and débridement.

Bacteria, such as staphylococci, can adhere particularly well to the implant surface, where they are protected from antibiotics.

All these wound complications can evolve into an acute infection if not cared for in an appropriate way. However, healing can be achieved by relatively simple means within a relatively short period. We do not recommend the term superficial wound infection, which is often used to refer to milder forms of infection.

2.3 Delayed/late first manifestations of infection (more than 2 weeks)

In the case of delayed first manifestation, the outbreak of infection is preceded by an insidious hidden infection that has spread unnoticed by the patient and all those treating him, possibly masked by the administration of non-specific antibiotics. There are certain bacteria (e.g., coagulase-negative staphylococci) which are responsible for this sort of slow development, while, occasionally, delayed contamination may occur. As a rule, it can be assumed that the infection has already established itself in a larger area of bone, requiring lengthier treatment and more radical intervention in order to achieve healing.

2.4 Additional essential definitions

Within the framework of infection after osteosynthesis the following terms appear crucial:

- **Implant-related infections:** If an infection gets in contact with an implant, **bacteria such as staphylococci can adhere particularly well to the implant surface, where they are protected from antibiotics.** Such infections, therefore, may flare up once the antibiotic treatment has been discontinued. Only a few antibiotics (e.g., rifampicin) or antiseptics are capable of destroying bacteria attached to the surface of an implant [2].

- **Osteomyelitis:** Infections can easily colonize necrotic bone. In the empty Haversian canals or osteocyte cavities, bacteria can evade the endogenous defense mechanisms, since these need a certain amount of space to build up a defense barrier. **The body can only eliminate infection by increased bone resorption and remodeling of vital areas.** As soon as a loose bone fragment has become a sequestrum there is little chance of complete resorption; such a dead fragment can only be rejected by fistulation. All defense mechanisms against infection are more successful within the bone marrow than in cortical bone. Cierny et al. [3] based their classification of osteomyelitis in adults on their knowledge of the major importance of bone necrosis and the more favorable prognosis for medullary infections. They differentiate type I (medullary osteomyelitis), type II (superficial osteomyelitis), type III (localized osteomyelitis) (see **Fig. 6.3-2**), and type IV (diffuse osteomyelitis). When considering exogenous, posttraumatic osteomyelitis, we prefer to define it in relation to the fracture fixation technique employed, since this is of greater importance [4] (**section 3.2**).
- **Chronic osteomyelitis:** This insidious condition can be diagnosed by its clinically slow progression and by specific histology with a more lymphoplasmocytic picture. The infection is chronic from the start in some cases.

- **Neglected osteomyelitis:** Untreated osteomyelitis may develop into protracted situations, characterized by chronic fistulation and chronic pain, which are difficult to treat. If the bacterial colonization persists, any treatment may be inadequate.
- **Infective arthritis:** Rapid recognition and immediate treatment of infective arthritis are decisive for its prognosis (**Fig. 6.1-8**). Late diagnosis and treatment, combined with even a slight malalignment of the articular surface, very soon lead to severe degenerative changes in the joint. Prompt revision of an adjacent osteomyelitis, on the other hand, contributes to the prevention of infective arthritis (**Fig. 6.1-7**).

3 Patients at risk

3.1 Extent of bone and soft-tissue damage in open and closed fractures

Direct injuries to a limb lead to extensive closed or open soft-tissue damage. This, in turn, carries a greater risk of soft-tissue and bone necrosis, on the one hand, and of contamination with pathogenic organisms on the other. The more extensive the damage to bone, the greater the risk of local bone necrosis and contamination when osteosynthesis is performed (**Fig. 6.1-1a**). Open fractures are particularly susceptible to infection (**chapter 5.1**). The analysis of a large consecutive series of ORIF recorded by the AO documentation from 1980–1988 disclosed an infection risk for closed fractures of 1.9%, for all open fractures of 6.2%, for III° open fractures

The body can only eliminate infection by increased bone resorption and remodeling of vital areas.

of 10.2% [5]. In a prospective study by Gustilo of 303 open fractures, infection occurred in 18 IIIB open fractures, corresponding to 44% of open segmental fractures with periosteal stripping and fragmentation of the bone [6].

3.2 Technique of fracture fixation

In general, it is important that the surgical approach for osteosynthesis be as direct as possible. However, bruised or open cutaneous areas must be carefully considered as potential risks (**chapters 1.4** and **5.1**). Vital muscle and periosteum must be preserved and left in contact with the bone as far as possible. Furthermore, every fracture fixation technique is associated with its own particular risk factors [4]. The following paragraphs describe osteomyelitis related to external fixation (pin tracks), plating, and intramedullary nailing.

3.2.1 Pin-track osteomyelitis

(**Fig. 6.1-1**)

Heat necrosis of cortical bone occurs after drilling with blunt drill bits or K-wires at excessive speed and power. Necrotic bone areas may also result from forced insertion of Schanz screws or Steinmann pins into inadequate holes or without predrilling (**Fig. 6.1-1b–d**). Necrotic fragments in the form of ring sequestra provide an excellent medium for bacteria, which migrate along the percutaneously inserted implant into the wound. Bone resorption around the implant can be seen on x-rays when the screw, pin, or nail becomes loose. Occasionally, chronic osteomyelitis reaching into the medullary canal may develop.

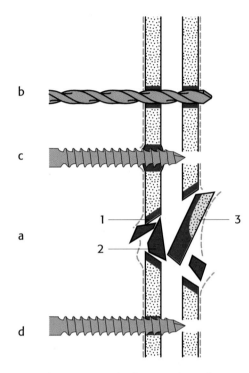

Fig.6.1-1: Complex fracture, pin-track osteomyelitis:
a) In complex fractures caused by direct trauma, we may find: 1) devitalized margins of the main fragments; 2) devitalized intermediate fragments; and 3) partially vital intermediate fragments still attached to the periosteum.
b) Reaming at excessively high speeds or with blunt drill bits produces heat necrosis in cortical bone.
c) Insertion of the Schanz screws or Steinmann pins with inadequate or no predrilling produces considerable heat and small, necrotic fragments, or ring sequestra.
d) Correct predrilling, correct placement of the Schanz screw.

3.2.2 Osteomyelitis in plating

(Fig. 6.1-2)

Even after correct application of a plate and preservation of the periosteum, devascularized areas will result at the interface between plate and bone. This circumscribed bone necrosis will be remodeled by "creeping substitution". When tissue handling during exposure and fracture reduction is poor, with unnecessary periosteal stripping of the fracture focus, additional damage to the vascularity of bone fragments will occur. If a contamination leads to infection, this will spread along the surfaces of implants and exposed bone, especially if instability develops. Necrotic and infected bone fragments will eventually be demarcated and sequestrated, with further loss of stability.

Subcutaneous and submuscular plate fixations produce different clinical symptoms when infection is present. Infection after subcutaneous plating may develop in case of disturbed wound healing, skin breakdown, hematoma, etc. Clinical diagnosis can and should be made early, while the implant may become exposed more easily. In case of submuscular or subfascial plate position (e.g., femur) an infection is often recognized late, as clinical signs are rarely apparent except for pain and fever. Ultrasound may help to detect fluid, which can then be aspirated for culture.

3.2.3 Osteomyelitis after intramedullary nailing

(Fig. 6.1-3)

Both unreamed and, even more so, reamed nailing lead to partial necrosis of the most central parts of the cortex [7]. However, the

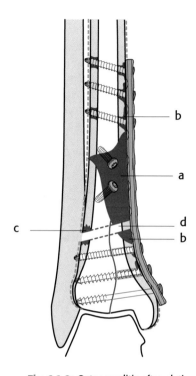

Fig. 6.1-2: Osteomyelitis after plating. Example: Tibial shaft fracture 42-B extending into the joint, correctly fixed with two 3.5 mm lag screws and 9-hole LC-DCP 4.5 without stripping the periosteum. An infection spreads along the implants and has its focus
a) in the devitalized butterfly fragment,
b) in local areas of devascularized bone under the plate,
c) in areas resulting from incorrect drilling,
d) in empty drill holes.

Both unreamed and reamed nailing lead to partial necrosis of the most central parts of the cortex.

periosteal blood supply remains in great part intact and contributes to cortical remodeling and fracture healing. Even if an infection spreads along the entire implant and medullary canal, periosteal bony bridging by external callus can be expected in many instances (**Fig. 6.1-9**). In nailing without reaming, cortical necrosis is less extensive than after reaming, but the bore dust which possibly promotes bone bridging is missing. In "open" nailing with surgical exposure of the fracture focus, additional periosteal stripping, loss of bone dust, and potential contamination must be taken into account. These are reasons to avoid open nailing whenever possible. Dull reamers and too large diameters may lead to heat necrosis and to obstruction of the Haversian canals. Dead bone prevents normal fracture healing and in case of infection may lead to an infected non-union which is especially hard to salvage [**8**, **9**].

3.3   General and local risk factors

The risk of an infection is increased by various factors, both general and local [**10**]. Local factors include venous stasis, occlusive arterial disease, extensive scarring, infectious skin lesions, neuropathy, chronic lymphatic edema, vasculitis, and radiation fibrosis. General factors include diabetes mellitus, renal and liver failure, chronic hypoxia, autoimmune diseases, malignancy, old age, immunosuppressive treatment, agranulocytosis, AIDS, and abuse of nicotine, alcohol, and drugs.

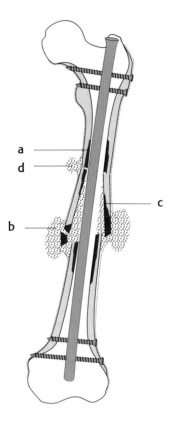

Fig. 6.1-3: Osteomyelitis after intramedullary nailing.
Example: Complex femur fracture stabilized by a closed, reamed, and locked intramedullary nail. This results in:
a) Devascularized inner cortex after reaming.
b) Reaming dust mixed with fracture hematoma.
c) Fracture fragments partially stripped from periosteum.
d) Infection spreading along the nail within the medullary cavity. Periosteal fracture healing by bridging callus formation is likely to occur despite infection.

4 Diagnosis of an acute infection

4.1 Clinical and laboratory findings

Clinical symptoms (redness, pain, fever) and laboratory findings (leukocyte count, CRP) often lead directly to the diagnosis. More frequently, however, and in spite of obvious local symptoms, there are no corresponding laboratory findings to support the clinical signs, which delays correct decision making (**Fig. 6.1-6–9**). Every surgeon has a tendency to underestimate unfavorable findings in his own cases. More experienced colleagues should, therefore, be consulted and, if there is real doubt, the wound should be revised.

Exceptionaly, an acute posttraumatic infection may develop into septicemia. Such a life-threatening situation must be dealt with aggressively, given that any metallic foreign body may be the focus.

4.2 Imaging procedures

In early first manifestation of an infection, imaging procedures play a minor role. However, faced with delayed first manifestations, there is a need to assess the extent to which the infection had already affected the bone or healing process of the fracture before symptoms became apparent. Accumulations of fluid (hematoma, seroma, abscess) are easily identified by ultrasound. The method is non-invasive, and reaches the deeper layers, especially of the thigh. Standard x-rays remain the most important source of information, as MRI and CT rarely provide more information in the early stage. Widening of the fracture gap as an indication of bone resorption, as well as loosening of implants, are signs of instability, possibly due to infection, while a lack of periosteal new bone formation may be a sign of absence of blood supply to bone and surrounding tissues. It is particularly important to identify the progress of bony bridging on one side and infection on the other (**Fig. 6.1-9**). Three-phase skeletal scintigraphy with technetium 99 may be of help in recognizing large areas of bone necrosis [10].

The size of acutely infected areas can be defined by infection scintigraphy with the patient's granulocytes labeled with indium or labeled antibodies against granulocytes [11]. Scintigraphic investigations are, however, reserved mainly for subacute cases. Since infection scintigraphy is based on labeling of granulocytes, chronic osteomyelitis may produce false negative results. Furthermore, with this method, hematogenic bone marrow is also displayed because of the labeled antibodies, leading to overshadowing.

4.3 Bacteriology and histology

In acute infection, the decision for surgical revision is generally taken without waiting for bacteriological evaluation. Adjuvant antibiotic treatment is started empirically and modified once the results of culture tests have been received (**section 5.3.1**). **We recommend that the bacteriological tests be based not only on liquid or aspirates (Video 6.1-1, Video 6.1-2) but also on specimens of tissue (blocks of 5–10 mm) from several infected sites (Video 6.1-3, Video 6.1-4, Video 6.1-5, Video 6.1-6).**

Bacteriology must include tissue samples from several sites.

Anaerobic pathogens will thereby be included [10]. Be aware of swabs taken from wound secretions, as they often include bacteria not responsible for the infection (e.g., *Pseudomonas aerugoinosa*). The most important bacteria responsible for posttraumatic infection are staphylococci. In protracted infections other pathogens may gain importance as a result of additional contamination from outside. The histological investigation of soft-tissue specimens has two objectives. If the bacteriological evaluation is negative, it is highly likely that a bacteriological etiology for the infection will

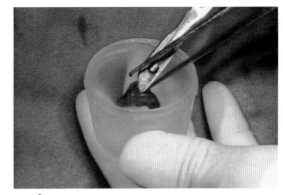

Video 6.1-3

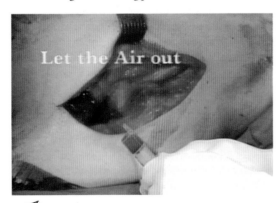

Video 6.1-1

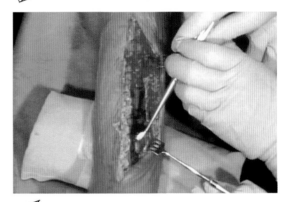

Video 6.1-4

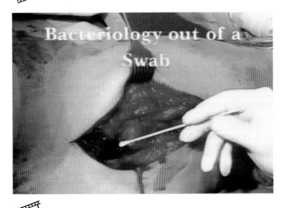

Video 6.1-2

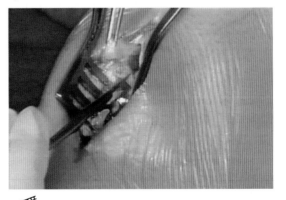

Video 6.1-5

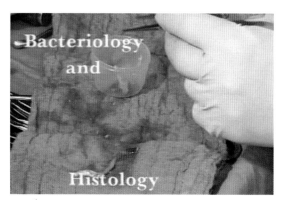

 Video 6.1-6

nonetheless be found. Furthermore, it is possible to determine histologically whether the acute infection is recent or has developed from a chronic infection.

The histological analysis of bone specimens is complex, takes long (decalcification), and has mainly scientific significance [12].

5   Treatment components

As a rule, an infection can be successfully treated by simple means if first manifestations appear early. However, if there are delayed first manifestations and the sequelae of infection on the bone are already apparent radiographically, more complex forms of treatment will be necessary for effective infection control and ultimate fracture healing.

5.1   Simple procedures

5.1.1   Débridement

Débridement consists of thorough removal of hematoma and necrotic soft tissue (wound margins, subcutaneous and muscular tissue), as well as dead bone splinters and sequestra, and excessive granulation tissue. Tissue specimens are taken from multiple sites and sent for bacteriological and histological investigation (**section 4.3**).

Débridement must include removal of all dead tissue (hematoma, soft parts, and bone).

5.1.2   Open wound treatment

Open wound treatment is particularly reliable, but rather slow. It prevents abscess formation and permits easy—even bedside—wound revision.

Antiseptic dressings reduce super-infection from outside, for example, in the case of an exposed, but stable plate (Fig. 6.1-6). A cannula is placed into the deepest part of the wound, which is irrigated four to five times a day with a tissue-compatible antiseptic solution, for example, Lavasept® (**section 5.3.2**). The dressing is changed once a day. Well granulating wound areas are covered with mesh graft or a rotation skin flap. Complete wound closure often occurs only after implant removal (**Fig. 6.1-6**).

Antiseptic dressings reduce super-infection from outside.

5.1.3   Closed wound treatment

This is the more risky but more direct way to wound healing. Deep sutures should be omitted, however, and efficient drainage with several wide-bore drains is necessary (**Fig. 6.1-4**). In addition, an irrigation-suction drainage with Ringer's solution or an antiseptic solution is

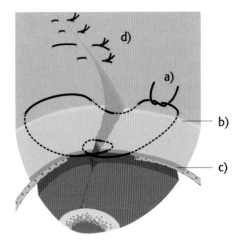

Fig. 6.1-4: Suture technique in infected wounds. Thick monofilament sutures (a) are used every 4–6 cm to secure the deeper levels of skin (b) and the fascia (c). Additional skin sutures (d) are placed between the deep sutures.

introduced for 2–4 days in order to prevent hematoma formation [13]. During irrigation-suction drainage, care must be taken that no retention of fluids occurs. This would require discontinuation of irrigation and sometimes even a revision. Some authors no longer irrigate and prefer non-resorbable or resorbable antibiotic or antiseptic carriers to raise the level of antibacterial agents in the debrided area (gentamicin beads, resorbable collagen sponges with antibiotics) [14].

5.1.4 Implant removal

As long as an implant provides stable fixation, fracture healing can take place despite the presence of a metallic foreign body, even an exposed plate, which should only be removed once bony bridging has occured. If, however, implants have become loose, they must be removed and replaced by another form of fixation, such as an external fixator (**Fig. 6.1-9**), a plaster cast, or an orthotic device, to provide stability which is necessary for further fracture and soft-tissue healing.

5.1.5 Arthroscopic joint irrigation in septic arthritis

At the slightest suspicion of septic arthritis, joint aspiration or preferably, arthroscopy should be performed to evaluate the involvement of the joint. Synovitis alone can be managed by antibiotic treatment (**section 5.3.1**). Depending on the severity of fibrinous deposits, arthrosopic or open synovectomy may be indicated. In case of clear infection, arthroscopic irrigation should be performed repeatedly (every 2 days) [15]. In severe arthritis, arthrodesis or joint resection may be unavoidable.

5.2 Complex measures

In the absence of bony bridging, a change of the fixation technique must be considered, usually to an external fixator. This may be combined with an additional procedure on bone (débridement, decortication, cancellous bone grafting). All necrotic tissue must be resected. If the resulting defect is large and segmental, callus distraction (as described by Ilizarov—see **chapter 6.3**) or bridging by a vascularized bone graft may be necessary (**chapter 6.3**). Options for soft-tissue coverage are discussed in **chapter 5.2**.

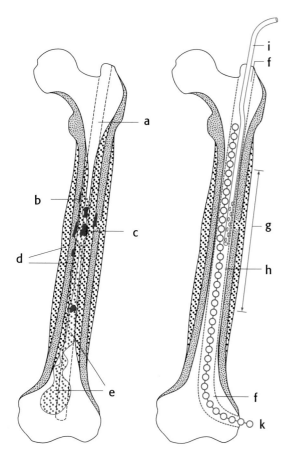

Fig. 6.1-5: Reaming of the medullary canal in chronic infection after nailing. Reaming of the medullary canal (a) leaves behind isolated necrotic areas of bone (b) which are partially sequestrated (c). The original cortex has been infiltrated by periosteal and endosteal bone regenerates (d). An intramedullary fistula has formed (e), which often spreads distally to form an abscess. In order to ream the medullary canal, it is opened from the proximal to the distal ends (f). If the central tunneling procedure is not entirely successful, a lateral window (g) is created. The aim of creating an ample reaming canal (h) supported by the thickened periosteum is to ensure that all necrotic fragments are removed. Overflow drainage without suction (i) is left in for a few days and a gentamicin-PMMA-chain (k) for 10 days.

5.2.1 Reaming of the medullary cavity

In case of infection of the medullary cavity, reaming of the canal is based on the assumption that there are areas of necrotic bone within the diaphysis (**Fig. 6.1-5**) which can be debrided and cleared from infection (**Video 6.1-7**). After nail removal, a distal opening is created to allow the debris from reaming and flushing to escape. A chain of gentamicin-PMMA-beads is inserted into the canal after it has been reamed to a diameter 2–3 mm larger than the removed nail. The PMMA-chain is removed after 10 days. In chronic infections, reaming must generally be even more radical [16].

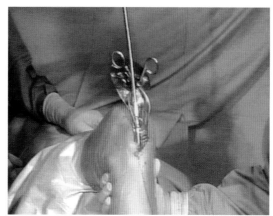

 Video 6.1-7

5.3 The use of antibiotics and antiseptics

(see **chapter 5.5**)

In posttraumatic osteomyelitis, antibiotics and antiseptics should only be considered as a useful supplement to radical operative intervention.

In posttraumatic osteomyelitis, antibiotics and antiseptics should only be considered as a useful supplement to radical operative intervention.

5.3.1 Antibiotics

Treatment with antibiotics is started, both therapeutically and as prophylaxis, during anesthesia (**chapter 5.5**). This does not prevent the intraoperative recovery of specimens for bacteriology. When the pathogens are unknown, it is recommended that treatment with a broad spectrum antibiotic starts preoperatively. This is later replaced by a specific antibiotic according to the sensitivity tests. Once started, treatment should be maintained for 6–12 weeks if the fracture is to consolidate with the implants *in situ*. Parenteral administration seems mandatory for the first 2–3 weeks for most antibiotics. Sometimes a port-a-cath implantation may facilitate intravenous application [**17**].

To be effective, antibiotics must be taken regularly and in adequate doses; only then is a sufficiently high concentration of antibiotics obtained in bone. The normalization of the CRP during treatment seems to confirm the effectiveness of the drug.

Implant-related infections: Staphylococci, in particular, once they have adhered to the surface of an implant, are able to survive in spite of appropriately chosen antibiotics. Currently, rifampicin is the only drug which will eliminate these pathogens at concentrations tolerable to the body. However, because of the danger of increased resistance, rifampicin may only be given in combination with other drugs, for example, ciprofloxacin. The efficacy of rifampicin has been demonstrated in a randomized study [**2**] (**chapter 5.5**).

5.3.2 Antiseptics

Antiseptics (originally carbolic spray) paved the way for modern surgery and their bactericidal properties are still indispensible for disinfecting surgeons' hands (alcohol, iodine preparations, chlorhexidine, etc.). These agents cannot be considered for treatment of the open wound or bone because of their tissue toxicity. Lavasept®, as a combination of a biguanide with polyethylglycol in aqueous solution, introduced by Willenegger and Good [**18**], has bactericidal properties without being toxic to soft tissue. It is used intraoperatively for prophylactic irrigation, except in joints. The bactericidal properties which alter the cell membrane have been proven for Lavasept®, even at very low concentrations. The substance is hardly resorbed because of the size of its molecules and only remains active on the surface. A local compromise is achieved with the antiseptic dressing, while a superinfection with new pathogens can be prevented. Clinical observations show the undisturbed development of healthy granulations which soon lend themselves to simple coverage with mesh grafts. The use of antiseptics intra-articularily is contraindicated, since the cells most capable of regeneration lie mainly on the surface. It is particularly important to note that serum albumins do not diminish the effect of Lavasept®, whereas they counteract the effect of iodine preparations within a short time.

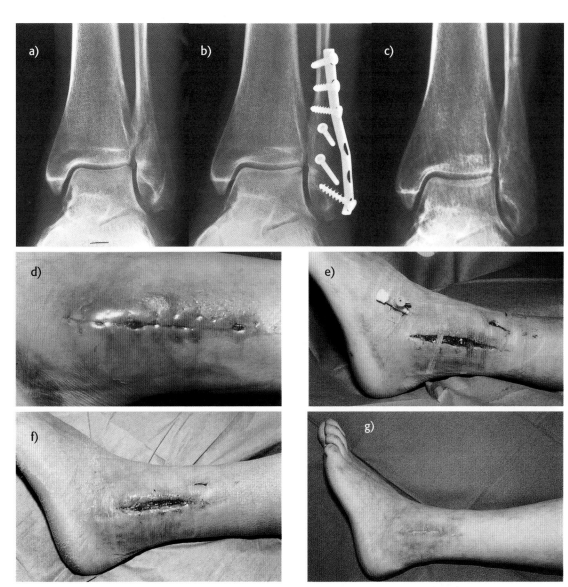

Fig. 6.1-6: Delayed first manifestation after subcutaneous plating:
a/b) Plate osteosynthesis of a multifragmentary malleolar fracture of the fibula type 44-B1.2.
d) Day 21: Infection with *Staphylococcus aureus*—leukocytes 18,500, CRP < 5. e) Débridement and antiseptic dressing of the open wound. A cannula was inserted per-cutaneously to the deepest point of the infected region. Irrigation four to five times a day with an anti-septic (Lavasept®) via the cannula to keep the wound moist. IV-cefazolin for 1 week, then ciprofloxacin for 4 weeks.
f) Plate removal after 6 weeks, uneventful wound healing.
c/g) One year follow-up: good functional result without osteoarthritis.

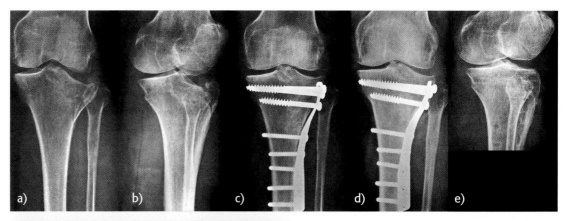

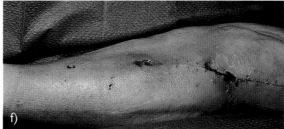

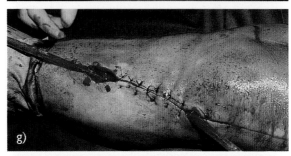

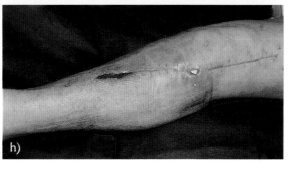

Fig. 6.1-7: Delayed first manifestation after a subcutaneous/submuscular plate osteosynthesis.
a/b) 63-year-old female suffering from a lateral fracture of the tibial plateau 41-B3.1.
c) Osteosynthesis on the same day.
f) Disturbed wound healing and infection with coagulase-negative staphylococci.
g) In spite of a normal CRP and in the absence of fever, a revision was performed on the twenty-fourth day. Débridement and open irrigation. Antibiotic treatment for 2 months (rifampicin, trimethoprim, and sulfamethoxazole), followed by healing (h) within 6 weeks.
d/e) One year after the operation, the patient was symptom-free.

6 Treatment concept in typical cases

6.1 Osteosynthesis in subcutaneous area

Débridement and assessment of stability, open wound treatment and antiseptic dressing (Fig. 6.1-6), or partial coverage and open drainage in the presence of adequate soft tissues (Fig. 6.1-7 and Fig. 6.1-8) are possible with the help of a local flap. Implants are removed after 6 (e.g., malleolar fractures) to 12 weeks (e.g., olecranon fractures).

6.2 Plate osteosynthesis in submuscular position

Débridement is accompanied by assessment of the stability of the plate fixation. In the absence of avital bone fragments, irrigation-suction drainage and wound closure are followed by antibiotics for 6–12 weeks. Implant removal as soon as solid bridging of fracture is confirmed. For infected pseudoarthroses or large bone defects see chapter 6.3.

6.3 Osteomyelitis after intramedullary nailing

If there are signs of bridging on x-ray assessment, but stability is lacking, abscess drainage is followed by antibiotics until bridging is achieved. After nail removal and reaming of the medullary cavity, antibiotics are continued for another 6 weeks. In the absence of signs of bridging, nail and sequestra are removed and reaming of the medullary cavity is followed by management as described in chapter 6.3.

6.4 Pin-track osteomyelitis in the presence of an external fixator

If there is suppuration along the Schanz screws, Steinmann pins, or transcutaneous wires, x-rays help to identify possible ring sequestra. The following regime is then followed: Remove or replace the implant, perform curettage, remove sequestra, and rinse with antiseptics. Administer antibiotics only in cases of simultaneous abscess revision and/or positive laboratory findings.

6.5 Concomitant arthritis

If findings from immediate aspiration are positive: bacteriology, arthroscopic joint revision, and antibiotics for 3–6 weeks. Repeated punctures every second day. After approximately 1 week, repeat arthroscopy and re-assess the situation.

7 Measures to prevent infections

7.1 General measures

The following measures help to prevent or reduce the number of infections:

- Regular disinfection of the hands with alcohol after every contact with a patient.

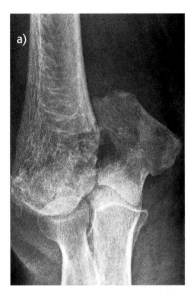
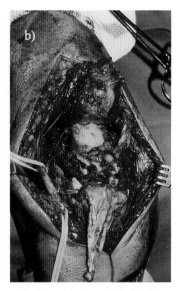
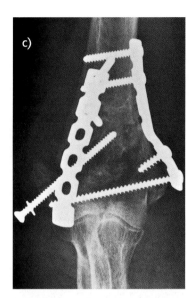

Fig. 6.1-8: Early first manifestation after plate osteosynthesis–posttraumatic arthritis.
a) Distal humeral fracture 13-C3.1 in an 83-year-old female with considerable osteoporosis.
b/c) Osteosynthesis on the fifth day with V-shaped transection of the triceps tendon. Instability of one screw.
d) Ten days later, pain, leukocytes 11,500, CRP 195. Débridement, joint closure, half-open irrigation. *Staphylococcus aureus*. Flucloxacillin introduced parenterally for 3 weeks, finally ciprofloxacin for 2 months.
e) Alleviation of the situation after 10 days.
f) After 2 years, obvious osteoarthritis, para-articular ossification and extension deficit. Despite arthrolysis at implant removal, flexion/extension remained at only 85-35-0, a condition arising from the combination of a comminuted fracture and posttraumatic arthritis.

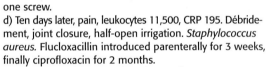
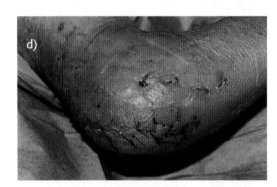
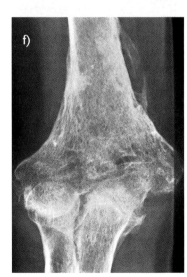
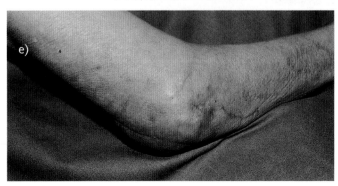

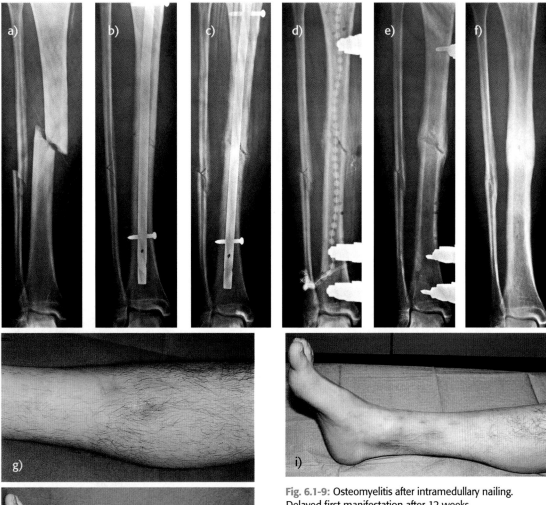

Fig. 6.1-9: Osteomyelitis after intramedullary nailing. Delayed first manifestation after 12 weeks.
a) Simple oblique fracture of the tibia, type 42-A2.2, after being hit by a falling trunk.
b) Fixation with a reamed universal nail, dynamically locked.
g) Temporary redness after about 9 weeks.
h) After 12 weeks, abscess formation and pain.
c) Radiologically, extensive callus bridging.
d) Nail removal, reaming of the medullary cavity (see **Fig. 6.1-5**) to 13.5 mm, external fixator and abscess revision (*Staphylococcus epidermidis*). Parenteral introduction of flucloxacillin for 2 weeks, clindamicin orally for 4 weeks, full weight bearing.
e) After 8 weeks external fixator about to be removed.
f/i) Two-year follow-up, patient working full-time as a laborer.

- Gloves must be worn to remove dressings; all dressings are disposed in separate bags. For further wound care etc., sterile gloves should be used.
- Dressings of secreting wounds should be so thick that the secretions do not penetrate. Otherwise, changes of such dressings have to occur more often.

7.2 Septic patients on the ward

Septic patients on the ward should be cared for in separate rooms that are thoroughly disinfected every time a patient is discharged from hospital.

7.3 Septic patients in the operating theater

Operations are performed in an operating theater reserved for this purpose or in a specially prepared room.

Barrier: The room is separated by a special barrier or warning sign. Inside, specially labeled shoes are worn and all waste, including disposable gowns, is handled separately.

At the end of the operation: The surgical team changes and leaves all potentially contaminated gear in the theater. The entire empty room is finally disinfected.

7.4 MRSA (methicillin-resistant staphylococci) and other problem pathogens

If MRSA is suspected or identified, a patient must be completely isolated in a separate room for the entire period of treatment or until bacteriology is negative. Nursing staff and visitors entering the room must wear masks, hospital gowns, gloves, and special slippers. Instruments must be handled according to special instructions and all potentially contaminated gear, linen, etc. must be handled separately as well.

8 Bibliography

1. **Willenegger H, Roth B** (1986) [Treatment tactics and late results in early infection following osteosynthesis]. *Unfallchirurgie;* 12 (5):241–246.
2. **Zimmerli W, Widmer AF, Blatter M, et al.** (1998) Role of rifampin for treatment of orthopedic implant-related staphylococcal infections: a randomized controlled trial. Foreign-Body Infection (FBI) Study Group. *Jama;* 279 (19):1537–1541.
3. **Cierny G, Mader JT, Penninck JJ** (1985) A clinical staging system for adult osteomyelitis. *Contemp Orthop;* 10:17–37.
4. **Burri C** (1975) *Post-traumatic osteomyelitis.* Bern Stuttgart Vienna: Hans Huber Publisher.
5. **Ochsner PE** (1992) [Prognosis and complications of open fractures]. *Helv Chir Acta;* 59 (1):129–141.

6. **Gustilo RB, Gruninger RP, Davis T** (1987) Classification of type III (severe) open fractures relative to treatment and results. *Orthopedics;* 10 (12):1781–1788.

7. **Klein MP, Rahn BA, Frigg R, et al.** (1990) Reaming versus non-reaming in medullary nailing: interference with cortical circulation of the canine tibia. *Arch Orthop Trauma Surg;* 109 (6):314–316.

8. **Ochsner PE, Baumgart F, Kohler G** (1998) Heat-induced segmental necrosis after reaming of one humeral and two tibial fractures with a narrow medullary canal. *Injury;* 29 (Suppl 2):B1–10.

9. **Baumgart F, Kohler G, Ochsner PE** (1998) The physics of heat generation during reaming of the medullary cavity. *Injury;* 29 (Suppl 2):B11–25.

10. **Mader JT, Ortiz M, Calhoun JH** (1996) Update on the diagnosis and management of osteomyelitis. *Clin Podiatr Med Surg;* 13 (4):701–724.

11. **Kaim A, Maurer T, Ochsner PE, et al.** (1997) Chronic complicated osteomyelitis of the appendicular skeleton: diagnosis with technetium-99m labelled monoclonal antigranulocyte antibody-immunoscintigraphy. *Eur J Nucl Med;* 24 (7):732–738.

12. **Böhm E** (1986) *Chronische posttraumatische Osteomyelitis, Morphologie und Pathogenese.* Berlin Heidelberg New York: Springer-Verlag.

13. **Pfister A, Ochsner PE** (1993) [Experiences with closed irrigation-suction drainage and simultaneous administration of an antiseptic]. *Unfallchirurg;* 96 (6):332–340.

14. **Klemm KW** (1993) Antibiotic bead chains. *Clin Orthop;* (295):63–76.

15. **Perry CR** (1996) Bone and joint infections. London: Martin Dunitz.

16. **Ochsner PE, Gösele A, Buess P** (1990) The value of intramedullary reaming in the treatment of chronic osteomyelitis of long bones. *Arch Orthop Trauma Surg;* 109 (6):341–347.

17. **Hunger T, Gösele A, Ochsner PE** (1993) Implantierbares Venenkathetersystem zur ambulanten Langzeit-Antibiotikatherapie bei chronischer Osteomyelitis. *Hefte Unfallchir;* 230:1032–1035.

18. **Willenegger H, Roth B, Ochsner PE** (1995) The return of local antiseptics in surgery. *Injury;* 26 (Suppl): 29–33.

9 Updates

Updates and additional references for this chapter are available online at:
http://www.aopublishing.org/PFxM/61.htm

6.2 Aseptic non-union

Michael D. McKee

1 Introduction

Failure of a fracture to heal prolongs the patient's disability and may have a greater negative impact on the quality of life than renal dialysis or ischemic heart disease [1]. Prompt attention to problems with healing will not only impact positively on the patient's life but will also decrease the potential for implant failure.

Delayed union occurs when a fracture heals more slowly than clinically expected for the site and the type of fracture in question. When a fracture has ceased to show any evidence of healing, non-union occurs, as indicated by persistent fracture lines, sclerosis at the fracture ends, a gap, and hypertrophic or absent callus. Unless there is bone loss, a non-union is usually declared between 6–8 months after the fracture. Since the "natural history" of most fractures is to heal, the treating surgeon must first consider why a delay has occurred. Failure of a fracture to unite is usually the result of a number of factors. Although any single one may predominate, **delayed or non-union is often multifactorial in nature** [2]. A careful investigation prior to surgical intervention will often reveal the solution to the problem [3].

2 Etiology of aseptic non-union

Whereas **disturbed vascularity and instability are the most important factors leading to a non-union,** others such as non-compliance and neuropathies may inhibit healing. Infection as a cause of non-union is dealt with in **chapter 6.3**.

2.1 Vascularity

All fractures disrupt the blood supply to the bone and soft tissue to some degree; the greater the energy, the greater the disruption. The location of the fracture, particularly if one fracture fragment gets its blood supply from an end artery (e.g., femoral head) is determinant. Surgical treatment may cause further vascular disruption. While it is still possible for a fracture that has one avascular or poorly vascularized segment to unite, it does so much more slowly than normal and may sometimes not do so at all. If both fragments are avascular, the fracture will most probably not unite. No amount of surgical manipulation of the mechanical environment will promote union unless either remodeling of the necrotic bone area or appo-

Disturbed vascularity and/or instability lead to aseptic non-union.

Delayed unions and non-unions have a multifactorial background.

sition of newly formed periosteal bone restores the local vascularity (see **Fig. 6.2-4**).

2.2 Instability

Plating of simple or wedge fractures without interfragmentary compression will lead to local instability and bone resorption at the fracture site. In such a situation, the plate will inhibit mechanical contact and healing between the fragments unless fatigue fracture of the plate occurs. In complex fractures fixed by plate or nail, most of the fragments may unite, leaving one fracture plane not united. It is a general phenomenon that a non-union is always limited to one plane of mechanical instability regardless of the classification of the original fracture and the initial treatment.

2.3 Non-compliance

It is the responsibility of the treating orthopedic surgeon to ensure that the care plan is compatible with the patient's personality and life style. The patient and surgeon must work cooperatively to assure the outcome. Inappropriate weight bearing, smoking, improper diet, and other shortcomings in behavior should be addressed [4] or taken into account when management is being planned.

2.4 Neuropathy

There appears to be a relationship between fracture healing and appropriate neurological function of the extremity. Diabetes, paraplegia, chronic alcoholism, spina bifida, syringomyelia, and leprosy may effect protective proprio-

ception, thereby limiting the ability of the patient to control weight bearing. Extensive soft-tissue damage of the affected area may lead to a loss of sensibility, compromising the already impaired healing response.

3 Classification and principles of treatment of non-union

The classification scheme described here is a well-established, straightforward description that guides the surgeon toward the most appropriate treatment strategy. Therefore, both the definition and the guidelines for treatment are mentioned within the same paragraph.

3.1 Delayed union

(**Fig. 6.2-1**)

Delayed union describes the situation where there are distinct clinical and radiological signs of prolonged fracture healing time. It is important to recognize the diagnosis of delayed union so that additional effort can be aimed at achieving fracture healing as fast as possible. Clinically, the fractured limb presents with local swelling, redness, and warmth, while mobilization or partial weight bearing is painful. Laboratory values such as ESR, C-reactive protein (CRP), and leukocyte counts are normal. The x-rays may show loosening of the implant. If the aim of the fracture fixation was absolute stability, then widening of the fracture gap and callus formation ("irritation callus") are signs of impending failure of fixation (**Fig. 6.2-1**).

In delayed union there are clinical and radiological signs of prolonged fracture healing.

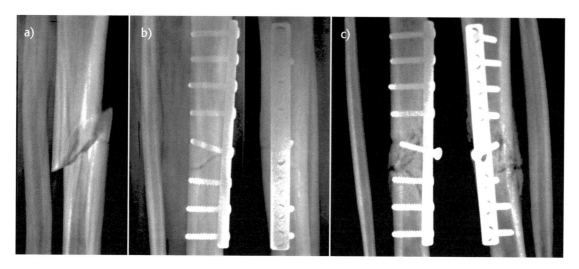

Fig. 6.2-1: Delayed union in a 19-year-old male.
a) Direct trauma in a motorcycle accident. Closed tibial fracture type 42-B2.
b) Neutralization plate with an interfragmentary lag screw of questionable value.
c) After 2 months pain, swelling, redness. Loosening of lag screw, widening of the fracture gap, and irritation callus. Decision for operative revision with decortication and compression plating.

The initial phase of treatment may be non-operative. Reducing the mechanical stress across the fracture site by decreasing weight bearing or applying a plaster cast for 6 weeks may direct the local response towards fracture healing. Repeated x-rays at 3–6 week intervals showing progression of healing are indicative of successful non-operative management. If during this phase there are signs of implant failure or a lack of healing response, then the treatment should be changed to an operative intervention. The patient should be forewarned about the possible need for an intervention whenever a delayed union is diagnosed. The type of operative intervention will depend on the etiology of the healing delay and the type and function of the existing fixation construct.

3.2 Diaphyseal non-union

3.2.1 Hypertrophic non-union

(**Fig. 6.2-2**)

Hypertrophic non-union is frequently localized in the lower extremities. Its development largely depends on an impaired mechanical stability. In well vascularized tissue, instability leads to local detachments of the periosteum, provoking additional new bone formation. Although the fracture is ready to unite, there is insufficient mechanical stability for the non-union to consolidate. The degree of instability may be such that the patient can use his leg but suffers pain when fatigued. In other

Hypertrophic non-union usually lacks stability.

Fig. 6.2-2: Well vascularized vital non-unions: All patterned areas mean vascularized bone, black = original cortex, red = at the moment of non-union.
a) Hypertrophic non-union (elephant foot), usually associated with some stability and mechanical irritation leading to excessive new bone formation.
b) Hypertrophic non-union (horse hoof), less prominent new bone formation in a less stable situation (see also **Fig. 6.2-3**).
c) Atrophic non-union. Due to marked instability there is resorption of original bone cortex leading to rounded ends.
⊖ = bone resorption

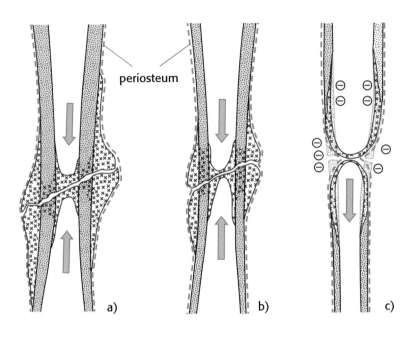

periosteum

a)   b)   c)

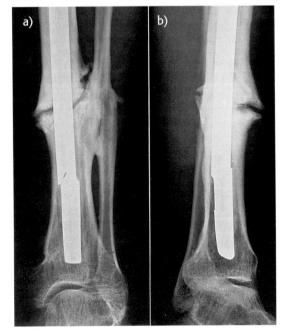

a)   b)

Fig. 6.2-3: Hypertrophic horse hoof non-union in a 36-year-old male 19 years after being run over by a truck.
a) Tibia 19 years after being fixed by intramedullary nail. Hypertrophic non-union with fatigue fracture of the nail.
b) Resorption around the nail indicates motion. Consolidated fibula with bridge to distal tibia prevents healing of tibia.

cases the patient may report constant pain when weight bearing and have some deformity (**Fig. 6.2-3**). According to the x-rays, either an elephant foot (**Fig. 6.2-2a**) or a horse's hoof shape is described (**Fig. 6.2-2b**, **Fig. 6.2-3**).

The most effective method of correcting a hypertrophic non-union is to improve the stability of the fracture site by compression plating or a reamed, locked intramedullary nail. **Mechanical stability leads to a calcification of the fibrous cartilage which can only then be penetrated by new vessels, finally allowing bony bridging and remodeling of the non-union site [5].** Bone grafting is not

Mechanical stability allows the fibrous cartilage to calcify and finally ossify after vascular penetration.

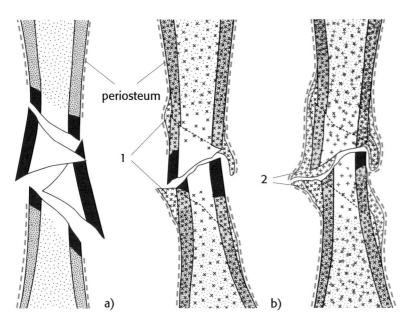

periosteum

1

2

a)   b)   c)

Fig. 6.2-4: Avascular/avital non-union.
a) Situation immediately following complex fracture. The red areas are devitalized. The dotted area remained viable.
b) Months later, the two intermediate fragments appear to be attached by callus (red, 1) to each main fragment, but there is no evidence of healing in the center of the fracture.
c) Even after years and and in spite of additional periosteal bone formation and some remodeling by creeping substitution (blue, 2) the non-union persists.

3.2.2 Avascular/avital non-union with/without bone loss

(**Fig. 6.2-4**)

usually necessary, although decortication ("shingling") may speed-up union (see section 4.2.1, **Decortication or osteoperiosteal petalling**). **Resection of a hypertrophic non-union must be regarded as an error,** since it removes bone tissue which is ready to bridge.

Hypertrophic non-union may also be managed using other methods such as fibular osteotomy combined with a walking cast, encouraging impaction that may lead to union. Prolonged immobilization in a plaster cast combined with electromagnetic fields or ultrasound action may also be helpful (see **section 4.5**). However, the ability to correct deformity and accelerate union (healing within 3–5 months) upholds the operative method as the current "gold standard".

Avascular non-union originates in the devascularization of the bone fragments adjacent to the fracture site due to injury and/or surgery. Avascular fragments may unite with vital bone elements, but unless additional measures are taken they will never unite with another avital fragment (**Fig. 6.2-4b**). Commencing at the vital main fragment, a remodeling process will slowly begin to revitalize the necrotic bone areas (**Fig. 6.2-4c**). Simultaneously, there may be an ongoing grinding process between the necrotic fragments at the non-union site leading to bone loss by resorption. Delay in recognition and treatment allows the abnormal remodeling process to result in shortening and osteopenia of the distal

Avascular non-union originates in the devascularization of the bone fragments.

Resecting a hypertrophic non-union is an error.

fragment due to non-use. This situation can be avoided by proper supervision during follow-up and prompt treatment. For the bone to heal, vital areas of contact must be created and mechanical stability must be provided. The treatment has to be planned according to the state of the local remodeling and the extent of the bone loss. Several options are available, including simple shortening, shortening combined with the shortening of the other limb, shortening with lengthening at a separate site (callus distraction see **chapter 6.3**), interposition of bone grafts (morcellized or structural), or a "bypass" as in a fibula-pro-tibia procedure (see section 4.2.1, **Cancellous autograft**).

3.2.3 **Atrophic non-union**

(see **Fig. 6.2-2c**)

In the upper extremities, atrophic non-union can typically occur as a vascularized non-union. The two bone ends at the site of the non-union undergo atrophy due to the absence of any force-transmission. The atrophic non-union is characterized by a lack of bony response in spite of being vascularized.

  This situation requires not only stabilization but also the addition of bone-inducing and conductive agents. Taking account of the local vascularity, the appropriate approach to dealing with the situation is decortication and bone grafting together with stabilization (preferably with a plate).

3.2.4 **Pseudarthrosis**

Persistent motion at a fracture site may result in the formation of a false joint where a fibro-cartilagenous cavity is lined with synovium producing synovial fluid. Such "synovial pseudarthroses" are commonly seen in the humerus, femur, and tibia and are usually vital, although they may at times appear atrophic. As well as a synovial cavity they often have an axial and/or rotational deformity. Corrective surgery consists of stabilization and correction of the deformity and possibly a bone graft (**Fig. 6.2-5**), as already outlined.

3.3 **Metaphyseal non-union**

Non-union in a diaphysis is different from non-union in a metaphysis in that it occurs in cancellous bone, usually with a small articular fragment, which may be difficult to fix and possibly also affected by osteoporosis (**Fig. 6.2-6**). Frequently, the only residual movement occurs in the non-union and not in the joint, so that any treatment must include a thorough arthrolysis. Stiffness of the neighboring joint may or may not be prominent. The non-union is either extra-articular or intra-articular, separating the joint in two parts.

4 **Treatment procedures**

4.1 **General remarks**

The primary objective in the treatment of a non-union is to eliminate pain and to achieve alignment by obtaining osseous consolidation as well as restoration of function of the injured limb. With the exception of non-unions with extensive bone loss or considerable areas of non-vital bone, consolidation can usually be

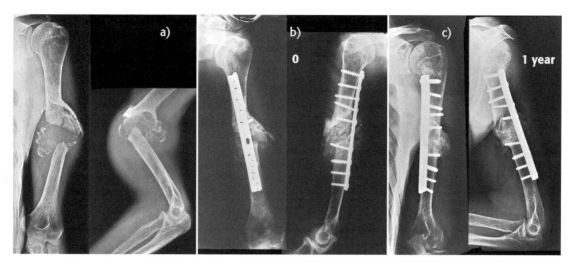

Fig. 6.2-5: Pseudarthrosis.
a) 49-year-old laborer working 100% in spite of an established pseudarthrosis of the left humerus for 15 years.
b) After resection of the synovia, a large cancellous autograft was placed into the gap and stabilized by a 10-hole broad DCP 4.5.
c) Full consolidation at 1 year follow-up with good function.

achieved in one operative step, with full weight bearing in 4–5 months. A detailed analysis of every case and a close personal contact with the patient, especially during the postoperative period, are essential to avoid further complications. Special precautions have to be taken in the case of neurological deficits in order to protect the patient from the consequences of inadvertent overuse (see **section 2.4**). As the rate of union achieved in most reported series of cases is over 95%, the operative reconstructive approach should generally be favored over more aggressive measures such as amputation, arthroplasty, or arthrodesis.

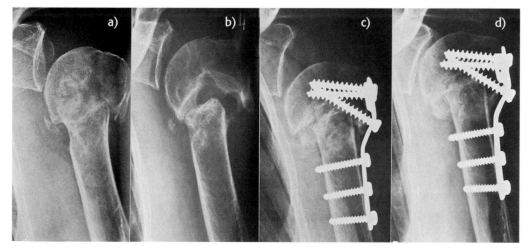

Fig. 6.2-6: Atrophic non-union in the metaphyseal area in a 78-year-old female.
a) Minimally displaced subcapital humeral fracture.
b) Eight months later atrophic non-union, limited function, and some pain.
c) Repair with T-plate and cancellous autograft plus tension banding using a resorbable cord.
d) Full consolidation with unlimited function after 1 year.

4.2 Diaphyseal non-union

The general guidelines for therapy of non-union have already been mentioned in **section 3**. In this section the details of the procedures are discussed.

4.2.1 Bone reconstruction

Bone reconstruction is only essential if there is a necrotic bone segment or a bone defect to be bridged. In cases where the viability of bone is questionable, reconstruction may be chosen as a precautionary measure. In the presence of a hypertrophic non-union, decortication may be indicated to add security (**Fig. 6.2-7** and **Fig. 6.2-9**).

Fig. 6.2-7: Musculo-periosteo-osteal decortication.
a) In areas of non-union the vascularization of the external part of the diaphysis depends largely on periosteal blood supply (green area).
b/c) Decortication with a sharp osteotome creates vascular periosteal bone fragments if they are kept large and well attached to the periosteum.

d) The area of decortication should extend 2–4 cm into healthy bone distal and proximal to the necrotic area to be bridged. The cancellous autograft should be placed deep to the decorticated lamellae.

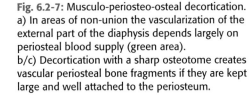

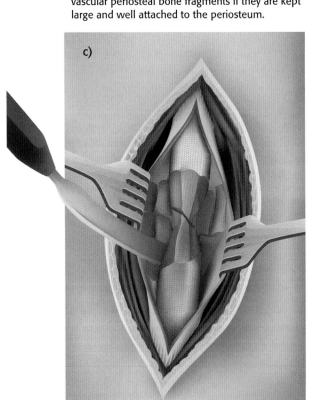

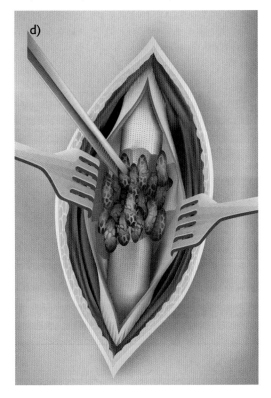

Decortication or osteoperiosteal petalling (shingling)

Decortication is the simplest and most effective way to expose a non-union without substantial devascularization. It expands the local cross-section of bone (**Fig. 6.2-7** and **Fig. 6.2-9**) [6]. In a diaphyseal non-union site, the periosteum is tightly attached to the adjacent muscles and subperiosteal bone (**Fig. 6.2-7a**), which receives its vascular supply from the extraosseous tissues. Chiseling of bone pieces from the outer aspect of the diaphyseal cortex preserves the vascular supply to the peripheral cortical bone via periosteal and muscular attachments bridging the non-union (**Fig. 6.2-7c/d** and **Fig. 6.2-9**). **This technique is used to enhance the healing response, creating a well vascularized bed.** Whenever a delayed union or non-union is approached from the periosteal side, this technique should be used to expose the site. It may be carried out circumferentially around the diaphysis to allow a correction of axial and rotational deformities without devascularizing the site. Shingling is of special help in atrophic and avascular non-union to provide a viable bed for the cancellous autograft. Decortication performed in the metaphyseal area may lead to some restriction of joint function.

Cancellous autograft

(**Fig. 6.2-8**)

The cancellous autograft, often in combination with decortication, is the most effective means of bypassing a necrotic bone area or a relatively limited bony defect with a bridge of vital bone (**Fig. 6.2-7**).

As "gold standard" for both biological and mechanical purposes, the autograft has the advantages of being osteogenic (a source of vital bone cells), osteoinductive (recruitment of local mesenchymal cells), and osteoconductive (scaffold for ingrowth of new bone). Biologically, it is far superior to allograft or currently available bone substitutes [7].

Cancellous bone graft is vascularized by the granulation tissue replacing the interfragmental hematoma. Within 6 weeks, the gaps between the cancellous bone fragments are vascularized and bridged by a network of woven bone. This woven bone is remodeled under the influence of force transmission [8].

The disadvantages of cancellous autograft include the morbidity associated with the harvesting and its limited supply. The most important harvesting areas are the anterior iliac crest (cancellous bone, corticocancellous grafts) (**Fig. 6.2-8a**), the posterior iliac crest (largest source of pure cancellous bone) (**Fig. 6.2-8b**), the greater trochanter and distal femur (both with increased fracture risk), and the proximal tibia (very soft bone in osteoporotic patients). Harvesting may lead to a substantial blood loss, requiring transfusion. Pure cancellous bone is the safest option in the presence of infection.

Callus distraction and free vascularized bone grafts

Osteogenesis by callus distraction (Ilizarov) and free vascularized bone graft should be taken into consideration when dealing with large (> 4–5 cm) segmental bone defects [9]. These situations are more frequent in infected non-unions (see **chapters 1.3** and **6.3**).

Cancellous autograft is osteogenic, osteoinductive, and osteoconductive.

Shingling is used to enhance the healing process.

For large defects, callus distraction or vascularized bone grafts are valid options.

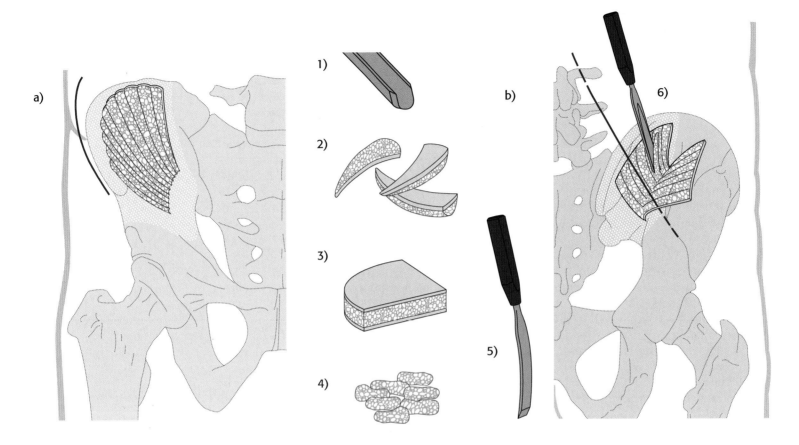

Fig. 6.2-8:
Harvesting of cancellous autograft from the pelvis.
a) From the anterior iliac crest.
Incision along the crest. Sharp dissection of the muscles
of the abdominal wall, lifting of the periosteum of the
inner wall of the iliac bone with a sharp rasp and
exposure with a retractor. In osteoporotic situations, use
of a U-shaped chisel (1) to remove corticocancellous
chips (2). Bicortical bone blocks (3) or pure cancellous
bone (4) may be harvested conserving the contours of
the iliac crest.
b) From the posterior iliac crest.
Splitting of the subcutaneous tissue and elevation of the
periosteum and the muscles from the outer surface of
the iliac bone. Elevation of the cortical layer with a curved
chisel (5) to harvest pure cancellous bone (6). The
greatest amount of cancellous bone is to be found in the
vicinity of the iliosacral joint.

Allografts and bone graft substitutes

Allograft and bone substitutes such as demineralized bone matrix, hydroxyapatite, tricalciumphosphate, as well as osteoinductive substances such as growth factors, bone morphogenic proteins (BMP), etc. are currently being intensively explored both experimentally and clinically, but have not yet proved to be significantly superior [10]. Most of these substances can contribute to the reconstruction of bone cavities due to their osteoinductive and/or conductive capacity, but they all require a vital environment in order to be effective. In the absence of living cellular elements and blood supply there is no possibility of any healing.

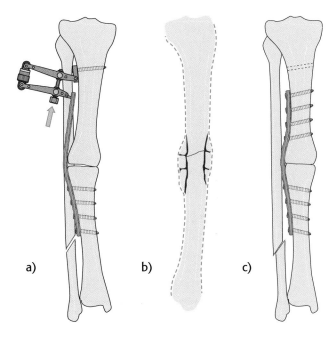

a)   b)   c)

Fig. 6.2-9: Tension band plating of a tibia with varus deformity and hypertrophic non-union.
a) Resection of a segment of the fibula distal to the non-union. Exposure of the lateral surface of the tibia and placement of a LC-DCP 4.5 anticipating valgization, minimal wedge resection laterally, and fixation of the plate to the distal tibia.
With the articulated tension device the non-union site is compressed and the tibia straightened.
b) Anterior and posterior decortication is optional.
c) Fixation of the plate proximally with four 4.5 mm cortex screws guarantees alignment.

Stabilization

Stabilization of a non-union provides the essential mechanical component to allow calcification of the fibrous cartilage within the non-union. This prepares the field for the development of a first bony bridge (see **section 3.2.1**). It has been proved as a basic AO experiment that in the presence of a sufficient stock and quality of bone, compression fixation alone, without resection of the non-union site, will guarantee healing [5].

Plating

The plate is probably the most adequate tool for the stabilization of a non-union. It allows interfragmentary compression, plus correction of any malposition and reconstructive (grafting etc.) measures, in a single procedure. Plates can be applied in metaphyseal as well as diaphyseal non-unions. In an oblique non-union stability can be increased by placing a lag screw across the non-union. More frequently, however, only axial compression is possible because of the transverse plane of the non-union and local bone quality. For optimal compression, the use of the tension device is strongly advisable (**Fig. 6.2-9**) as the excursion of DCP or LC-DCP plate holes is usually too short to generate the level of compression required. For the best position of the plate, the tension side of the bone (convex side of a deformity) should be considered. This is especially true in the presence of concomitant deformities (**Fig. 6.2-9**). In cases where a wave plate is used to bridge the non-union, a cancellous bone graft between the plate and the bone may enhance healing (**Fig. 6.2-10**) [11]. One disadvantage of plating may be the need for partial weight bearing for 2–5 months depending on the healing progress.

Mechanical stabilization of a non-union is essential.

The plate is the most adequate and versatile implant to stabilize an aseptic non-union.

Fig. 6.2-10: Wave plate principle. It consists of two components:

1. The distance between the narrow bony bridge between the two main fragments and the laterally lifted plate increases the functional diameter of the non-union site and, therefore, greatly improves the local stability.

2. The distance between the plate and the non-union allows placement of autografts all around the non-union site.

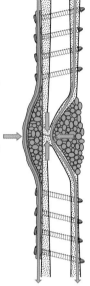

Intramedullary nailing

(**Fig. 6.2-11**)

Intramedullary nailing has its main application in diaphyseal non-unions of the lower extremity. The tight fit of the nail due to reaming the non-union site without exposing it, the rotational stability of dynamic interlocking allowing for axial compression from weight bearing, and an increase in periosteal blood flow are important factors in promoting union. To introduce the guide wire for the reamer, the marrow cavity must usually be opened with the hand reamer, while the fibrous scar tissue plus the reaming debris are a good combination which functions like a bone graft. Nailing has few advantages in the upper extremities and thin unreamed nails are not suitable, as they provide insufficient stability.

External fixation

In most aseptic non-unions external fixation brings little advantage. It may be applied in the presence of poor soft-tissue conditions, or in complex multiplanar deformities near joints, where a single-stage correction appears difficult and hazardous. Its main application is where there is considerable loss of length to be bridged by callus distraction, which is, however, rare in aseptic non-union (see **chapter 6.3**).

4.3   Metaphyseal non-union

Surgery usually consists of a limited local decortication avoiding devascularization of the joint fragment, correction of the deformities, and mechanical adaptation of the main fragments with fixation by interfragmentary compression using one or two plates. Bone grafting may be necessary. Careful arthrolysis of intra-articular adhesions is often necessary but must not compromise vascularity. In the postoperative period, forced motion must, however, be avoided until healing is achieved. The treatment of a non-union of the femoral neck requires a Pauwels osteotomy, which consists of a valgization of the proximal femur in order to realign the non-union perpendicular to the resultant forces of the hip. A vital femoral head is a precondition [12] (for technique and planning see **chapter 2.4**).

4.4   Treatment in special situations

Arthrodesis/arthroplasty: In general, these options should be considered when fixation of a periarticular non-union is impossible due to loss of bone, poor bone quality, or irreparable joint damage.

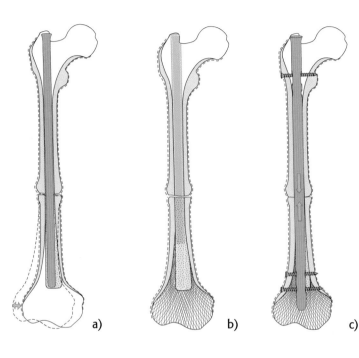

Fig. 6.2-11: Hypertrophic non-union after conventional nailing of the femur.
a) Instability is increased by a too short unlocked nail creating a resorption cavity in the distal femur.
b) After removal of the nail, additional stability can be gained by over-reaming creating a cylindrical cavity proximal and distal to the non-union site.
c) Introduction of a thicker and longer nail into the as yet untouched and unreamed distal metaphysis with dynamic interlocking.

Amputation may be indicated when an extremity distal to the avascular non-union is of poor quality (disturbed neurovascular situation, restricted joint movement, and considerable deformity). The pros and cons of a time-consuming reconstruction must, therefore, be extensively discussed with the patient and his family, and evaluated with respect to the possibility of a rapid rehabilitation.

4.5 Adjuvant treatment

Electromagnetic stimulation and, more recently, ultrasound have been extensively applied and advocated to stimulate bone healing. They do appear to generate a certain physical (thermal) effect at the fracture or non-union site [13, 14], but the actual agent responsible for the final outcome is still questionable and real evidence is lacking.

5 Conclusion

The successful treatment of a non-union may be one of the most rewarding procedures that a surgeon can perform. When dealing with these challenging problems, careful planning and a systematic approach will improve the results. Prior to embarking on its reconstruction, it is of paramount importance to understand and evaluate the reasons why a particular fracture has failed to unite. While personal experience and expertise are most crucial for success, no single technique or implant is ideal for every situation, or for every surgeon.

6 Bibliography

1. **McKee MD, Yoo D, Schemitsch EH** (1998) Health status after Ilizarov reconstruction of post-traumatic lower-limb deformity. *J Bone Joint Surg [Br]*; 80(2):360–364.

2. **Rosen H** (1988) Treatment of nonunion: General principles. In: Chapman WM, editor. *Operative Orthopaedics*. Philadelphia: Lippincott-Raven: 489–509.

3. **Weber BG, Cech O** (1976) *Pseudarthrosis. Pathophysiology, biomechanics, therapy, results*. Bern: Huber.

4. **Ueng SW, Lee MY, Li AF, et al.** (1997) Effect of intermittent cigarette smoke inhalation on tibial lengthening: experimental study on rabbits. *J Trauma*; 42(2):231–238.

5. **Schenk RK, Müller ME, Willenegger H** (1968) [Experimental histological contribution to the development and treatment of pseudarthrosis]. *Hefte Unfallheilkd*; 94:15–24.

6. **Judet PR , Patel A** (1972) Muscle pedicle bone grafting of long bones by osteoperiosteal decortication. *Clin Orthop*; 87:74–80.

7. **Goldberg VM, Stevenson S, Shaffer JW** (1989) Bone and cartilage allografts: biology and clinical applications. In: Friedlaender GE, editor. *Biology of autografts and allografts*. Park Ridge, IL: American Academy of Orthopedic Surgeons.

8. **Verburg AD, Klopper PJ, van den Hoof A, et al.** (1988) The healing of biologic and synthetic bone implants. An experimental study. *Arch Orthop Trauma Surg*; 107 (5):293–300.

9. **Weiland AJ, Moore JR, Daniel RK** (1983) Vascularized bone autografts. Experience with 41 cases. *Clin Orthop*; (174):87–101.

10. **Cook SD, Baffes GC, Wolfe MW, et al.** (1994) The effect of recombinant human osteogenic protein-1 on healing of large segmental bone defects. *J Bone Joint Surg [Am]*; 76 (6):827–838.

11. **Ring D, Jupiter JB, Sanders RA, et al.** (1997) Complex nonunion of fractures of the femoral shaft treated by wave plate osteosynthesis. *J Bone Joint Surg [Br]*; 79 (2):289–294.

12. **Müller ME** (1991) Reconstructive surgery of bone. In: Müller ME, Allgöwer M, Schneider R, Willenegger H, et al., editors. *Manual of internal fixation*. 3rd ed. Berlin Heidelberg: Springer-Verlag.

13. **Sharrard WJW** (1990) A double-blind trial of pulsed electromagnetic fields for delayed union of tibial fractures. *J Bone Joint Surg [Br]*; 72 (3):347–355.

14. **Kristiansen TK, Ryaby JP, McCabe J, et al.** (1997) Accelerated healing of distal radial fractures with the use of specific, low-intensity ultrasound. A multicenter, prospective, randomized, double-blind, placebo-controlled study. *J Bone Joint Surg [Am]*; 79 (7):961–973.

7 Updates

Updates and additional references for this chapter are available online at:
http://www.aopublishing.org/PFxM/62.htm

6.3 Chronic infection and infected non-union

Eric E. Johnson

1 Introduction

Osteomyelitis is an infection of bone (osteon) and marrow (myelon) (see **chapter 6.1**). Chronic osteomyelitis has its source either in a neglected acute infection or it may slowly develop as the delayed first manifestation of a missed infection (see **chapter 6.1**). **Devitalized bone fragments within this infected environment become sequestra, which cause persistence of chronic infection.** Granulation tissue develops and is eventually transformed into a layer of dense fibrous tissue. This membrane isolates the host from the infected area and acts as a barrier around the sequestra and devitalized bone. Periosteal new bone formation around the periphery of the infected area produces an involucrum that further walls off the infection (**Fig. 6.3-1**). Today, this rarely happens because of the intermittent administration of antibiotics, by which the process is slowed down but without leading to bone healing.

Bacteria react to the host's attempts at eradication by releasing a variety of virulent factors. Glycocalyx (slime), a hydrated muco-polysaccharide layer, covers avascular material, for example, necrotic bone or metal implants.

This slime protects the bacteria in a sessile state increasing their resistance to destruction by a factor of 500 [1]. This results in an increased bacterial surface adherence isolating them from the effects of antibiotics, antibodies, and immune-directed phagocytosis. This is the basis for the difficulty in eliminating implant-related infections. The most common organisms cultured in chronic osteomyelitis are staphylococcus aureus and epidermidis. Both of these species can form a biofilm-protective layer of glycocalyx [2]. As a consequence, chronic osteomyelitis with persistent drainage and sequestra formation is resistant to eradication by long-term antibiotics alone. **Furthermore, all patients with chronic osteomyelitis must be considered as potential MRSA (methicillin-resistant *Staphylococcus aureus*) carriers who require special isolation.** Surgical intervention is the only effective method to eliminate such infection and promote healing. Most gram-negative bacteria do not have a biofilm-forming capacity, with the exception of pseudomonas aeruginosa [3].

In the presence of infection, devitalized fragments become sequestra.

Every patient with chronic osteomyelitis is a potential carrier of MRSA!

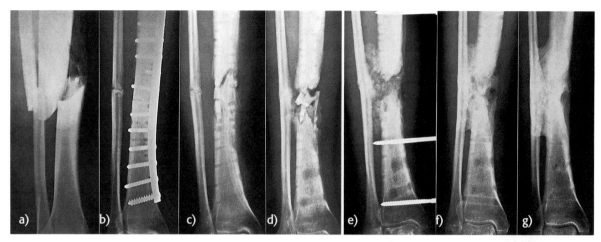

Fig. 6.3-1: Development of an infected non-union, and its treatment in a 49-year-old male.
a/b) Plate osteosynthesis of an open tibial fracture type 42-A1.2. Several empty drill holes indicate that the surgeon had some problems during surgery.

c) Four months later, and after plate removal, sequestration of an entire segment of the tibia seems to occur. The periosteal new bone formation adjacent to the diaphysis indicates the presence of some vital callus.
d) Complete sequestration of the necrotic segment after 10 months.
e) Thorough débridement, external fixation, and cancellous bone graft as a second step procedure.
f) Six months later, full weight bearing.
g) Full consolidation after 2 years in a slight varus position.

2 Classification of osteomyelitis

2.1 Classification according to the anatomical localization

(Fig. 6.3-2)

Chronic osteomyelitis may be classified according to its localization within bone [4]. This classification is based on the importance of bone necrosis and the more favorable prognosis of medullary infections. It has its origins in the treatment of hematogenous osteomyelitis. Four entities are differentiated: type I (medullary), type II (superficial), type III (localized), and type IV (diffuse osteomyelitis).

2.2 Classification according to the implant

Classification according to the implant involved has the advantage of being more specific for chronic postoperative osteomyelitis [5]. We can distinguish between pin-track osteomyelitis, plate osteomyelitis (either superficial or deep), and osteomyelitis after medullary nailing (see **chapter 6.1**).

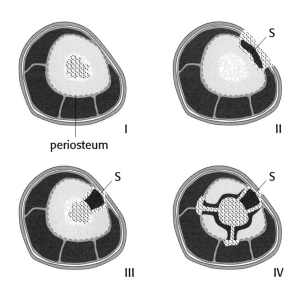

Fig 6.3-2:
Anatomical classification of adult osteomyelitis according to Cierny and Mader [4]:
Type I: Medullary osteomyelitis. Infection within the medullary cavity, usually without involvement of the epiphyseal area.
Type II: Superficial osteomyelitis involving the outer cortical area, the subcutaneous tissue, and the skin. The infection resides within an isolated area consisting of cortical sequestra (S) and granulation tissue (red dotted) (**Fig 6.1-6**).
Type III: Localized osteomyelitis involving full thickness of cortex and the adjacent medullary canal. Pin-track infections (**Fig. 6.1-1**) and plate infections may be examples (**Fig. 6.1-2**).
Type IV: Diffuse osteomyelitis as a fully developed disease of the entire bone. It involves the cortex and the medullary cavity as well, leading to an extensive devitalization of bone (red).

3 Diagnosis of chronic infection and infected non-union

3.1 Clinical and laboratory findings

The diagnosis of chronic osteomyelitis is rarely difficult. Chronic drainage, pain, erythema, and (rarely) edema are typical clinical findings. Drainage is often intermittent and localized in an area of scar tissue, limiting the possibilities of revision. On the other hand, we should know the extent of the infection, the degree of bone necrosis, the localization of sequestra and the overall condition and function of the limb involved. Comorbidities and other factors that affect the outcome must be thoroughly assessed. Laboratory values such as the ESR, C-reactive protein (CRP), or leukocyte counts are more often negative than positive. If positive, they are helpful in monitoring the treatment plan, but negative findings do not mean that the disease cannot progress.

3.2 Imaging techniques

(see **chapter 6.1**)

A complete series of x-rays, from the original fracture to the current state, is helpful for the analysis of an infected non-union. Necrotic areas are usually recognized by a lack of new bone formation adjacent to them, while sequestra are very dense and appear completely isolated (**Fig 6.3-1**) from the surrounding bone. Today, CT and MRI are the best methods to determine the extent of the disease

A complete x-ray series from the inital fracture to the current aspect is helpful.

and the location of sequestra. Consultation with a musculoskeletal radiologist is very beneficial in deciding which investigation would be helpful, especially in the presence of metal implants. CT scan may be preferred to demonstrate sequestration underneath a periosteal new bone formation (**Fig. 6.3-3**) [6], while MRI gives more information on soft-tissue involvement.

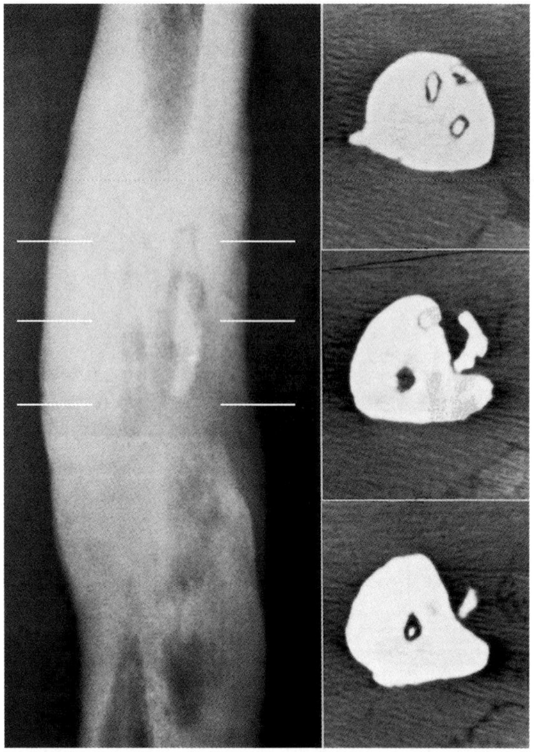

Prior to any surgical reconstruction the affected limb, as well as the whole patient, must be carefully assessed.

Fig. 6.3-3: CT analysis searching for sequestration in a 31-year-old male.
Six years after complex femoral fracture with early infection after ORIF. Sinus producing MRSA (methicillin-resistant *Staphylococcus aureus*). Part of the sequestrated femoral diaphysis is encapsulated in periosteal new bone formation.

Frequently, a three-phase skeletal scintigraphy or special infection scintigraphy, for example, with radioactive indium, as well as scintigraphy with labeled antibodies against granulocytes, can be of additional help [7–10].

3.3   Bacteriology and histology

The bacteriological analysis should be based on several tissue samples of bone and granulation tissue from different areas affected by the infection (see **chapter 6.1**). Swabs taken from the fistula or superficial drainage are not usually adequate in determining the agent, as there may be contamination with other bacteria. A histological work-up may be helpful in case of negative bacterial cultures.

3.4   Condition of the affected limb and of the patient

In order to evaluate the benefits and the risks of any reconstruction, the limb distal to infected focus must be carefully assessed. The vascularity and the sensibility of the foot and the function of the joints must be tested and correlated with the needs and expectations of the patient. The pros and cons of a reconstruction of the limb or of an amputation, supported by a detailed treatment plan, must be discussed with the patient and his relatives.

There are physical as well as psychological aspects to be considered. Patients who have been non-weight bearing for many years and are expected to have a prolonged period of reconstruction and rehabilitation may not have the energy or motivation to cooperate.

4 Principles of treatment

The principles of the management of chronic osteomyelitis and infected non-unions are similar and consist of:

- Eradication of the infection by means of surgery combined with antibiotics.
- Creation of a viable and stable soft-tissue environment.
- Reconstruction, alignment, and stabilization of the skeleton.

Every case of osteomyelitis is to be considered individually, since there is no standard procedure which can be routinely applied.

4.1 Débridement

All dead tissues, especially dead bone, all implants (except those providing stability), old suture material, and sinuses have to be resected. To prevent the creation of additional necrotic bone areas, care must be taken to avoid any stripping of the vascularized periosteum. The resection of necrotic bone which is in contact with vital bone is the most difficult step. Dead bone does not show any bleeding points; it is very brittle when chiseled off (**Fig. 6.3-4**). In areas of cancellous bone the dead tissue is best removed with a high-speed burr until bleeding is encountered (**Fig. 6.3-5**). Intramedullary débridement in a diaphysis is best done by gentle intramedullary reaming (see **chapter 6.1, Fig. 6.1-5**). Sometimes a second look may be considered. **In case of instability it is essential to provide fixation in spite of the infection.**

Fig. 6.3-4: Local débridement of an infected non-union.

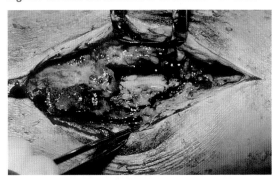

a) The non-union is covered with granulation tissue stained with methylene blue.

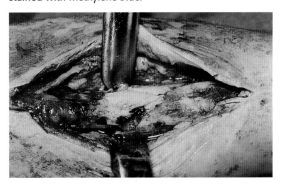

b) After resection of the granulation tissue, the necrotic bone adjacent to the non-union contrasts distinctly with the living bone.

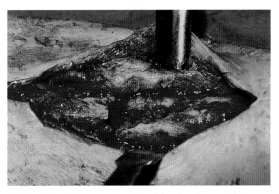

c) After débridement only living-bleeding bone is left.

Stabilization of the bone is essential in spite of infection.

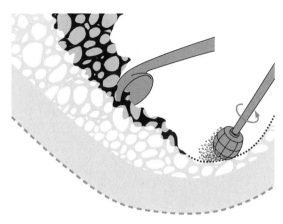

Fig. 6.3-5:
Débridement of a medullary cavity. Cross-section of a diaphysis. Dead, not bleeding bone (red) is curetted and rounded with a high-speed burr.

4.2 Stabilization

The aim of stabilization is:
- To bring about bony bridging.
- To allow functional aftertreatment.
- To allow easy wound care and to support the eradication of infection.
- To allow later reconstructive surgery if necessary.

Stepwise or staged procedures may be required depending on the extent of infection and degree of stability.

4.2.1 External fixation

External fixation is the standard method in infected non-union.

External fixation is the standard method of stabilization in infected non-union. It must follow the general rules of external fixation (see **chapter 3.3.3**). In septic surgery, external fixation may need to remain for up to a year or more. To satisfy this demand, the chosen frame should be constructed more rigidly than in an acute fracture. The risk of pin-track infection is higher than usual. It may be necessary to replace one or more pins during the course of treatment. There are basically two fixation systems applicable: the Ilizarov-type ring fixator with thin wires or a simpler frame built from the tubular system with Schanz screws.

Tubular system (Fig. 6.3-6): This has the advantage of allowing free access for wound care and eventual plastic reconstructive surgery. Its simplicity allows the system to be adapted to most clinical situations. Monotube systems may sometimes be easier to place but are less versatile.

Ilizarov fixator: The circular arrangement of rings together with multiple thin pretensioned wires, which can be placed individually, allows for compression and lengthening, as well as a gradual correction of axial deformities [11]. Wires are also reported to have fewer "pin-related" problems.

4.2.2 Plates, nails

If in infected non-unions the original implants (plates and nails) are no longer effective, they have to be removed. New internal fixation carries a higher risk of recurrence of infection. However, in special cases (femur, humerus) internal fixation may be considered again in combination with adequate protection by antibiotics. The choice of implant is usually dependent on the aim of obtaining an optimally functional limb.

4.3 Reconstruction of bone

As a rule, all measures for obtaining bony bridging are much safer if carried out after a

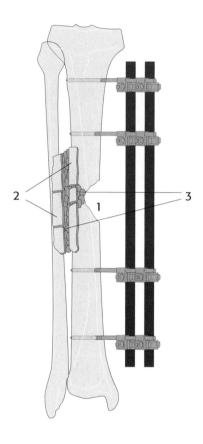

Fig. 6.3-6: Infected non-union without loss of length in a tibia. Decortication and cancellous bone graft in infected non-union—dorsal view. Overview after external fixation.

1 Area debrided from medial aspect will be covered with muscle flap or free vascularized flap.
2 Decortication, from posterior or lateral aspects, of the fibula and the lateral and dorsal aspect of the tibia.
3 Placement of autogenous cancellous bone graft.

Care must be taken not to injure the anterior tibial artery and veins and the nervus peroneus profundus.

complete débridement. In problem cases, reconstruction of bone defects should be done as a second step (**Fig. 6.3-7**). Healing is more reliable if the reconstructive measures are sited in an area of vital tissues with healthy skin covers.

4.3.1 Decortication-autogenous cancellous bone graft

The technique of decortication is described in the chapter on aseptic non-union (**chapter 6.2, Fig. 6.2-7**). It is performed over a distance of about 2 cm proximal and distal to the involved

area (**Fig. 6.3-7**). Cancellous bone is harvested, preferably from the anterior or posterior iliac crest. Dense pieces of cancellous bone are morselized which allows for quicker vascularization with minimal risk of sequestration (**Fig. 6.3-7**). In the lower leg, a posterolateral or central placement of the graft into a vital bed avoids the infected focus (**Fig. 6.3-6**) [12]. In the humerus or femur the best position of the graft depends mainly on the defect and the soft-tissue envelope. **If a bone graft has to be applied to an area where the soft tissue is defective, the establishment of a healthy soft-tissue cover should precede grafting.**
In intramedullary infections (**chapter 6.1, Fig 6.1-5**), a tube temporarily placed into the reamed medullary canal can be of help in introducing the cancellous graft [13].

Bone grafts have a better chance of surviving in a "healthy" soft-tissue environment.

Fig. 6.3-7:
Débridement, decortication, and cancellous autograft combined with distraction and secondary compression.
a) Infected non-union with sequestra (1) and new periosteal bone formation (2).
b) Débridement, external fixation, and distraction of about 5 mm.
c) Decortication leaving the decorticated bone pieces in connection with the adjacent muscles; cancellous autograft.
d) 6 weeks later, woven bone interlaces the cancellous bone graft and the decorticated bone lamellae. Compression about 6 weeks later to accelerate remodeling of the bone graft and callus formation.

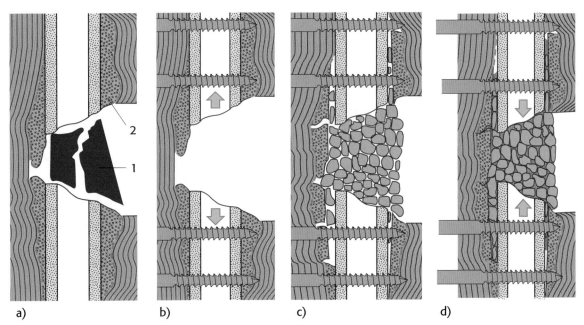

a)   b)   c)   d)

4.3.2   Open bone graft (Papineau) [14]

Open bone grafting is a method with a long tradition, which often achieves bony bridging and soft-tissue coverage at the same time. Its main disadvantage is the need for a relatively large amount of bone to fill in a relatively small defect.

4.3.3   Callus distraction (Ilizarov)

Ilizarov [11] has introduced the technique of gradual callus distraction by osteotomy in order to restore limb length or to bridge a defect (**Fig. 6.3-8** and **Fig. 6.3-9**). The great advantage of the method is that while callus distraction corrects the length of the bone, the soft tissues are distracted as well, thereby minimizing the need for additional reconstruction. After

extensive local resection of the necrotic bone followed by external fixation, a transverse corticotomy is performed away from the defect, preferably close to a metaphysis. The corticotomy is performed either a week after the débridement or—in low-grade infections—at the same time. Distraction is not commenced for 10 days, but the gap is kept at a distance of 1 mm. Thereafter, the newly formed callus is slowly distracted at a rate of 1 mm per day in four to five steps evenly distributed over 24 hours. Partial weight bearing is usually allowed. The progress of the distraction, callus maturation, and correction of any irregularity are monitored by x-rays. When the planned length is reached, weight bearing is gradually increased. Full weight bearing is usually achieved 4–6 months after closure of the defect. As the docking sites have a tendency to delayed union, decortication and bone grafting of these areas may be required, or

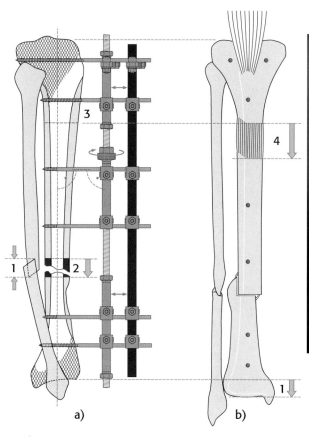

Fig. 6.3-8:
Segmental bone transport using the tubular system.
a) Bone transport system combined with a unilateral external fixator mounted anteriorly on a tibia with distal defect. There is shortening as judged by the overlap of the fibula (1). Resection of the infected non-union (2) and proximal corticotomy (3). Gradual distraction of 1 mm per day in four to five steps.
b) The lengthening (4) compensates the tibial shortening plus the resection distance. Consolidation of the distraction area and at the docking site.

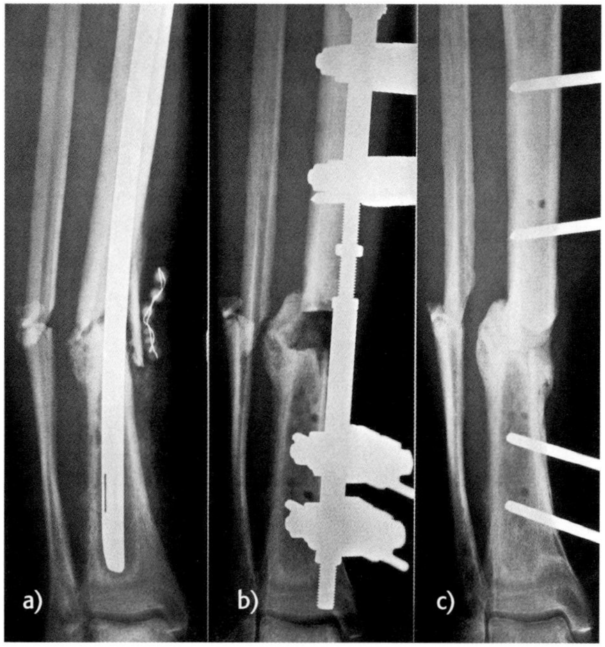

Fig. 6.3-9:
Clinical example of **Fig. 6.3-8**. 28-year-old male.
a) Infected non-union 5 months after intramedullary nailing of a closed tibial fracture. Sequestration and periosteal new bone formation.
b) Resection, osteotomy of the fibula, and installation of a transportation system.
c) Healing in the docking site after 9 months.

sometimes an internal fixation is needed. Bone transport may be painful; it therefore requires a commitment by both the patient and the physician. The patient has to be seen weekly during the distraction period, and physiotherapy should be instituted early to mobilize the adjacent joints. In trauma cases neurological problems due to overstretching of the nerves are rare.

Callus distraction over an intramedullary nail may reduce the period of external fixation but is not without hazards, especially in case of previous infections [15, 16].

4.3.4 **Free vascularized bone graft**

Free vascularized bone grafts (fibula, iliac crest) are especially suitable for the bridging of bone defects longer than 10 cm [17, 18]. The advantage is that, after bony integration at the host site, they undergo gradual hypertrophy, slowly adapting their size and structure to the local needs. However, it may take years until full loading is possible, which requires long-term protective measures, especially in the lower extremity. Because of the relatively small diameter of the grafts, they are more suitable for forearm and humerus (**Fig. 6.3-9**). In the tibia, one has to consider double grafting, using the contralateral fibula first and, as a second step, the ipsilateral fibula [19]. Because of the big difference of size (graft vs. defect site) the method is of restricted value in the femur.

4.4 **Soft-tissue coverage**

Hypertrophic infected non-unions are relatively stable and asymptomatic, with intermittent draining.

As a rule, soft-tissue coverage without complete débridement is useless. In case of a second look it is advisable to leave the wound open with some antiseptic spacer in order to prevent superinfection (see **chapter 6.1**). In unexposed small defects with good granulation tissue covering the bone, split skin grafts may be sufficient. In more complex situations, local muscle flaps (e.g.,gastrocnemius flap), fasciocutaneous flaps, or free vascularized flaps are needed [20, 21] as outlined in **chapter 5.2**.

4.5 **Antibiotics—antiseptics**

Antibiotics are always to be considered as being complementary to surgery. Their systemic administration has to follow strict rules in order to achieve a therapeutic concentration in the bone (see **chapter 6.1**). The special situation of implant-related infections has to be respected. For topical application, chains of beads impregnated with antibiotics may be useful. They offer a high concentration of antibiotics, usually gentamicin, at the infection focus for a couple of days. They also can serve as spacers for further bone grafting procedures [22, 23]. Antiseptics have their main application in antiseptic dressings and in irrigation-suction drainage (see **chapter 6.1**).

5 **Treatment concepts of typical cases**

5.1 **Hypertrophic infected non-union (relatively stable)**

Hypertrophic infected non-unions, by their description indicate adequate blood supply as evidenced by the excessive callus formation on x-rays. These non-unions frequently possess only a draining sinus and are relatively asymptomatic. The patients are able to function quite well, as instability is minimal. Hypertrophic infected non-unions frequently have an angular and/or rotational deformity due to muscle imbalance or weight bearing.

Treatment: Débridement of the focus can usually be combined with definitive soft-tissue cover because of the limited area of infection. External fixation will correct a deformity and provide stability while a cancellous autograft can be performed after curetting of the infected focus. Consolidation can be observed within 4–6 months. After removal of the external fixation, a brace may be advisable for a few months.

5.2 Avital and unstable infected non-union

Instability and non-viable bone are the classical features of an infected non-union. There is little or no evidence of any attempt at healing, the bone looks osteopenic or sclerotic and there is often associated shortening, joint contracture, limb atrophy, and chronic pain.

Treatment: The treatment of this more complex condition should occur in stages. Thorough débridement is combined with external fixation. Next, the resulting defect has to be assessed. Some shortening may be acceptable to gain stability, while reconstructions of 2–3 cm are possible with local bone grafting (**Fig. 6.3-1** and **Fig. 6.3-7**). There exists, however, a risk of secondary angulation in reconstructions based purely on cancellous autografting, especially in the lower leg. In small tibial defects, the graft is usually placed posteriolaterally between fibula and tibia (**Fig. 6.3-6**). In the femur and humerus, grafting may be combined with plate fixation once the local situation appears to be safe.

5.3 Avital infected non-union with segmental bone defect

With segmental bone loss and avital bone ends, severe dystrophy of the bone and soft tissues occurs due to disuse of the limb.

Treatment: Any attempt at reconstruction has to be preceded by a thorough débridement. A segmental bone loss exceeding 3–5 cm can usually not be bridged successfully by cancellous bone graft. It is, therefore, advisable to use the callus-distraction method for defects up to 10–20 cm if there is an experienced surgeon

available (**Fig. 6.3-8** and **Fig. 6.3-9**). **The advantage of callus distraction is the creation of a new bone segment which, once matured, has similar shape and strength to the original bone.** The problem of soft-tissue cover can usually be solved at the same time. On the other hand, the procedure may be painful and time-consuming. If the bone loss is situated in the forearm or the humerus, vascularized grafts have to be considered (**Fig. 6.3-10**). In the lower extremity, if the defect exceeds 8–12 cm, vascularized bone grafting competes, as a method, with callus distraction.

New bone formed by callus distraction has, once matured, good strength and similar shape to the original bone.

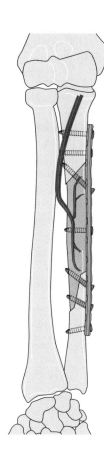

Fig. 6.3-10:
Vascular fibular graft in infected non-union of the ulna stabilized with a plate. Well-adapted diameter of the fibula to that of the ulna.

5.4   Chronic infection

5.4.1   Chronic infection after plate osteosynthesis

In chronic infection after plate osteosynthesis, plate removal and thorough débridement are advocated once the bone has consolidated. In case of an insufficient bony bridge, external fixation is advised. Using CT scan, a thorough analysis of the bone structures can then be performed. During a secondary revision, any remaining necrotic areas should be debrided.

5.4.2   Chronic infection after medullary nailing

Intramedullary nailing may lead to bony consolidation even in the presence of infection. Often, however, there remains an infected area within the medullary cavity, with or without a sinus (see **Fig. 6.1-5**). The best treatment is gentle reaming and flushing of the medullary canal. Because the vascularity comes mostly from the periosteum, there is little risk of permanent damage (see **Fig. 6.1-5**). In infections years after the removal of the nail, the medullary cavity is quite often filled with endosteal new bone. Reaming can only then be performed after removal of this bone through a cortical window.

5.4.3   Recurrence of osteomyelitis after several years

Any osteomyelitis can recur even after decades of "quietness". Clinical manifestations are pain, tenderness, swelling, fever, and even abscess formation. It may be difficult to see any pathology on standard x-rays, but CT scan, scintigraphy, or MRI may demonstrate a sequestrum worthy of removal. Systemic antibiotics are also usually helpful as a supplement to surgery.

6   Bibliography

1.   **Dendrinos GK, Kontos S, Lyritsis E** (1995) Use of the Ilizarov technique for treatment of non-union of the tibia associated with infection. *J Bone Joint Surg [Am]*; 77 (6):835–846.
2.   **Masterson EL, Masri BA, Duncan CP** (1997) Treatment of infection at the site of total hip replacement. *J Bone Joint Surg [Am]*; 79:1740–1749.
3.   **Ekkernkamp A, Muhr G, Josten C** (1996) [Infected pseudarthrosis]. *Unfallchirurg*; 99 (12):914–924.
4.   **Cierny G, Mader JT, Pennick JJ** (1985) A clinical staging system for adult osteomyelitis. *Contemp Orthop*; 98:17–37.
5.   **Burri C** (1975) *Posttraumatic osteomyelitis.* Bern Stuttgart Vienna: Hans Huber Publisher.
6.   **Ochsner PE, Sokhegyi A, Petralli C** (1990) [The value of computerized tomography in the assessment of chronic osteomyelitis. A radiological, histological, and clinical correlation study]. *Z Orthop Ihre Grenzgeb*; 128 (3):313–318.
7.   **Esterhai JL, Jr., Goll SR, McCarthy KE, et al.** (1987) Indium-111 leukocyte scintigraphic detection of subclinical osteomyelitis complicating delayed and non-union long bone fractures: a prospective study. *J Orthop Res*; 5 (1):1–6.

8. **Kaim A, Maurer T, Ochsner P, et al.** (1997) Chronic complicated osteomyelitis of the appendicular skeleton: diagnosis with technetium-99m labeled monoclonal antigranulocyte antibody-immunoscintigraphy. *Eur J Nucl Med;* 24 (7):732–738.

9. **Nepola JV, Seabold JE, Marsh JL, et al.** (1993) Diagnosis of infection in ununited fractures. Combined imaging with indium-111-labeled leukocytes and technetium-99m methylene diphosphonate. *J Bone Joint Surg [Am];* 75 (12):1816–1822.

10. **Seabold JE, Nepola JV, Conrad GR, et al.** (1989) Detection of osteomyelitis at fracture non-union sites: comparison of two scintigraphic methods. *AJR Am J Roentgenol;* 152 (5):1021–1027.

11. **Ilizarov GA** (1990) Clinical application of the tension-stress effect for limb lengthening. *Clin Orthop;* (250):8–26.

12. **Toh CL, Jupiter JB** (1995) The infected non-union of the tibia. *Clin Orthop;* (315):176–191.

13. **Ochsner PE, Hugli RW** (1995) [The value of intramedullary boring and intramedullary splinting in revision of infected pseudarthroses]. *Unfallchirurg;* 98(3):145–150.

14. **Lortat-Jacob A, Koechlin P, Benoit J, et al.** (1977) [Failures and limitations of the Papineau technique. A report of 54 cases]. *Rev Chir Orthop Reparatrice Appar Mot;* 63 (7):667–666.

15. **Barbarossa V, Brunner UH, Claudia BF** (1993) Advances in osteogenesis. *Injury;* 24 (Suppl 2).

16. **Brutscher R, Cordey J, Eggers C** (1994) Treatment of bone defects in traumatology by means of autologous bone grafts and callus distraction. *Injury;* 25 (Suppl 1).

17. **de Boer HH, Wood MB, Hermans J** (1990) Reconstruction of large skeletal defects by vascularized fibula transfer. Factors that influenced the outcome of union in 62 cases. *Int Orthop;* 14 (2):121–128.

18. **Yajima H, Tamai S, Mizumoto S, et al.** (1993) Vascularized fibular grafts in the treatment of osteomyelitis and infected non-union. *Clin Orthop;* (293):256–264.

19. **Banic A, Hertel R** (1993) Double vascularized fibulas for reconstruction of large tibial defects. *J Reconstr Microsurg;* 9 (6):421–428.

20. **Salimbeni-Ughi G, Santoni-Rugiu P, de Vizia GP** (1981) The gastrocnemius myocutaneous flap (GMF): an alternative method to repair severe lesions of the leg. *Arch Orthop Trauma Surg;* 98 (3):195–200.

21. **Strauch B, Vasconez LO, Hall-Findlay E** (1990) *Grabb's Encyclopedia of Flaps.* Boston Toronto London: Little Brown and Company.

22. **Cattaneo R, Catagni M, Johnson EE** (1992) The treatment of infected non-unions and segmental defects of the tibia by the methods of Ilizarov. *Clin Orthop;* (280):143–152.

23. **Klemm KW** (1993) Antibiotic bead chains. *Clin Orthop;* (295):63–76.

7 Updates

Updates and additional references for this chapter are available online at:
http://www.aopublishing.org/PFxM/63.htm

6.4 Malunion

René K. Marti, Flip P. Besselaar,
Ernst L.F.B. Raaymakers

1 Principles and philosophy

The term malunion in an adult patient is not clearly defined and its natural history in different localizations is not well known. The classification of malunions is based on the localization, i.e., intra-articular, metaphyseal, and diaphyseal. Furthermore, they can be defined as simple (one plane) or complex (several planes and translation) deformities. **However, some malalignments are better tolerated and compensated by the neighboring joints than others** (e.g., malunions of the upper extremity are much better tolerated than those of the weight-bearing lower extremity and at the lower leg valgus is more acceptable than varus). This means that there are both absolute and relative indications to correct deformities and leg length discrepancies.

1.1 Leg length discrepancies

The indication to perform an operative correction of a leg length discrepancy is not absolute and cannot be expressed in centimeters. Decisions must be made on an individual basis. The intertrochanteric shortening by osteotomy is a very safe operation; corrections of up to 5 cm can be expected to have a low complication rate [1]. The same is true for the intertrochanteric single/one-step lengthening of up to 3.5 cm which, however, is only indicated when other corrections at hip level are also necessary. The Wagner lengthening device, using Ilizarov's principles, allows safe diaphyseal lengthening of more than 5 cm by callus distraction. The combination of intertrochanteric shortening on one side and diaphyseal lengthening on the other is a very elegant method of correcting differences of more than 8 cm.

1.2 Intra-articular malunion

Painful and disabling articular incongruency leading to progressive arthritic changes with instability, is an absolute indication for surgery, particularly in the lower extremity. The decision as to whether secondary reconstruction, extra-articular correction

Some malunions are better tolerated and compensated by neighboring joints than others.

Painful and disabling articular incongruency is an absolute indication for surgery.

The indication to perform an operative correction of a leg length cannot be expressed in centimeters.

osteotomy, arthrodesis, or arthroplasty is performed depends on

- the local situation,
- the function of the joint,
- the age of the patient, and on
- socio-economic factors.

In young patients with severe joint destruction, arthrodesis is still the method of choice. The technique of fusion should allow for a total joint replacement at a later stage (hip, knee).

1.3 Metaphyseal malunion

In the absence of pain and functional disability there is only a relative indication to correct a metaphyseal malunion. Such a situation should be discussed individually, taking particular account of the long-term prognosis. The fact that procedures at this level are technically relatively easy may also influence decision making. Both open and closed wedge techniques have their own specific indications. The plate is the implant of choice, whereas external fixation and intramedullary nailing are rarely indicated.

1.4 Diaphyseal malunion

In the presence of malunion in the shaft, the main question is the level of a corrective osteotomy. The primary goal is to restore anatomy and function, however, the condition of the soft tissues and the bone at the level of the deformity may be a high risk factor. Biomechanically, the deformity itself is often unproblematic if the center of hip, knee, and ankle joint are in correct line to one another (Mikulicz). A simple

In diaphyseal malunion the primary goal is to restore anatomy and function.

diaphyseal malunion can be corrected in the metaphyseal area where the healing potential is much greater. At the proximal tibia, two-plane metaphyseal osteotomies may be indicated to restore the normal inclination of the joint. In case of diaphyseal deformity and shortening, correction can be combined using a lengthening device.

2 Decision making and planning

Any correction of a malunion has to be planned carefully [2]. Three dimensional thinking is of great importance but the ability to improvise may also be required. Good quality standard x-rays of the affected and the healthy limb, including both joints, are needed. For intra-articular corrections, conventional x-ray techniques in different directions form a good basis. CT imaging including 3-D reconstructions may be helpful but are not absolutely necessary. After evaluating the soft-tissue and bone condition at the level of the deformity, the first drawings of the different possible constructions are made to obtain correct alignment of the extremity. The level of the osteotomy must then be decided on (at the deformity or in a virgin area). Sometimes a double osteotomy has to be considered.

3 Reduction and fixation techniques

3.1 Choice of implant

In contrast to acute fracture treatment, the principles of stable internal fixation are still fully valid for corrective osteotomies. Interfragmentary compression is the key to safe healing, especially in sclerotic and poorly vascularized bone. Compression is best achieved by plates, by special techniques of external fixation and, exceptionally, with an intramedullary nail. If the soft tissues are not at risk, plates, especially the angled blade plates, are ideal for axial compression of metaphyseal osteotomy surfaces. It is important to use the removable compression device, which allows dynamic compression of the deformity before any screws are inserted.

The external fixator can adequately compress the osteotomy surfaces only if a frame construct is used. To avoid soft-tissue irritation that limits functional aftertreatment, this fixation technique should be restricted to the tibial plateau and supramalleolar osteotomies.

Stabilization of osteotomies by an intramedullary nail is restricted to the shaft. Reaming the canal is also necessary to obtain a long nail-bone contact and to increase stability in all directions. In cases where hardware is still *in situ*, there must be good reasons for switching from one implant system to the other. With a plate still in place, the approach will be a direct one and it is usually both logical and safe to stabilize the osteotomy with a plate again.

3.2 Metaphyseal and diaphyseal osteotomies

In the metaphyseal area, the osteotomy should be close enough to the joint where the cortex is already thin, so as to break or crack it without causing displacement. The constantly cooled oscillating saw should, therefore, not go all the way across the bone. Small drill holes may complete the cut while a large chisel helps break the cortex for an open wedge osteotomy. In the case of a rotational correction or a closed wedge osteotomy, a complete osteotomy is necessary; this also requires a more rigid osteosynthesis.

In the diaphyseal area, corrective osteotomies have a tendency to slow or delayed healing. A decortication, producing vital bone pieces at the level of the osteotomy, is advisable and may also help loosen the typically tight attachments of the periosteum and the adjacent muscles to the bone.

The principles of stable internal fixation are still fully valid for corrective osteotomies.

In the diaphyseal area, corrective osteotomies have a tendency to slow or delayed healing.

4 Specific osteotomies—indication and technique

4.1 Clavicle

A fracture of the clavicle almost always heals in a well-tolerated malunion. Shortening and angulation, causing brachialgia and local symptoms, are rare (ca. 2%). A lengthening osteotomy leading to an enlargement of the subclavicular space can relieve any impingement of neurovascular structures. The plate (e.g., LC-DCP 3.5) has to be carefully contoured to the surface of the bone or to a slightly waved plate. A primary cancellous graft might be indicated (see **Fig. 6.4-7**).

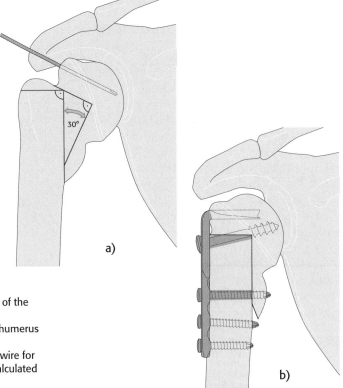

a)

b)

4.2 Humerus

4.2.1 Proximal humerus

Rotator cuff avulsions and other malunions of the proximal humerus can lead to an impingement syndrome which limits shoulder motion. Subcapital osteotomies or reconstruction osteotomies to decompress the rotator cuff can be performed using tension band techniques and small angulated plates. The standard deltopectoral approach (see **Fig. 4.2.1-5**) can be used for such osteotomies and/or an arthrodesis.

Varus or rotational malunions lend themselves to subcapital correction osteotomies (**Fig. 6.4-1**).

Malunion of the greater tuberosity usually causes an impingement during abduction. After identification of the supraspinatus and the infraspinatus tendon insertions, a 1 mm wire loop is placed through the Sharpey's fibers using a cannulated needle. The greater tuberosity is then osteotomized and pulled distally. After testing the shoulder mobility, the reduced fragment is secured with a lag screw and one or two tension band wires.

Fig. 6.4-1: Varus malunion of the proximal humerus.
Deformity of the proximal humerus after subcapital fracture.
a) Placement of the guide wire for the plate, respecting the calculated correction.
Osteotomy along the contours of the humeral shaft, carving of the place for the shaft allowing a correction of 30° valgus.
b) Impaction of an angled blade plate for adolescents or a 4-hole, 40 mm, 90° angled blade plate 4.5 with cannulated blade and impaction of the distal fragment. Compression with pointed reduction forceps. Further compression with dynamic cortex screws, followed by two lag screws, cancellous bone screws, and cortex screws for interfragmentary compression.
Clinical case: 62-year-old female.
c) Preoperative.
d) Postoperative.
e) Late control after 2 years.

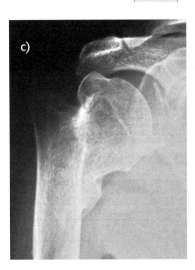

c)

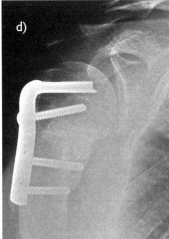

d)

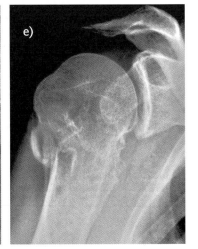

e)

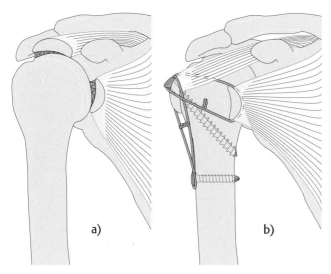

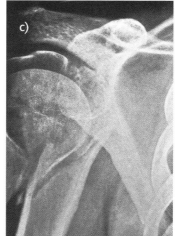

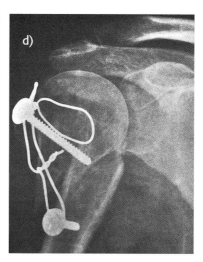

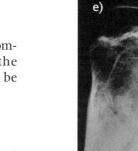

In malunited four-part fractures, the anatomical relationship between the center of the humeral head and the tuberosities should be restored (**Fig. 6.4-2**).

Fig. 6.4-2: Malunited four-part fractures.
a) Malunited four-part fracture, interposition of both tuberosities.
b) Deltopectoral exposure, identification of the rotator cuff muscles, osteotomy of the tuberosities and reinsertion by tension bands wires fixed to screws.
Clinical case:
c) Malunited four-part fracture; painful stiff joint 5 months after the accident.
d) Osteotomy and reinsertion of the two tuberosities, restoring the rotator cuff.
e) Excellent shoulder function after 13 years. Slight impingement symptoms treated by local infiltrations.

4.2.2   Humeral shaft

Although quite frequent, malunited humeral shaft fractures rarely require correction, whereas malrotation is easily corrected by subcapital osteotomy.

4.2.3   Distal humerus

The most frequent malunions are varus and valgus deformities. After failed arthrolysis, loss of elbow extension can be another indication for an osteotomy [3]. The radial approach with rigid plate fixation is a safe procedure in both open and closed wedge techniques. Intra-articular osteotomies of the distal humerus are rarely indicated and not without risk to the joint function.

In the presence of an ulnar nerve irritation, the medial approach with neurolysis of the ulnar nerve is indicated. A transposition of the nerve is usually not necessary.

Malunited humeral shaft fractures rarely require correction, but malrotation is easily corrected by subcapital osteotomy.

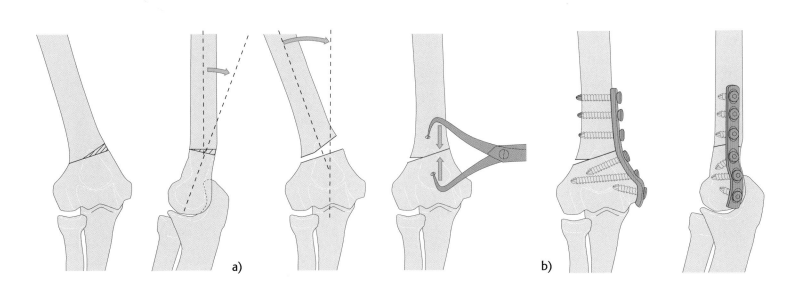

Fig. 6.4-3: Varization-extension osteotomy of the distal humerus in valgus and flexion deformity.
a) Ulnar approach, dissection of the ulnar nerve. Wedge osteotomy proximal to the fossa olecrani with mediodorsal basis of the wedge.
b) Contouring of a DCP 3.5 to the ulnar side of the humerus and fixation by compressing the osteotomy.
c) AP and lateral x-rays preoperative and after 2 months.

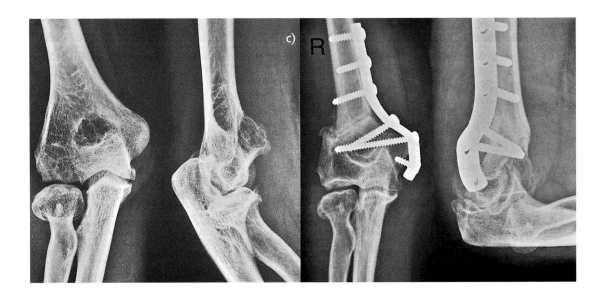

In one-plane deformities, the oblique osteotomy (**Fig. 6.4-3**) creates a bigger surface and an optimal stability using the lag screw-neutralization plate principle. In multi-plane correction osteotomies a stepwise wedge resection is recommended, allowing temporary reduction by pointed reduction forceps to check the elbow function (**Fig. 6.4-3b**).

4.3 Forearm

4.3.1 Proximal radius and ulna

Unreduced radial head in malunited Monteggia fractures: Corrective osteotomy of the ulna may lead to the spontaneous reduction of the radial head; however, the functional results are not always satisfactory.

4.3.2 Forearm shaft

The forearm bones have to be considered in their function as a joint, where even a slight malalignment of one of the two bones disturbs pronation and supination, as well as elbow and wrist function. In the shaft, angulation osteotomies restore the physiological distance and bow between ulna and radius; dissection of the interosseus membrane may be necessary

Supination or pronation contractures limiting the use of the forearm can be neutralized by a rotation osteotomy of the ulna, thus creating a more functional position of the forearm.

4.3.3 Wrist

Malunions following fractures of the distal radius are frequent but often well tolerated by elderly patients. In the young patient, meta-physeal osteotomies of the radius may be indicated. Depending on the direction of deformation with dorsal or palmar shortening, the correction osteotomy produces an open or closed wedge with a bone graft. For stabilization, plates 3.5 of varying shapes are used [4, 5] (**Fig. 6.4-4**).

Shortening of the ulna alone is indicated in the presence of minor axis deviation of the distal radius. Beware of irritation or compression

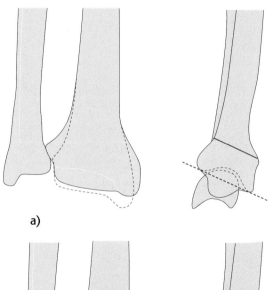

a)

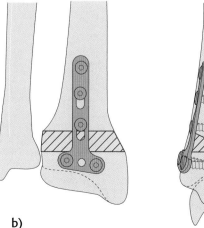

b)

Fig. 6.4-4: Malunion after fracture of distal radius.
a) Dorsal angulation and shortening.
b) Dorsal approach, transverse open wedge osteotomy of the radius, correction of all the deformation (extension, ulnar/radial adduction) using a small laminar spreader, interposition of iliac graft. The intrinsic stability is excellent; internal fixation with a small plate and two screws in the distal segment. The dorsal open wedge osteotomy compensates the overlength of the ulna.

Contractures limiting the use of the forearm can be neutralized by a rotation osteotomy of the ulna.

of the median nerve! Intra-articular osteotomies may be performed for malunions of single intra-articular fragments of the radius. Functional aftertreatment is the rule.

4.4 Femur

4.4.1 Proximal femur

In the presence of a malunion of the proximal femur with a normal hip function, the intertrochanteric osteotomy restores the biomechanical situation in all planes [1, 6–9]. Special indications may be the correction of leg length discrepancies by shortening or lengthening.

In general, the indications for surgery in malunion of the proximal femur are varus and rotational deformities in combination with shortening leading to limping and overuse of the neighboring joints.

Preoperative planning is based on AP and lateral x-rays of the proximal femur, and the calculation of all correction angles, including the gain of leg length by valgization (open or closed wedge osteotomy). The valgization should restore the biomechanical balance, but on the other hand, to avoid an abduction contracture the amount of correction is limited by the current hip function (**Fig. 6.4-5**).

The universal implant is the condylar plate. Depending on the amount of valgization, a 95° angled blade plate can easily be bent to any desired angle, the 120° and 130° angled blade plates being useful for special indications (malunion and non-union of the femoral neck).

The interlocking nail does not allow a precise correction of complex deformities but may be indicated for purely rotational deformities.

The aftertreatment is usually functional with 8 weeks of partial weight bearing.

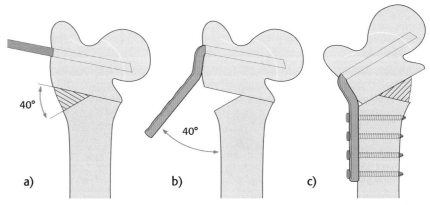

a)   b)   c)

Fig. 6.4-5: Intertrochanteric valgization osteotomy for varus deformity after a lateral femoral neck fracture. Lateral approach, placement of K-wires for the control of anteversion, rotation, and the calculated angle for the seating chisel.
a) Introduction of the seating chisel, osteotomy more or less parallel to the chisel creating a great bony surface, stepwise removal of a lateral wedge.

b) Use of a 120° angled blade plate after repeated reduction using the seating chisel as lever arm until the calculated correction is achieved without creating an abduction contracture.
c) Stabilization of the osteotomy under compression. The medial defect is then filled with the removed wedge.

Three-dimensional subtrochanteric lengthening of combined malunion including shortening (Fig. 6.4-6)

The indication for surgery is leg length discrepancy in combination with other malalignments of the proximal femur. This osteotomy is technically demanding and experience in individual shaping of plates is required.

Fig. 6.4-6: Three-dimensional subtrochanteric osteotomy of the proximal femur (valgization, rotation, lengthening).
a) Placement of the seating chisel and adaptation of the osteotomy plane respecting the desired corrections.
b) Distraction with a strong laminar spreader with the plate *in situ*.
c) Interposition of corticocancellous bone grafts (ipsilateral iliac crest), internal fixation with adapted condylar plate 95° or a 6-hole hip plate.
Clinical case:
d) Slight varus, shortening, and extreme malrotation after intramedullary nailing of a femoral shaft fracture in a 24-year-old female.
e) 50° derotation, 10° valgization, and 1.6 cm lengthening; stable fixation with condylar plate.
f) Consolidated corrective osteotomy after implant removal.

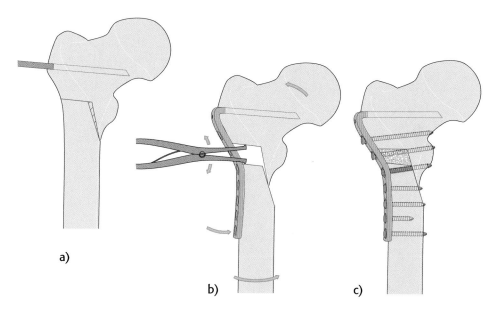

a)

b)

c)

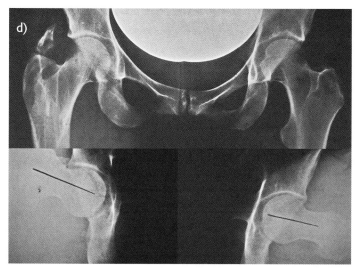

d)

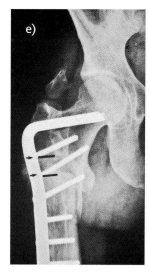

e)

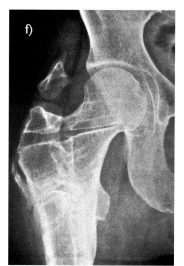

f)

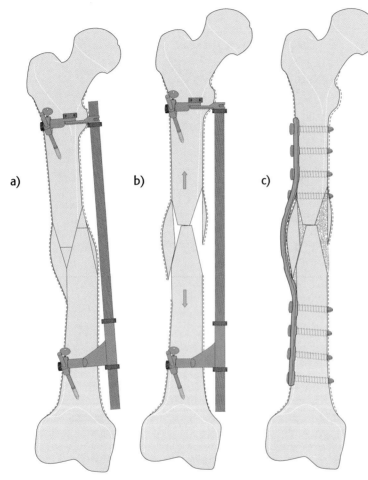

a)   b)   c)

Fig. 6.4-7: Correction and lengthening osteotomy of a malunited femoral shaft fracture.
a) Decortication of the region of shortening specially on the dorsal aspect (linea aspera) and fixation of the distraction apparatus ventrolateral outside the area of the future plate.
b) Oblique osteotomy and distraction of the fragments until the desired length is achieved. Osteotomy of the tips of the fragments and adaptation on the level of the transverse osteotomy.
c) Tension band plate (wave plate) compressing the osteotomy with a tension device. Autogenous bone graft if the contact area is small and the decorticated fragments do not provide a sufficient bone bridge.

Lengthening and reduction can be difficult; temporary interposition of artificial bone blocks may be helpful before interposition of the autogenous graft [9].

Subtrochanteric shortening of relative overlength [1, 9]

This is a low risk operation for shortening of up to 5 cm; we observed only one non-union in 70 cases. Preoperative planning is extremely important. The plate has to fit the greater trochanter and the femur exactly in order to achieve adequate contact and to avoid risk of fracture of the lesser trochanter.

4.4.2 Femoral shaft

Indication for surgery: Diaphyseal malunions with serious shortening caused by a fracture healed with overlap of the shaft fragment (Fig. 6.4-7).

Correction osteotomies at the level of the deformity can be stabilized by plates and nails [1]. Normally, the old fracture area is sclerotic, making nailing difficult and even dangerous. Where a nail is already *in situ* axial corrections can hardly be achieved by renailing.

The decortication approach stimulates healing of transverse, oblique, and stepwise lengthening osteotomies.

4.4.3 Distal femur

Indication for surgery: Malunions in valgus, varus, ante, or recurvation deformities, and, exceptionally, rotation deformities.

There are two techniques to correct malunions of the distal femur. In both the open and closed wedge technique the rather thin contralateral cortex should remain intact so as to create some intrinsic stability. The hip plate 90° with a displacement potential of 10–20 mm is the ideal implant for medial application in valgus deformities, while the condylar plate fits exactly to the lateral side of the distal femur for varus, antecurvation/recurvation and rotational malunions. Both can be used for the open wedge technique [1].

The techniques for osteotomy to correct varus and valgus deformity are illustrated in **Fig. 6.4-8**.

Aftertreatment:

Postoperative positioning of the knee in 90° flexion and early exercise (a CPM machine is helpful) are recommended as is partial weight bearing for 6–8 weeks.

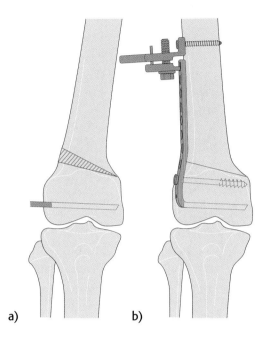

a)   b)

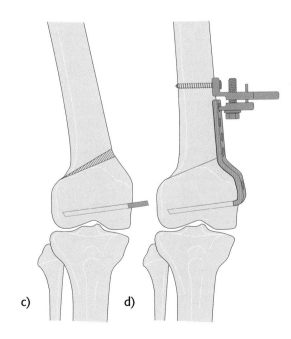

c)   d)

Fig. 6.4-8: Correction osteotomies of the distal femur.
a/b) Valgization osteotomy.
Supine position, sterile draping of the whole leg including iliac crest, possibility of bending the knee up to 90°. Atraumatic approach in front of the lateral intermuscular septum, positioning K-wire through the joint and under the patella. Introduction of the seating chisel respecting the planned correction with a condylar plate 95°.
a) Long, oblique, closing wedge osteotomy. Careful osteoclasis of the contralateral cortex with oscillating saw, small drill holes, and chisels. Removing the wedge, secure the osteotomy with two pointed reduction forceps before introducing the plate.
b) Full compression in closed wedge-type osteotomies using the compression device.
c/d) Varization osteotomy.
The same positioning of the patient as in a/b, approach through the medial septum, identical oblique osteotomy and osteoclasis, stabilization with a hip plate 90°.

Pitfalls and complications:

Displacement of the contralateral cortex is avoided by careful introduction of the plate, especially the hip plate on the medial side. The 90° plate is chosen, with the adequate displacement distance (10–15–20 mm). Delayed unions and non-unions are extremely rare.

4.5 Tibia

4.5.1 Proximal tibia

Indications for surgery are deformities of the proximal tibia in all three planes, intra-articular malunions after monocondylar fractures, as well as residual joint impaction in combination with ligamentous instability.

Preoperative planning is difficult but very important. It is done on the basis of AP, lateral, and oblique views, as well as CT-scan reconstruction in intra-articular deformities.

General considerations: Posttraumatic malalignments and deformities of the tibial head are corrected with open wedge technique to compensate the lost bony substance and to tension the loosened ligaments. This is valid for valgus (most frequent), varus, and recurvatum, but also for monocondylar and complex intra-articular malalignments. To achieve full correction, an osteotomy of the fibula is almost always indicated, but this seldom needs to be fixed. In the particular situation of a *genu recurvatum* with a normal femoropatellar joint, the technical principles are the same, but, in general, the osteotomy starts below the tuberosity, otherwise a reorientation of the patella is necessary.

Functional aftertreatment with partial weight bearing for about 8 weeks is the rule.

Intra-articular malunions with circumscribed impaction of the joint surface can be elevated and buttressed in combination with an open-wedge varization osteotomy. Weight-bearing forces are thereby transferred to the less damaged part of the joint.

Valgus deformity is progressive due to unicompartmental degenerative changes after fracture or meniscectomy. The correction may be bicondylar or unicompartmental (**Fig. 6.4-9**), depending on the extent of the malunion.

Pitfalls and complications:

Intra-articular osteotomy, as a single procedure, is rarely indicated. In most cases, axial correction by open wedge of the tibial head is added. A slight overcorrection of the axis is of great importance in order to eliminate extreme forces on the partially destroyed compartment. This means a correction to 0° in varization osteotomy, or to a slight hypervalgus in valgization osteotomy.

The aim of all osteotomies is to delay arthrodesis or joint replacement.

4.5.2 Tibial shaft

The indication to correct a malunion at the level of the diaphysis depends on the localization, the bone configuration, and the soft-tissue conditions. This also applies to the choice of fixation. A reamed nail (without tourniquet) can provide excellent stability allowing early weight bearing. The tension band plate has clear advantages if the intramedullary canal is obliterated by sclerotic callus formation [1] (see **section 4.4.2**).

Valgus deformity is progressive due to unicompartmental degenerative changes after fracture or meniscectomy.

The aim of all osteotomies is to delay arthrodesis or joint replacment.

Fig. 6.4-9: Unicondylar osteotomy of the proximal tibia. In supine position straight parapatellar approach. Lateral arthrotomy, identification of the old fracture line with small chisels, and drill holes.
a) Osteotomy of the lateral condyle along the old fracture line, and osteotomy of the head of the fibula.
b) Careful introduction of a small laminar spreader and elevation of the osteotomized condyle avoiding intra-articular dislocation by temporary fixation with a pointed reduction forceps or transverse K-wires. Interposition of wedge-shaped corticocancellous autograft and fixation with L-plate.
c) Clinical example of a secondary dislocation of the lateral condyle and of the head of the fibula in a 52-year-old female resulting in considerable valgus malunion.
d) Monocondylar osteotomy and osteotomy of the fibular head, graft interposition, and fixation with L-plate.
e) 17-year follow-up with only slight arthritic changes.

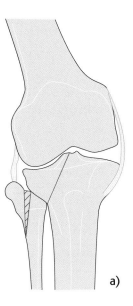 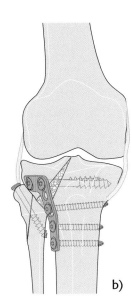 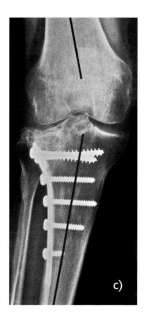 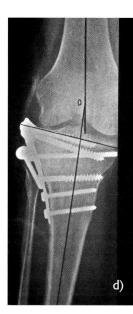 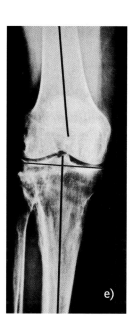

a) b) c) d) e)

4.5.3 Distal tibia

Indications for surgery are:

- Symptomatic malalignment after asymmetric closure of the growth plate in ankle fractures in children.
- Malunions of pilon fractures with good ankle function.
- Rotational deformities after fractures of the lower leg.

Intra-articular malunions can sometimes be an indication for a joint reconstruction.

Varus deformities: The usual method of correction is the open wedge osteotomy with plate fixation or external fixator depending on soft-tissue conditions (Fig. 6.4-10).

4.6 Ankle

In younger patients arthritic changes are well tolerated where there is perfect alignment.

Even in the presence of arthritic changes reconstruction can often delay secondary arthrodeses or prosthetic replacement for many years.

Valgus deformities are easier to manage by closed wedge osteotomy because of the fibula.

The alternative to this surgery is fusion or prosthetic replacement. **In younger patients, an attempt at reconstruction should be made. The results can be amazing; arthritic changes are well tolerated where there is perfect alignment.**

The diagnosis of malunion of a malleolar fracture is facilitated by the observation of the lateral joint line and the talar tilt (**Fig. 6.4-11a/b**). **Even in the presence of arthritic changes, malunited ankle fractures are a good indication for reconstruction and can often delay secondary arthrodeses or prosthetic replacement for many years [10, 11].**

Fig. 6.4-10: Correction of a supramalleolar varus deformity with external fixation.
The soft-tissue situation at the supramalleolar region allows transfixion with Steinmann pins. This method is excellent for total or partial closed wedge corrections and rotation osteotomies.
a) Introduction of the first Steinmann pin parallel to the joint line, the second one respecting the desired correction. Resection of a total or partial wedge. Osteotomy of the fibula of the resection type.
b) Compression osteotomy using the small lateral wedge medially.

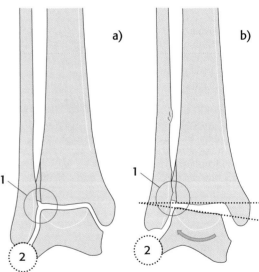

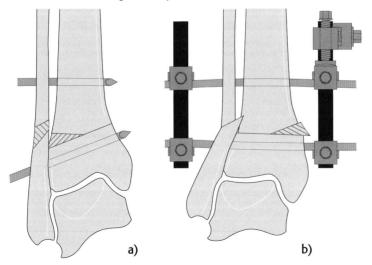

a)   b)

Fig. 6.4-11: Shortening of the fibula after malleolar fracture.
a) Characteristics of a normal ankle joint: (1) regular joint line (Shenton-line) without interruption at the level of the syndesmosis, (2) a circle fits exactly at the tip of the external malleolus and the processus lateralis of the talus.
b) After shortening and malrotation of the fibula, the Shenton-line is interrupted (1), the circle (2) does not fit anymore. A lateral tilt and external rotation of the talus is usually the consequence (arrow).

Shortening of the fibula in type C fractures often leads to talar shift and tilt and sometimes malrotation. Furthermore, malunion of the posterior malleolus in a proximal position can be present. By correction of length and rotation of the fibula, and exceptionally by osteotomy of the posterior malleolus, the ankle mortise can be restored (**Fig. 6.4-12a-d**) (see also **chapter 4.9**).

Fig. 6.4-12: Correction osteotomy of the malunited fibula after ankle fracture.
a) Malunion after type C fracture with shortening of the fibula, talar tilt, and shift (see also **Fig. 6.4-1a**).
Lateral approach and capsulectomy. Exposure and excision of the syndesmotic scar tissue. Sometimes the medial joint space has to be cleared of interposed fibrin or scar tissue.
b) Transverse osteotomy of the fibula, fixation with a DCP 3.5 or one-third tubular plate 3.5 in slight valgus at the distal fibula. Lengthening and rotation of the fibula using the articulated tension device or the laminar spreader as a distractor.
c) Reduction of the external malleolus into the incisura tibiae until the articular cartilage of distal tibia, fibula, and talus are congruent.
d) Fixation of the plate filling the defect with cortico-cancellous bone. A malunited posterior malleolus can be inspected and osteotomized through the lateral arthrotomy or by an osteotomy of the medial malleolus.

4.7 Calcaneus, mid foot, Lisfranc

The indication to perform an osteotomy of a malunited fracture of the calcaneus is rare. The treatment of choice is a corrective arthrodesis of the damaged subtalar joint. The same treatment applies to deformation of the navicular bone, the cuboid, and the Lisfranc joint.

5 Combined malunions

Multiple shaft fractures of the same limb may lead to multiple malunions which compensate each other in the sense that the centers of hip, knee, and ankle are in line. Especially in young individuals, the indication to perform a double correction osteotomy is based on the inclination of the knee joint in the sagittal and/or frontal plane, as well as in rotation. In preoperative planning, level, type of osteotomy, and fixation have to be considered in respect of the soft-tissue situation, the function, and the esthetic aspect.

The indication to perform an osteotomy of a malunited fracture of the calcaneus is rare.

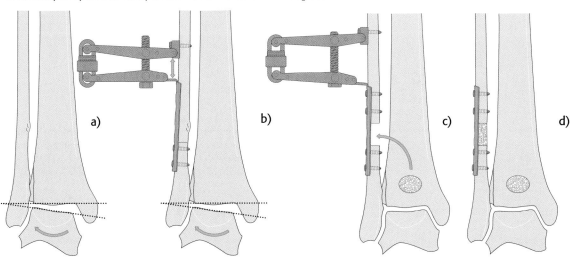

a) b) c) d)

6 Conclusions

The indication for a corrective osteotomy in posttraumatic cases depends on the individual disability.

Surgeons should be aware of their technical limitations.

In conclusion, the indication for a corrective osteotomy in posttraumatic cases depends on the individual disability. The natural history of the deformity should be respected. Advantages and disadvantages of prophylactic osteotomy should be discussed with the patient. The surgeon is responsible for precise planning; he should be aware of his technical limitations, be able to treat the complications, and to predict the end result.

7 Bibliography

1. **Müller ME, Allgöwer M, Schneider R, et al.** (1979) Osteotomies. In: *Manual of Internal Fixation*. Berlin Heidelberg New York: Springer-Verlag.

2. **Mast J, Jakob R, Ganz R** (1989) Osteotomies. In: *Planning and Reduction Technique in Fracture Surgery*. Berlin Heidelberg New York: Springer-Verlag: 12–15.

3. **Marti RK, Ochsner PE, Bernoski FP** (1981) [Correction osteotomy of the distal humerus in adults (author's transl)]. *Orthopade;* 10 (4):311–315.

4. **Fernandez DL** (1982) Correction of post-traumatic wrist deformity in adults by osteotomy, bone-grafting, and internal fixation. *J Bone Joint Surg [Am];* 64 (8):1164–1178.

5. **Fernandez DL, Jupiter JB** (1995) Malunion of the Distal End of the Radius. In: *Fractures of the Distal Radius*. Berlin Heidelberg New York: Springer-Verlag: 263–315.

6. **Pauwels F** (1984) Biomechanical Principles of Varus/Valgus Intertrochanteric Osteotomy (Pauwels I and II) in the Treatment of Osteoarthritis of the Hip. In: Schatzker J, editor. *The Intertrochanteric Osteotomy*. Berlin Heidelberg New York Tokyo: Springer-Verlag: 3–23.

7. **Bombelli R** (1976) *Osteoarthritis of the Hip*. Berlin Heidelberg New York: Springer-Verlag.

8. **Schatzker J** (1984) *The Intertrochanteric Osteotomy*. Berlin Heidelberg New York Tokyo: Springer-Verlag.

9. **Marti RK** (1993) Osteotomies in posttraumatic deformities following fractures of the proximal femur. In: Marti RK, Dunki JP, editors. *Proximal Femoral Fractures, Operative Techniques and Complications.* London: Medical Press Ltd.: 573–587.

10. **Weber BG** (1981) Lengthening osteotomy of the fibula to correct a widened mortice of the ankle after fracture. *Int Orthop;* 4 (4):289–293.

11. **Marti RK, Raaymakers EL, Nolte PA** (1990) Malunited ankle fractures. The late results of reconstruction. *J Bone Joint Surg [Br];* 72 (4):709–713.

8 Updates

Updates and additional references for this chapter are available online at:
http://www.aopublishing.org/PFxM/64.htm

6.5 Algodystrophy

Lijckle van der Laan & Rene J. A. Goris

1 Introduction

Algodystrophy is a complication occurring in an extremity after operation or minor trauma. This syndrome may induce severe disability and intractable pain. In a prospective study of 829 algodystrophy patients the syndrome developed in 65% after trauma (mostly fracture), in 19% after operation, in 2% after an inflammatory process, in 4% after various other enhancing factors (such as intramuscular or intravenous injection), while in 10% no factor was identified [1]. The reported incidence of algodystrophy after a Colles' fracture varies from 7–37%, and for a tibial shaft fracture is 30%. Examples of minor operations which may initiate algodystrophy are carpal tunnel release and arthroscopy. The various acronyms used for algodystrophy, depending on the country concerned, the specialty treating the patient, or the different factors are confusing. Most frequently used denominations are causalgia, reflex sympathetic dystrophy, postinfarction sclerodactylia, Babinsky-Froment sympathetic paralysis, Pourfour du Petit syndrome, Sudeck's atrophy, or peripheral trophoneurosis. In the differential diagnosis of algodystrophy the following diseases have to be excluded: phlebothrombosis, arterial insufficiency, infection or an inflammatory condition, compartment syndrome, carpal or tarsal tunnel syndrome, rheumatological disorders, and neurological illness, such as polyneuropathy.

2 Pathophysiology

In 1864, causalgia was firstly reported by Weir Mitchell who described in detail the signs and symptoms of the syndrome in soldiers wounded by a gunshot during the American Civil War. The name algodystrophy was introduced by the neurosurgeon Leriche in 1916, who suggested that an increased activity of the sympathetic system was involved in the pathogenesis of this syndrome. Livingston suggested that activation of the nociceptors leads to excitation of the internuncial pool of neurones of the spinal cord with induction of an increased activation of the efferent sympathetic system. The subsequent vasoconstriction, with ischemia of the tissues, may stimulate the nociceptors with re-excitation of the spinal cord, resulting in a "vicious circle". Recently, the "increased efferent sympathetic" theory has been replaced by the hypothesis that an upregulated sensitivity of

Most common acronyms of algodystrophy:
- Causalgia
- Reflex sympathetic dystrophy
- Sudeck's atrophy
- Complex regional pain syndrome

α-adrenergic receptors for catecholamines may induce algodystrophy. This total reversal is based on the reportedly reduced concentrations of norepinephrine and neuropeptide Y in the algodystrophic extremity, as compared to the unaffected side [2] and on the increased numbers of α_1-adrenoreceptors in the skin of algodystrophy patients as compared to normal individuals. The recently reported double-blind, randomized studies of sympathetic blockade versus placebo [3, 4], in which no difference in treatment outcome is described, is also a reason for refuting the sympathetic theory.

In 1942, Sudeck formulated a totally different theory, suggesting an exaggerated regional inflammatory response of an extremity to injury or operation in the pathogenesis of algodystrophy. In extremities affected by acute algodystrophy an increased uptake of Indium-111-immunoglobin G as compared to the contralateral unaffected extremities is measured by using Indium-111-immunoglobin G scintigraphy. This technique is an established method for recognizing infectious and inflammatory foci. Another support for the inflammatory theory is the therapeutic effect of anti-inflammatory drugs such as corticosteroids or of local application of the free radical scavenger dimethyl sulfoxide (DMSO) [5, 6]. Light and electron microscopic analysis of skeletal muscle biopsies of chronic RSD patients showed various abnormalities which are compatible with free radical-induced changes.

Finally, it has been theorized that algodystrophy is triggered by various predisposing psychosocial factors; emotional instability, depression, anxiety, and life events may provoke algodystrophy. A critical review of the relevant literature, however, reveals no evidence in support of predisposing psychosocial factors [7, 8].

In 1993, the International Association for the Study of Pain renamed algodystrophy Complex Regional Pain Syndrome (CRPS), to be neutral in respect of the various theories of the pathogenesis of this complex disease. This term is not generally used.

3 The signs and symptoms

Based on a prospective study of 829 algodystrophy patients [1], we defined the following diagnostic criteria of algodystrophy:
1. At least four out of five of the following:
   - unexplained diffuse pain,
   - difference in skin color (red or blue discoloration) compared with the other extremity,
   - diffuse edema,
   - difference in skin temperature (warm or cold) compared with the other extremity,
   - limited active range of motion.
2. Appearance or increase in severity of the above signs and symptoms after using the extremity.
3. The above signs and symptoms present in an area larger than the area of primary injury or operation and including the area distal to the primary injury.

In the acute phase of algodystrophy Veldman et al. reported hyperhidrosis in 57% of the patients and changed growth of hair in 54% as sympathetic signs. From the onset of the disease various neurological symptoms may appear in the affected extremity, for example: hypersthesia (typically with a glove-like or stocking-like distribution), hyperpathy, incoordination, tremor, involuntary movements, muscle spasms, and paresis.

In the chronic phase of the disease the neurological symptoms may still be present while the inflammatory signs diminish. The paresis and exercise limitation of the affected extremity may be explained by the reported decreased oxygen consumption and/or altered energy metabolism of the affected extremity as compared to the unaffected limb [9, 10].

In conclusion, algodystrophy, in the acute phase, is characterized by signs and symptoms of inflammation, and may affect all structures and functions present in an extremity.

4 X-ray and bone scintigraphy

In 1900 Sudeck described the radiological appearance of algodystrophy. The changes start as a patchy osteoporosis within the small bones of the hands or feet and within the distal metaphysis of forearm or tibial bones. X-ray as well as three phase technetium bone scan has a low sensitivity and low specificity in recognizing algodystrophy. Algodystrophy remains mainly a clinical diagnosis.

5 Treatment

In accordance with the variety of theories regarding the pathogenesis of algodystrophy, various therapeutic regimens are used. However, independent of the kind of therapy, **it is generally accepted that whatever the treatment, the best results are obtained when algodystrophy is diagnosed early and treated immediately**.

During the last 15 years, we have progressively adapted our treatment schedule for algodystrophy to new knowledge and increasing experience.

5.1 Free radical scavenger treatment

Patients with severe, acute algodystrophy are treated via a central venous catheter with the free radical scavenger mannitol (10%, 1000cc/24 hours) for a period of one week. Care should be taken in patients with renal failure, as hyperosmolarity may occur. When renal function is normal, osmolarity is not significantly increased. Subsequently, these patients are treated with local application of dimethyl sulfoxide cream 50% on the skin of the affected area. Application is performed five times daily and continued for approximately 2–3 months. Less severe cases of algodystrophy are initially treated with dimethyl sulfoxide cream. This is the major part of our treatment schedule and is based on a prospective crossover study performed in our department in 1985 [6]. In this study, the treatment with dimethyl sulfoxide cream resulted in significantly greater improvement of the algodystrophy as compared to the placebo treatment. In the prospective, randomized and double-blind study (dimethyl sulfoxide vs. placebo) of Zuurmond et al. similar results are reported [5]. Subsequently, the patients are treated with the free radical scavenger N-acetyl cysteine (3 times 600 mg/day orally) until the signs and symptoms of algodystrophy disappear or become stabilized in an intractable situation.

In the acute phase algodystrophy has signs of inflammation affecting all structres and functions of an extremity.

Whatever the treatment the best results are obtained with immediate onset after an early diagnosis.

5.2 Vasodilation treatment

A minority of algodystrophy patients have cold skin from the onset of the disease as compared to the unaffected side. Special attention is necessary because these patients are more at risk of a poor outcome, have a higher incidence of recurrence of algodystrophy [11], and more frequently require an amputation because of severe complications [12]. Therefore, this group is in addition treated early and rigorously with the above-mentioned free radicals in combination with peripheral vasodilators such as verapamil "retard" (240 mg once or twice/day orally), ketanserin (2 times 20 or 40 mg/day per os), or pentoxyfiline (2 times 400 mg/day per os) to optimize perfusion of the affected extremity. Verapamil is the most recognized medication. When the skin temperature remains cold despite the vasodilators, sympathetic blockade is performed at an early stage.

5.3 Attention to painful trigger points

Typically muscular exercises induce or increase the inflammatory symptoms.

In about 50% of the algodystrophy patients a "trigger point" is present. A trigger point is defined as a specific painful area within the affected algodystrophy extremity, in which the pain does not directly result from algodystrophy. Examples are: carpal tunnel syndrome, tendinitis of the scapular insertion of the biceps, neuroma, trigger finger, epicondylitis lateralis or medialis, anterior metatarsalgia, "jumpers knee", or tendinitis of the patella tendon. Our hypothesis is that these trigger points may induce, sustain, or worsen the algodystrophy, possibly by a local process of neurogenic inflammation. During the treatment of algodystrophy, these trigger points are identified and given specific treatment, which may include the operative removal of a neuroma, local injection of bupivacaine followed by methylprednisolone for tendinitis [13], or providing an orthosis for immobilization of a painful joint. Retrospective analysis of bupivacaine and methylprednisolone injection of the shoulder in algodystrophy patients who had a tendinitis of one or both biceps muscles, resulted in permanent relief of complaints in 48%, temporary or moderate relief in 42%, no difference in 4%, and increase of complaints in 1%; in 3% the results were not documented [13].

5.4 Physical therapy

Muscular work is accompanied by an increase in oxygen consumption and may induce free radical production. **It is almost pathognomonical of algodystrophy patients that muscular work induces or increases the inflammatory signs and symptoms, especially pain, within the affected extremity** [1]. For this reason, we advise algodystrophy patients to exercise their affected extremity actively, but only below their pain threshold. In our department physical therapy is started when the acute inflammatory algodystrophy signs and symptoms have largely disappeared. Treatment consists of mobilizing the affected joints below the pain threshold. Aggressive physical therapy induces an increase of algodystrophy complaints and may be torture for the patient.

5.5 Chronic algodystrophy

Patients with chronic algodystrophy are treated similarly, following the schedule outlined above. However, the free radical scavengers therapy will be used for one month and may be prolonged as long as improvement continues. In the chronic phase we advise treatment of the severe pain complaints by anesthesiologists.

5.6 Algodystrophy with severe disability

Some cases of algodystrophy are resistant to any of the modes of treatment presently known. In these patients, a completely different approach is necessary to address their severe disability. Such an approach should include proper pain medication, and providing an orthosis, a wheelchair, and/or adaption of their home situation, as appropriate.

6 Bibliography

1. **Veldman PH, Reynen HM, Arntz IE, et al.** (1993) Signs and symptoms of reflex sympathetic dystrophy: prospective study of 829 patients. *Lancet;* 342 (8878):1012–1016.

2. **Drummond PD, Finch PM, Smythe GA** (1991) Reflex sympathetic dystrophy: the significance of differing plasma catecholamine concentrations in affected and unaffected limbs. *Brain;* 114 (Pt 5):2025–2036.

3. **Ramamurthy S, Hoffman J** (1995) Intravenous regional guanethidine in the treatment of reflex sympathetic dystrophy/causalgia: a randomized, double-blind study. Guanethidine Study Group. *Anesth Analg;* 81 (4):718–723.

4. **Jadad AR, Carroll D, Glynn CJ, et al.** (1995) Intravenous regional sympathetic blockade for pain relief in reflex sympathetic dystrophy: a systematic review and a randomized, double-blind crossover study. *J Pain Symptom Manage;* 10 (1):13–20.

5. **Zuurmond WW, Langendijk PN, Bezemer PD, et al.** (1996) Treatment of acute reflex sympathetic dystrophy with DMSO 50% in a fatty cream. *Acta Anaesthesiol Scand;* 40 (3):364–367.

6. **Goris RJ, Dongen LM, Winters HA** (1987) Are toxic oxygen radicals involved in the pathogenesis of reflex sympathetic dystrophy? *Free Radic Res Commun;* 3 (1–5):13–18.

7. **Bruehl S, Carlson CR** (1992) Predisposing psychological factors in the development of reflex sympathetic dystrophy. A review of the empirical evidence. *Clin J Pain;* 8 (4):287–299.

8. **DeGood DE, Cundiff GW, Adams LE, et al.** (1993) A psychosocial and behavioral comparison of reflex sympathetic dystrophy, low back pain, and headache patients. *Pain;* 54 (3):317–322.

9. **Heerschap A, den Hollander JA, Reynen H, et al.** (1993) Metabolic changes in reflex sympathetic dystrophy: a 31P NMR spectroscopy study. Muscle Nerve; 16 (4):367–373.

10. **Goris RJ** (1991) Tissue oxygen utilization. In: Gutierrez G, Vincent JL, editors. *Conditions associated with impaired oxygen extraction.* Berlin: Springer-Verlag.

11. **Veldman PH, Goris RJ** (1996) Multiple reflex sympathetic dystrophy. Which patients are at risk for developing a recurrence of reflex sympathetic dystrophy in the same or another limb [see comments]. *Pain;* 64 (3):463–466.

12. **Dielissen PW, Claassen AT, Veldman PH, et al.** (1995) Amputation for reflex sympathetic dystrophy. *J Bone Joint Surg [Br];* 77 (2):270–273.

13. **Veldman PH, Goris RJ** (1995) Shoulder complaints in patients with reflex sympathetic dystrophy of the upper extremity. *Arch Phys Med Rehabil;* 76 (3):239–242.

7   Updates

Updates and additional references for this chapter are available online at:
http://www.aopublishing.org/PFxM/65.htm

Glossary

Chris L. Colton
with acknowledgements to
Stephan M. Perren

The inclusion of a glossary may seem superfluous in a work for surgeons. Nevertheless, it may be helpful in clarifying certain confusions and misnomers that can creep into common parlance. It is hoped that it may be of use to some of those readers whose native tongue is not English. The editors, therefore, decided that it would be more helpful to include it.

abduction: Movement of a part away from the midline, e.g., abduction at the shoulder moves the arm away from the trunk and out to the side. At the thumb, it describes movement of the digit forward from the anatomical position, away from the palm. This is because in evolutionary terms, the thumb of the primitive hand lies in the same plane as the fingers and abduction carries it sideways away from the midline, as the arm abducts at the shoulder. In man, to allow human grasp, the thumb has rotated through 90° from its atavistic alignment.

adduction: Movement of a part towards the midline, e.g., adduction at the hip joint moves the leg toward the midline and adduction of both legs would press the knees together or cross the legs.

algodystrophy: Alternatively known as Reflex Sympathetic Dystrophy or Sudek's atrophy—see **chapter 6.5**, also **fracture disease**.

allograft: Graft of tissue from another individual of the same species, who is genetically different from the recipient. Bone is generally transplanted without revascularization. Histocompatibility studies, essential in organ transplantation, are not necessary in bone allografting.

anaerobic: Those metabolic processes which are not dependent on oxygen. Anaerobic organisms can, therefore, thrive in tissues which are hypoxic or anoxic.

anastomosis: A junction between two vessels or other tubular anatomical structures.

anatomical position: The reference position of the body—standing facing the observer, with the palms of the hands facing forward.

anatomical reduction: The exact adaptation of fracture fragments (hairline adjustment). It will result in complete restoration of the normal anatomy. While overall stability does not depend on precise reduction, precise reduction more reliably results in stability and increased strength of fixation. It is more important in articular fractures than in diaphyseal fractures—see also **stability of fixation**.

ankylosis: Fusion of a joint by bone or a tight fibrous union, occurring spontaneously as a result of a disease process, e.g., following septic arthritis (pyarthrosis).

angulation: The orientation of one body (e.g., bone fragment) in such a manner that the two parts meet at an angle rather than a straight line. The standard surgical convention is that the angulation is characterized by describing the deviation of the distal part from its anatomical position. For example, at a Colles's fracture, the distal radial fragment is dorsally (or posteriorly) angulated, even though the apex of the deformity points anteriorly; similarly a tibial fracture whose apex angulation points backward should be referred to as angulated anteriorly, as the distal part is indeed angulated anteriorly from its anatomical position.

anterior: The front aspect of the body in the anatomical position. If A is in front of B in the anatomical position, then A is said to be anterior to B.

antibiotic: Any drug, such as penicillin, produced by certain fungi, bacteria, and other organisms, which can inhibit the growth of, or destroy, microorganisms. They are used for the prevention or treatment of infections.

antibody: A substance produced by the host's immune system, in response to the detection of an **antigen**. The antibody is specifically elaborated to attack and destroy only the antigen which stimulated its production—antigen specific.

antigen: Component of a foreign biological substance (transplanted tissue, invading virus, etc.), which stimulates the host's immune system to attack that foreign substance by elaborating **antibodies** which destroy the antigen and in so doing may result in damage to the "invader".

antiseptic: Originally the surgical strategy for avoiding postoperative sepsis by applying to the wound bactericidal chemicals, as in the carbolic acid aerosol described and used by Joseph Lister in the late 19th century—the era of antiseptic surgery. Now a term used for non-biological chemicals which have topical bactericidal properties.

arthritis: Literally, an inflammatory condition of a diarthrodial (synovial) joint. It may be septic or aseptic. The former may be blood-borne (hematogenous), as in children, or it may follow penetration of the joint by wounding or surgery. Aseptic arthritides are usually of the rheumatoid type (including Reiter's syndrome, psoriatic arthropathy, etc.) or due to degenerative change (see **osteoarthritis**).

arthrodesis: Fusion of a joint by bone as a planned outcome of a surgical procedure.

articular fracture–partial: Only part of the joint is involved while the remainder remains attached to the diaphysis.

articular fracture–complete: The entire articular surface is separated from the diaphysis.

autograft: Graft of tissue from one site to another within the same individual (homograft).

avascular necrosis (often abbreviated as AVN): Bone which has been deprived of its blood supply dies. In the absence of sepsis, this is called avascular necrosis (aseptic necrosis). The dead bone retains its normal strength until the natural process of revascularization by "creeping substitution"—see **blood supply**—starts to remove the dead bone, in preparation for the laying down of new bone. Loaded areas may then collapse—segmental collapse. This occurs in the femoral head and the talus more frequently than at other skeletal sites.

avulsion: Pulling off, e.g., a bone fragment pulled off by a ligament or muscle attachment is an avulsion fracture.

bactericidal: Capable of killing bacteria.

biocompatibility: The ability to exist in harmony with, and not to injure, associated biological tissues or processes.

biological (biologically respectful) internal fixation [1]: In any internal fixation there is always a skilful balance to be struck between the degree of surgical stabilization produced and the biological insult caused by the necessary surgical exposure. The balance will be judged by an experienced surgeon. Biological fixation utilizes a technique of surgical exposure and fixation which favors the preservation of the blood supply and thereby optimizes the healing potential of the bone and soft tissues. It provides sufficient stability for multifragmentary fractures to heal in correct length and alignment. It relies on a rapid biological reaction (early callus formation) for the protection of the implants from mechanical failure (fatigue or loosening). See **chapter 1.2**.

biopsy: The surgical removal of a piece of tissue for histological examination, usually undertaken to establish a diagnosis.

blood supply to cortical bone (restoration of): Cortical bone which has been completely deprived of its blood supply for any extended period of time dies. It may become revascularized either by ingrowth of blood vessels without marked widening of the Haversian canals [2], or by newly formed Haversian canals which result from the penetration of osteons. Such osteonal remodeling is a process with a marked lag period and a slow speed (0.1 mm/day according to Schenk [3]). When aseptic necrotic bone is revascularized by resorption and replacement with newly formed, vascular bone, the term creeping substitution is often applied. See **vascularity** and **avascular necrosis**.

bone graft: Bone removed from one skeletal site and placed at another. Bone grafts are used to stimulate bone union and also to restore skeletal continuity where there has been bone loss—see **allograft, autograft, xenograft**.

broad spectrum: Refers to antibiotics which are active against a wide range of different organisms.

butterfly fragment: Where there is a fracture complex with a third fragment which does not comprise a full cross section of the bone (i.e., after reduction there is some contact between the two main fragments), the small wedge-shaped fragment, which may be spiral, is occasionally referred to as a butterfly fragment—see **wedge fracture**.

buttress: When there is impaction of bony fragments (e.g., at the distal metaphysis of the tibia in pilon injuries) a defect remains after fracture reduction. An implant used to maintain the reduction "out to length" by resisting the compressive loads tending to re-impact the fragments is functioning as a buttress.

callus: A tissue complex formed at a site of bony repair. Following a fracture it makes a gradual and progressive transition through a series of tissue types—hematoma → granulation tissue → fibrous tissue (or fibrocartilagenous tissue) → calcified tissue → remodeling into woven bone, gaining in stiffness as it does so. Callus formation is the response of living bone to any irritation—chemical [4], infective, mechanical instability [5], etc. In internal fixation with absolute stability, where direct (callus-free) bone healing is expected, the appearance of callus is a sign of unexpected mechanical instability (formerly referred to as "irritation" callus) and will alert the surgeon to a failure of the original mechanical objective. Callus is welcome as a repair tissue in all treatment methods where relative fracture stability has been the planned goal.

cancellous bone: Is the spongy trabecular bone found mostly at the proximal and distal bone ends in contrast with the dense cortical bone of the shafts. Cancellous bone has a much larger surface area per unit volume and is, therefore, more readily available to its blood supply, as well as to osteoclasts for resorption. Its large surface/volume ratio also offers more surface for invading blood vessels attempting to re-vascularize dead cancellous bone, and this is an advantage when cancellous bone is used for grafting.

caudad: Literally "tailward". If A is nearer to the "tail", or coccyx, than B, then A is caudad of B. Usually confined to the axial, rather than the appendicular, structures—see **cephalad**.

caudal: Pertaining to the tail, or tail region, e.g., caudal epidural injection.

cephalad: Literally "headward". If A is nearer to the head than B, then A is cephalad of B. Usually confined to the axial, rather than the appendicular, structures—see **caudad**.

chemotherapy: Treatment of malignant lesions with drugs that impair, or stop, their cellular proliferation.

chondrocytes: The active cells of all cartilage, whether articular cartilage, growth cartilage, fibrocartilage, etc. They produce the chondral matrix, both its collagen and the mucopolysaccharides of the ground substance.

cis cortex: See **near cortex**.

compartment syndrome: See **muscle compartment**.

complex fracture: Fracture in which after reduction there is no contact between the main fragments.

compound fracture: The British school has long referred to fractures with an overlying, communicating wound of the integument as "compound" fractures, the opposite being simple fractures. No fracture should be regarded as simple, and the use of the archaic word "compound" does not convey the important clinical distinction. The term is now largely superseded by "open fracture".

compression screw: See **lag screw**.

compression: The act of pressing together. It results in deformation (shortening like a spring) and improvement or creation of stability. Compression is used (1) to provide stability of fixation where motion-induced resorption must be prevented, and (2) to protect the implants and to improve their efficiency by unloading them. Unloading is achieved through restoration of the load-bearing capacity of the bone. Any fixation taking advantage of the loadbearing capacity of fracture fragments can withstand load without mechanical failure, or temporary micro-motion, within the fracture. This is the main reason for using careful reduction and application of compression. Compression, furthermore, helps to restore dynamic loading of the bone fragments, a process for which stable contact of the fracture fragments is a prerequisite.
If the implant (screw, plate) bridging the fracture is applied under tension, then the fracture locus undergoes an equivalent amount of compression. The compression is used to help stabilize the fracture. We have not observed any "magic biological effect" of compression.

contact healing: Occurs between two fragment ends of a fractured bone, at circumscribed places that are maintained in motionless contact. The fracture is then repaired by direct internal remodeling. Contact healing may be observed additionally where the gap is only a few micrometers wide.

coronal: This is a vertical plane of the body passing from side to side, so that a coronal bisection of the body would cut it into a front half and a back half. It is so called because at a coronation, the crown (*corona* in Latin) is held with a hand on either side as it is lowered onto the royal head; the line joining the hands is in the "coronal" plane.

cortex: See **cortical bone**.

cortical bone: The dense bone forming the tubular element of the shaft, or diaphysis (middle part) of a long bone. The term is also applied to the dense, thin shell covering the cancellous bone of the metaphysis. The term is generally used interchangeably with cortex.

corticotomy: A special osteotomy where the cortex is surgically divided but the medullary content and the periosteum are not injured.

CPM—continuous passive motion: The use of apparatus to move a joint through a controlled range of motion has been shown to enhance articular cartilage healing after injury and to promoted soft tissue recovery after surgery. Salter et al. and Sheperd [6, 7], and others have demonstrated that the use of passive motion machines for continuous periods is necessary for cartilage repair. The indiscriminate

use of CPM machines for other indications can lead to muscle wasting and should be combined with other techniques of physical therapy.

creeping substitution: See **blood supply**.

cytoplasm: The non-nuclear substance of a cell.

debricolage: A French term signifying the process of mechanical failure of an internal fixation prior to the onset of solid bone healing.

débridement: Literally the "unbridling" of a wound. Strictly speaking it refers to the extension of a wound and the opening up of the planes of the injured tissue, usually in the context of open fractures, as described by Ambrose Paré in the 16th century. It is usually used in the context of open fractures. It has come to be understood as the opening up of a wound or pathological area (e.g., bone infection) together with the surgical excision of all avascular, contaminated, infected, or other undesirable tissue.

deformity: Any abnormality of the form of a body part.

delayed union: See **non-union, union, pseudarthrosis.** Failure of any given fracture to achieve bony continuity within the period predicted for a fracture of that type and location. Serial examinations reveal slow, but continuing, progress of the healing process. Delayed union, like **union** is a surgical judgment and cannot be allocated a specific time period.

diaphysis: The cylindrical, or tubular, part between the ends of a long bone, often referred to as the shaft.

direct healing: A type of fracture healing observed with absolutely stable (rigid) internal fixation. It is characterized by:
1. Absence of callus formation specific to the fracture site.
2. Absence of bone surface resorption at the fracture site.
3. Direct bone formation, without any intermediate repair tissue.

Direct fracture healing was formerly called "primary" healing, a term avoided today so as not to imply any grading of the quality of fracture healing. Two types of direct healing are distinguished, namely **contact healing** and **gap healing**.

dislocation: A displacement, usually traumatic, of the components of a joint such that no part of one articular surface remains in contact with the other. The term subluxation applies when there is partial contact between the two surfaces.

displacement: Out of place. A fracture is displaced if the fragments are not perfectly anatomically aligned. Displacement may be linear (or translational)—as when one fragment shifts sideways in relation to another—angular, rotational, or axial—when the displacement results in shortening along an axis. The term "dislocation" is sometimes misused to describe displacement. Dislocation is reserved for joint malalignment—see **dislocation**.

distal: Away from the center of the body, more peripheral. For example, the hand is distal to the elbow, the phalanges are distal to the metacarpals. In certain instances, it means nearer the end than the beginning; for example, in the digestive system the stomach is distal to the esophagus, or in the urinary tract the bladder is distal to the ureter.

dorsal: Pertaining to the back—or dorsum—of the body in the anatomical position. An exception is the foot; the top of the foot, even though it faces forward in the anatomical position, is called the dorsum.

ductility: The attribute of an implant material which characterizes its tolerance to **plastic deformation**.

dynamization: The process whereby mechanical load transferred across a fracture locus can be increased at a certain stage to enhance bone formation or to promote "maturation" of the healing tissues. An example would be the reduction in stiffness of an external fixation by either loosening some clamps, reducing the number of pins, or moving the tubular construct further from the bone. Early dynamization, i.e., before solid bridging of the bone, can result in stimulation of callus formation. The value of late dynamization is debatable.

elastic deformation: See **plastic deformation**.

endosteal: The adjective derived from endosteum, which means the interior surface of a bone, e.g., the wall of the medullary cavity.

energy transfer: When tissues are traumatized, the damage is due to energy that is transferred to the tissues. This is most commonly due to the transfer of **kinetic energy** from a moving object (car, missile, falling object, etc.). The greater the amount of energy transferred to the tissue, the more extensive the damage.

epiphysis: The end of a long bone which bears the articular component. The epiphysis develops from the cartilaginous element between the joint surface and the growth plate—see **metaphysis**.

extension: The movement of an articulation that causes the relationship between the part above the joint and the part below the joint to become straighter.

extensor: Adjective from the noun "extension". The muscles which cause extension of a part are its extensor muscles; the surface of a part where those muscles are found is sometimes called the extensor surface.

external fixation: The technique of skeletal stabilization, which involves the implantation into bone of pins, wires, or screws that protrude through the integument and are linked externally by bars or other devices.

extra-articular fracture: Does not involve the articular surface, but may be intracapsular.

far cortex: The cortex more distant from the operator. Sometimes called the *trans* cortex. In plating and tension band wiring, a defect has more important consequences in the far rather than in the near cortex. This difference is due to the inability of a defective far cortex to resist compressive forces.

fasciocutaneous: A term describing tissue flaps which include the skin, the subcutaneous tissues, and the associated deep fascia as a single layer.

fasciotomy: The surgical division of the investing fascial wall of an osseofascial muscle compartment, usually to release pathologically high intracompartmental pressure—see **muscle compartment**.

fibrocartilage: Tissue consisting of elements of cartilage and of fibrous tissue. This may be a normal anatomical entity, such as certain intra-articular structures (menisci, triangular fibrocartilage of the wrist, the symphysis pubis) or constitute the repair tissue after lesion of the articular cartilage.

fixation, flexible: Traditionally, internal fixation according to the AO method has meant absolutely stable (rigid) fixation, using close adaptation and compression. Recently, a less stable fixation (flexible fixation using splinting plates, nails, or fixators) has been observed to yield very good results under conditions in which the fragments are well vascularized. Given best preservation of the viability of the fragments, flexible fixation induces abundant and rapid callus formation. Recall that the combination of instability and compromise of the biology of the fracture locus is deleterious. See **biological internal fixation**.

flexion: The movement of an articulation that causes the relationship between the part above the joint and the part below the joint to become more angulated.

flexor: Adjective from the noun "flexion". The muscles which cause flexion of a part are flexor muscles; the surface of a part where those muscles are found is sometimes called the flexor surface.

floating knee: Isolation of the knee joint from the remainder of the skeleton by fractures of the femur and the tibia in the same limb.

fracture disease: A condition characterized by disproportionate pain, soft-tissue swelling, patchy bone loss, and joint stiffness [8]. Fracture disease can best be avoided by that scheme of fracture management most likely to produce skeletal integrity whilst permitting early active motion of the part (early functional rehabilitation) [9]. Linked terms are algodystrophy, reflex sympathetic dystrophy (RSD), Sudeck's atrophy—see **chapter 6.5**.

fracture locus (injury zone): Locus derives from the Latin word for "place". It is used in our context to describe the biological unit comprising the fracture fragments and the immediately associated soft tissues, all of which function together to produce healing of the injury.

fracture: A loss of continuity (breakage), usually sudden, of any structure resulting when internal stresses produced by load exceed the limits of its strength. The complexity and displacement of the fracture depend largely on the energy build-up in the structure prior to fracture; the shape of the fracture planes (transverse fracture, spiral fracture, avulsion, impaction, etc.) is related to the nature of the load-compressive, bending, torsional, shear, or any combination of these.

frontal: Pertaining to the front of the body in the anatomical position. That part of the skull forming the forehead is the frontal bone. The frontal plane of the body, parallel to the front, is the same as the coronal plane (see above).

Galeazzi injury: A fracture of the radial shaft associated with a dislocation of the inferior radioulnar joint. Its first description is attributed to Galeazzi [10]. Sometimes referred to as the "reversed Monteggia".

gap healing: The healing process taking place between two fragment ends kept in stable relative position with a small gap between them. Gap healing progresses in two phases: (1) the filling of the gap with lamellar bone of different orientation than the bone of the fragments, (2) the subsequent remodeling of the newly filled bone from within the gap into the fragments (plugging) or crossing from one fragment through the newly filled bone into the other fragment (remodeling).

gliding hole: When a fully threaded screw is used as a lag screw, the cortex under the screw head should not engage the screw threads. This can be accomplished by over-drilling the near cortex screw hole to at least the size of the outer diameter of the screw thread.

gliding splint: A splint (such as an unlocked intramedullary nail) which allows for axial shortening. Such a splint provides the possibility for the re-establishment of bony coaptation under conditions of fragment end shortening due to bone surface resorption.

goal of fracture treatment: According to Müller et al. [11], the goal of fracture treatment is to restore optimal function of the limb in respect to mobility and load-bearing capacity. The goal is, furthermore, to prevent early complications, such as reflex sympathetic dystrophy, fracture disease, or Sudeck's atrophy and, in the case of polytrauma, multiple system organ failure, as well as late sequelae, such as posttraumatic arthrosis.

Haversian system: The cortical bone is composed of a system of small channels (osteons) about 0.1 mm in diameter. These channels contain the blood vessels and are remodeled after a disturbance of the blood supply to bone. There is a natural turnover of the Haversian systems by continuous osteonal remodeling; this process is part of the dynamic and metabolic nature of bone. It is also involved in the adaptation of bone to an altered mechanical environment

healing: Restoration of the original integrity. The healing process after a bone fracture lasts many years, until internal fracture remodeling subsides. For practical purposes, however, healing is considered to be complete when the bone has regained its normal stiffness and strength.

hematogenous: Blood-borne.

heterograft: See **allograft** and **xenograft**.

814

homograft: See **allograft** and **autograft**.

horizontal: Parallel with the horizon.

hypovolemia: A state where the circulating blood volume is reduced. This can lead to shock.

hypoxia: A state where the oxygen level in the arterial blood, or in other tissue, is pathologically reduced.

impacted fracture: A fracture in which the opposing bony surfaces are driven one into the other, resulting often in an inherent fracture stability and usually a degree of angulation.

indirect healing: Bone healing as observed in fractures treated either with relative stability, or left untreated. Callus formation is predominant, the fracture fragment ends are resorbed, and bone formation results from a process of transformation of fibrous and/or cartilaginous tissue into bone—see **callus**.

inferior: Literally below or lesser than. In the anatomical position, if A is lower than B, A is inferior to B. The opposite is **superior**.

inoculation: The instillation, either accidental or deliberate, of microorganisms into body tissues or into a culture medium.

interfragmentary compression: Static compression applied to a fracture plane imparts a high degree of stability to the fragments and thus reduces micromotion and strain. Bone surface resorption does not then occur. There is no demonstrable proof that interfragmentary compression, per se, has any effect upon internal remodeling of the cortical bone [12].

intramedullary nail—locked or unlocked: An intramedullary nail provides some degree of stability, mainly as a result of its (flexural) stiffness. An unlocked nail will allow the fragments to slide together along the nail; the fracture must, therefore, be provided with a solid support against shortening—see **gliding splint**. For the treatment of multifragmentary fractures, where there is axial instability (the fear of collapse into a shortened position), the nail can be interlocked above and below the fracture locus to prevent this shortening and also to reduce rotational displacement. This is achieved by locking bolts traversing a locking hole prepared in the nail and passing through the cortex on either side of the nail. If the locking hole is round and matches the size of the locking bolt, then static locking has been achieved. If the locking hole is elongated in the nail's long axis, the possibility of a limited excursion of axial movement is achieved, whilst preserving the rotational control—so-called dynamic locking.

ischemia: Pathological absence of blood flow.

kinetic energy—see **energy transfer**: The energy stored by a body by virtue of the fact that it is in motion. As energy cannot be destroyed, when a moving object is slowed or stopped, its kinetic energy is converted into other energy. If a moving object strikes a slower or stationary object, it imparts some of its kinetic energy to the body that it strikes. This may accelerate the other body (or parts of it), causing damage, or produce other energy transfer effects such as heat production—the sparks seen when a metal bullet hits a rock, for example. Kinetic energy is calculated according to the formula $E = mv^2/2$, where m is the mass of the moving object and v its velocity.

lag screw technique: Produces interfragmentary compression by driving the bone fragment beneath a screw head against another fragment in which the screw threads obtain purchase The compression produced by a screw so inserted acts directly within the fracture surface and is, therefore, very efficient. A screw designed specifically for this purpose, being only partially threaded, is a lag screw, or shaft screw. A fully threaded screw used with an over-sized hole in the near cortex to prevent thread purchase in the near fragment (a **gliding hole**) is strictly speaking not a lag screw but a threaded screw used with a lag technique; it is, nevertheless, often loosely termed a lag screw. Interfragmentary compression will be reduced by engagement of the screw threads with the walls of the gliding hole. Anchorage in the near fragment can be avoided by the use of a shaft screw. This technique is also required to maintain efficient compression when a screw is inserted through the plate and across a fracture plane in an inclined position.

lateral: Literally, of, or toward, the side. The side of the body in the anatomical position is the lateral aspect or surface. If

A is nearer the side of the body than B (further from the midline), then A is lateral to B. The opposite is **medial**.

lymphedema: Accumulation of edema fluid in the tissues as a result of poor drainage of the lymph, usually due to the incompetence, or obstruction, of the lymphatic vessels.

malunion: Consolidation of a fracture in a position of **deformity**.

matrix: Literally, a place or medium in which something is bred, produced, or developed. In cartilage it is the substance between the chondrocytes. It consists of a network of collagen fibers interspersed with a "jelly" of waterlogged mucopolysaccharide macromolecules (complex organic chemicals in large molecular chains).

medial: Literally, of, or toward the middle, or median. The inner side of a part with the body in the anatomical position is the medial aspect or surface. If A is nearer the middle, or center-line, than B, then A is medial to B. The opposite is **lateral**.

metaphysis: The segment of a long bone located between the end part (**epiphysis**) and the shaft (**diaphysis**). It consists mostly of cancellous bone within a thin cortical shell.

methylmethacrylate: A chemical substance, the monomer of which can be induced to polymerize, producing a hard plastic. It can be a form of bone cement (polymethylmethacrylate or PMMA), but in a different polymerized form it produces Perspex.

microvascular: Pertaining to microscopic blood vessels. Microvascular tissue transfer is related to the technical need for an operating microscope to perform the anastomoses (see **anastomosis**).

midline: The center line of the body in the anatomical position.

Monteggia injury: A displaced ulnar fracture associated with a dislocation of the radial head from its articulation with the capitellum. First described in the 19th century by Monteggia [13], an Italian physician.

Morse cone: Is a cone whose walls are very steep and almost parallel. When a screw whose head with an appropriate undersurface is inserted in a corresponding plate hole, the screw locks rotation and inclination when the surgeon begins to tighten it. The three effects are:
1. The connection is stable,
2. Self-locking prevents stripping of the bone thread even in very soft bone.
3. The axial pull of the plate screw is minimal allowing for construction of the internal fixator principle.

The Morse cone connection is the basic element on the PC-Fix.

multifragmentary fracture: A term usually reserved for fractures that have one or more dissociated intermediate fragments. See also **complex fracture**.

muscle compartment: An anatomical space, bounded on all sides either by bone or deep fascial envelope, which contains one or more muscle bellies. The relative in-elasticity of its walls means that if the muscle tissue swells, the pressure in the osseo-fascial envelope can increase to levels which cut off the flow of blood to the muscle tissue, resulting in its severe compromise or death—so-called muscle compartment syndrome.

near cortex: The cortex near the operator and on the side of insertion of an implant. Sometimes called the *cis* cortex, it is usually a term used in relation to plating, interfragmentary screw fixation, and tension band wiring. In respect to bending, the convex near cortex contributes little to stability of fixation. When—for example, in wave plate application—the distance between the plate and the near cortex is increased, the bone and the repair tissues gain better leverage.

neutralization: An implant (plate, external fixator, or nail) that functions by virtue of its stiffness is said to "neutralize" the effect of the functional load. The implant carries a major part of the functional load and thus diverts loads away from the fracture locus and may serve to protect a more vulnerable element of a fixation complex. An example is where a spiral fracture has been reduced and fixed with interfragmentary screws, and then a plate is applied to protect the primary screw fixation from potentially disruptive functional loads. The use of such a protection, or "neutralization", plate will allow earlier functional aftercare than if the screw fixation had been left unsupported. It does not actually "neutralize", but does minimize, the effect of the forces (see **protection**).

non-union: See **union, pseudarthrosis, delayed union.** Non-union is failure of bone healing. A fracture is judged to be ununited if the signs of non-union are present when a sufficient time has elapsed since injury, during which the particular fracture would normally be expected to have healed by bony union. That period will vary according to fracture location and pathoanatomy.

The signs of non-union include persisting pain and/or tenderness at the fracture sight, pain and/or mobility on stressing the fracture site, and inability progressively to resume function. Slight warmth may be detected if the fracture site is subcutaneous. Radiographs will be likely to show failure of re-establishment of bony continuity.

When a fracture has been fixed internally, loosening and/or breakage of the implant may indicate the instability of a non-union. If a non-union has resulted from a mechanical environment at the fracture locus that is not conducive to bone healing, despite good fracture biology and osteogenic response, a *hypertrophic* ("elephant's foot") non-union occurs—the solution to this is a mechanical one.

If a non-union has resulted from impaired biological response at the fracture locus, an *atrophic* non-union occurs—the solution to this is biological enhancement, usually with mechanical support.

opposition: The action of opposing one part to another; if the pulp of the thumb is placed in contact with the pulp of a finger, the movement, or action, of the thumb is that of opposition.

ORIF: A widely used abbreviation for open reduction and internal fixation (**osteosynthesis**).

osteoarthritis: This is a condition which affects diarthrodial (synovial) joints and is characterized by loss of articular cartilage, reactive subchondral bone sclerosis (sometimes with subchondral cysts), and the formation of peripheral bony outgrowths—osteophytes. The primary lesion is degeneration of the articular cartilage as a consequence of infection, trauma, overuse, congenital skeletal anomaly, or as part of the aging process.

osteoblast: Cells that form new bone.

osteoblastic: Producing bone.

osteoclast: Cells that destroy bone. Osteoclasts rest in the Howship lacunae (small wells within the bone surface). They are typically found at the tip of the remodeling **osteons**, but also in all sites where bone is being removed by physiological processes.

osteolytic: Resorbing, destroying, or removing bone.

osteomyelitis: An acute or chronic inflammatory condition affecting bone and its medullary cavity, usually the result of bone infection. This may be a blood-borne infection (hematogenous osteomyelitis)—usually in children or in the immunocompromised, or follow an open fracture (posttraumatic osteomyelitis). The acute form, if diagnosed early and treated vigorously, can heal with no residual effects. If the diagnosis is delayed or treatment neglected, then the infection and the consequent interference with the local vascularity, can result in dead bone (which may separate to form one or more sequestra—see **sequestrum**) that remains infected in the long term because the defence mechanisms have no vascular access to it. The treatment of chronic osteomyelitis is surgical and includes wide excision of all dead and infected tissue, the identification of the responsible organism, and the delivery, both locally and systemically, of appropriate antibacterial agents.

osteon: The name given to the small channels which combine to make up the Haversian system in cortical bone.

osteopenia: An abnormal reduction in bone mass. This may be generalized, as in some bone diseases, or localized, as a response to inflammation, infection, disuse, etc.—see **osteoporosis**.

osteoporosis: A reduction in bone mass. It is a natural aging process but may be pathological. It can result in pathological fracture (most fractures of the femoral neck in the elderly are due to osteoporosis plus minimal trauma)—see **osteopenia** and **pathological fracture**.

osteosynthesis: A term coined by Albin Lambotte [14] to describe the "synthesis" (derived from the Greek for making together, or fusing) of a fractured bone by a surgical intervention using implanted material. It differs from "internal fixation" in that it also includes external fixation.

osteotomy: Controlled surgical division of a bone.

overbending (of plate): See **prebending**.

palmar: Pertaining to the palm of the hand, e.g., the palmar fascia, the palmar aspect of the fingers.

pathological fracture: A fracture through bone which is abnormal as a result of a pathological process. It may be the result of the application of a force less than that which would be required to produce a fracture in a normal bone.

periosteal: Adjective derived from **periosteum**.

periosteum: The inelastic membrane bounding the exterior surface of a bone. The periosteum plays an active part in the blood supply to cortical bone, in fracture repair, and in bone remodeling. It is continuous with the perichondrium—the membrane that bounds the periphery of the physis.

pilot hole: If a fully threaded screw is to function as a lag screw, it must be anchored near its tip, within a threaded hole in the far bone fragment. The original drill hole, which is made prior to tapping of the thread in the bone, is called the pilot hole. Within the bone fragment near the head of the screw, the thread should not obtain purchase but should glide (**gliding hole**). A pilot hole is also prepared when inserting a Schanz screw or a Steinmann pin.

pin loosening: The pins of external fixator frames serve to stabilize the fragments of a fracture by linking the bone to the frame. Stability depends, among other things, upon the contact between pin and bone (pin–bone interface). Pin loosening occurs when bone surface resorption at the pin-bone interface takes place due to excessive cyclical loading of the bone. Stability is thereby reduced. However, pin loosening is less important in respect of loss of stability than in respect of its deleterious effect in promoting pin-track infection.

plantar: Pertaining to the sole of the foot, i.e., the surface of the foot which is "planted" on the ground. Examples are the plantar fascia, and the plantar surfaces of the toes. Plantar flexion is a movement at the ankle that moves the foot downward, or in a plantar direction.

plastic deformation: If an object is deformed within those limits that allow it to regain its original form once the deforming force is removed, it is said to have undergone elastic deformation. If the force is increased above the upper level for elastic deformation, permanent deformity (known in engineering terms as "set") is produced. When the deforming force is removed, the object cannot return to its original form. Plastic deformation, in the shape of a young, growing bone can occur without fracture following the application of a deforming force. The alteration in shape does not "rebound" to the original as the bone has been stressed beyond its elastic limit, but not to the point of breaking.

polytrauma: Multiple injury to one or more body systems or cavities. An Injury Severity Score (ISS) of more than 16 is usually taken to indicate polytrauma.

position screw: One which is inserted between two bones, or two bone fragments, having thread purchase in both so that the relative position of the two pieces of bone at the time of screw insertion is maintained. An example is the fibulotibial screw (diastasis screw) sometimes inserted to hold the fibula in its correct orientation to the tibia, after disruption of the inferior tibiofibular syndesmosis. A position screw does not compress the bones together, but maintains their anatomical relationship.

posterior: The back of the body in the anatomical position is the posterior surface. If A is nearer to the back of the body in the anatomical position than B, then A is posterior to B. Equivalent to dorsal, except in the foot, where the dorsum is anterior in the anatomical position—see **dorsal**.

prebending of plate: Precisely contoured plates, when loaded using either the external compression device or the DCP principle, produce asymmetrical compression, i.e., the near cortex is more compressed than the far cortex. Indeed, the latter may not be compressed at all and, in certain cases, can even be distracted. To achieve stabilization against both torque and bending, compression at the far cortex is even more important than at the near cortex. To provide uniform compression across the whole width of the bone, including the far cortex, the plate is applied after contouring with an additional bend of the plate segment bridging the fracture. The bend is such that the midsection of the plate is slightly elevated from the surface of the reduced fracture, prior to fixation to the bone and the application of compression. Pre-bending is an important tool to increase stability in small and/or osteoporotic bones—see **osteopenia**.

precise reduction: See **anatomical reduction**.

preload: The application of interfragmentary compression keeps the fragments together until a tensile force is applied, exceeding the compression (preload).

pronation: The movement of rotating the forearm so that the palm of the hand faces backward from the anatomical position. Pronation is also sometimes used to describe a movement of the foot into inclination away from the midline, otherwise called eversion; so that a pronated foot would bear more weight on its medial border than on its lateral border.

prophylactic: Preventive.

protection: While the term "neutralization" has often been used in plate and screw fixation, the term "protection" should replace it. In reality true neutralization cannot be achieved. In plate fixation the plate reduces the load placed upon the interfragmentary screw fixation. It therefore protects the screw fixation from overload—see **neutralization**.

proximal: Nearer to the center of the body in the anatomical position. The opposite of distal. Thus, the elbow is proximal to the wrist. In certain instances, it means nearer the beginning than the end; for example, in the digestive system the stomach is proximal to the ileum, or in the urinary tract the kidney is proximal to the bladder.

pseudarthrosis: See **delayed union**, **non-union**, **union** literally means "false joint". When a non-union is mobile and allowed to persist for a long period, the ununited bone ends become sclerotic and the intervening soft tissues differentiate to form a crude sort of synovial articulation. The term is often loosely and incorrectly used to describe all non-unions. Occasionally, a pseudarthrosis (in the sense of a false articulation) may be deliberately created surgically. As for example, in excision arthroplasty of the hip or excision of a segment of the distal ulnar shaft, in combination with fusion of the inferior radio-ulnar joint—the Kapandji procedure. Excision of the radial head is another example of surgical pseudarthrosis.

pure depression: An articular fracture in which there is depression alone of the articular surface without split—see **impacted fracture** and **pure split**.

pure split: An articular fracture in which there is a longitudinal metaphyseal and articular split, without any additional osteochondral lesion.

radial preload: To prevent external fixator **pin loosening**, the contact zone (interface) between the implant and bone can be pre-loaded, i.e., a static compressive force is applied. Hitherto, preloading was achieved by applying a permanent bending moment to the pins, within their elastic range. Currently, the pins are designed with a thread and shank that automatically generate radial preload—a tight, compressive fit produced by insertion of a pin slightly larger than the drill hole. The effect of radial preload is to minimize pin loosening and to seal the pin track so that a potential infection cannot reach the medullary cavity from outside. The amount of misfit between the hole diameter and the pin diameter should not exceed 0.05–0.1 mm. Such a precise geometric discrepancy can only reliably be ensured by using self-cutting tips—see **preload**.

radiotherapy: Treatment of pathological conditions, usually malignant, with ionizing radiation. It has been recommended in low dosage to discourage heterotopic bone formation.

reduction: The realignment of a displaced fracture.

reflex sympathetic dystrophy (RSD): One of the names given to algodystrophy—see **chapter 6.5** and **fracture disease**.

refracture: A fracture occurring after the bone has solidly bridged, at a load level otherwise tolerated by normal bone. The resulting fracture line may coincide with the original fracture line, or it may be located remote from the original fracture, but within the area of bone that has undergone changes as a result of the fracture and its treatment.

relative stability: See **stability of fixation**.

remodeling (of bone): The process of transformation of external bone shape (external remodeling), or of internal bone structure (internal remodeling, or remodeling of the Haversian system).

resorption (of bone): The process of bone removal includes the dissolution of mineral and matrix and their uptake into the cell (phagocytosis). The cells responsible for this process are **osteoclasts**.

rigid fixation: A fixation of a fracture which allows little or no deformation under load—see **stability of fixation**.

rigid implants: In general implants are con–sidered to be rigid when they are made of metals. The implant geometry is more important than the physical stiffness of the material. Most implants made of metal are much more flexible (less rigid) than the corresponding bone.

rigidity: This term is often used synonymously with stiffness. Some, for example Timoshenko [15], feel that its use should be confined to considerations of shear (e.g., at the interface of plate and bone).

sagittal: Literally, pertaining to an arrow (*sagitta* is Latin for arrow); so called because an arrow fired into the body would normally strike from the front and would thus pass in a sagittal direction. Bisection of the body in the sagittal plane would divide it into left and right halves.

second look: The practice, in open fracture treatment, following débridement, of surgically inspecting the injury zone again at 48–72 hours, to permit re-evaluation of the tissue excision and to conduct further débridement if indicated.

segmental: If the shaft of a bone is broken at two levels, leaving a separate shaft segment between the two fracture sites, it is called a "segmental" fracture complex.

sequestrum: A piece of dead bone lying alongside, but separated from, the osseous bed from which it came. It is formed when a section of bone is deprived of its blood supply and the natural processes create a cleavage between the dead and the living bone. A sequestrum may be aseptic (sterile), as, for example, beneath a plate when there has been massive periosteal stripping and then a plate with a high contact "footprint" applied, killing the underlying bone. This is especially seen if a plate has been applied to the cortex at the same time as a reamed intramedullary nail has been inserted. Infected sequestra are formed in chronic osteomyelitis—see **osteomyelitis**.

shear: A shearing force is one which tends to cause one segment of a body to slide upon another, as opposed to tensile forces, which tend to elongate, or shorten, a body.

shock: A state of reduced tissue perfusion, usually due to a fall in intravascular pressure secondary to **hypovolemia**, overwhelming sepsis (gram-negative shock, or "red" shock), or allergic anaphylaxis.

simple (single) fracture: A disruption of bone (diaphyseal, extra-articular, articular) with only two main fragments.

splinting: Reducing the mobility at a fracture locus by coupling a stiff body to the main bone fragments. The splint may be external (plaster, external fixators) or internal (plate, intramedullary nail).

split depression: A combination of split and depression in an articular fracture—see **pure split** and **pure depression**.

spontaneous fracture: One that occurs without adequate trauma, usually in abnormal bone—see **pathological fracture**.

spontaneous healing: The healing pattern of a fracture without treatment. Solid healing is observed in most cases, but malunion frequently results. This is how animal fractures normally heal in the wild.

stability of fixation: This is characterized by the degree of residual motion at the fracture site after fixation (i.e., very little or no displacement between the fragments of the fracture). In technical terms, stability describes the tendency to revert to a condition of low energy, but this strict definition is not adhered to in the lingua franca of fracture surgery.

stability, absolute: The compressed surfaces of the fracture do not displace under applied functional load. The definition of absolute stability applies only to a given time and at a given site: some areas of a fracture may displace in relation to each other while other areas of the same fracture locus may not; different areas may also exhibit different displacements at different times. Practically, the only method of achieving absolute stability consists in the application of **interfragmentary compression**. The compression results in stability by preloading the fracture interface and by producing friction [16].

stability, relative: An internal fixation construct that allows small amounts of motion in proportion to the load applied. This is the case with a fixation that depends exclusively on the stiffness of the implant (such as a nail, or plate, bridging a multifragmentary fracture segment). The residual deformation or displacement is inversely proportional to the stiffness of the implant. Such motion is always present, but usually harmless, in nail fixation. According to the philosophy of the AO group, plate fixation is more reliable if motion can be prevented, but never at the expense of the biology of the fracture locus—see **biological fixation**.

stiffness: The resistance of a structure to deformation. Under a given load, the higher the stiffness of an implant the smaller its deformation, the smaller the displacement of the fracture fragments, and the lower the strain generated in the repair tissue. Excessive tissue strain can interfere with healing. The stiffness of a structure is expressed as its Young's modulus of elasticity.

stiffness and geometrical properties: The thickness of a structure affects deformability by its third power. Changes in geometry are, therefore, much more critical than changes in material properties—

a fact often overlooked by non-engineers. Thus, if flexible fixation is a goal, it can be achieved more effectively and in a more controlled manner by small changes of implant dimension than by using a "less rigid" material.

strain: Relative deformation of a material, for example, repair tissue. Motion at the fracture site in itself is not the important feature, but the resulting relative deformation, which is called strain (dL/L), of the healing tissues. As strain is a ratio (displacement of fragments divided by width of fracture gap), very high levels of strain may be present within small fracture gaps even under conditions where the displacement may not be perceptible.

strain induction: Tissue deformation—among other things—may result in induction of callus. This would be an example of a mechanically-induced biological reaction. For those reactions triggered by strain, such as callus formation and bone surface resorption, the concept of a lower limit of strain, the minimum strain, is to be considered.

strain tolerance: This determines the tolerance of the repair tissues to mechanical conditions. No tissue can be formed under conditions of strain which exceed the levels of strain at which the tissue will rupture because of excessive elongation. Above such a critical level, strain will disrupt the tissue once formed, or will prevent its formation.

strength: The ability to withstand load without structural failure. The strength of

a material can be expressed as ultimate tensile strength, bending strength, or torsional strength. The local criterion for failure of bone, or of implants, is measured in units of force per unit area: stress, or (equivalent) deformation per unit length (strain), or elongation at rupture.

stress protection: This term, initially used to describe bone reaction to reduced functional load [17], is used today mainly to express the negative aspects of any stress relief of bone. The basic assumption is that bone, deprived of its necessary functional stimulation by a reduction in its mechanical load, becomes less dense and thus less strong (Wolff's law). Stress protection is often used synonymously with stress shielding, i.e., in a purely mechanical sense. It is often used to characterize bone loss, implying a negative connotation to stress shielding. With regard to the internal fixation of cortical bone, stress protection seems not to play an important role, compared with vascular considerations—see **stress shielding**. The early bone loss seen deep to a plate, which has in the past been attributed to stress protection, can better be explained on the basis of a denial of blood supply to the underlying cortex, due to the pressure of the "footprint" of the plate. The resultant necrotic bone is then remodeled by osteons, which originate from the well vascularized, adjacent cortex. This remodeling process is associated with temporary osteoporosis. Investigations of late bone loss under clinical conditions of internal fixation in the human, using quantitative computed tomography, show very little residual bone loss at the time of implant removal

[18]. In summary, bone may react to unloading, but this plays a minor role in internal fixation of cortical bone fractures.

stress riser: In any body subject to deformation, stress will be generated within its material. If any part of the body is weaker than the rest, there will be a concentration of stress (high mean stress) at this place. If an implant is notched by inappropriate handling, the area of damage will act as a stress riser and produce the risk of fatigue failure with cyclical loading. If a hole is drilled in a bone and then left empty, this too will result in high mean stress and the risk of fracture. With the exception of the LC-DCP, with its even strength, most plate holes represent weaker points on the plate than the solid sections between the plate holes: in a fixation with such a plate, where a screw hole has been left unfilled in the fracture zone, the empty hole acts as a stress riser and also produces the risk of fatigue failure, or bending under high functional load.

stress shielding: When internal fixation relies upon screws and plates, the stability of the construct is achieved mainly by the interfragmentary compression exerted by the lag screws. Lag screw fixation alone is very stable, but generally provides little security under functional load. A plate providing protection (or neutralization) is therefore often added. The function of such a plate is to reduce the levels of peak load passing through the lag screw fixation. Protection is provided by virtue of the stiffness of the plate. The plate shields the fracture's primary fixation with screws—see **neutralization** and **protection**.

Sudeck's atrophy: One of the names given to algodystrophy—see **chapter 6.5** and **fracture disease**.

superior: Literally, above, or better than. In the anatomical position, if A is higher than, or above, B, then A is superior to B. The opposite is **inferior**.

supination: The movement of rotating the forearm that causes the palm of the hand to face forward, that is restoring the hand to the anatomical position. Supination is also sometimes used to describe a movement of the foot into inclination toward the midline, otherwise called inversion; a supinated foot would bear more weight on its lateral border than on its medial border.

synovectomy: Excision of the synovial membrane.

systemic: Refers to any route for drug, or fluid, administration, other than via the gastrointestinal tract, and usually by injection.

tension band: An implant (wire or plate) functioning according to the tension-band principle: when the bone undergoes bending load, the implant, attached to the bone's convex surface, resists the tensile force. The bone, especially the far cortex, is then dynamically compressed. The plate is able to resist very large amounts of tensile force, while the bone best resists compressive load: this bone-implant composite, therefore, is ideally suited to resist the bending force.

threaded hole: Discussed in conjunction with **pilot hole**.

tibial intercondylar eminence: The area of the proximal tibia lying between the medial and lateral tibial plateaux, which is non-articular and bears the attachments of the horns of the two menisci, and of the tibial ends of the anterior and posterior cruciate ligaments, to the anterior and posterior tibial spines.

toggling: This term is used to describe the slight movement (or play) which can occur between a hole in an intramedullary nail and the screw or bolt which passes through it, since the tolerances of the assembly do not permit an exact fit.

torque: The moment produced by a turning or twisting force. As an example: torque is applied to drive home and tighten a screw. The moment is equal to the product of lever arm (in meters) and force (in Newtons) producing torsion and rotation about an axis (the unit of torque in Nm).

torus: A geometrical body in the shape of a solid ring that in cross section is circular or elliptical—such as an inflated tire inner tube. It is a term used in architecture to described the circumferential bulge seen at the top and bottom of classical columns. It has been applied to the "wrinkle" or "buckle" appearance seen in the compression cortex of angular fractures of young children's bones (torus fracture).

toxins: Poisonous chemicals. Some pathogenic organisms release powerful toxins when they multiply and some when they die.

trabecula (pl. trabeculae): A solid bony strut of cancellous bone. Literally, a small beam or bar.

track: Describes the path created surgically through tissues by the insertion of an external fixator pin. In that context, the word "track" should be used (in the sense of its meaning the mark, or trail, left by the passage of anything—Oxford English Dictionary).

tract: Literally, a treatise or document (often religious), an anthem, an extent of territory, or an anatomical structure comprising mixed tissues organized to serve a specific physiological function (spinothalamic tract, urinary tract, etc.). It is commonly misapplied in discussing external fixator pins—see **track**.

***trans* cortex:** See **far cortex**.

transverse: Across. Transverse bisection of the body in the anatomical position would divide it into upper and lower halves. Not the same as horizontal, which means parallel with the horizon. Thus, if the body were lying flat on its back (supine), horizontal would be the same as the coronal plane (see above), but if the body were standing, in the anatomical position, horizontal would be in the transverse plane. In other words, horizontal is always related to the horizon, whereas the anatomical planes (coronal, frontal, sagittal, transverse) always relate to the anatomical position.

translation: Displacement of one bone fragment in relation to another, usually at right angles to the long axis of the bone—see **displacement**.

union: Strictly speaking, union means "as one"—as in marital union, a workers' union, even national groups, e.g., the United States. Equally strictly, if a fracture is fixed so that the bone functions as a single unit, then it has been surgically "united" (**osteosynthesis**); the bone is not, however, healed. Bone healing is a process initiated by fracture and continuing until the bone is restored to its final state by remodeling—this may take years. We speak loosely of a fracture being united, but this is not a discrete event. What we are saying is that a healing fracture has reached the point in the process of union when the experienced surgeon estimates that it can withstand normal functional loads for that patient. Union is, therefore, a judgment, usually based upon a synthesis of temporal, clinical, and imaging information. This calls into question the validity of "time to union", which is reported in so much of the surgical literature as a parameter for the judgment of the comparative efficacy of different treatments.

valgus: Deviation away from the midline in the anatomical position. Thus, genu valgum is a deformity at the knee where the lower leg is angled away from the midline (knock knee). By convention, any deformity, or deviation, is described in terms of the movement of the distal part.

varus: Deviation toward the midline in the anatomical position. Thus, genu varum is a deformity at the knee where the lower leg is angled toward the midline (bow leg). By convention, any deformity, or deviation, is described in terms of the movement of the distal part.

vascularity: That property of a tissue which reflects the extent to which it has, or does not have, a blood supply. A tissue is said to be vascularized if its intrinsic network of blood vessels is connected to the main circulatory system. Blood vessels may be shut off temporarily from the circulatory system. If the connection to the main circulation is permanently interrupted, or if the vessels present are not functioning, e.g., obliterated by thrombosis, the tissue is said to be avascular, or devascularized. We consider a tissue to be non-vascular if there are normally no functioning vessels, as in hyaline cartilage

vertical: Upright, perpendicular to horizontal. Derives from vertex—the top, as in the vertex of the skull.

wave plate: If the central section of a plate is contoured to stand off the near cortex over a distance of several holes, it leaves a gap between the plate and the bone, which (a) preserves the biology of the underlying bone, (b) provides a space for the insertion of a bone graft, and (c) increases the stability because of the distance of the "waved" portion of the implant from the neutral axis of the shaft. Such plating is useful in non-union treatment.

wedge fracture: Fracture complex with a third fragment in which, after reduction, there is some direct contact between the two main fragments—see **butterfly fragment**.

xenograft: A graft of tissue from an individual of one species to a recipient (host) of another species.

Bibliography

1. **Mast J, Jakob R, Ganz R** (1989) *Planning and reduction techniques in fracture surgery.* Berlin Heidelberg New York: Springer-Verlag.
2. **Pfister U** (1980) *Morphologische, histologische und biomechanische Untersuchungen nach Marknagelung der Tibia.* AO Research Institute, Davos Platz.
3. **Schenk R** (1987) Fracture healing. In: Lane JM, editor. *Cytodynamics and histodynamics of primary bone repair.* New York: Churchill Livingstone.
4. **Küntscher G** (1970) *Das Kallus-Problem.* Stuttgart: Enke.
5. **Hutzschenreuter P, Perren SM, Steinemann S, et al.** (1969) Some effects of rigidity of internal fixation on the healing pattern of osteotomies. *Injury;* 1 :77–81.
6. **Salter RB, Simmonds DF, Malcolm BW, et al.** (1980) The biological effect of continuous passive motion on the healing of full-thickness defects in articular cartilage. An experimental investigation in the rabbit. *J Bone Joint Surg [Am];* 62 (8):1232–1251.
7. **Mitchell N, Shepard N** (1980) Healing of articular cartilage in intra-articular fractures in rabbits. *J Bone Joint Surg [Am];* 62 (4):628–634.
8. **Lucas-Championniére J** (1907) Les dangers de l'immobilisation des membres-fagilité des os-altération de la nutrition du membre-conclusions pratiques. *Rev Méd Chir Pratique;* 78 :81–87.
9. **Allgöwer M** (1978) Cinderella of surgery-fractures? *Surg Clin North Am;* 58 :1071–1093.
10. **Galeazzi R** (1934) Über das besondere Syndrom bei Verletzungen im Bereich der Unterarmknochen. *Arch Orthop Unfallchir;* 35 :557–562.
11. **Müller ME, Allgöwer M, Willenegger H** (1963) *Technik der operativen Frakturenbehandlung.* Berlin Heidelberg New York: Springer-Verlag.
12. **Matter P, Brennwald J, Perren SM** (1974) Biologische Reaktion des Knochens auf Osteosyntheseplatten. *Helv Chir Acta;* 12 (Suppl) (1).
13. **Monteggia GB** (1814) *Instituzioni Chirurgiche;* 5 :130.
14. **Lambotte A** (1907) *L'intervention opératoire dans les fractures recentes et anciennes.* Bruxelles: Lamertin.
15. **Timoshenko S** (1941) *Strength of materials.* Princeton: Van Nostrand.
16. **Perren SM** (1991) Basic Aspects. In: Müller ME, Allgöwer M, Schneider R, et al., editors. *Manual of Internal Fixation.* 3rd ed. Berlin Heidelberg New York: Springer-Verlag.
17. **Allgöwer M, Ehrsam R, Ganz R, et al.** (1969) Clinical experience with a new compression plate "DCP". *Acta Orthop Scand;* 125 (Suppl): 45-63.
18. **Cordey J, Schwyzer HK, Brun S, et al.** (1985) Bone loss following plate fixation of fractures? *Helv Chir Acta;* 52 :181–184.

Updates

Updates and additional references are available at:
http://www.aopublishing.org/PFxM/glossary.htm

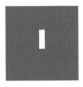

Index

Index of video sequences: see page **859**.
<u>Underlined</u> page numbers refer to entries in the **Glossary**.

854

temporary transfixation to radius 354–355
ulnar ligament 313
ulnar nerve 297, 302, 314–317, 320, 321, 329, 362, 367, 370
   decompression in distal radial fractures 370
ulnar nerve irritation 787
ulnar neurapraxia 321
ulnar palmar corner exposure 369–370
ulnar styloid process
   fixation in distal radial fractures 377
   internal fixation 367
ulnar variance 364
ulnocarpal ligament 364–365
ultrasound
   aseptic non-union 765
   children 682
unicortical screws 162, 165–166, 249, 250
union 822
universal nail 195–196
unreamed solid nail
   humeral shaft fractures 297
   tibial fractures 530, 531–532, 533, 538
upper arm
   soft-tissue damage 654–663
upper limb
   reconstruction of injuries 84
   soft-tissue damage 654–656

V

vaginal examination
   acetabular fractures 419–420
valgization, femur 790
valgus 462, 822
valgus deformity 93
valgus osteotomy
   femoral neck fractures 452–453

vanadium 38
vancomycin 705, 708
varus 462, 822
varus deformity 93
varus malalignment 483
varus malrotation 483
vascular bypass surgery 87–88
vascular injuries 87
   open fractures 637–638
vascular intraluminal shunts
   temporary 638
vascularity 822
vasodilators
   peripheral 804
vena cava filters 717, 718
venous return 716
venous thrombosis
   risk in soft-tissue repair 654
ventilation, maintenance 82
verapamil 804
Virchow's triad 714, 715
Volkmann's fracture 567, 578
Volkmann's fragment 579–580
Volkmann's triangle 569, 570

W

Wagner lengthening device 783
walking caliper
   patellar-tendon-bearing (PTB) 553
warfarin 717
washers 163–164
wave plate 226, 822
   diaphyseal non-union 763, 764
wedge
   cutting 135
wedge fractures 52, 94
   bridge plate 123

weight bearing
   delay 716
   postoperative 726–727
window
   preoperative planning 132, 135
wire
   bending forces 191
   breaking 191
wiring. See K-wire fixation
wound
   cleaning 724
   closed 741
   complications 734
   condition 59
   dressing 724, 741
   hematoma 734
   infections 703
   irrigation 741
   types 60
wound closure 646–648
   soft-tissue damage 650, 652–653
wound contamination
   polytrauma 669
   soft-tissue injuries 66, 67
wound débridement
   open fractures 625
   physiological 61
wound edge necrosis 734
wound healing
   disturbed 733, 734
wound surgical extension 627–628
wounds, surgical 723
wrist
   bridging external fixation 244
   malunion 789–790
   range of movement 345
   rehabilitation 370–371
   soft-tissue damage 656
   x-rays 361–362
wrist fixator 377

X

Z

Video

All video sequences with label "AO..." are taken from original AO instruction videos. They were digitized by AO Media Services.

Non-AO videos

- Chapter 3.3.1, Intramedullary nailing:
  © C. Krettek
- Chapter 4.5, Acetabular fractures:
  © J.M. Matta
- Chapter 5.7
  Postoperative management:
  © Spital Davos
- Chapter 6.1, Acute infection:
  © U. Müller, P.E. Ochsner

CD-ROM users will find the videos for the chapters 1.1 through 4.5 on disk 1 and videos for chapters 4.6.1 through 6.5 on disk 2. DVD-ROM users will find all video sequences on one disk.

A message from AO Publishing

Language

US-English spelling is used throughout the whole publication to conform to MeSH (Medical Subject Headings) and facilitate easier electronic search.

Bibliography

The source of our bibliography is the National Library of Medicine's Medline. Whenever a title of an article is set in [brackets], it indicates the original article was published in a language other than English. In such cases we took the Medline translation, which may differ slightly from the translation provided by the original publisher. For most chapters the Editorial Board decided not to print more than 20 references. The full reference lists submitted by the authors are at the reader's disposal on the Internet page accessible by hyperlink at the end of each chapter. Where available, the titles of the publications in their original language are added to each citation.

Convention of citations: The AO style follows the principles outlined in the NLM (National Library of Medicine) and the AMA (American Medical Association). To clarify: the number after the name of the Journal represents the volume followed by the issue number in (brackets).

Videos

Video sequences were deliberately kept short to better coordinate and complement the steps described in the text. It should be noted that voice-over for such short footage was not feasible. The complete teaching videos with voice-over are available on our DVD-ROM update:
ISBN 3-13-131021-9 (GTV)
ISBN 1-58890-098-3 (TNY)

How to use the electronic book

The CD-ROM contains a file called PFxM.pdf. This file is in Adobe's portable document format (PDF) and contains all the pages of the printed book, enhanced by the capabilities of linked documents on a computer.

To work with the file you need the **Acrobat® reader** which is also provided on the CD-ROM. (To install the reader please refer to the installation guide.)

open document...
print... (updated chapters only)

view stack:
previous view
next view

standard views:
actual size (100%)
fit in window
fit to width

show/hide bookmarks & thumbnails
hand tool (navigation)
zoom in/out
text selection tool

navigation: go to
...first page
...previous page
...next page
...last page

text search

The figure shows the Acrobat reader main window with a typical page of the electronic book.

Bookmarks mirror the structure of the book. Jump to any section by a mouse click. **Thumbnails** give a small view of each page and allow quick browsing through the whole volume. Select a given page by clicking on its thumbnail.

To jump to a specific page in the book, type in the **page number** in the bottom menu or use the scroll bar to the right.

To select a view, use the standard view buttons in the tool bar or type in the **zoom factor** in the menu field at the bottom bar.

You may switch between a single page view or a view with facing pages, as in the printed book.

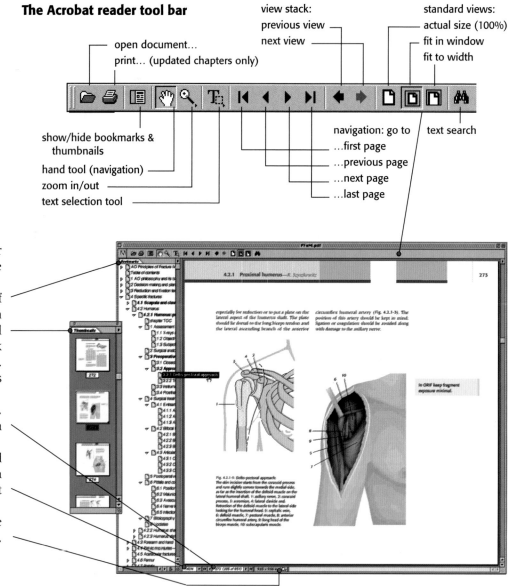

Links

Links to figures not located on the current page can be activated by a single mouse click. (The cursor changes when moved over the link.) Clicking on the number next to the target figure brings you back to the citation in the text.

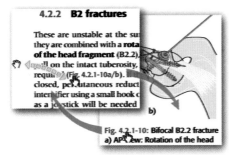

Internet links

The links in the reference list lead to the abstract in the Medline data base of Medscape. You need to have an internet browser and internet access to use this option. The first time you activate an internet link, Acrobat prompts you to select a browser on your computer.

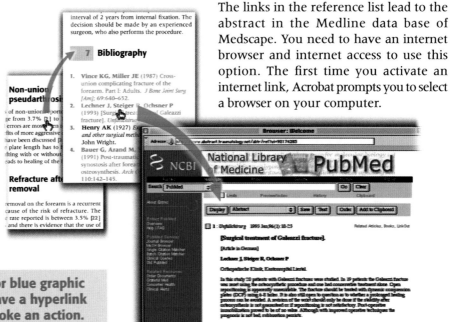

Letters typed in blue or blue graphic elements in general have a hyperlink to a destination, or evoke an action.

Hierarchic navigation links

A click on a subsection number leads to the next section above. By clicking on a section number you are led to the table of contents of the current chapter. The main chapter number is a link to the table of contents of the book. The main table of contents can also be easily accessed by a click into the blue header bar on top of each page. There you will also find a quick link to the index.

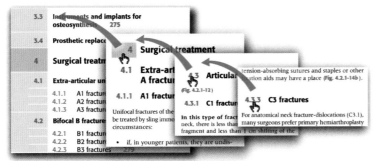

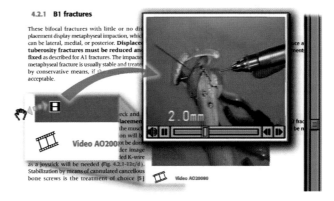

Videos

When moving the cursor over a video still it changes into a film icon. Click once and the video is shown in a separate window. Stop and restart it using the corresponding control buttons in this window or quit with **Esc**.

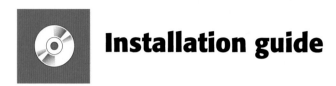

Installation guide

To work with the electronic version, you will require Apple QuickTime 5.0 or higher. If you have it installed, no further action is required, otherwise install the required software.

Installation Microsoft Windows

1. To install QuickTime for Windows, start the program "QuickTimeInstaller.exe" located in the "QuickTime" folder on the CD-ROMs and DVD-ROM. When asked by the Apple QuickTime installer to enter a serial number, do so if you have one, otherwise just click "cancel". The Pro version of QuickTime provides you with video editing functions which are not necessary for the use of the AO PFxM.
2. Restart your computer.

Installation Mac OS

1. To install QuickTime, start the program "QuickTime Installer" located in the "QuickTime" folder on the CD-ROMs and DVD-ROM. When asked by the Apple QuickTime installer to enter a serial number, do so if you have one, otherwise just click "cancel". The Pro version of QuickTime provides you with video editing functions which are not necessary for the use of the AO PFxM.
2. Restart your computer.

After successful installation start the PFxM electronic publication by double-clicking "PFxM.PDF" on the CD-ROM/DVD-ROM "PFxM2001".

For Internet connection you will need either Netscape Navigator or Microsoft Internet Explorer, both version 4.0 or higher (not supplied).

In case you are facing difficulties while running video clips, please download the latest version of QuickTime from the Internet: http://www.apple.com/quicktime/

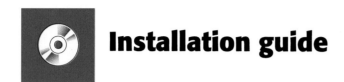# Installation guide

To work with the electronic version, you will require Apple QuickTime 5.0 or higher. If you have it installed, no further action is required, otherwise install the required software.

Installation Microsoft Windows

1. To install QuickTime for Windows, start the program "QuickTimeInstaller.exe" located in the "QuickTime" folder on the CD-ROMs and DVD-ROM. When asked by the Apple QuickTime installer to enter a serial number, do so if you have one, otherwise just click "cancel". The Pro version of QuickTime provides you with video editing functions which are not necessary for the use of the AO PFxM.
2. Restart your computer.

Installation Mac OS

1. To install QuickTime, start the program "QuickTime Installer" located in the "QuickTime" folder on the CD-ROMs and DVD-ROM. When asked by the Apple QuickTime installer to enter a serial number, do so if you have one, otherwise just click "cancel". The Pro version of QuickTime provides you with video editing functions which are not necessary for the use of the AO PFxM.
2. Restart your computer.

After successful installation start the PFxM electronic publication by double-clicking "PFxM.PDF" on the CD-ROM/DVD-ROM "PFxM2001".

For Internet connection you will need either Netscape Navigator or Microsoft Internet Explorer, both version 4.0 or higher (not supplied).

In case you are facing difficulties while running video clips, please download the latest version of QuickTime from the Internet: http://www.apple.com/quicktime/